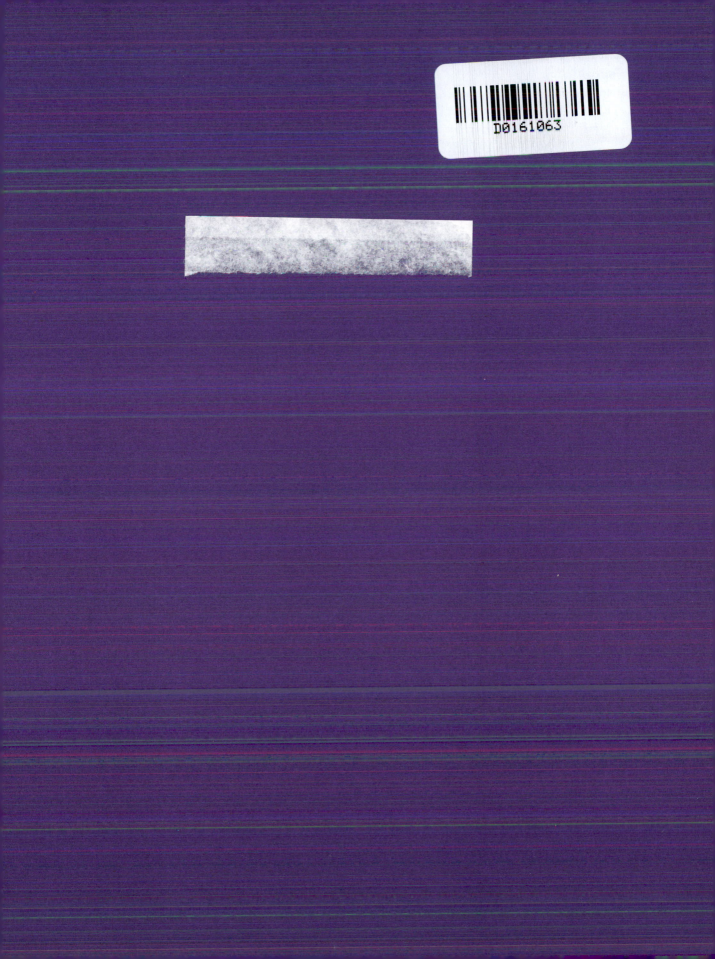

ATHLETIC INJURY ASSESSMENT

ATHLETIC INJURY ASSESSMENT

James M. Booher, Ph.D., A.T.,C., R.P.T.

Professor, Department of Health, Physical Education, and Recreation
South Dakota State University
Brookings, South Dakota

Gary A. Thibodeau, Ph.D.

Chancellor and Professor of Biology
University of Wisconsin—River Falls
River Falls, Wisconsin

Third Edition

with 788 illustrations

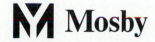

St. Louis Baltimore Boston Chicago London Madrid Philadelphia Sydney Toronto

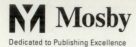
Mosby
Dedicated to Publishing Excellence

Publisher: Alison Miller
Editor-in-Chief: James Smith
Acquisitions Editor: Vicki Malinee
Developmental Editor: Kristin Shahane
Project Manager: Carol Sullivan Wiseman
Production Editor: Florence Achenbach
Designer: Betty Schulz
Cover Photo: Bill Leslie Photography, Inc.
Cover Design: GW Graphics & Publishing

This book is based on research, recommendations, and suggestions of athletic trainers, physicians, and other health professionals currently active in the field of sports medicine. The authors and publisher disclaim responsibility for any adverse effects or consequences resulting from the misapplication or injudicious use of the information contained within this text.

Credits for all illustrations and photos used by permission appear after the index.

THIRD EDITION

Printed in the United States of America
Composition by University Graphics, Inc.
Printing/binding by Maple-Vail Book Manufacturing Group

Mosby–Year Book, Inc.
11830 Westline Industrial Drive
St. Louis, MO. 63146

Library of Congress Cataloging in Publication Data
Booher, James M.
    Athletic injury assessment / James M. Booher, Gary A. Thibodeau. -
- 3rd ed.
      p.   cm.
    Includes bibliographical references and index.
    1. Sports—Accidents and injuries—Diagnosis.   2. Physical
    diagnosis.   I. Thibodeau, Gary A., 1938-   .   II. Title.
    [DNLM: 1. Athletic Injuries—diagnosis.   2. Sports Medicine.   QT
260 B724a 1993]
    RD97.B65   1993
    617.1′027—dc20
    DNLM/DLC
    for Library of Congress   93-31531
                                                                        CIP

        95 96 97 / 9 8 7 6 5 4 3 2

Preface

The third edition of *Athletic Injury Assessment* continues to be specifically designed for use by athletic trainers, coaches, and other individuals who have the medical responsibility for the physically active. It is a comprehensive text on assessment techniques and procedures that are essential to properly evaluate athletic related injuries and conditions. This text is designed to be used in athletic training curricula and advanced athletic training coursework, as well as provide a reliable, ready resource of assessment skills.

NEW TO THIS EDITION

In addition to updating and improving the existing materials from the first two editions, the following new features were added to the third edition:

1. This text discusses all athletic injuries/illnesses listed in *Competencies in Athletic Training,* a manual by the National Athletic Trainers Association, which lists all the competencies and criteria required for educational programs in athletic training. With this addition, at least 90 more conditions are discussed. Each injury/illness is marked with the icon ❖.
2. Four-color pages of skin diseases and conditions have been added, making these more readily visualized.
3. Chapter 9, Psychology of Injury, was added to cover this important aspect of injury management in more depth.
4. Head and Face Injuries was divided into two separate chapters to more adequately cover these important body areas.
5. Illustrations of surface anatomy were added to each chapter covering an area of the body.
6. The athletic injury assessment portion of each chapter was revised. The secondary survey is divided into History, Observation, and Physical Examination procedures. Physical examination is subdivided into palpation, movement procedures, neurological evaluations, and circulatory evaluations.
7. Neurological evaluations include a more in-depth discussion of sensory functions, motor functions, and reflexes.

ORGANIZATION AND CONTENT FEATURES

The 22 chapters of *Athletic Injury Assessment* are grouped into six organizational units. Unit I includes an introduction to the profession of athletic training and information on dealing with the body as a whole. Chapters 3, 4, 5, and 6 provide an overview of the structure and function of the skeletal, articular, muscular, and nervous systems. These chapters furnish an essential review of basic anatomical information necessary to adequately and accurately evaluate athletic injuries.

Unit II covers athletic-related trauma and is concerned with how the body responds to detrimental traumas or stresses associated with athletic activity and the development of related signs and symptoms. Recognizing and evaluating the signs and symptoms associated with athletic trauma are the bases of assessment. Chapter 7 discusses the body's basic responses to trauma and environmental conditions. Chapter 8 discusses and illustrates the various types of athletic-related injuries and conditions. Chapter 9 is concerned with the psychology of an injury.

The athletic injury assessment process is discussed in Unit III. Athletic trainers are continuously evaluating and reevaluating athletic-related trauma, and the more highly skilled they become in the assessment process, the more accurate and successful they become in managing athletic injuries. Chapter 10 discusses various factors related to the evaluation of athletic injuries, and Chapter 11 presents a rational approach to the athletic injury assessment process.

The final three units of this text are concerned with athletic injuries occurring to various areas of the body. Unit IV discusses athletic injuries of the axial region, which includes the head, face, spine, and torso. This area of the body is presented first because of the vital organs within this region and the possibility that injuries involving these organs can be life-threatening. Unit V is concerned with athletic injuries to the most frequently injured area of the body, the lower extremities. The final section of this text, Unit VI, is concerned with athletic injuries occurring to the upper extremities.

LEARNING AIDS

Some of the unique pedagogical features incorporated into each chapter of this text include the following:

1. Chapter objectives provide an overview of the topics to be examined and reinforce important chapter goals.
2. Prolific use of illustrations (line drawings and photographs) provides the student with a visual review of the procedures, functional tests, and

assessment techniques discussed. Additionally, many photographs of specific athletic injuries and related types of trauma are included to provide a broad base of exposure to the world of sports medicine.

3. Each chapter covering athletic injuries to an area of the body provides:
   - A review of functional anatomy of the region
   - Common mechanisms of athletic injury
   - Athletic related injuries and conditions
   - Associated signs and symptoms
   - Sequencing of athletic injury assessment procedures
   - List of indicators for medical referral
   - Assessment procedure checklist outlining the process

4. Key terms are highlighted in **boldface** and defined clearly and concisely within the chapter and in the glossary.

5. Each chapter includes a bibliography of current reference resources and suggested additional readings.

6. The icon ✣ marks all athletic related injuries/illnesses listed in the National Athletic Trainers Association competency manual.

James M. Booher

Gary A. Thibodeau

Acknowledgments

Throughout the writing of this edition we have been fortunate to have benefited from the experience, suggestions, and enthusiastic support of many physicians, athletic trainers, and health professionals active in the sports medicine field. For their thoughtful suggestions and constructive criticism, we would also like to thank the publisher's reviewers:

Leah Putman, New Mexico State University, M.A., A.T.,C., L.A.T.
Barrie Steele, University of Idaho, M.S., A.T.,C.
Gordon Stoddard, University of Wisconsin-Madison, M.ED., A.T., C.
Karen Toburen, Southwest Missouri State University, Ed.D., A.T., C.
Carol Zweifel, Washington State University, M.S., A.T., C.

A special thanks to James E. Lidstone, Ed.D., South Dakota State University, for contributing Chapter 9 to this edition. We also extend our appreciation to the students enrolled in our athletic training curriculum who gave freely of their time as subjects and photographers throughout the preparation of this edition.

Contents

Unit I   Introduction and Anatomic Basis for Athletic Injury Assessment

1   Introduction to athletic injury assessment, 2
Sports Medicine, 3
Athletic Training, 3
    Prevention, 6
    Recognition and Evaluation, 7
    Management and Treatment, 8
    Rehabilitation, 8
    Organization and Administration, 8
    Education and Counseling, 8

2   The body as a whole, 11
Somatotype, 11
Body Composition, 12
    Body Fat Distribution Patterns, 13
    Assessing Body Composition, 14
Generalizations about Body Structure, 17
    Bilateral Symmetry, 17
    Body Regions, 18
    Anatomic Position, 18
    Directional Terms, 18
    Body Planes (Sections), 19
    Abdominopelvic Quadrants and Regions, 19
    Surface Anatomy, 22

3   Osteology, 25
Functions of the Skeleton, 25
Classification of Bones, 26
Features of a Typical Bone, 27
Bone Markings, 28
Organization of the Skeleton, 31
    Axial Skeleton, 34
    Appendicular Skeleton, 39
Differences Between Male and Female Skeletons, 48
    Skeletal System: Lifespan Differences, 48

4   **Arthrology, 50**
     Classification of Joints, 50
        Synarthroses, 51
        Amphiarthroses, 52
        Diarthroses, 52
        Range and Type of Movement in Diarthroses, 57

5   **Myology, 65**
     General Functions, 66
     Muscles and Bony Levers, 66
        Lever Systems, 66
     Anatomy of Skeletal Muscles, 68
        Size and Shape, 68
        Fiber Arrangement, 68
        Connective Tissue Components, 69
        Nerve Tissue, 70
     Microscopic Anatomy, 72
        Types of Skeletal Muscle Contraction, 72
     Muscle Action, 74
     How Skeletal Muscles Are Named, 75
     Origins, Insertions, Functions, and Innervations of Representative Muscles, 75
        Muscle Strength, 84

6   **Neurology, 88**
     The Nervous System, 89
        Organs and Divisions, 89
        Receptors, 91
        Cells, 91
     Neurologic Assessment, 97
        Cerebrum, Cerebellum, and Cranial Nerve Assessment, 98
        Spinal Nerves, 99
        Nerves Plexuses, 104
     The Sensory System, 112
        Sensory System Tests, 113
        Reflex Status Tests, 113

Unit II   **Athletic-Related Trauma**
7   **The body's response to trauma and environmental stress, 118**
     Body's Response to Physical Trauma, 118
        Acute Inflammatory Process, 120
        The Immediate Care of Athletic Injuries, 125
        Follow-up Treatment Procedures, 126
        Chronic Inflammation, 127
        Summary, 128
     Shock, 128
        Types of Shock, 128
     Body's Response to Thermal Exposure, 130
        Physiologic Basis of Heat Exposure, 130

Heat-Related Conditions, 134
Preventive Measures, 136
Summary, 139
Body Response to Cold Exposure, 140
Physiologic Basis of Cold Exposure, 140
Cold-Related Conditions, 142
Summary, 144

8   Athletic injuries and related skin conditions, 146
Skin, 147
Visual Inspection, 147
Color, Temperature, and Texture, 147
Anatomy and Structure, 147
Accessory Organs, 149
Functions, 150
Exposed Athletic Injuries, 150
Open Wounds, 150
Common Skin Lesions, 155
Unexposed Athletic Injuries, 167
Contusions, 168
Strains, 171
Sprains, 172
Dislocation, 174
Fractures 177

9   Psychological aspects of injury, 182
Pre-Disposition to Injury, 183
Life Stress Events, 183
Personality Factors, 184
Situational Factors, 184
Attitudes, 185
Self-Concept and Self-Esteem, 186
Preventive Measures, 187
Psychological Consequences of Injury, 187
The Grief Response, 187
Perceptions of Injury, 188
Fear, 189
Alienation, 189
Depletion of Coping Resources, 190
Psychological Considerations in Treatment and Rehabilitation, 190
The Athlete as Human Being, 190
Social Support, 190
Psychological Rehabilitation Strategies, 191

Unit III   Athletic Injury Assessment Process

10   Factors related to athletic injury assessment, 196
Athletic Injury Assessment Considerations, 197
When to Assess, 197
Where to Assess, 197

Personal Assessment Skills, 197
Referral Skills, 199
Plan of Action, 199
Summary, 200
Athletic Injury Assessment Process, 200
Anatomy, 200
Athletic Injuries, 201
Evaluative Techniques, 201
Signs and Symptoms, 201
Diagnostic Procedures, 201
Radiology, 202
Laboratory Evaluations, 214
Electroencephalography, 214
Electrocardiography, 214
Echocardiography, 214
Electromyography, 220
Arthroscopy, 220
Pulmonary Function Tests, 222
Summary, 222

11   Assessment procedures, 223
Primary Survey, 223
Airway, 224
Breathing, 225
Circulation, 226
Secondary Survey, 227
History, 230
Observation, 234
Physical Examination, 237
Evaluation of Findings, 245

Unit IV   Athletic Injuries of the Axial Region

12   The unconscious athlete, 250
Unconsciousness, 250
Causes of Unconsciousness in Athletic Activity, 251
Athletic Injury Assessment Process, 251
Primary Survey, 251
Airway, 252
Breathing, 252
Circulation, 253
Secondary Survey, 255
History, 256
Observation, 256
Physical Examination, 260
Evaluation of Findings, 264

13 Head injuries, 266
Head Injuries, 266
  Scalp, 267
  Skull, 268
  Brain, 270
Athletic Injury Assessment Process, 278
  Primary Survey, 278
  Secondary Survey, 279
    History, 279
    Observation, 282
    Physical Examination, 283
    Evaluation of Findings, 287

14 Face injuries, 290
Anatomy of the Face, 290
  Jaw, 292
  Nose, 295
  Ear, 298
  Teeth, 301
  Eye, 305
  Evaluation of Findings, 313

15 Spine injuries, 316
Anatomy of the Spine, 316
  Intervertebral Discs, 316
  Ligaments of the Vertebral Column, 317
  Spinal Cord, 318
  Spinal Nerves, 318
  Muscles Acting on the Vertebral Column, 320
  Cervical Spine, 321
  Thoracic Spine, 324
  Lumbar Spine, 326
  Sacrum and Coccyx, 329
Athletic Injury Assessment Process, 330
  Primary Survey, 331
  Secondary Survey, 331
    History, 333
    Observation, 334
    Physical Examination, 339
    Evaluation of Findings, 351

16 Throat, chest, abdomen, and pelvis injuries, 354
Throat (Anterior Neck), 354
  Neck Muscles, 355
  Anatomic Structures of the Neck, 355
Throat Injuries and Conditions, 357
Chest, 358
  Topographic Anatomy of the Thorax, 358
  Thoracic Viscera, 362

Lungs and Pleura, 363
Mechanism of Pulmonary Ventilation, 363
Chest Injuries and Conditions, 364
Chest Wall, 364
Intrathoracic Injuries, 366
Conditions Affecting the Respiratory Tract, 367
Abdomen and Pelvis, 369
Anatomic Mapping, 369
Surface Anatomy, 369
Muscles of the Abdominal Wall, 370
Abdominal and Pelvic Anatomy, 371
Abdominal Injuries and Conditions, 371
Abdominal Wall, 371
Intra-abdominal Injuries, 373
Gastrointestinal Conditions, 375
Additional Abdominal Conditions, 377
Eating Disorders, 378
The Genitalia, 378
Male, 378
Female, 380
Genitalia Injuries and Conditions, 381
Menstrual Dysfunctions, 381
Sexually Transmitted Diseases, 383
Athletic Injury Assessment Process, 384
Primary Survey, 384
Secondary Survey, 384
History, 385
Observation, 386
Physical Examination, 387
Evaluation of Findings, 390

Unit V   **Athletic Injuries of the Lower Extremities**

17   **Foot, ankle, and leg injuries, 398**
Anatomy of the Foot and Ankle, 398
Accessory Bones, 401
Arches, 401
Joints, 402
Foot Types, 403
Ankle Joint, 406
Ankle Ligaments, 407
Foot and Ankle Injuries/Conditions, 407
Foot Conditions, 409
Contusions, 410
Strains, 410
Sprains, 411

Dislocations, 414
Fractures, 414
Anatomy of the Leg, 416
Tibia and Fibula, 416
Tibiofibular Joints, 416
Muscles of the Leg, 417
Circulation and Nerve Supply, 425
Leg Injuries, 426
Contusions, 426
Strains, 427
Fractures, 430
Athletic Injury Assessment Process, 432
Secondary Survey, 433
History, 433
Observation, 436
Physical Examination, 437
Evaluation of Findings, 454

18   Knee injuries, 457
Anatomy of the Knee, 457
Movements, 457
Structures, 458
Athletic Injury Assessment Process, 474
Secondary Survey, 474
History, 475
Observation, 476
Physical Examination, 478
Evaluation of Findings, 506

19   Thigh and hip injuries, 509
Anatomy of the Thigh and Hip, 509
Hip Joint, 510
Articular (Fibrous) Capsule, 511
Ligaments, 512
Muscles, 512
Movements, 512
Injuries to the Thigh and Hip, 519
Contusions, 519
Strains, 522
Sprains, 523
Dislocations, 524
Fractures, 524
Athletic Injury Assessment Process, 525
Secondary Survey, 525
History, 526
Observation, 527
Physical Examination, 528
Evaluation of Findings, 539

Unit VI   Athletic Injuries of the Upper Extremities

20   **Shoulder injuries, 544**
    Anatomy of the Shoulder, 544
        Sternoclavicular Joint, 546
        Acromioclavicular Joint, 547
        Glenohumeral Joint, 548
        Shoulder Muscles, 550
        Brachial Plexus, 554
        Anatomic Relationships, 544
    Injuries to the Shoulder, 555
        Contusions, 556
        Strains, 556
        Sprains, 558
        Dislocations, 560
        Fractures, 561
        Other Conditions of the Shoulder, 562
    Athletic Injury Assessment Process, 563
        Secondary Survey, 564
        History, 564
        Observation, 565
        Physical Examination, 567
        Evaluation of Findings, 587

21   **Elbow and forearm injuries, 589**
    Anatomy of the Elbow, 589
        Articular Capsule and Collateral Ligaments, 591
        Synovial Membrane and Subcutaneous Bursae, 592
        Elbow Muscles and Movements, 593
        Muscles of the Forearm, 595
        Interosseous Membrane, 596
    Injuries to the Elbow and Forearm, 598
        Contusions, 598
        Strains, 599
        Sprains, 600
        Dislocations, 601
        Fractures, 601
        Nerve Involvement, 603
    Athletic Injury Assessment Process, 604
        Secondary Survey, 604
        History, 605
        Observation, 606
        Physical Examination, 607
        Evaluation of Findings, 618

22   **Hand and wrist injuries, 621**
    Anatomy of the Wrist, 622
        Carpals, 623
        Distal Radioulnar Articulation, 624
        Radiocarpal Articulation, 624

Midcarpal Articulations, 624
Carpometacarpal Articulations, 625
Ligaments, 625
Anatomic Snuffbox, 626
Injuries to the Wrist, 626
Contusions, 627
Strains, 627
Sprains, 628
Dislocations, 628
Fractures, 629
Carpal Tunnel Syndrome, 630
Anatomy of the Hand, 630
Metacarpals, 631
Phalanges, 631
Metacarpophalangeal Articulations, 631
Interphalangeal Articulations, 632
Palmar Region, 632
Dorsal Region, 632
Fingers, 632
Muscles of the Hand, 632
Sensory Innervation of the Hand, 633
Motor Innervation of the Hand, 633
Injuries to the Hand, 633
Contusions and Abrasions, 635
Lacerations and Punctures, 636
Infections, 637
Strains, 637
Sprains, 638
Dislocations, 639
Fractures, 640
Athletic Injury Assessment Process, 641
Secondary Survey, 641
History, 642
Observation, 642
Physical Examination, 643
Evaluation of Findings, 654

Glossary, 657-683

UNIT I

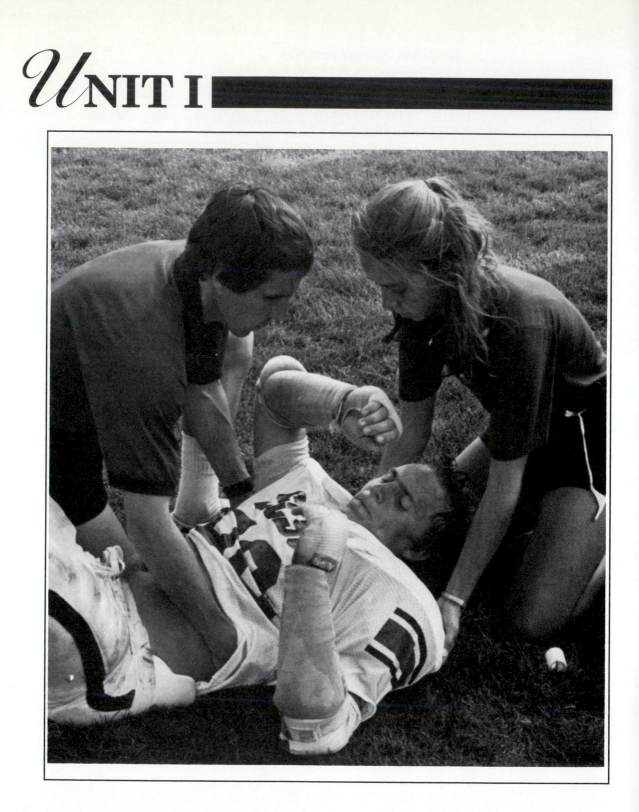

Introduction and Anatomic Basis for Athletic Injury Assessment

Athletic injury assessment is the comprehensive evaluation of an athletic injury. Assessment skills are necessary for all who are responsible for the medical care of athletes. Competency and proficiency in assessing athletic injuries requires many skills, including knowledge, technique, and experience. This unit provides an introduction to the profession of athletic training and the importance of athletic injury assessment (Chapter 1), as well as a basic review of the essential anatomic characteristics of the human body as they relate to athletic injury assessment.

Chapter 1 introduces the student to the concept of athletic injury assessment. In addition to material covered in Chapter 1 and the development in Chapter 2 of an appreciation for the physical characteristics of the whole body, this unit highlights the anatomy of the four major organ systems of most direct importance to those interested in athletics and the assessment of athletic injuries—bones, articulations (joints), muscles, and nerves.

1 **Introduction to athletic injury assessment**
2 **The body as a whole**
3 **Osteology**
4 **Arthrology**
5 **Myology**
6 **Neurology**

CHAPTER 1

Introduction to athletic injury assessment

After you have completed this chapter, you should be able to:
- Define the terms *sports medicine* and *athletic training*.
- List the professional disciplines that contribute to the health and performance of the athlete.
- List the specific contributions and functions of the athletic trainer as a provider of services and health care support for athletes.
- Discuss the competencies necessary for an individual to become a certified athletic trainer.
- Discuss the relationship of athletic injury assessment to each of the other major duties or functions of the certified athletic trainer.

Athletic injury assessment is of paramount importance for anyone who is responsible for the well-being of athletes. The assessment process is the first step in a series of steps to properly care for an athletic injury. The information gained during the assessment process provides the basis for decisions concerning referral to medical assistance, appropriate follow-up care, effective treatment procedures, productive rehabilitation techniques, and efficient functional testing. Assessment is the cornerstone of effective management of athletic injuries by athletic trainers and physicians but is often carried out by coaches and others accepting the responsibility for the medical care of athletes. This chapter will discuss the importance of the athletic injury assessment process, as well as the growing field of sports medicine and the profession of athletic training.

It is inevitable that injuries will always be associated with physical activity and athletics. The risk of injury is much higher in some sports, such as those requiring contact or collision, but it is inherent to all athletic activity. Although the majority of athletic injuries are relatively minor, the potential for serious and possibly life-threatening injuries is constantly present. The incidence of serious and life-threatening conditions associated with athletic activity has decreased over the years as a result of the delineation of causative factors and subsequent rule modifications in many sports and vast improvements and increased sophistication in all facets of sports medicine and athletic training. In spite of this increased sophistication, there has been an overall increase in the number of athletic injuries; this is primarily due to an increase in the number of participants, the intensity of modern training techniques, and the growth of athletic activities.

Today a wider selection of athletic activities, physical fitness programs, and sports are available to a larger cross-section of the population than ever before. Interest in physical activities and athletics continues to increase, and participation is no longer limited to high school, college, amateur, and professional athletes. A greater number of organized athletic programs are available to children in junior high school and upper elementary grades. Youth sports competitions, recreational programs, intramural activities, and sports for the disabled and all age groups are increasing in popularity. The number of participants in all areas continues to increase dramatically. The development of many women's athletic programs is another factor that has greatly changed the number of sports activities and opportunities for participation. Because of all these developments, there are greater opportunities for persons of all ages to participate in recreational and competitive activities.

People are becoming more health and fitness conscious than ever before. This awareness has produced an increased interest in the benefits of physical fitness. More people are participating in lifetime activities, such as walking, jogging, bicycling, swimming, golf, and tennis. People today have more leisure time as a result of many factors, including shorter work weeks, mechanization, and time-saving devices. Many people are using this additional leisure time to participate in recreational activities requiring some degree of physical exertion.

Whatever the reason for the dramatic increase in the number of participants and activities available, injuries are a reality at every level of participation and in every type of program. Participants in all forms of athletic activity are subjected to many stresses and forces that can result in injury. It is important to remember that injuries to athletes are essentially no different from those suffered by nonathletes. A sprained ankle can result in the same severity of damage whether it is sustained by a competitive athlete, a weekend jogger, or a business person. However, the demands in terms of evaluation, treatment, rehabilitation, and return to activity are normally significantly greater for the competitive athlete.

SPORTS MEDICINE

Just as there have been tremendous increases in participation and interest in athletics, there have been corresponding increases in interest, knowledge, and understanding concerning all aspects of the medical management of athletic-related injuries and conditions. **Sports medicine** is the phrase that is used to describe this vast network of medical and paramedical management. Sports medicine is multidisciplinary and encompasses all phases of medical concerns relating to athletic activity: biomechanical, psychological, nutritional, environmental, pathological, and physiological. It is an umbrella term that includes all medical and paramedical professionals who are concerned with and provide expertise aimed at enhancing the performance and health care of individuals (Figure 1-1).

The field of sports medicine has seen phenomenal growth in recent years, as evidenced by the number of professional associations designating sports medicine as a subspecialty; the vast amounts of literature, research, and educational experiences now available; the number of professional journals that are now devoted entirely to sports medicine; and the number of medical clinics specializing in sports medicine that are emerging throughout the country. Sports medicine is a rapidly growing, dynamic field. The knowledge and techniques gained benefit not only competitive athletes and the vast legion of fitness buffs but also everyone else involved in athletic and nonathletic activities. One of the subspecialties of sports medicine is athletic training.

ATHLETIC TRAINING

Athletic training provides a wide array of health care support services for athletes.

Athletic training has been defined as "the art and science of prevention and management of injuries at all levels of athletic activity." The provider of athletic training services is an **athletic trainer.** The profession of athletic training and the position of the athletic trainer on the sports medicine team have developed to meet a demand for a professional highly skilled in the evaluation, management, and care of athletic injuries. As long as there has been athletics, there has generally been someone designated to manage or care for athletes who become injured. In the past this position of responsibility was generally filled by a coach, teacher, student, or other interested person. Now most of these positions at the collegiate and professional levels are being filled by a certified athletic trainer (ATC). However, much of the responsibility for the medical care of athletes, particularly at the high school level, will continue to remain with the coach until the need for highly skilled athletic trainers at all levels of participation is

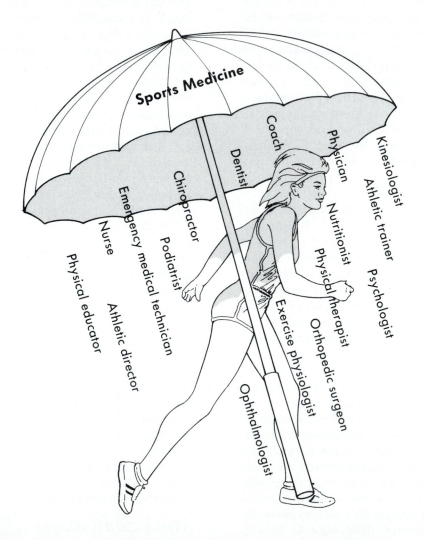

FIGURE 1-1
Sports medicine is an umbrella term and includes all professionals who are concerned with enhancing the performance and health care of individuals.

recognized. Currently, approximately 45% of all certified athletic trainers work at the college or professional level, 20% work in high school athletic programs, and 32% work in hospital-based or private sports medicine clinics. Many of these athletic trainers in clinics also cover a high school athletic program. There are more certified athletic trainers now administering to high school athletes than ever before. However, there remains a small percentage of high schools in the United States that employ an athletic trainer. Athletes at schools without athletic trainers are more likely to experience injuries that go unrecognized or untreated.

Compared with other allied health professions, athletic training is quite young. The National Athletic Trainer's Association (NATA) was founded in 1950. The profession of athletic training has undergone explosive growth in the past 5 years, and NATA has become one of the fastest growing allied health care associations in the country.

Qualifications and requirements to become an athletic trainer have also grown and evolved over the years. In 1969, guidelines were developed for those institutions offering athletic training curricula to obtain NATA approval. At that time only two schools were able to meet all of the requirements needed for approval. In 1993, over 90 schools offered NATA-approved curricula at the undergraduate or graduate level. In June 1990, the American Medical Association (AMA) formally recognized athletic training as an allied health profession. Now all programs that provide athletic training education must seek accreditation through the AMA's Committee on Allied Health Education and Accreditation.

In 1970 a certifying procedure for athletic trainers was established and has been continually upgraded and improved. To become an athletic trainer a person must have a college degree that fulfills specific educational requirements and practical experiences. On successful completion of these requirements the candidate must then take a national certifying examination, which includes a written examination, a written simulation, and an oral/practical examination. This examination is designed to ensure that the candidate meets the minimal standards and competencies required to become a certified athletic trainer. In addition to obtaining the initial certification, athletic trainers must also earn a designated number of continuing educational units to maintain their certified status.

The NATA Board of Certification (NATABOC) conducted role delineation studies in 1982 and 1990. The results of these studies serve as the basis for development of competencies identified as those necessary for effective functioning as an entry level certified athletic trainer. These competencies are categorized into six major "domains" that comprise the role of the certified athletic trainer: (1) prevention, (2) recognition and evaluation, (3) management/treatment and disposition, (4) rehabilitation, (5) organization and administration, and (6) education and counseling. The competencies identified within each of these major domains are further classified into behavioral objectives: (1) cognitive (knowledge and intellectual skills), (2) psychomotor (manipulative and motor skills), and (3) affective (attitudes and values). Each of these areas is important, and all are interrelated. The athletic trainer must develop knowledge and competency in each category to provide athletes with optimal medical care. In addition to the competencies, the role delineation studies identified a list of athletic injuries and illnesses with which an athletic trainer may be confronted and should know about. Each of these injuries/illnesses is discussed in this textbook and indicated by boldface and an icon.

An athletic trainer must be able to combine medical and scientific information in the areas of anatomy, physiology, kinesiology, psychology, physiology of exercise, health, physics, nutrition, and first aid with a wide array of complex practical skills. In addition, he or she must also have a sincere interest in athletics and in working with athletes and must possess communication and leadership skills. The athletic trainer is

TABLE 1-1

Competencies in Athletic Training

Prevention	Recognition and evaluation	Management and treatment
Preparticipation examination	Primary survey	Immediate first aid
Medical history	Airway	Ice
Physical examination	Breathing	Compression
Fitness screening	Circulation	Elevation
Proper conditioning	Secondary survey	Rest
Protective equipment	History	Follow-up treatment
Selection	Observation	Therapeutic modalities
Fitting	Physical examination	Exercise programs
Maintenance	Palpation	Protective techniques
Safety supervision	Movement procedures	Taping
Facilities	Neurological	Splinting
Equipment	evaluation	Padding
Preventive techniques	Circulatory evaluations	Supporting
Taping	Evaluation of findings	Immobilizing
Padding	Medical referral	Assessment of techniques
Bandaging	Treatment application	Evaluation of the effects of treatment
Bracing		procedures on signs and symptoms
Observing athletes		
Recognizing problems and minor		
injuries		
Hygiene		
Rest		
Diet		
Assessment techniques		
Recognizing injury		
Determining severity of injury		
Observation when returned to		
activity		
Emergency care procedures		
Supplies		
Plan of action		
Immediate care		
Rehabilitation strategies		
Prevent reinjury		
Strengthen previously injured		
area		
Monitoring environmental		
conditions		

no longer a "jack of all trades, master of none," but a professional who must be proficient in many varied skills. Today's athletic trainer is more scientific and knowledgeable about the many aspects of health care for athletes. The athletic trainer has become a vital member of the sports medicine team responsible for coordinating and providing health care for athletes. The primary competencies or proficiencies necessary to become a certified athletic trainer are briefly discussed and are listed in Table 1-1.

Prevention

The best method of managing and caring for athletic injuries is to prevent them from occurring; therefore much of the athletic trainer's time and effort is devoted to preventing injuries. Numerous factors, briefly discussed in this section, are important in the prevention of athletic injuries. A thorough preparticipation evaluation does not guarantee that an athlete will participate injury free, but it does affirm that there is no discernible clinical reason to preclude participation.

Rehabilitation	Organization and administration	Education and counseling
Range of motion	Maintain records	Previous injuries and present status
Muscular strength	Injuries	Medical history
Muscular endurance	Treatment	Requirements of each sport
Coordinated movements	Facilities	Health topics
Functional activities	Inspection	Knowledge of health education
Cardiovascular endurance	Safety	Sports psychology
Assessment techniques	Sanitation	Social and personal problems
Evaluation of effects of	Equipment and supplies	Knowledge of available professionals
rehabilitation program	Purchasing	Knowledge of situation requiring
	Maintaining	consultation
	Health care services	Referral procedures
	Team coverage	Knowledge of team or family physician
	Organization	Instructing student trainers
	Communication	Continuing education
	Policies and procedures	
	Emergency support services	

Proper conditioning is the preventive medicine of athletics. Athletic trainers often work in conjunction with coaches in establishing preseason, in-season, and off-season conditioning programs. Another facet of athletic injury prevention in which the athletic trainer is involved is the selection, fitting, and maintenance of protective equipment. An athletic trainer may also be responsible for checking the safety of facilities and apparatus required for athletic activity.

More familiar preventive tasks performed by athletic trainers include the application of protective taping, padding, bandaging, braces, and other devices. Athletic trainers must also constantly observe their athletes. If recognized early, minor problems can often be treated with minimal inconvenience to the athlete and no significant decrease in performance. Early recognition and effective treatment prevent most minor injuries from becoming severe and disabling. An injury that is properly recognized and managed effectively generally does not become more severe, and the potential for reinjury is decreased. In addition, athletic trainers are often asked to counsel athletes and coaches in the areas of diet, rest, and sanitation.

Recognition and Evaluation

Athletic trainers must possess a high level of proficiency in assessment skills to accurately recognize and evaluate the nature and severity of an athletic injury. Athletic trainers are normally at the location or playing field where an injury occurs and have to handle the emergency care. They must be able to recognize and deal with conditions such as severe head or spine injuries, hemorrhaging, shock, heat illness, or choking. Athletic trainers must be prepared to administer cardiopulmonary resuscitation, apply emergency splinting, or supervise the transportation of an injured athlete.

The athletic injury assessment process is based on a scientific method that involves (1) recognition and statement of the problem, (2) collection of data about the problem, and (3) creation and testing of hypotheses to solve the problem. An athletic trainer's initial assessment creates the foundation, or data base, for the ensuing procedures. When an athletic injury or related condition occurs, data related to the incident are collected through the systematic steps of history, observation, and physical examination, each of which may include various techniques and procedures. From the data collected, the athletic trainer must determine and initiate the appropriate course of action. This includes emergency medical care, follow-up treatment procedures, transportation, medical referral, rehabilitation strategies, or return to athletic activity. Once action has been taken, the athletic trainer must continually evaluate the results of this action. Is the athlete getting better or worse? Why? What can be done to improve or enhance the athlete's recovery? The athletic trainer should then modify or adjust the plan of action accordingly. Assessment and reassessment are ongoing processes in athletic training. The assessment process is discussed in more detail in Unit III, and assessment procedures are discussed throughout this text.

Management and Treatment
Athletic trainers must be skilled in various management and treatment procedures. These include (1) administering immediate first aid, (2) providing therapy to promote healing and recovery, (3) applying protective techniques to support and protect an injured area, and (4) referring an injured athlete for further medical assistance when necessary. Athletic trainers can have a dramatic effect on the overall recovery of an injured athlete by the proper use of treatment procedures. The goal is to return the injured athlete to activity as soon as possible without risking further injury. The treatment of an athletic injury is a three-step process: (1) examination of the signs and symptoms, (2) application of treatment routines, and (3) assessment of the effects of these techniques on the signs and symptoms of the injury. This cycle continues throughout the treatment process; that is, assessment, treatment, and reassessment. If an athlete is to return to optimum physical activity in a minimal amount of time, there can be no delay in an accurate assessment and a properly instituted treatment program.

Rehabilitation
Rehabilitation is the restoration of normal form and function after an injury. Athletic

rehabilitation is the reconditioning of an injured athlete to his or her highest level of function in the shortest possible time. This level of function is generally higher than that of a nonathlete. Athletic trainers must be skilled in developing programs to effectively rehabilitate an athlete in a minimal amount of time. Depending on the nature and the conditions surrounding the injury, rehabilitation requires a progressive, systematic program that develops range of motion, muscular strength and endurance, coordinated movements, functional activities, and circulorespiratory endurance. Although each of these phases overlap, maximal development of any phase requires prior development of the preceding phases. Rehabilitation also includes total body conditioning/maintenance occurring concurrently with restoration of the injured area so the athlete can meet the physical demands of athletic activity when returning to participation. During rehabilitation, repeated assessment techniques should be performed to evaluate progress and adjust the program as needed.

Organization and Administration
Organization and administration of the athletic training program are often overlooked aspects of an athletic trainer's responsibilities. Athletic trainers must plan, organize, evaluate, and implement procedures and policies necessary to provide their athletes with the most effective health care available. To aid in efficient health care delivery, athletic trainers must maintain accurate and detailed records to document injuries, treatments, and other services rendered to the athletes under their care. Selecting, purchasing, maintaining, and instructing others in the use of equipment and supplies necessary for operation of a training room are also the athletic trainer's responsibilities.

Education and Counseling
The final function of an athletic trainer to be discussed is the role of educator and counselor to the athlete and student athletic trainer. Athletic trainers need to have the skill and knowledge necessary to instruct students in the competencies required to be-

come professional athletic trainers. This responsibility requires that the athletic trainer keep abreast of current sports medicine issues and also be able to convey this information to others. Another facet of education and counseling skills required is the athletic trainer's ability to recognize situations that require consultation with other health care professionals regarding an athlete's social or personal problem. This involves skill in assessing an athlete's need for professional consultation and referral of the athlete to the appropriate professional. To be effective in this area, an athletic trainer must possess effective communication skills. These communication skills enable the athletic trainer to interact with athletes, parents, coaches, administrators, physicians,

and other professionals concerning various health-related topics.

To summarize, athletic trainers must develop knowledge and competency in each of these duties or functions to provide optimal medical care to athletes. Note that assessment or evaluation skills are listed and discussed under each of these categories. Athletic injury assessment is a necessary and extremely important skill for anyone who has medical responsibilities for athletes. Indeed, planning an athlete's medical care based on an accurate assessment is the foundation of current athletic training practices. Athletic injury assessment affects each of the other major duties or functions of an athletic trainer (Figure 1-2). This textbook specifically addresses this important function of

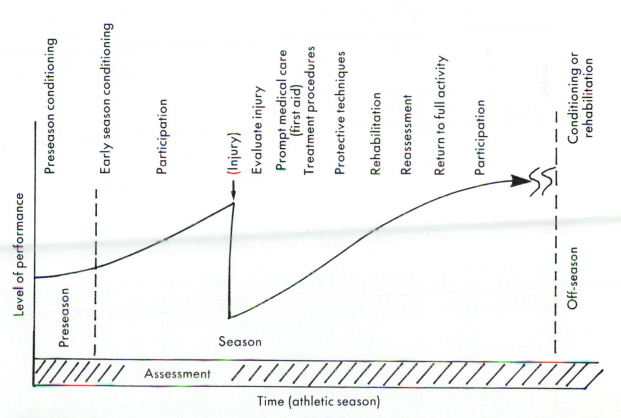

FIGURE 1-2
Effect of an athletic injury on performance.

athletic training—assessment of athletic injuries.

REFERENCES

Cadwell F: Epidemiology takes its place on the sports medicine team, *Phys Sportsmed* 13(3):135, 1985.

DiNitto LM: Sports medicine: many options available for adding the athletic trainer to the high school staff, *Interscholastic Athletic Administration* 14(2):22, 1987.

Emerick CE, Schrader JW: Back to reality: athletic training at the high school level, *Ath Train* 16(3):180, 1981.

Gieck J: The athletic trainer and counselor education, *Ath Train* 12(2):58, 1977.

Hage P: Medical care for athletes: are coaches getting the message? *Phys Sportsmed* 10(11):159, 1982.

Hage P, Moore M: Medical care for athletes: what is the coaches role? *Phys Sportsmed* 9(5):140, 1981.

Howe WB: Primary care sports medicine: a part-timer's perspective, *Phys Sportsmed* 16(1):102, 1988.

Kegerreis S: Health care for student athletes, *JOPER* 50(6):78, 1979.

Kelley EJ, Miller SJ: The need for a certified athletic trainer in the junior-senior high schools, *Ath Train* 11(4):180, 1976.

National Athletic Trainers' Association: *Professional preparation in athletic training*, Champaign, 1982, Human Kinetics, Inc.

Powers HW: The organization and administration of an athletic training program, *Ath Train* 11(1):14, 1976.

Rogers CC: Does sports medicine fit in the new health care market? *Phys Sportsmed* 13(1):116, 1985.

Rowe PJ, Miller LK: Treating high school sports injuries—are coaches/trainers competent? *JOPER* 62(1):49, 1991.

Vereschagin KS: Expanding sports medicine's role in primary care, *Phys Sportsmed* 21(5):121, 1993.

Vinger PF, Hoerner EF: *Sports injuries; the unthwarted epidemic,* Boston, 1982, John Wright-PSG, Inc.

Whieldon TJ, Cerny FJ: Incidence and severity of high school athletic injuries, *Ath Train* 25(4):344, 1990.

SUGGESTED READINGS

Arnheim DD, Prentice WE: *Principles of athletic training,* ed 8, St Louis, 1993, Mosby.
An excellent comprehensive text covering all aspects of athletic training. The first chapter discusses the development and growth of athletic training and sports medicine.

Lombardo JA: Sports medicine: a team effort, *Phys Sportsmed* 13(4):72, 1985.
The author describes why sports medicine is not reserved for only the physician but depends on various professional groups to add their expertise to the sports medicine team.

National Athletic Trainers' Association: *Competencies in athletic training,* 1992, The Association.
Competencies in this manual have been identified as those necessary for effective functioning as an athletic trainer. The list of competencies was developed by the National Athletic Trainers' Association as a result of role-delineation studies completed in 1982 and 1990. This manual is a must for every student working toward becoming a certified athletic trainer.

O'Shea ME: *A history of the National Athletic Trainers' Association,* 1980, The Association.
A comprehensive history of the growth and development of the National Athletic Trainers' Association.

CHAPTER 2

The body as a whole

After you have completed this chapter, you should be able to:

- Explain the relationship of accurate athletic injury assessment to the systematic observation of the athlete as a whole person.
- Describe the use of basic somatotyping techniques as a mechanism to quantify subjective physical characteristics.
- Explain mechanisms used to determine body composition and discuss their importance in athletic injury assessment.
- List and define the principal directional terms and body sections (planes) employed in describing the body and the relationship of its parts.
- List the major body areas that comprise the axial and appendicular divisions of the body.

Proficiency and knowledge in athletic injury assessment procedures depend on much more than good technique and a thorough understanding of anatomy in the area of injury. Assessment begins with systematic and deliberate observations of the person as a whole. Athletes are certainly more than the sum of their parts, and the adage "know your athlete" is as important to the athletic trainer as it is to the coach.

In studying and perfecting the techniques for assessment of an athletic injury to specific body parts or areas, it is all too easy to think of each part in isolation from the body as a whole. Always remember that you are dealing with an injured person and not just an injured knee, elbow, or shoulder. Having a complete and detailed information base or profile on an athlete before an injury is immensely helpful in making an accurate assessment of an injury should the need arise. Information presented in this chapter is intended to help you view the athlete, healthy or injured, as a whole person. Material covered includes a brief introduction to the concept of body type (somatotype) and composition and some generalizations on the organization of the body and the language of anatomy.

SOMATOTYPE

Even an untrained eye can see that there are a variety of athletic body types or physiques. Certain physiques dominate particular sports or positions within sports. For example, a cross-country runner tends to have a small, lean body, whereas a defensive end in football tends to be quite large and muscular. The classification of the body according to physique is known as **somatotyping.** Early work in somatotyping was

11

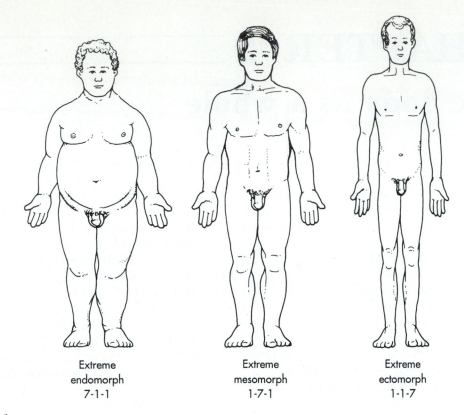

Extreme
endomorph
7-1-1

Extreme
mesomorph
1-7-1

Extreme
ectomorph
1-1-7

FIGURE 2-1
Examples of the extreme somatotypes. Note the almost total dominance of a single somatotype component in each type of physique.

done by Sheldon, who classified the body into three categories: the **endomorph,** the **mesomorph,** and the **ectomorph** (Figure 2-1). The endomorphic body type is characterized by a roundness and softness of the body, the mesomorphic individual has a very muscular physique with heavy bones, and the ectomorphic athlete's characteristics are small bones and a lean body. To quantify the description of the prevalence of the three components, a rating scale is used. Each component is rated on a scale of one to seven, with one being the least and seven indicating a strong amount of the component. When the description is written out, it is expressed in the following order: endomorph-mesomorph-ectomorph. Therefore, if the rating is 3–6–1, an athlete has predominately mesomorphic body qualities, with some endomorphic qualities and few, if any, ectomorphic characteristics.

In addition to the Sheldon somatotyping system, another method has been developed by Heath and Carter. The Heath-Carter somatotype includes anthropometric measurements in addition to visual assessment of the athlete. Therefore it is a more objective method. The Heath-Carter somatotype can also be used with women, as well as men. Somatotyping is used most frequently in research investigations that attempt to identify which physiques are most successful at particular athletic activities.

BODY COMPOSITION

The assessment of body composition is more valuable to the athletic trainer than somatotyping. The assessment of body composition is used to identify what percentage of the body is made up of lean tissue (fat-free mass) and what percentage is fat. During the last decade, there has been increased interest in the assessment of body composition in physiological and nutritional research, as well as in sports medicine. Body composition is an important aspect of physical fitness and has become a focus for many wellness programs. Body composition analysis can also serve a variety of purposes in athletics. One use is to set minimal weight guidelines for sports with weight classes such as wrestling. For example, experts agree that 5% body fat is the lowest acceptable level for athletes competing in wrestling. Another use is to monitor athletes as they try to lose or gain weight. As the athlete loses weight, it is important that the weight loss comes from excess fat and not lean muscle mass. When trying to gain weight, the athlete wants to increase muscle mass and not fat. A third use for body composition assessment is to determine whether an athlete is "overweight" or "overfat." To determine if an athlete is overweight, many people look to height-weight charts. A height-weight chart gives an average weight for a given height. One must remember, however, that many athletes are well above the average weight because of an increase in muscle mass, not fat. An athletic trainer will have a more accurate assessment about whether or not an athlete needs to lose weight by determining what percentage of the total body weight is fat. Many generalized fitness programs for young adults often suggest body-fat percentages of 15% to 18% for men and 22% to 29% for women. However, the percentages of fat typical of athletes in training is less. It should be stressed that there is no single percentage of fat that can be singled out as optimal. Each athlete is unique, and optimal body fat levels are often independent of body weight. Further, variances within a normal range are also related to age and gender. Good records showing rate of fatigue and performance data on an athlete are helpful in determining what percentage of body fat is ideal for that individual.

Body Fat Distribution Patterns

Increasing numbers of athletic trainers are participating as members of health care de-livery teams who assist community agencies, school districts, and corporations in developing fitness, stress reduction, and wellness programs. Knowledge of an individual's somatotype and body composition can provide health care professionals and educators with vital information useful in such areas as disease screening procedures, programs designed to identify individuals who may be "at risk" for developing certain diseases, and for predicting performance capability in selected physical education and sports programs.

Researchers have discovered that individuals (especially endomorphs) who have large waistlines and are "apple-shaped," or fattest in the abdomen, have a greater risk for heart disease, stroke, high blood pressure, and diabetes than individuals with a lower "pear-shaped" distribution pattern of fat in the hips, thighs, and buttocks. Endomorphic individuals of the same height and weight but with a lower, or pear-shaped, body fat distribution pattern develop these diseases in larger numbers than mesomorphs and ectomorphs but less frequently than endomorphs with an apple-shaped, or high body fat, distribution pattern. This information explains the rekindled interest in somatotype analysis. Although always an area of research interest, it was considered by practicing athletic trainers as largely "historical" and of relatively little practical importance. These new research findings, however, have modified a growing number of clinical screening procedures to include somatotype identification procedures, body composition studies, and analysis of body fat distribution patterns. Individuals "at high risk" can be advised to watch closely for signs of diseases now known to be associated with body shape.

Gender, exercise, diet, dominance (i.e., right, left), and heredity all play a role in determining body shape, symmetry, and fat content. Although body shape is not gender specific, men are more likely than women to be apple-shaped and are therefore more at risk for diseases now associated with this higher body fat distribution pattern. In apple-shaped individuals, abdominal fat is stored deep in abdominal tissues, whereas in the pear-shaped physique, most excess fat is located just below the skin near the body surface.

The *waist-to-hip ratio* is now used with assessment of somatotype to evaluate the risk of individuals developing diseases we know are related to body fat distribution patterns. Endomorphs with an "apple shape" are at highest risk. To determine the waist-to-hip ratio, the hips are measured at their widest point around the buttocks and the waist is measured at the level of the umbilicus. To obtain the ratio, divide the waist measurement by the hip size. A ratio greater than 1.0 for men and 0.8 for women places the person "at risk" for diseases associated with a high body, or apple-shaped, fat distribution pattern. In men the risk factor appears if the waist size exceeds the hip measurement; in women, risk increases significantly if the waist size exceeds 80% of the hip measurement.

Assessing Body Composition

Currently there are many methods available for assessing body composition, but none are wholly satisfactory for all purposes. The ideal method for assessing human body composition would be relatively inexpensive, require little inconvenience for the subject, be operated by an unskilled individual, and yield highly accurate and reproducible results. No method available meets all these criteria. Laboratory methods such as neutron activation, absorptiometry, isotope dilution, computed tomography (CT) scan, and magnetic resonance imaging (MRI) are accurate but expensive, cumbersome, or require sensitive instrumentation and highly trained technicians. These methods are used primarily in research settings. In the athletic setting, there is often a compromise between cost, ease of operation, and reliability. Following is a brief description of common techniques used to assess body composition.

Underwater weighing

The gold standard by which body composition estimates are judged is *underwater weighing* (Figure 2-2). The common method for underwater weighing is to weigh the athlete in air and in water and estimate the lungs' residual volume. From these measurements, the density of the body is deter-

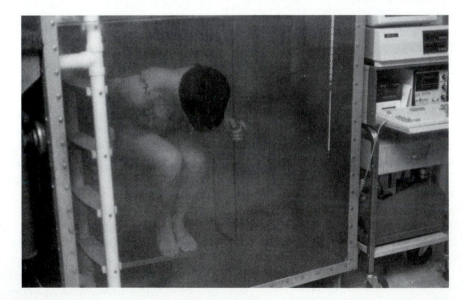

FIGURE 2-2
Determining the body composition by using underwater weighing.

mined. Once the body density is known, the value can be placed into an equation to determine what percentage of body weight is fat. In an athletic training setting, the regular use of underwater weighing may be inconvenient because it requires extensive equipment, cooperation of the athlete while submerged, and time. For a more detailed explanation of underwater weighing, including equations, refer to exercise physiology texts.

Skinfold measurements

A practical alternative to underwater weighing is estimating body composition by measuring selected skinfold sites (Figure 2-3). With practice, this method is reliable and fairly accurate. *Skinfold measurements* are practical, require little equipment, do not involve any learning on the part of the athlete, and the athletic trainer can become proficient fairly quickly. As with other indirect determinations of body composition there is inevitably some error, approximately ±3%. It is important to remember that this is an estimation of body composition and that it may not be exactly representative of the amount of fat in the body.

Equations that are used to predict body density from skinfold measurements tend to be population specific. That is, they work best with individuals who most closely resemble the subjects who were used to deter-

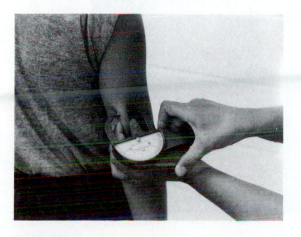

FIGURE 2-3
Obtaining skinfold measurement data.

mine the equation. If an inappropriate equation is selected, there will be a much greater chance of underestimating or overestimating the athlete's percentage of body fat. Some generalized equations have been developed for men (Jackson and Pollock, 1978) and women (Jackson, Pollock, and Ward, 1980) that have worked well with young adults. In addition to selecting the appropriate equation, it is important that the person measuring the skinfolds has some experience and an accurate skinfold caliper to determine the athlete's percentage of fat most accurately.

Another method using skinfolds is to sum the scores from the various sites and use this score to represent a relative degree of fatness. As the athlete trains or undertakes a weight control program, the changes in the sum of the skinfolds are monitored. The skinfold sites commonly measured are the triceps, subscapular, suprailiac, abdominal, and anterior thigh.

When measuring a skinfold, the thickness of two layers of skin and the underlying fat are measured. It is standard practice to measure the skinfolds on the right-hand side of the body. To measure a skinfold, grasp a fold of skin and subcutaneous fat but not the underlying muscular tissue. The skinfold should follow the natural contour of the fat fold. Once the skinfold has been grasped, the skinfold caliper should be placed perpendicular to the fold, approximately 1 cm from the thumb and forefinger holding the skinfold. The caliper should be read 1 to 2 seconds after the application of pressure. The skinfold thickness is recorded to the nearest 0.5 cm. Multiple measurements at each site are recommended with an average of two to five trials. To become proficient at using skinfold calipers, athletic trainers must practice this skill.

After the appropriate equation has been selected and the skinfold sites have been measured, the body density is determined. After the body density has been calculated, this value is placed into an equation to determine body fatness. The two equations most frequently used are those determined by Siri [f = (4.95/D) − 4.5] and Brozek [f = (4.57/D) − 4.142]. Both equations were developed for use with young adult men; however, they have been used extensively with women, athletes, children, and the elderly. Lohman has proposed a different equation to estimate body fat from density in boys and girls before they reach puberty. The equation is [f = (5.3/D) − 4.89]. This change was proposed because the total body water and bone mineral content in children is lower than in adults.

Much of the research in body composition involves college-aged men who are well hydrated as subjects. There is a need for more research to determine the sources of variation in fat-free body weight in children, women, athletes, and the elderly. Also, the effects of various stages of hydration on body composition need to be determined. Research so far has revealed that the density of fat-free body weight in children and the elderly is less than that found in young adult men. Another variation to be considered, especially when measuring skinfolds, is that with increasing age, a greater proportion of fat is deposited internally as opposed to subcutaneous fat. For example, in young adults

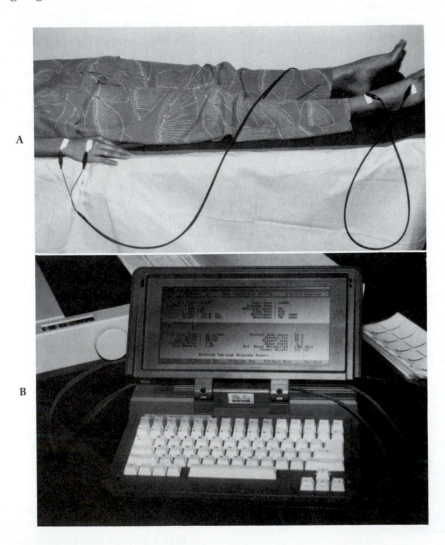

FIGURE 2-4
Determining the body composition by using bioelectrical impedance. **A,** Application of surface electrodes on athlete and **B,** body composition information displayed on screen before being printed.

approximately 50% of total body fat is subcutaneous, whereas the remainder is internal.

Bioelectrical impedance

There has been considerable interest in **bioelectrical impedance** as an inexpensive, safe, portable method of estimating body composition (Figure 2-4). This method is designed to detect changes in electrical impedance between electrodes placed on the body. The basic underlying concept is that lean tissue, which has a high water content, conducts electricity easily, whereas fat tissue resists the flow of electricity. Consequently, impedance to the flow of electric current will be directly related to the level of body fat. This technique involves placing electrodes on the hands and feet, introducing a painless, localized electrical signal, and determining the impedance or resistance to the current's flow. Using an equation, the impedance value is then converted to body density, which in turn is converted to percent body fat.

A factor affecting the accuracy of bioelectrical impedance analysis is the maintenance of normal hydration levels. Dehydration or overhydration affects the normal concentrations of electrolytes, which will affect the electrical current flow. Therefore this method provides more accurate estimates of body composition when measurements are made under normal levels of hydration.

The advantage of the bioelectrical impedance system is that it is fairly easy to use. As this type of system becomes more refined, it may become more accurate for estimating fat percentages.

GENERALIZATIONS ABOUT BODY STRUCTURE

Bilateral Symmetry

Bilateral symmetry is one of the most obvious of the external organizational features in humans. To say that humans are bilaterally symmetric simply means that the right and left sides of the body are mirror images of each other (Figure 2-5). An impor-

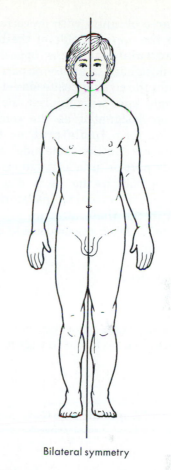

Bilateral symmetry

FIGURE 2-5
Bilateral symmetry. As a result of this organizational feature the right and left sides of the body are mirror images of each other.

tant feature of bilateral symmetry is balanced proportions. There is a remarkable correspondence in size and shape when comparing similar anatomic parts or areas on opposite sides of the body. However, right or left dominance influences muscle strength and mass on the dominant side. Repetitive exercise of prominent muscle groups on an athlete's dominant side can result in localized asymmetric development.

Assessment of injury, especially to an extremity, often requires careful comparison of the injured with the noninjured side. Minimal swelling or deformity on one side of the body is often apparent only to the trained observer who routinely compares a suspected area of injury with its corresponding part on the opposite side of the body. The term **contralateral** means "opposite" and is used to designate an anatomic part or region on the uninjured or opposite side of the body. If the right knee were injured, the left knee would be designated as the contralateral knee. The term **ipsilateral,** on the other hand, means "on the same side" and refers to a body part or area situated on the same side of the body as the injury. For example, if reference is made to ipsilateral muscle spasms in the thigh after an injury to the right knee, those spasms would be in the right thigh.

Body Regions

The body as a whole can be divided into **axial** and **appendicular** divisions. These primary divisions are subdivided as follows and should be reviewed in Figure 2-6.

Axial and Appendicular Body Regions

Axial

Head
   Skull (cranium)
   Face
Neck
Trunk
   Thorax
   Upper Back
   Lower Back
   Abdomen
   Pelvis

Appendicular

Upper extremity
   Shoulder
   Arm
   Elbow
   Forearm
   Wrist
   Hand and fingers
Lower extremity
   Buttocks
   Thigh
   Knee
   Lower leg
   Ankle
   Foot and toes

Anatomic Position

When assessing an athletic injury it is necessary to use precise terms to describe body parts or areas and the relationships that exist between them. To avoid misunderstanding when using terms that describe direction or location on the body, a standardized anatomic position has been adopted. In the **anatomic position** the body is erect and facing forward, as in Figure 2-6, *A*. Note the position of the arms at the side of the body with the palms of the hands turned forward (forearms supinated).

Directional Terms

When the body is in the anatomic position, the following directional terms can be used to describe the location of one body part in relation to another. Refer to Figure 2-6.

- **Superior**: Toward the head end of the body; upper (the eyes are superior to the mouth)
- **Inferior**: Away from the head end of the body; lower (the bladder is inferior to the stomach)
- **Anterior** (ventral): Front (the eyes are located on the anterior surface of the head)
- **Posterior** (dorsal): Back (the shoulder blades are located on the posterior side of the body)
- **Medial**: Toward the midline of the body (the great toe is located at the medial side of the foot)
- **Lateral**: Away from the midline of the body (the little toe is located at the lateral side of the foot)
- **Proximal**: Nearer the point of attachment of an extremity to the trunk or the point of origin of a part (the elbow is proximal to the wrist)
- **Distal**: Farther from the point of attachment of an extremity to the trunk or the point of origin of a part (the hand is located at the distal end of the forearm)
- **Superficial**: Nearer the surface (the skin of the arm is superficial to the muscles below it)
- **Deep**: Farther from the body surface (the humerus of the arm is deep to the muscles that surround it)

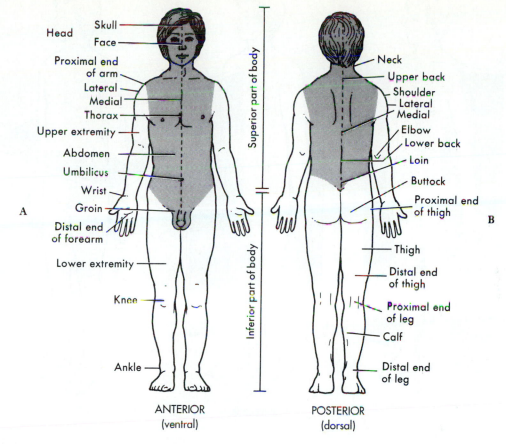

Head — Skull
Face

A

Proximal end
of arm
Lateral
Medial
Thorax
Upper extremity
Abdomen
Umbilicus
Wrist
Groin
Distal end
of forearm
Lower extremity
Knee
Ankle

Superior part of body

Inferior part of body

Neck
Upper back
Shoulder
Lateral
Medial
Elbow
Lower back
Loin
Buttock
Proximal end
of thigh

B

Thigh
Distal end
of thigh
Proximal end
of leg
Calf
Distal end
of leg

ANTERIOR
(ventral)

POSTERIOR
(dorsal)

FIGURE 2-6
The anatomic position showing axial and appendicular subdivisions. **A**, Anterior view and **B**, posterior view. Directional terms are used in describing a number of body regions.

Body Planes (Sections)

To visualize the internal organs, it is necessary to cut, or section, the body into component parts for study. The body is a three-dimensional structure and as such can be divided by three standard planes, or sections, of reference (Figure 2-7). Each plane is oriented at right angles to the two remaining planes as they pass through the body.

The **coronal (frontal) plane** runs from side to side. It cuts the body or any of its parts into anterior and posterior (front and back) portions.

The **sagittal plane** runs from front to back. This lengthwise plane divides the body into right and left portions.

The **transverse (horizontal) plane** is a crosswise cut or section that divides the body or any of its parts into superior and inferior (upper and lower) portions.

Abdominopelvic Quadrants and Regions

Clinicians and other allied health personnel generally divide the abdominal area into quadrants (Figure 2-8) to more easily describe and locate organs in the abdominopelvic cavity. To accomplish this, the umbilicus is intersected by two planes, or sections. The sagittal plane is intersected at the umbilicus by a horizontal or transverse section or cut. As a result, the two sections divide the abdomen into right and left su-

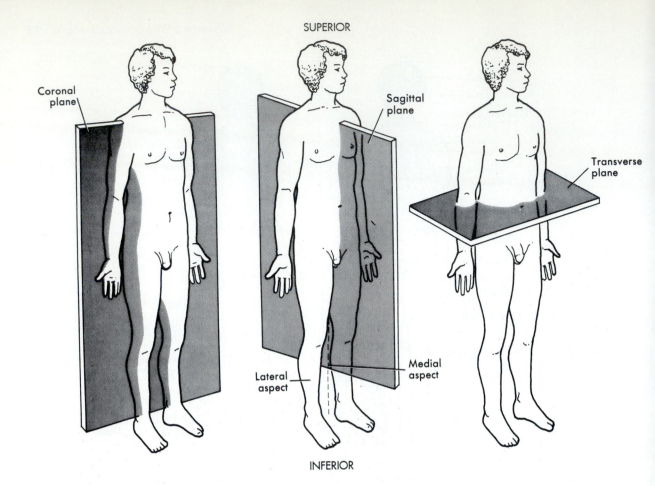

FIGURE 2-7
Body planes or sections.

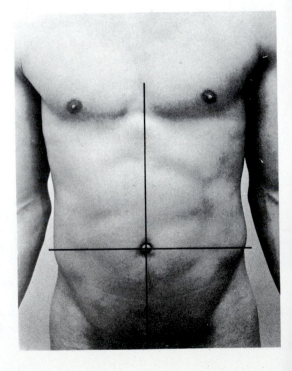

FIGURE 2-8
Subdivision of the abdominal area into four quadrants. Sagittal and transverse planes intersect at right angles at the umbilicus.

20

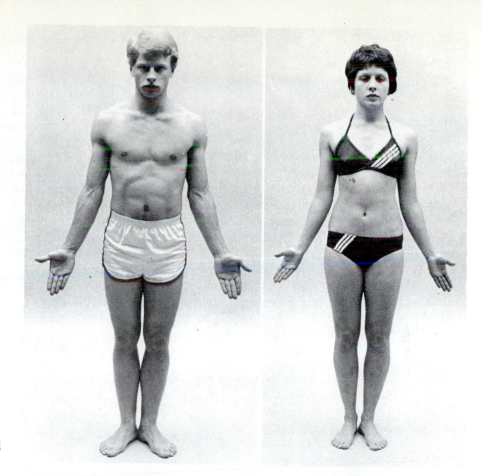

FIGURE 2-9
The human body viewed from the front.

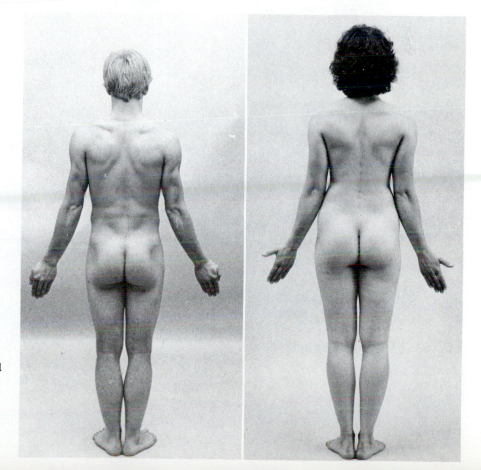

FIGURE 2-10
The human body viewed from behind. Note the differences in fat distribution. In the female loin area, fat extends from the buttocks to the waist.

perior (upper) quadrants and right and left inferior (lower) quadrants.

Surface Anatomy

The study of human anatomy often begins with visual inspection of the form and markings of the body surface. An appreciation of body form and symmetry is critically important in athletic injury assessment, and the need to sharpen observational skills cannot be overemphasized. With that end in mind, carefully inspect and compare the male and female forms in Figure 2-9. Differences in body form between men and women are strikingly evident. Note, however, that the axial and appendicular portions of the body and the divisions of each region are easily identifiable in both sexes.

The smooth, more rounded contours of the female form result in large part from accu-

mulation of more fat below the skin surface of the body as a whole than is typical of the male form. In addition, the bony framework is generally smaller and more delicate in women. In areas such as the buttocks, breasts, hips, flanks, and outer thighs, accumulation of fatty tissue is particularly noticeable in the female. In women the gluteal fat merges into the fat of the loin area so that the buttocks appear to extend almost to the waist (Figure 2-10). As a result, women tend to have a relatively large abdominal surface area and a lower center of gravity than men.

Carefully note and compare differences in appearance of the extremities. In the female the arm is more cylindric, in the male, flatter from side to side. The female thigh tends to be shorter and more conical than the male thigh. Note the obvious difference in defini-

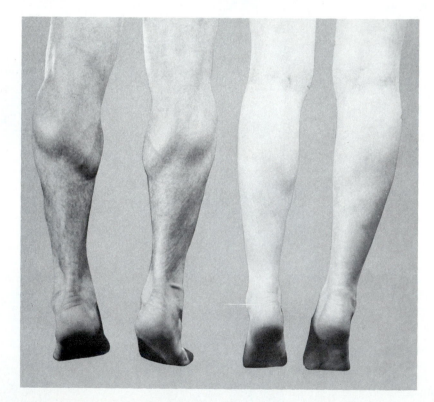

FIGURE 2-11
Differences in definition of calf musculature between a male and a female athlete.

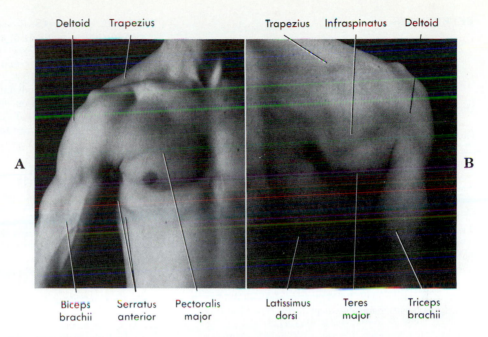

FIGURE 2-12
Surface anatomy of the **A**, anterior and **B**, posterior shoulder area.

tion of the calf muscles between the sexes in Figure 2-11. Even in women with powerfully developed musculature, the even layer of fatty tissue just below the skin surface tends to confer a smoother form and appearance.

Careful attention to surface anatomy using both observation and palpation techniques can provide the athletic trainer with extremely valuable information in the assessment of injury. It is particularly important in understanding the skeletal and muscular systems and in arthrology—the specialized area of anatomy that deals with joints, or articulations. A knowledge of surface body landmarks is often essential for accurate application of assessment techniques and will be stressed in the chapters that follow.

Almost every bone in the skeletal system can be palpated. Often by identifying the shape and placement of a bone as a whole or by locating specific bone markings, other anatomical structures can be identified. Further, knowledge of how muscles attach to bones coupled with correct identification of their surface appearance or palpable shape provides the athletic trainer with a basis for assessment of range of motion and joint function. In addition to bones and muscles, many other anatomical structures, including certain blood vessels, nerves, and even internal organs, can be identified directly from surface markings. Other structures, although not themselves visible on the body surface, can be located using an external landmark such as the umbilicus as a point of reference.

The surface anatomy of the anterior and posterior shoulder area is shown in Figure 2-12. Chapter 20 addresses assessment of injury in this important area. To develop proficiency in the necessary shoulder assessment techniques requires knowledge of both surface anatomy and of the deeper structures involved.

REFERENCES

Baumgartner AN, Chumlea WC, Roche AF: Bioelectric impedance for body composition, *Exer Sport Sci Rev* 18:193, Baltimore, 1990, Williams & Wilkins.

Carter JEL: *The Health-Carter somatotype method,* San Diego, 1972, San Diego State College.

Damon A and others: Predicting somatotype from body measurements, *Am J Phys Anthropol* 20:461, 1962.

Goss CM, editor: *Gray's anatomy,* ed 29, Philadelphia, 1980, Lea & Febiger.

Hollinshead WH: *Textbook of anatomy,* ed 3, New York, 1974, Harper & Row.

Jackson AS and others: Generalized equations for predicting body density of women, *Med Sci Sports Exerc* 12(3):175, 1980.

Jackson AS, Pollock ML: Generalized equations for predicting body density of men, *Br J Nutri* 40:497, 1978.

Lohman TG and others: Methodological factors and the prediction of body fat in female athletes, *Med Sci Sports Exerc* 16(1):92, 1984.

Lohman TG and others: Relationships of somatotype to body composition in college-aged men, *Ann Hum Biol* 5:174, 1978.

Lukaski HC: Methods for the assessment of human body composition: traditional and new, *Am J Clin Nutr* 46:537, 1987.

Malina RM: Bioelectric methods for estimating body composition: an overview and discussion, *Hum Biol* 59(2):329, 1987.

McMinn RMH, Hutchings RT: *Color atlas of human anatomy,* Chicago, 1984, Year Book Medical Publishers, Inc.

Nash HL: Body fat measurement: weighing the pros and cons of electrical impedance, *Phys Sportsmed* 13(11):124, 1985.

Oppliger RA and others: Body composition of collegiate football players: bioelectrical impedance and skinfold compared to hydrostatic weighing, *JOSPT* 15(4):187, 1992.

Pearman A and others: Comparison of hydrostatic weighing and bioelectric impedance measurements in determining body composition pre- and postdehydration, *JOSPT* 9(5):451, 1989.

Pollock ML, Jackson AS: Research progress in validation of clinical methods of assessing body composition, *Med Sci Sports Exerc* 16(6):606, 1984.

Stamford B: Somatotypes and sports selection, *Phys Sportsmed* 14(7):176, 1986.

Sterner TG, Burke EJ: Body fat assessment: a comparison of visual estimation and skinfold techniques, *Phys Sportsmed* 14(4):101, 1986.

Vannini V, Pogliana G, editors: *The color atlas of human anatomy,* New York, 1981, Crown Publishers, Inc.

SUGGESTED READINGS

Body composition: a round table, *Phys Sportsmed* 14(3):144, 1986.

A panel of four specialists, experienced in body composition research, discuss topics concerning body composition assessment.

Brodie DA: Techniques of measurement of body composition; Part I, *Sports Med* 5:11, 1988.

Reviews various methods used to estimate body density.

Hyner GC and others: Assessment of body composition by novice practitioners after a short intensive training session, *J Sports Med* 26:421, 1986.

Compares body composition measurements taken by novice practitioners to those taken by experienced technicians. Results suggest that, with minimal training, novice practitioners can estimate body fat reliably and with acceptable accuracy.

Thibodeau GA, Patton KT: *Anatomy and physiology,* ed 3, St. Louis, 1993, Mosby–Year Book.

An excellent comprehensive textbook of anatomy and physiology.

Thorland WG and others: Validity of anthropometric equations for the estimation of body density in adolescent athletes, *Med Sci Sports Exerc* 16(1):77, 1984.

Study compares 142 adolescent male and 133 adolescent female athletes to determine the validity of available anthropometric equations for estimating body density. Results identified several equations that would potentially be best used for screening approximate body density levels among young athletes.

CHAPTER 3

Osteology

After you have completed this chapter, you should be able to:
- List and describe the generalized functions of the skeletal system.
- Identify the major anatomical structures found in a typical long bone.
- Discuss the importance of the major types of bone markings in athletic injury assessment.
- Discuss the importance of externally palpable bony landmarks.
- Identify the two major subdivisions of the skeleton and list the bones found in each subdivision.
- Describe the differences between male and female skeletons.

A thorough understanding of the underlying anatomy of an injured area is an absolute prerequisite for the successful assessment of athletic injuries. Therefore an adequate review of appropriate anatomy will always precede discussion of specific assessment techniques introduced in subsequent chapters of the text. The intent is to provide the necessary anatomic detail required to understand and execute specific assessment procedures immediately before practical application of that information. Chapters 3, 4, 5, and 6 are intended only to provide a general overview of bones, joints, muscles, and nerves—the body areas most often involved in athletic injuries.

The human skeleton is a joined framework of living organs called bones. The skeleton lies buried within the muscles and other soft tissues, thus providing a support structure for the body.

The adult skeleton is composed of 206 separate bones. Rare variations in the total number of bones in the body may occur as a result of certain anomalies, such as extra ribs or from failure of certain small bones to fuse in the course of development.

FUNCTIONS OF THE SKELETON

The skeleton has five principal functions. The first three listed are of particular interest to athletic trainers.

Protection

Bones protect vital and delicate soft tissue structures from injury. Obvious examples include the brain encased within the skull, or the heart and lungs protected by the rib cage.

Support

The skeleton provides the support necessary to safely maintain an upright posture. A number of unique skeletal support mechanisms, for example, make it possible to run or jog without subjecting the body to undue stress and potential injury.

Movement

Bones serve as points of attachment for muscles. As the muscles contract and shorten, force is applied to the bones, which then act as levers. The joints, or articulations, between bones serve as pivot points, or fulcrums, that permit actual movement to occur.

Mineral storage

The skeleton serves as a massive storage reservoir for minerals, especially the salts of calcium and phosphorus. In the event of increased demand or inadequate intake of calcium or phosphorus, the body can activate complex regulatory mechanisms that result in transfer of one or both of these important salts from bone (osseous tissue) to the blood. Maintaining a normal blood level of calcium is particularly important because of calcium's role in blood clot formation, muscle contraction, and nerve impulse conduction.

Hemopoiesis

Hemopoiesis is the process of blood cell formation. It occurs in red bone marrow in the sternum and ribs, in the bodies of the vertebrae, and in the proximal ends of the femur and humerus.

CLASSIFICATION OF BONES

Bones may be divided into five groups for study purposes. Bones in the four most common groups (long, short, flat, and irregular) are illustrated in Figure 3-1.

Long bones

Long bones of the body often serve as levers. If pulled by contracting muscles, these bones make movement of the body possible. Examples of long bones are the humerus, radius, and ulna of the arm and the femur, and the tibia and fibula of the leg.

Short bones

The carpal bones of the wrist are typical short bones. As a group, short bones tend to be cube shaped and are generally found in areas in which only very limited motion is required. Their principal function is to provide strength.

Flat bones

Flat bones consist of parallel, platelike layers of hard or compact bone separated by a

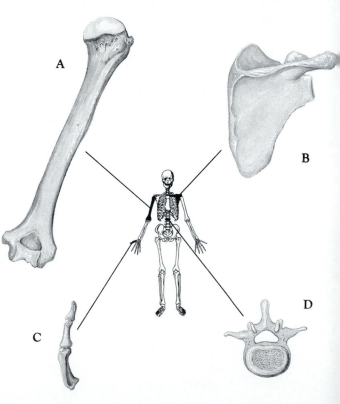

FIGURE 3-1
Types of bones. Examples of bone types include: **A**, long bones (humerus); **B**, flat bones (scapula); **C**, short bones (phalanx); and **D**, irregular bones (vertebra).

thin layer of spongy or cancellous bone tissue. These bones provide large areas for muscle attachment and in general serve a protective function. The bones of the skull (such as frontal and parietal) and the shoulder blades (scapulae) are good examples of flat bones.

Irregular bones

Bones that have obvious peculiarities in their shape are placed in this classification. Unique in their appearance and function, these bones must be studied individually. Examples include the pelvic bones, certain bones of the skull such as the ethmoid, and the ossicles of the ear.

Sesamoid bones

The patella, or kneecap, is the largest and most definitive of the sesamoid bones. As a group, these small and rounded or triangular bones develop within the substance of tendons or fascial tissue and are found adjacent to joints. They are named for their fancied resemblance to sesame seeds.

FEATURES OF A TYPICAL BONE

Every bone in the skeleton is a unique organ—a distinct structural unit. However, as a group, long bones uniformly possess many of the features of bones in general. For this reason, the major anatomic features of a "typical" long bone are often described before the study of individual bones in the skeleton. A long bone consists of the following structures visible to the naked eye: diaphysis, or shaft; epiphyses; articular cartilage; periosteum; marrow (*medullary*) cavity; and endosteum. Identify each of these parts in Figure 3-2 as you read the following paragraphs.

Diaphysis

The **diaphysis** is the long, shaftlike portion of the bone. The hollow, cylindric shape of the diaphysis provides strong support without cumbersome weight. Functionally, it can be compared to a length of strong metal tubing. The walls of the diaphysis are formed from hard, dense, compact bone.

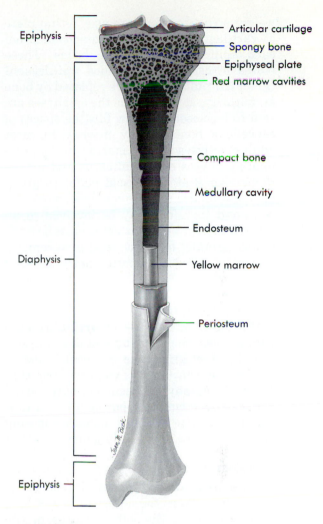

FIGURE 3-2
Diagram of the structural features of a typical long bone.

Epiphyses

The **epiphyses** are the extremities, or ends, of long bones. They enter into the formation of joints and, because of their somewhat bulbous shape, provide generous space for muscle attachments. Note the appearance of the bone in the epiphysis in Figure 3-2, *B*. Like a sponge, it is permeated by innumerable small spaces—hence its name: spongy, or cancellous, bone. Because of the porous nature of this bone and because the epiphyses have only a thin layer of dense, compact bone over their outer surface, they are light-weight structures for their size. A thin plate of cartilage separates the diaphysis from each epiphysis in growing bones. These plates of cartilage are called **epiphyseal (growth) plates.** They are replaced by bone at maturity, at which time the epiphyses are said to be closed. Marrow fills the spaces of cancellous bone—yellow marrow in most adult epiphyses but red marrow in the proximal epiphyses of the humerus and femur. Remember that epiphyseal plates in growing children are the weakest links along the bone and therefore may be involved in an athletic injury. Young athletes must be evaluated carefully for epiphyseal involvement, especially after traumatic injury to long bones.

Articular cartilage

A thin layer of **hyaline** or **articular cartilage** covers the joint surfaces of epiphyses. This layer of gristlelike material is firmly fixed to the thin layer of compact bone that covers the epiphyses. Resiliency of the articular cartilage cushions jars and blows that might otherwise erode or damage opposing epiphyseal bone surfaces in joints.

Periosteum

The **periosteum** is a dense, fibrous membrane that covers the outer surface of long bones except at the joint surfaces of the epiphyses, where articular cartilage forms the covering. The periosteal membrane is composed of an outer fibrous layer and a deep, more cellular layer close to the bone surface. Many of the periosteum's outer fibers (Sharpey's fibers) penetrate the underlying bone, welding these two structures together. In addition, muscle tendon fibers interlace with periosteal fibers, thereby anchoring muscles firmly to bone. The deep cellular layer of the periosteum contains numerous blood vessels and bone-forming cells called osteoblasts. These specialized cells are essential for normal bone growth and for repair of bones after an injury. Blood vessels pass from the deep cellular layer of the periosteum to supply nutrients to both bone and marrow. This fact helps explain the very se-

rious nature of periosteal avulsion injuries. If the periosteum is stripped from bone as a result of injury, the resulting decrease in blood supply may cause death of underlying and adjacent bone. Such injuries are often more serious in terms of potential for bone loss than fractures.

Marrow (medullary) cavity

The **marrow cavity** is a tubelike hollow in the diaphysis of long bones. In the adult it contains yellow or fatty marrow.

Endosteum

The **endosteum** is a fibrous membrane that lines the marrow cavity of long bones. Specialized bone-destroying cells, osteoclasts, are found in this membrane. In the growth years, maintenance of appropriate shape and proportion in long bones is possible only by constant remodeling. Concomitant activity of bone-building (osteoblast) cells in the periosteum and bone-destroying (osteoclast) cells in the endosteum is required. As osteoblasts add bone to the diaphysis under the periosteum, osteoclasts excavate the marrow cavity proportionately, resulting in maintenance of a relatively constant relationship between the circumference of the shaft and the diameter of the marrow cavity.

BONE MARKINGS

All bones exhibit surface markings that, if identified correctly, can provide a wealth of useful and functional information. Bone markings are functional in the sense that they provide information concerning the relationships that exist between bones, joints, muscles, tendons, blood vessels, nerves, and the body as a whole. Examples include markings that help to join one bone to another, to provide for attachment of muscles, or to serve as passageways for blood vessels or nerves. Bone markings that can be felt, or palpated, through the skin are especially useful to the athletic trainer in assessment of injury.

In many cases the location of a specific "externally palpable bony landmark" is one of the first steps in the assessment process.

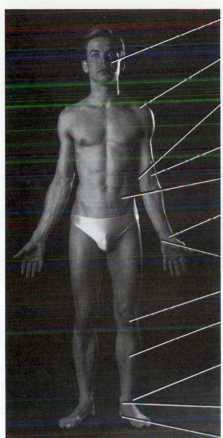

Zygomatic bone

Acromion process of scapula

Medial epicondyle of humerus

Lateral epicondyle of humerus

Iliac crest

Styloid process of radius

Styloid process of ulna

Patella

Anterior border of tibia

Lateral malleolus of fibula

Medial malleolus of tibia

Calcaneus

FIGURE 3-3
Palpable bony landmarks.

Instruction in the location and identification of these unique skeletal landmarks occur as assessment techniques are presented in subsequent chapters of the text. There are externally palpable bony landmarks throughout the body (Figure 3-3). Many skull bones, such as the cheek or zygomatic bone, can be palpated. The medial and lateral epicondyles of the humerus, the olecranon process of the ulna, and the styloid process of the ulna and the radius at the wrist can be palpated on the upper extremity. The highest corner of the shoulder is the acromion process of the scapula.

When you put your hands on your hips, you can feel the superior edge of the ilium, called the *iliac crest*. The anterior end of the crest, called the *anterior superior iliac spine*, is a prominent landmark used often as a clinical reference. The medial malleolus of the tibia and the lateral malleolus of the fibula are prominent at the ankle. The calcaneus, or heel bone, is easily palpated on the posterior aspect of the foot. On the anterior aspect of the lower extremity, examples of palpable bony landmarks include the patella, or kneecap; the anterior border of the tibia, or shin bone; and the metatarsals and phalanges of the toes. Try to identify as many of the externally palpable bones of the skeleton as possible on your own body. Using these as points of reference will make it easier to visualize the placement of other structures that cannot be touched or palpated through the skin.

Although the anatomic terms used to de-

TABLE 3-1

Bone Markings

Marking	Description	Example
Processes (including elevations and projections)		
Processes that form joints		
Head	A rounded projection beyond a narrow neckline	Head of femur
Condyle	A rounded projection that usually articulates with another bone	Medial or lateral condyle of femur
Facet	A small flat or nearly flat surface	Articular facet of a vertebra
Processes to which muscles, tendons, or ligaments attach		
Tubercle	A small, rounded projection	Rib tubercles
Tuberosity	A large, rounded projection	Ischial tuberosity of hipbone
Trochanter	A very large projection	Greater trochanter of femur
Spine (spinous process)	A sharp, slender projection	Spinous process of vertebra
Epicondyle	A projection located above a condyle	Medial epicondyle of humerus
Crest	A prominent, narrow, ridgelike projection on a bone	Iliac crest of hipbone
Line	A ridge of bone less prominent than a crest	Linea aspera of femur
Process	Any prominent projection	Mastoid process of temporal bone
Suture	A line of union between bones	Sagittal suture between parietal bones of skull
Cavities (depressions) (including openings and grooves)		
Fossa	A hollow or depression	Mandibular fossa of temporal bone
Sinus	A cavity, or hollow space, within a bone	Frontal sinus
Foramen	A hole in a bone	Foramen magnum in base of skull
Meatus	A tubelike passageway within a bone	External auditory meatus of temporal bone
Sulcus (groove)	A furrow, or groovelike, depression on a bone	Intertubercular groove of humerus
Fovea	A very small pit or depression	Fovea capitis of femur

TABLE 3-2

Bones in the Axial Division of the Skeleton

Area	Number of bones
Skull	
Cranium	8
Face	14
	22
Vertebral column	
Cervical vertebrae	7
Thoracic vertebrae	12
Lumbar vertebrae	5
Sacrum	1 (5 fused bones)
Coccyx	1 (3 to 5 fused bones)
	26
Sternum	1 (3 fused bones)
Manubrium	
Body	
Xiphoid process	
Ribs	12 pairs
Hyoid	1
Ear ossicles	
Malleus	2
Incus	2
Stapes	2
	6
TOTAL	80 Bones

TABLE 3-3

Bones in the Appendicular Division of the Skeleton

Area	Number of bones
Shoulder girdle	
Clavicle	2
Scapula	2
	4
Upper extremities	
Humerus	2
Ulna	2
Radius	2
Carpals	16
Metacarpals	10
Phalanges	28
	60
Hip girdle	
Os coxae	2
Lower extremities	
Femur	2
Fibula	2
Tibia	2
Patella	2
Tarsals	14
Metatarsals	10
Phalanges	28
	62
TOTAL	126 Bones

scribe bone markings are not always consistent, they can be divided into two groups: (1) **processes** (including elevations and projections), and (2) **cavities** or depressions (including openings and grooves). Table 3-1 describes and gives examples of many terms in common use.

If available, an articulated skeleton will prove to be especially useful as you complete this chapter. If skeletal material is not routinely available for study, ready access to a well-illustrated reference textbook of anatomy is recommended.

ORGANIZATION OF THE SKELETON

The 206 bones of the adult skeleton are grouped into two subdivisions, namely, the axial skeleton (80 bones) and the appendic-

ular skeleton (126 bones). The axial skeleton includes 6 tiny middle ear bones and the 74 bones that form the upright axis of the body, including the skull, vertebral column, and thorax (sternum and ribs). The 126 bones of the appendicular skeleton form the appendages and girdles that attach them to the axial skeleton. Included are the bones in the shoulder girdles, arms, wrists, and hands, and the bones in the hip girdles, legs, ankles, and feet. Bones in each component of the axial and appendicular subdivisions of the skeleton are listed in Tables 3-2 and 3-3.

Locate as many of the major bones of the axial and appendicular subdivisions of the skeleton listed in Tables 3-2 and 3-3 as you can in Figures 3-4 and 3-5.

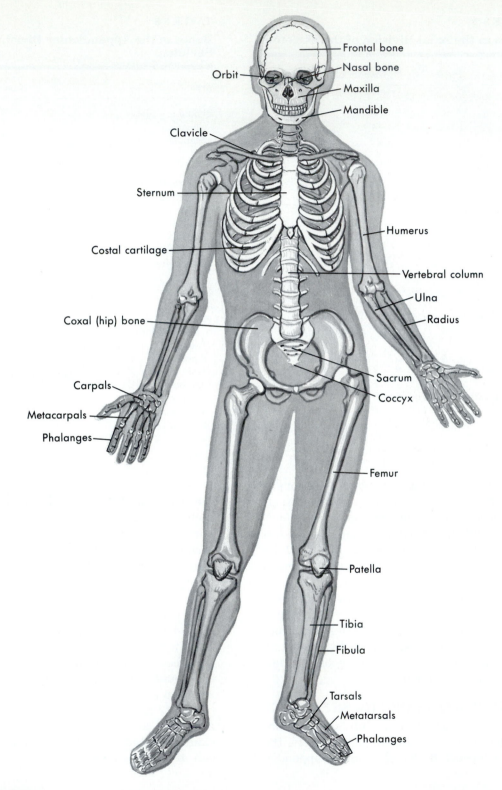

FIGURE 3-4
Skeleton, anterior view.

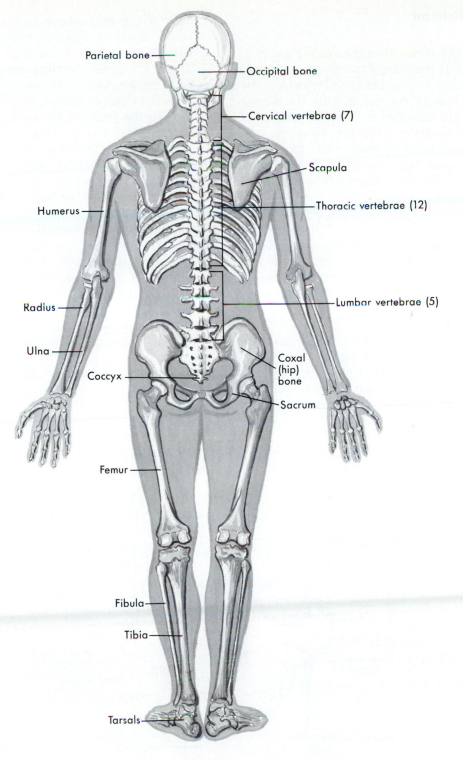

Parietal bone

Occipital bone

Cervical vertebrae (7)

Scapula

Humerus

Thoracic vertebrae (12)

Radius

Lumbar vertebrae (5)

Ulna

Coxal (hip) bone

Coccyx

Sacrum

Femur

Fibula

Tibia

Tarsals

FIGURE 3-5
Skeleton, posterior view.

Axial skeleton

Skull

Twenty-two bones form the skull (Figures 3-6 to 3-8). It consists of two major divisions: the cranium, or brain case, (8 bones) and the face (14 bones). For convenience the six ear ossicles are classified in Table 3-2 as part of the axial skeleton. They are, however, generally considered by anatomists as a separate group of bones rather than as a component of the skull proper. The single, U-shaped hyoid bone lies just below the skull, imbedded in the musculature of the tongue. The hyoid is the only bone in the body that does not articulate with any other bone. Names, locations, and brief descriptions of the cranial bones, face bones, ear ossicles, and hyoid are given in Table 3-4.

Vertebral column

The vertebral column (backbone or spine) of an adult consists of 26 separate bony segments or vertebrae. They form a strong, flexible, curved column that extends from the base of the skull above to the bony pelvis below. Each vertebra is named and numbered according to its location (Figure 3-9). There are seven cervical vertebrae in the neck region, twelve thoracic vertebrae behind the chest or thorax, five lumbar vertebrae in the small of the back, and a single sacrum and coccyx. The cervical thoracic and lumbar vertebrae are often called "true" or movable vertebrae, whereas the sacral and coccygeal portions of the spine are referred to as "false" or fixed vertebrae.

Note in Figure 3-9 that four curves can be identified in the normal vertebral column when it is viewed from the side. Located in the cervical, thoracic, lumbar, and sacral regions of the spine, these curves increase both the strength and resilience of the column and help to maintain balance in the upright position. In addition to serving as an axis for bearing weight, the vertebrae surround and protect the spinal cord and emerging spinal nerves (Table 3-5).

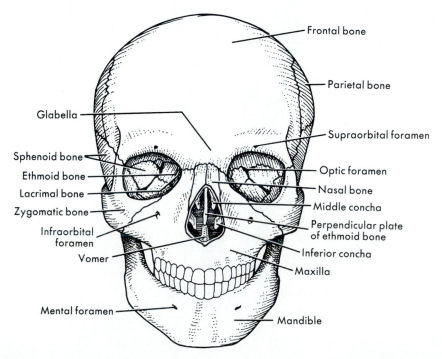

FIGURE 3-6
Skull viewed from the front.

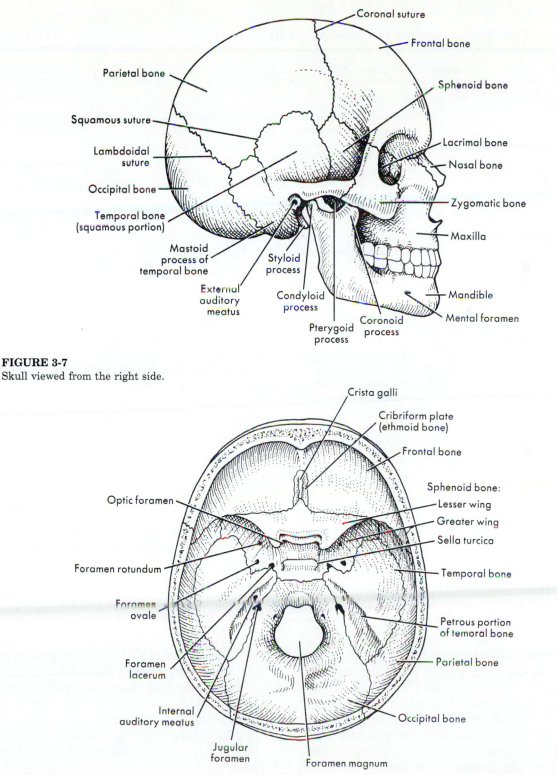

FIGURE 3-7
Skull viewed from the right side.

FIGURE 3-8
Floor of the cranial cavity.

TABLE 3-4

Bones of the Skull, Including Ear Ossicles and Hyoid Bone

Name	Number	Description
Cranial bones		
Frontal	1	Forehead bone; also forms front part of floor of cranium and most of upper part of eye sockets; cavity inside bone above upper margins of eye sockets (orbits) called *frontal sinus;* lined with mucous membrane
Parietal	2	Form bulging topsides of cranium
Temporal	2	Form lower sides of cranium; contain *middle* and *inner ear structures; mastoid sinuses* are mucosa-lined spaces in *mastoid* process, the protuberance behind ear; *external auditory canal* is tube leading into temporal bone
Occipital	1	Forms back of skull; spinal cord enters cranium through large hole *(foramen magnum)* in occipital bone
Sphenoid	1	Forms central part of floor of cranium; pituitary gland located in small depression sphenoid called sella turcica *(Turkish saddle)*
Ethmoid	1	Complicated bone that helps form floor of cranium, side walls and roof of nose and part of its middle partition (nasal septum), and part of orbit; contains honeycomb-like spaces, the *ethmoid sinuses; superior* and *middle turbinate bones* (conchae) are projections of ethmoid bone; form ledges along side wall of each nasal cavity
Facial bones		
Nasal	2	Small bones that form upper part of bridge of nose
Maxillary	2	Upper jawbones; also help form roof of mouth, floor, and side walls of nose and floor of orbit; large cavity in maxillary bone is *maxillary sinus*
Zygoma (malar)	2	Cheek bones; also help form orbit
Mandible	1	Lower jawbone
Lacrimal	2	Small bone; helps form medial wall of eye socket and side wall of nasal cavity
Palatine	2	Form back part of roof of mouth and floor and side walls of nose and part of floor of orbit
Inferior turbinate	2	Form curved "ledge" long inside of side wall of nose, below middle turbinate
Vomer	1	Forms lower, back part of nasal septum
Ear ossicles		
Malleus	2	Malleus, incus, and stapes are tiny bones in middle ear cavity in temporal bone; malleus means "hammer"—shape of bone
Incus	2	Incus means "anvil"—shape of bone
Stapes	2	Stapes means "stirrup"—shape of bone
Hyoid bone	1	U-shaped bone in neck at base of tongue

Thorax (sternum and ribs)

The thorax (Figure 3-10) is a bony, cagelike structure that resembles a flattened cone in shape, being broad below and quite narrow on top. It is formed by the sternum and costal cartilages anteriorly, the ribs laterally, and the thoracic vertebrae posteriorly. The floor of the thorax is formed by the diaphragm. The thorax encloses and protects the lungs, heart, and other life-sustaining structures of the chest cavity. It also supports the bones of both shoulder girdles and the upper extremities (Table 3-5).

Sternum. The dagger-shaped sternum (Figure 3-10) consists of three parts: the upper "handle" portion or manubrium; the middle "blade" portion, the body or gladiolus; and a lower tip called the xiphoid process.

Ribs. There are 12 pairs of ribs in humans (Figure 3-10). The first seven pairs (1 through 7) are called true or *vertebrosternal*

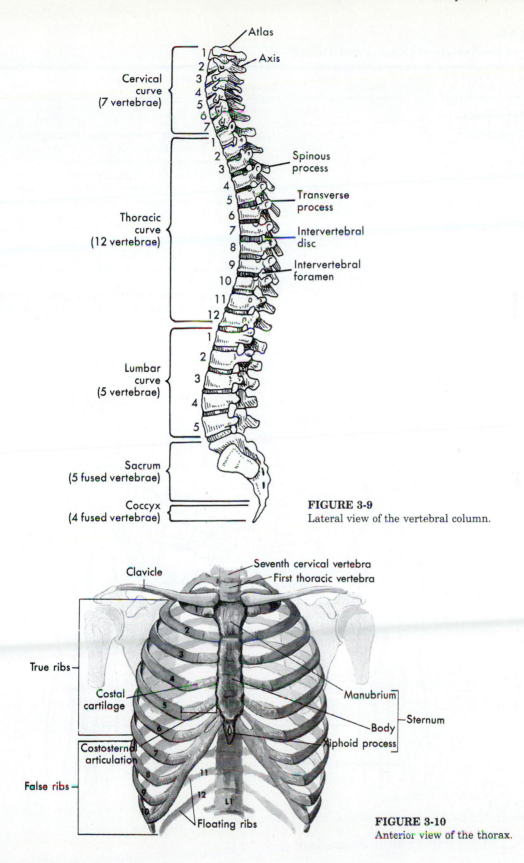

Atlas

Axis

Cervical
curve
(7 vertebrae)

1
2
3
4
5
6
7

Spinous
process

1
2
3
4
5
6
7
8
9
10
11
12

Thoracic
curve
(12 vertebrae)

Transverse
process

Intervertebral
disc

Intervertebral
foramen

Lumbar
curve
(5 vertebrae)

1
2
3
4
5

Sacrum
(5 fused vertebrae)

Coccyx
(4 fused vertebrae)

FIGURE 3-9
Lateral view of the vertebral column.

Clavicle

Seventh cervical vertebra
First thoracic vertebra

True ribs

Costal
cartilage

Manubrium

Body

Xiphoid process

Sternum

Costosternal
articulation

False ribs

Floating ribs

L1

FIGURE 3-10
Anterior view of the thorax.

TABLE 3-5

Bones of the Vertebral Column and Thorax

Name	Number	Description
Vertebral column		
Cervical vertebrae	7	Upper seven vertebrae, in neck region; first cervical vertebra called *atlas;* second called *axis*
Thoracic vertebrae	12	Next twelve vertebrae; ribs attach to these
Lumbar vertebrae	5	Next five vertebrae; those in small of back
Sacrum	1	In child, five separate vertebrae; in adult, fused into one
Coccyx	1	In child, three to five separate vertebrae; in adult fused into one
Thorax		
True ribs	14	Upper seven pairs; attach to sternum by way of *costal cartilages*
False ribs	10	Lower five pairs; lowest two pairs do not attach to sternum, therefore, called *floating ribs;* next three pairs attach to sternum by way of costal cartilage of seventh ribs
Sternum	1	Breastbone; shaped like a dagger; lower end of sternum bone called *xiphoid process*

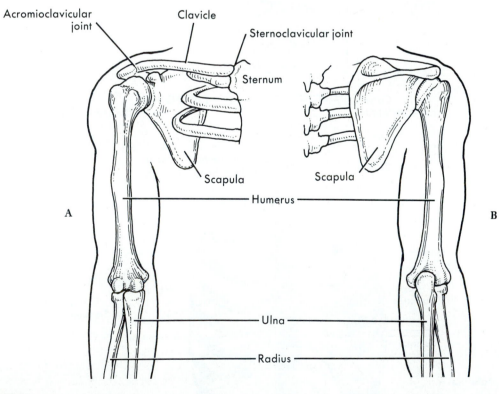

FIGURE 3-11

Right shoulder girdle and upper extremity. **A,** Anterior view; **B,** posterior view.

TABLE 3-6
Bones of the Upper Extremities

Name	Number	Description
Upper extremities		
Clavicle	2	Collarbones; only joints between shoulder girdle and axial skeleton are those between each clavicle and sternum
Scapula	2	Shoulder blades; scapula plus clavicle forms *shoulder girdle; acromion process*—tip of shoulder that forms joint with clavicle; *glenoid cavity*—arm socket
Humerus	2	Upper arm bone
Radius	2	Bone on thumb side of lower arm
Ulna	2	Bone on little finger side of lower arm; *olecranon process*—projection of ulna known as elbow or "funny bone"
Carpal bones	16	Irregular bones at upper end of hand; anatomic wrist
Metacarpals	10	Form framework of palm of hand
Phalanges	28	Finger bones; three in each finger, two in each thumb

ribs because they articulate *directly* with the sternum through their costal cartilages. The remaining five pairs of ribs (8 through 12) are called false ribs. The eighth, ninth, and tenth rib pairs are also referred to as *vertebrochondral* ribs because they articulate with the sternum *indirectly* by fusion of their costal cartilages to the cartilages of the rib pairs above them. The eleventh and twelfth rib pairs do not articulate in any way with the sternum. They are called "floating ribs."

Appendicular Skeleton
Shoulder girdle and upper extremities
The shoulder girdles are formed by two pairs of bones; the clavicles (collar bones) are anterior and the scapulae (shoulder blades) are posterior. Together these bones serve to attach each upper extremity to the axial skeleton. The mechanism of attachment that exists between the shoulder girdles, upper extremities, and axial skeleton provides for maximal mobility. As you learn to assess injury in this area, the price paid for this high degree of mobility (joint disarticulations) will become apparent. It should be stressed that the articulation between clavicle and sternum (sternoclavicular joint) is the only bony joint that exists between the shoulder

girdle and the axial skeleton (Figure 3-11). For the athletic trainer this is an extremely important and practical anatomic fact. It helps to explain the high incidence of clavicular fractures in contact sports, especially those that occur when an athlete uses the arm to break a fall.

Each upper extremity is attached to the shoulder girdle by articulation between the head of the humerus and the scapula. There is no direct bony articulation between the axial skeleton and the upper extremities. Each upper extremity contains 30 bones and consists of the humerus (brachium, or upper arm), radius and ulna (forearm), carpals (wrist), metacarpals (palm), and phalanges (fingers and thumb). Table 3-6 includes names, locations, and brief descriptions of these bones.

Humerus (Figure 3-12). The humerus is the largest and longest bone of the upper extremity. It forms the bony framework of the upper arm (brachium). The humerus articulates with the scapula proximally and with both the radius and ulna distally.

Radius and ulna (Figure 3-13). The radius is located on the thumb, or lateral, side of the forearm. It articulates with the humerus proximally and with the carpals of the wrist distally. Its companion, the ulna,

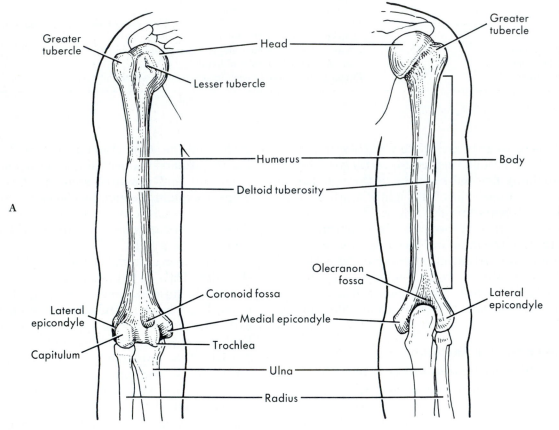

FIGURE 3-12
Right humerus and elbow joint. **A**, Anterior view; **B**, posterior view.

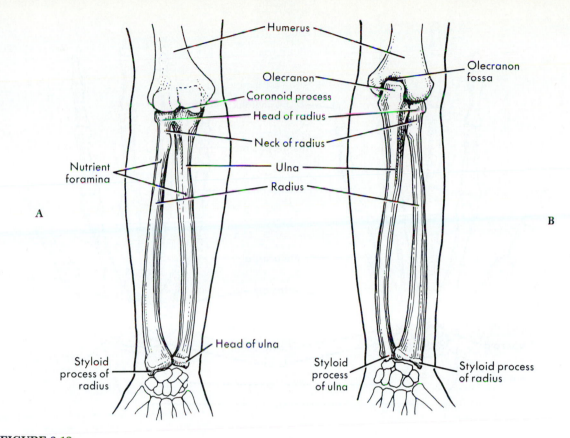

FIGURE 3-13
Right ulna and radius. **A**, Anterior view; **B**, posterior view.

is found on the little finger, or medial, side of the forearm. It also articulates with the humerus proximally, but distally it articulates with a fibrocartilaginous disc and not with the carpal bones of the wrist directly.

Carpals, metacarpals, and phalanges (Figure 3-14). The eight carpal, or wrist, bones are arranged in two irregular rows, each containing four bones. Only the pisiform is easily identifiable. It projects posteriorly from the little finger, or medial, side of the wrist. The pisiform is a good example of an externally palpable bony landmark.

In the anatomic position the arms are at the sides, with the palms of the hands turned forward (Figure 2-6). In this position the five metacarpals that make up the framework of the palm of the hand are numbered in ascending order. Metacarpal number 1 is on the most lateral, or thumb, side of the hand; metacarpal number 5 is the most medial and articulates with the little finger. The phalanges form the bony framework of the fingers and thumb. There are 14 phalanges in each hand—three in each finger and two in the thumb.

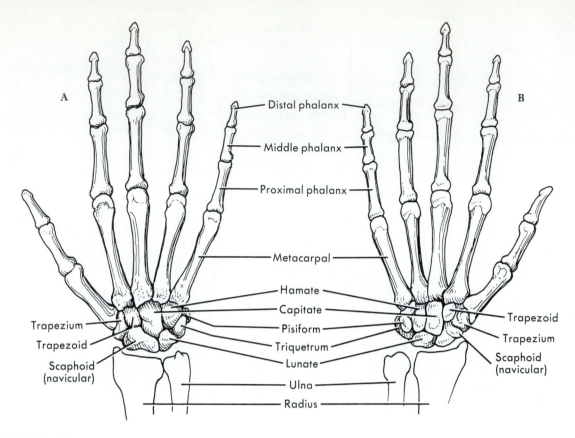

A

B

Distal phalanx

Middle phalanx

Proximal phalanx

Metacarpal

Hamate

Capitate

Pisiform

Triquetrum

Lunate

Ulna

Radius

Trapezium

Trapezoid

Scaphoid
(navicular)

Trapezoid

Trapezium

Scaphoid
(navicular)

FIGURE 3-14
Right wrist and hand. **A**, Dorsal view; **B**, palmer view.

Hip girdle and lower extremities

Strong ligaments bind the right and left hip bones (os coxae, or innominate bones) together to form the hip or pelvic girdle. The hip girdle is a circular base that supports the trunk and, unlike the shoulder girdle, serves as a very stable point of attachment for the lower extremities. Although athletic trainers deal with shoulder disarticulations all too frequently, a dislocated hip is seldom seen as a result of athletic injury. The mechanism of attachment that exists between the hip girdle, lower extremities, and axial skeleton provides for *maximum stability*. The lower extremities are very firmly attached to the hip girdle on each side by articulation between the head of the femur and a deep, cup-shaped depression in each innominate (hip) bone called the acetabulum.

Each lower extremity contains 30 bones and consists of the femur, patella, tibia and fibula, tarsals, metatarsals, and phalanges (Figure 3-15). Table 3-7 includes names, locations, and brief descriptions of these bones.

Femur (Figure 3-16). The thighbone, or femur, is the longest and one of the strongest bones in the skeleton. Located between the hip and knee, it articulates above with the acetabular socket in each innominate bone and below with the tibia and patella, or kneecap.

Tibia and fibula (Figure 3-17). The tibia, or shin bone, is the larger, stronger, and more medially and superficially located of the two lower leg bones. Because of its superficial location, the tibia is often subjected to painful "bone bruises." The upper (proxi-

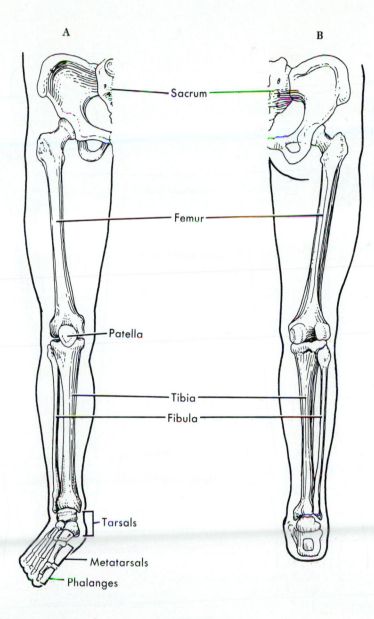

FIGURE 3-15
Right pelvic girdle and lower extremity. **A**, Anterior view; **B**, posterior view.

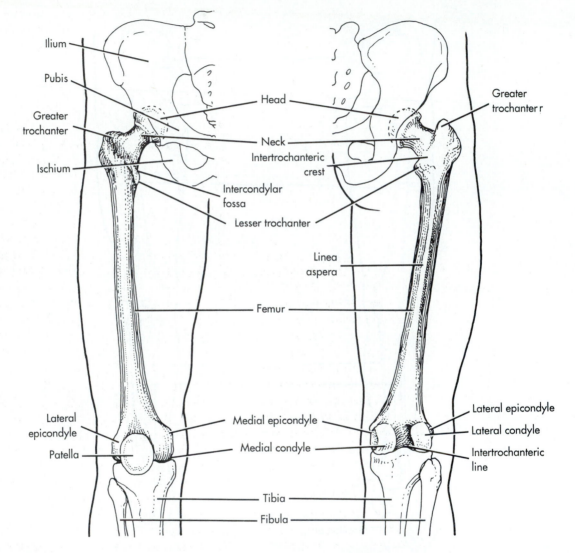

FIGURE 3-16
Right femur showing proximal (hip) and distal (knee) articulations. **A**, Anterior view; **B**, posterior view.

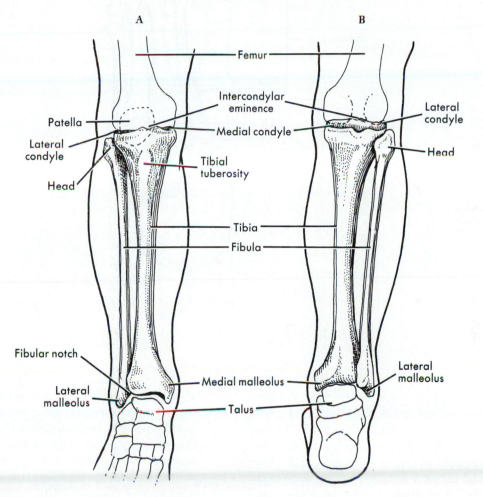

FIGURE 3-17
Right tibia and fibula. **A,** Anterior view; **B,** posterior view.

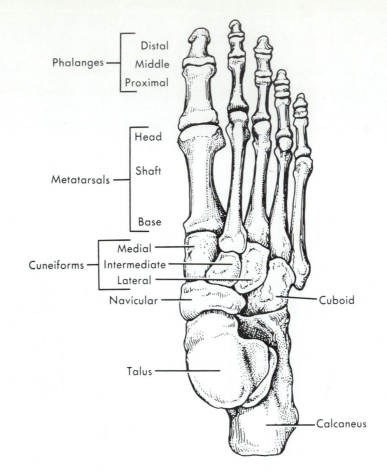

FIGURE 3-18
Bones of right foot viewed from above.

mal) end, or epiphysis, of the tibia expands to form two condyles that articulate with and bear the weight transmitted by the femur. The fibula is parallel with the tibia but does not enter into formation of the knee joint and is not a weight-bearing bone of the lower leg. The distal epiphysis of the fibula projects downward into a pointed process called the lateral malleolus. It is this process that forms the prominent outer surface of the ankle.

Tarsals, metatarsals, and phalanges (Figure 3-18). The basic structure of the ankle and foot is similar in many ways to that of the wrist and hand. The most prominent structural differences noted in the ankle and foot are adaptations that increase stability or provide a strong base for support

of weight. The largest and strongest of the seven tarsal bones is called the calcaneus, or heel bone. It is the calcaneus that transmits the weight of the body to the ground. The bones of the feet are held together in such a way as to form springy lengthwise and cross-wise arches (Figure 3-19). Strong ligaments and leg muscle tendons normally hold the foot bones firmly in these arched positions. Unfortunately, these arches sometimes weaken, causing a condition aptly called fallen arches, or flatfeet (Figure 3-19, *B*).

Note in Figure 3-18 that the tarsal bones consist of cuneiforms (three), navicular, talus, cuboid, and calcaneus. The five metatarsals of the foot are numbered from medial to lateral, with the first metatarsal extending to the base of the great toe. The tarsals

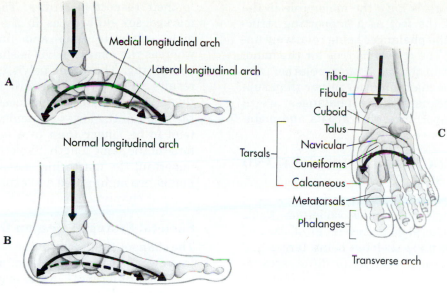

FIGURE 3-19

Arches of the foot. **A,** Longitudinal arch. Medial portion formed by calcaneus, talus, navicular, cuneiforms, and three metatarsals; lateral portion formed by calcaneus, cuboid, and two lateral metatarsals. **B,** "Flatfoot" results when there is a weakening of tendons and ligaments attached to the tarsal bones. Downward pressure by the weight of the body gradually flattens out the normal arch of the bones. **C,** Transverse arch in the metatarsal region of the right foot.

TABLE 3-7

Bones of the Lower Extremities

Name	Number	Description
Lower extremities		
Os Coxae	2	Hipbones; *ilium*—upper flaring part of pelvic bone; *ischium*—lower back part; *pubic bone*—lower front part; *acetabulum*—hip socket; *symphysis pubis*—joint in midline between two pubic bones; *pelvic inlet*—opening into *true pelvis,* or pelvic cavity; if pelvic inlet is misshapen or too small, infant skull cannot enter true pelvis for natural birth
Femur	2	Thigh or upper leg bones; *head of femur*—ball-shaped upper end of bone; fits into acetabulum
Patella	2	Kneecap
Tibia	2	Shinbone; *medial malleolus*—rounded projection at lower end of tibia
Fibula	2	Long slender bone of lateral side of lower leg; *lateral malleolus*—rounded projection at lower end of fibula
Tarsal bones	14	Form heel and back part of foot
Metatarsals	10	Form part of foot to which toes attach; tarsal and metatarsal bones so arranged that they form three arches in foot; *inner longitudinal arch* and *outer longitudinal arch,* both of which extend from front to back of foot, and transverse or *metatarsal arch* that extends across foot
Phalanges	28	Toe bones; three in each toe, two in each great toe

and metatarsals have the major role in the function of the foot as a supporting structure, with the phalanges being relatively unimportant. The reverse is true for the hand. Recall that in the hand, manipulation (mobility) is the main function rather than support. Consequently, the phalanges are of primary importance, the carpals and metacarpals are secondary.

DIFFERENCES BETWEEN MALE AND FEMALE SKELETONS

Both general and specific differences exist between male and female skeletons (Table 3-8). The general difference is one of size and weight, the male skeleton being larger and heavier. Examples of specific differences include the angle of articulation between certain bones in the extremities and the angle of attachment of the extremities as a whole

to their respective girdles. There are also marked sex differences in the pelvis. The male pelvis is deep and funnel-shaped, whereas the female pelvis is shallow, broad, and flaring. The wider pelvis in the female results in a greater inward slant of the thighs from the hips to the knees. In general, the bones of the lower extremity in the male tend to be longer than in a female with a torso of the same length. Skeletal differences important to mastering assessment techniques are highlighted and explained in subsequent chapters.

Skeletal System: Lifespan Differences

The changes that occur in the body's skeletal framework over the course of a lifespan result from differences in the maturation and completion of ossification of different bones during different periods of development and

TABLE 3-8

Comparison of Male and Female Skeletons

Portion of skeleton	Male	Female
General form	Bones heavier and thicker Muscle attachment sites more massive Joint surfaces relatively large	Bones lighter and thinner Muscle attachment sites less distinct Joint surfaces relatively small
Skull	Forehead shorter vertically Mandible and maxillae relatively larger Facial area more pronounced Processes more prominent	Forehead more elongated vertically Mandible and maxillae relatively smaller Facial area rounder, with less pronounced features Processes less pronounced
Pelvis		
Pelvic cavity	Narrower in all dimensions Deeper Pelvic outlet relatively small	Wider in all dimensions Shorter and roomier Pelvic outlet relatively large
Sacrum	Long, narrow, with smooth concavity (sacral curvature); sacral promontory more pronounced	Short, wide, flat concavity more pronounced in a posterior direction; sacral promontory less pronounced
Coccyx	Less movable	More movable and follows posterior direction of sacral curvature
Pubic arch	Less than a 90° angle	Greater than a 90° angle
Symphysis pubis	Relatively deep	Relatively shallow
Ischial spine, ischial tuberosity, and anterior superior iliac spine	Turned more inward	Turned more outward and further apart
Greater sciatic notch	Narrow	Wide

from structural changes in bone, cartilage, and muscle tissues. For example, the resilience of incompletely ossified bone in infants and toddlers allows their bones to withstand the mechanical stresses of childbirth and learning to walk with relatively little risk of fracturing, but young athletes are at risk of epiphyseal fractures in long bones that have not fully ossified. Exercise has a beneficial effect on bone density and strength throughout life. In the absence of disease, the density of bone and cartilage in the young to middle-aged adult permits the carrying of great loads. Unfortunately, the reduced activity of many older individuals contributes to loss of bone density in later adulthood and can make a person so prone to fractures that simply walking or lifting with moderate force can cause bones to crack or break. The loss of skeletal tissue density may result in a compression of weight-bearing bones that causes a loss of height and perhaps an inability to maintain a standard posture. Degeneration of skeletal muscle tissue in late adulthood may also contribute to postural changes and loss of height. Fortunately, with proper nutrition and exercise, the trabeculae of spongy bone are able to change their orientation to become arranged along lines of stress, and their orientation therefore differs between individual bones according to the nature and magnitude of the applied load. Lifespan skeletal changes that contribute to injury will be highlighted when appropriate in the discussion of assessment techniques throughout the text.

REFERENCES

Bassett CA and others: Pulsing electromagnetic field treatment in ununited fractures and failed arthrodeses, *JAMA* February, 1982.

Beck EW: *Mosby's atlas of concise functional human anatomy,* St Louis, 1982, C.V. Mosby Co.

Bourne GW, editor: *The biochemistry and physiology of bone,* ed 2, New York, 1972, Academic Press, Inc.

Garn S: Bone loss and aging. In Garn S: *The physiology and pathology of human aging,* New York, 1975, Academic Press, Inc.

Hogan L, Beland I: Cervical spine syndrome, *Am J Nurs* 76(7):1104, 1976.

Maffulli N and King JB: Effects of physical activity on some components of the skeletal system, *Sports Med* 13(6):393, 1992.

Thomsen DE: Electrifying biology, *Sci News* 127(16):268, 1985.

Zuidema GD, editor: *The Johns Hopkins atlas of human functional anatomy,* ed 2, Baltimore, 1980, The Johns Hopkins University Press.

SUGGESTED READINGS

Caplan AI: Cartilage, *Sci Am* 251(4):84, 1984.
   Concise, well-written article that explains the multiple functions of cartilage. Development, structure, and aging are explained.

Gray H: In Clemente CD, editor: *Anatomy of the human body,* Philadelphia, 1985, Lea and Febiger.
   Advanced and lavishly illustrated text of human anatomy. Authoritative and comprehensive. Osteology coverage is excellent.

Murray PDF: *Bones,* New York, 1985, Cambridge University Press.
   Comprehensive and detailed overview of osteology. Excellent correlation between complex written material and related artwork.

Orwold ES and others: The effect of swimming on bone mineral content, *Clin Res* 35(1):194A, 1987.
   Easy-to-read presentation of current research supporting theory of increased bone density in both men and women swimmers. Methodology involved dual-energy CT scans of vertebrae and single-beam photon absorptiometry of the radius in subjects over age 40.

Vaughan JM: *The physiology of bone,* ed 3, New York, 1981, Oxford University Press.
   Comprehensive, well-written, and readable review of bone physiology. Developmental determinants and importance of vascular and nutritional factors receive careful treatment.

CHAPTER 4

Arthrology

After you have completed this chapter, you should be able to:
- Describe the classification of joints using structural features or potential for movement as distinguishing criteria.
- List the joint types in each major classification.
- Identify the major anatomic features of a typical synovial joint.
- List and describe the specific types of diarthrotic or synovial joints.
- Explain range of motion (ROM) and types of movement in diarthroses.
- Explain how to measure ROM subjectively and objectively.
- List and define the terms used to describe angular, rotatory, and special movements in joints.

Arthrology is a specialized area of anatomy that deals with the study and description of joints, or articulations. By definition a joint, or articulation, exists where two or more skeletal components, whether bone or cartilage, come together or meet. For the athletic trainer the practical importance of acquiring a basic understanding of arthrology cannot be overemphasized. This information is important in understanding how joints normally function and in providing a basis for understanding the nature of joint injuries. Athletes are almost universally characterized by an ability to execute complex, highly coordinated, and purposeful movements. Without joints between bones the controlled and graceful movement of the athlete would be impossible; the body would be a rigid, immobile hulk. Simply stated, it is the existence of joints between bones that makes movement of body parts possible. This chapter provides an overview of the classification, structure, and function of joints, or articulations. The anatomy of individual joints is presented in subsequent chapters of the text and precedes discussion of techniques employed in the assessment of specific joint injuries.

CLASSIFICATION OF JOINTS

Joints are classified into three major groups or types using structural features or potential for movement as distinguishing criteria (Table 4-1). For the athletic trainer, a system of joint classification using degree of movement is clearly the more functional and appropriate method. On this basis, three joint classes can be identified: **synarthroses** (immovable joints), **amphiarthroses** (slightly movable joints), and **diarthroses** (freely movable joints). If structural criteria are

TABLE 4-1

Primary Joint Classification

Functional name	Structural name	Degree of movement permitted	Example
Synarthroses	Fibrous	Immovable	Sutures of skull
Amphiarthroses	Cartilaginous	Slightly movable	Pubic symphysis
Diarthroses	Synovial	Freely movable	Shoulder joint

used for classification, these three joint classes are called, in the same order, fibrous, cartilaginous, and synovial.

Synarthroses

There are three basic types of synarthrotic, or immovable, joints (Figure 4-1).

Syndesmosis

This type of synarthrotic joint is characterized by the presence of a dense fibrous membrane that binds the articular bone surfaces very closely and tightly to each other. Ligaments play an important role in restriction of movement in these joints. The articulation between the distal ends of the tibia and fibula is a good example of a syndesmosis.

Suture

True sutures are found only in the skull. As a group, sutures are not characterized by the

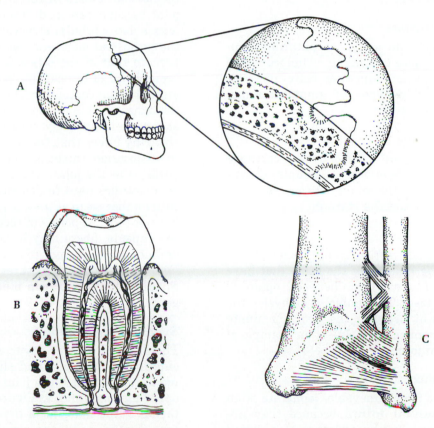

FIGURE 4-1

Types of synarthrotic joints. **A**, Suture (coronal suture); **B**, gomphosis (root of tooth in socket); **C**, syndesmosis (distal tibiofibular articulation).

substantial fibrous membranes or dense ligaments seen in syndesmoses. Instead, the adjoining bone margins are united into rigid, immovable joints by a series of jagged, interlocking processes. The sagittal suture between the two parietal bones of the skull is a good example of this joint type.

Gomphosis

A gomphosis is a synarthrotic, or fibrous, joint in which a conical peg or projection fits into a socket. Articulations between the roots of the teeth and sockets of the jaw bones are the only examples of this type of joint in the body. The fibrous type of membrane between the root of the tooth and its socket is called the **periodontal membrane.** Successful replacement of teeth that have been knocked out as a result of injury is possible if this membrane remains relatively undamaged.

Amphiarthroses

Slightly movable joints, or **amphiarthroses,** have a pad of hyaline or fibrocartilage located between adjoining bony surfaces. There are two types of amphiarthrodial joints (Figure 4-2).

Synchondrosis

In this type of joint a pad of hyaline cartilage joins one bone to another. Examples of synchondroses are the joints between rib pairs 1 through 10 and the sternum.

Symphysis

Symphyses are articulations, generally located in the midline of the body, that have a pad of fibrocartilage between opposing bone surfaces. The pubic symphysis, the midline joint between the two innominate bones in front (anteriorly), is an example of this type of joint.

Diarthroses

Diarthrotic (freely movable) joints are often called **synovial joints** because they are characterized by the presence of a closed cavity, called the synovial or joint cavity, between the bones. As a group, the diarthrotic, or synovial, joints include by far the majority of the body's articulations. Because they are the most mobile of the three types of joints, they are functionally the most important. They also have the most complex structure and are most vulnerable to athletic injuries.

Structural features

Refer to Figure 4-3 to identify the following structural features of synovial joints.

Fibrous joint capsule

In movable joints a tough but flexible sleeve-like structure called the **joint capsule** helps to hold the articulating bones together. The capsule encloses a space or cleft that exists between the opposing bone surfaces. Note in Figure 4-3 that the joint capsule consists of two layers: a tough, fibrous, outer layer called the fibrous capsule of the joint and a more cellular inner layer called the synovial membrane. Fibers in the outer layer of the joint capsule run in different directions to form a dense tubular structure that connects the periosteal membrane of one bone in the joint to that of the other. The resulting fibrous layer of the capsule has great tensile strength that completely encases the ends of the bones and binds them to each other. This structure is uniquely constructed to resist shearing forces that would otherwise result in dislocation (luxation) of opposing bone surfaces at the joint. The term *subluxation* is sometimes used to describe partial dislocations that occur if the capsule is stretched but not torn. At points of recurring stress in the capsule, fibers may become oriented in definite parallel bands to form *intracapsular ligaments*. These structures provide additional stability and help bind the bones together.

Synovial membrane

The deep, or cellular, layer of the joint capsule forms the moist and slippery synovial membrane. It lines the joint space between opposing bones and, as Figure 4-3 shows, attaches to the margins of the articular cartilage. Functionally, the synovial membrane secretes synovial fluid, or synovia, which serves to lubricate the joint and provide nourishment for the articular cartilage. The

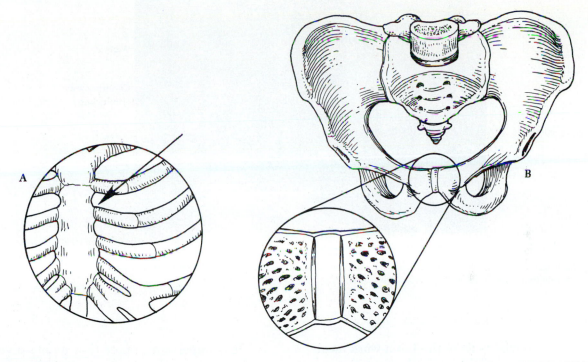

FIGURE 4-2
Types of amphiarthrotic joints. **A**, Sychondroses (articulation between true ribs and sternum);
B, symphyses (symphysis pubica).

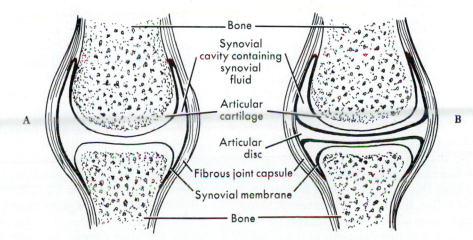

FIGURE 4-3
Section through diarthrotic joints. **A**, Without, and, **B**, with an intervening articular disc in the
joint cavity.

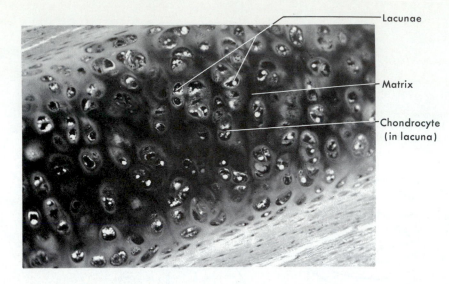

Lacunae

Matrix

Chondrocyte
(in lacuna)

FIGURE 4-4
Micrograph of hyaline cartilage. Note the absence of blood vessels in the gel-like matrix of this
unique avascular tissue.

term synovial is from the Latin word meaning "with egg" because it resembles egg white in consistency and appearance. Synovial fluid varies in amount from less than 0.1 ml to over 3.0 ml in different joints of the body. Quantity depends on joint size and potential for movement.

Articular cartilage

In Chapter 3 the presence of a specialized type of articular cartilage was included as one of six anatomic features common to long bones as a group. Articular, or **hyaline,** cartilage (Figure 4-4) is a unique type of connective tissue. It consists of specialized cells called **chondrocytes** and a firm, gel-like intercellular matrix. Note in Figure 4-4 that very few fibers are present in hyaline cartilage and that the chondrocytes reside in little spaces called **lacunae.** The intercellular matrix that surrounds the chondrocytes is similar to a fairly firm, smooth plastic and, if kept lubricated, is superbly adapted for coating the articulating ends (epiphyses) of bones in movable joints. Tough, collagenous fibers anchor articular cartilage to the underlying bone and adjacent periosteal membrane.

It is important to note that no blood vessels penetrate the gel-like matrix of hyaline (articular) cartilage. It is said to be **avascular.** For cells in cartilage tissue to survive without a direct blood supply, nutrients and oxygen must pass through the matrix bed by diffusion from synovial fluid. Diffusion over such distances is a slow and generally inefficient way to transfer nutrients to cells. Indeed, in tissues other than cartilage it is not possible to sustain cell life if the normal blood supply is cut off. It is the unique diffusion mechanism of nutrient transfer in cartilage, however, that explains how bits of this tissue that detach from articulating bone surfaces by injury not only survive but also grow and increase in size. These small but sometimes troublesome bits of cartilage derive their nutrients by diffusion from the synovial fluid in the joint space.

In addition to the thin layer of hyaline cartilage that covers the articulating bone surfaces in movable joints, pads of fibrocartilage may lie between the bones and divide the joint cavity (Fig. 4-3, *B*). These pads of fibrocartilage are called **articular discs,** or **menisci.** They provide an additional "cushion" between the articulating ends of the

TABLE 4-2
Classification of Synovial Joints

Types	Examples	Structural features	Movements
Uniaxial			
Hinge	Elbow joint	Spool-shaped process fits into concave socket	Around one axis; in one plan Flexion and extension only
Pivot	Joint between first and second cervical vertebrae	Arch-shaped process fits around peglike process	Rotation
Biaxial			Around two axes, perpendicular to each other; in two planes
Saddle	Thumb joint between first metacarpal and carpal bone	Saddle-shaped bone fits into socket that is concave-convex-concave	Flexion, extension in one plane; abduction, adduction in other plane; opposing thumb to fingers
Condyloid (ellipsoidal)	Joint between radius and carpal bones	Oval condyle fits into elliptical socket	Flexion, extension in one plane; abduction, adduction in other plane
Multiaxial			
Ball and socket	Shoulder joint and hip joint	Ball-shaped process fits into concave socket	Around many axes Widest range of movements; flexion, extension, abduction, adduction, rotation, circumduction
Gliding	Joints between adjacent vertebrae; joints between carpal and tarsal bones	Relatively flat articulating surfaces	Gliding movements without any angular or circular movements

bones and help stabilize the joint. Fibrocartilage, as the name implies, contains a larger number of collagenous fibers imbedded in the matrix than is typical of hyaline. The direct blood supply to fibrocartilage is little better, however, than that of the hyaline variety. Torn or damaged fibrocartilage in a joint often does not heal properly and must be removed by surgery. In most instances, only the damaged portion must be removed, thus saving as much of the structure as possible.

Types of diarthroses

Diarthrotic (synovial) joints are grouped or subdivided on the basis of (1) the kind of movement each joint is capable of performing and (2) the shape of the surfaces of the adjacent articulating bones. Table 4-2 lists the six types of diarthroses that can be grouped into three categories according to axial movement.

Uniaxial joints. Uniaxial joints (Figure 4-5) permit movement in only one plane and around a single axis. There are two types of uniaxial joints: *hinge* and *pivot*.

Hinge joints such as the elbow permit movement only about one axis, which passes through the joint from side to side. Only flexion and extension occur in hinge joints. Because they allow movement in only one plane, hinge joints are those most often involved in athletic injuries.

Typically, the single axis of *pivot* joints is vertical. In this type of uniaxial joint, movement is limited to rotation. In pivot joints a type of bony ring on one bone rotates around a pivot point on another bone. For example,

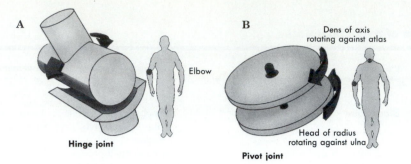

FIGURE 4-5
Uniaxial joints. **A**, Hinge joint (elbow); **B**, pivot joint (atlantoaxial joint).

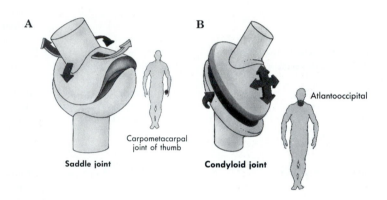

FIGURE 4-6
Biaxial joints. **A**, Saddle joint (carpometacarpal joint of thumb); **B**, Condyloid joint (atlantooccipital joint).

the first cervical vertebra, or atlas, acts as a bony ring that rotates around a conical pivot process called the **dens** on the second cervical vertebra, or axis. This joint permits you to turn (rotate) your head from side to side. The head of the radius rotating against the ulna is another example of a pivot joint.

Biaxial joints. In biaxial joints (Figure 4-6), movement occurs in two planes and around two axes that are at right angles to each other. Flexion and extension are allowed around one axis and abduction and adduction around the second axis. There are two types of biaxial joints: *saddle* and *condyloid*.

The articular surface of one bone in a *saddle* joint is concave in one direction and convex in the other, whereas the articular surface of the remaining bone is exactly the opposite (Figure 4-6, *A*). The opposing saddle-shaped surfaces fit neatly together, permitting flexion and extension around one axis and abduction and adduction around the other. The carpometacarpal joint at the base of the thumb is the only saddle joint in the body. Articulation occurs between the proximal end of the metacarpal bone of the thumb and the carpal bone named the trapezium.

Condyloid joints are those in which an oval condyle fits into an elliptic socket or cavity. This type of articular surface permits angular movement in two planes, but no axial rotation. In short, it permits biaxial movement. Example: condyles of the occipital bone fit into elliptical depressions of the atlas.

Multiaxial joints. Multiaxial joints (Figure 4-7) have two or more axes of rotation and permit movement in three or more planes. There are two types of multiaxial joints: *ball-and-socket* and *gliding*.

Ball-and-socket joints are those in which a ball-shaped head of one bone fits into a

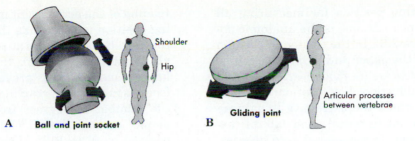

FIGURE 4-7
Multiaxial joints. **A,** Ball and socket joint (shoulder, hip); **B,** Gliding joint (articular processes between vertebrae).

concave socket or depression of another bone. Of all the joints in our bodies, ball-and-socket joints permit the widest and freest range of movements in almost any direction or plane. Movements in this type of joint include flexion, extension, abduction, adduction, rotation, and circumduction. Examples are the shoulder and hip joints.

Gliding joints are numerous and almost always small. Articular surfaces in these joints are either flat, nearly flat, or slightly curved. They include most of the joints between the carpal and tarsal bones and also all the joints between the articular processes of the vertebrae. These joints allow only the simplest kind of slight displacement motion between their articular surfaces. Gliding movements occur in all planes.

Range and Type of Movement in Diarthroses

Range of motion (ROM)

Diarthrotic, or synovial, joints are often referred to as "freely movable joints." Such a description, of course, applies only to the normal direction and ROM available at any particular joint. Even for the most supple athlete there are distinct and necessary limitations to joint mobility.

The normal type and range of joint movements are influenced primarily by four factors: (1) the shape of the articular, or joint, surfaces; (2) the restraining effects of the joint capsule; (3) the number, type of attachment, and tautness of ligaments; and (4) the effect of muscles that may act as fixators to stabilize the joint. In addition, there is also

frequent and sometimes considerable variation in the range of movement among individuals.

The terms *range of motion* and *flexibility* are not synonymous, although athletes who exhibit limited or excess flexibility have related changes in joint ROM. Good flexibility is highly desirable and increases ROM within optimal limits, thus reducing the potential for injuries such as muscle strains and tendinitis, whereas hyperflexibility predisposes an athlete to suffer dislocations and subluxations. Considerable variability in the degree of flexibility occurs between individuals and between the various joints in the body. A number of subjective tests such as the sit and reach can be used to assess flexibility, or actual ROM can be measured using a Leighton Flexometer or goniometer as explained in the paragraphs that follow.

Measurement of ROM

The measurement of joint ROM is an important component of a comprehensive physical examination of the extremities and spine. This enables an athletic trainer to accurately measure dysfunction, as well as gauge treatment and rehabilitative progress. Repeated observations and measurement of ROM are performed throughout the athletic injury assessment process. Correct interpretation of this important assessment step requires knowledge of the normal type and range of motion available at each joint in the absence of injury. This information is provided in each of the chapters concerning assessment of a body area in Units IV, V, and VI.

The starting position for measuring all ROMs, except rotations, is the anatomic position (Figure 2-6). In the anatomic position the joints of the upper and lower extremities are at zero degrees for flexion-extension and abduction-adduction. For rotation, the body position in which the extremity is halfway between medial (internal) and lateral (external) rotation is considered zero degrees. The amount of motion available at any specific joint is then measured in degrees from the zero starting position. The ROM can be measured actively or passively. In active movements the athlete voluntarily moves the joint or body part through its ROM, and in passive movements the athletic trainer moves the part with the muscles relaxed. Normally, active and passive ROM should be about equal.

There are two ways to measure joint ROM: (1) the subjective method and (2) the objective method. The subjective method is used to observe the available joint movement and estimate the approximate ROM. This method is frequently used by an athletic trainer as he or she compares the ROM available between the injured and the uninjured side or collates the observed ROM to what is considered normal for that specific joint. With practice and experience, athletic trainers can become fairly accurate at estimating ROM subjectively.

A more accurate method of determining ROM is to actually measure the available motion objectively. This is accomplished by using an instrument called a **goniometer.** A goniometer consists of two rigid shafts that intersect at a hinge joint. A protractor is fixed to one shaft so that motion can be read directly from the scale in degrees. The axis of the goniometer should coincide with the appropriate axis of motion of the joint being measured. This point can be determined by moving the joint through the ROM and visually estimating the site of rotation. The shafts of the goniometer should be aligned parallel to the long axis of the limb segments that are associated with the joint being measured (Figure 4-8). One of these segments must be stabilized for an accurate

reading of the actual joint motion. The starting position is defined as the point at which the movable segment is at zero degrees (usually anatomic position). If the athlete has limited motion that prevents him or her from assuming the starting position, record the number of degrees from zero. For example, normal flexion of the elbow is expressed as 0° to 150°. If the athlete cannot straighten the elbow, the reading might be 15° to 150°. If the athlete has excessive mobility beyond the starting position, the reading is expressed as a negative value from the zero position. In the previous example this would be termed *hyperextension* and the reading for the elbow might now be −10° to 150°. With practice and experience, athletic trainers can become very accurate at measuring joint ROM with a goniometer.

Kinematic chains

In our extremities, the series of bones connected by joints form a linkage system. In engineering, this sequence of links and joints is called a **kinematic chain.** In the human body this kinematic chain can be an open or closed system. An **open kinematic chain** occurs when the distal end of the extremity is not fixed and allows a joint to function independently without necessarily causing motion at another joint. Examples would be waving your hand or raising your foot off the ground. In a **closed kinematic chain** the distal end of the extremity is fixed, and motion at one joint will cause predictable movement in adjacent joints. Examples would be doing pushups or knee bends. Motion must occur in several joints simultaneously for these activities to result. A change in function or structure of one joint in the system can effect the function of the adjacent joints. For example, limited motion in an injured knee may cause an athlete to compensate at the hip and/or ankle joints when walking. This is an important concept in rehabilitation. Exercises that are closed kinematic chain activities are more functional than open chain activities. Exercises that emphasize strengthening of the entire kinematic chain should be incorporated

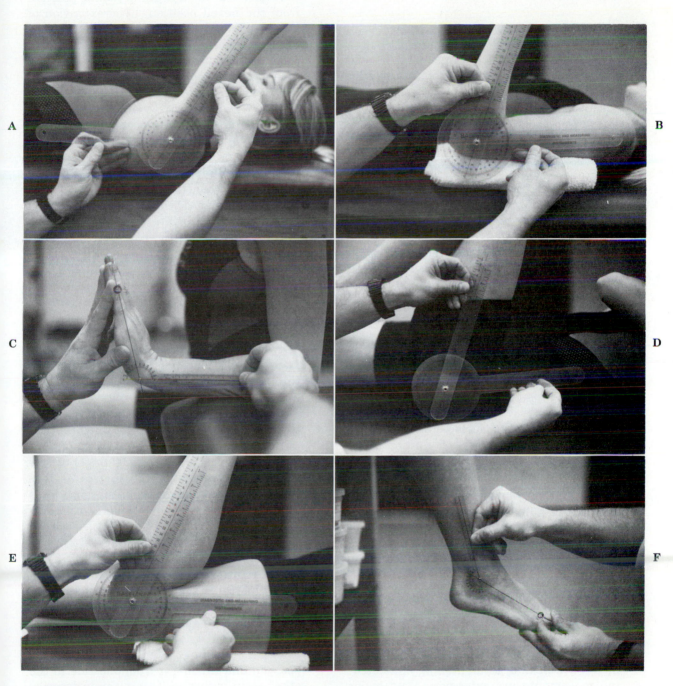

FIGURE 4-8
Using a goniometer to measure the joint ROM of the **A**, shoulder; **B**, elbow; **C**, wrist; **D**, hip; **E**, knee; and **F**, ankle.

rather than an exercise that isolates a single segment.

Types of movement

Although we have the ability to perform a single movement at a single joint at one time, most coordinated types of body activity occur only as a result of simultaneous or successive movements at many joints. Articulating bones in synovial joints, acting in conjunction with other joints, are capable of moving in many directions, along different axes of rotation, and through different planes of reference in the body. The various types of combined joint movements that occur as a result of such activity can be categorized or grouped as follows: (1) *angular* if there is a change in the angle between bones; (2) *rotation and circumduction* if there is movement of a bone around its own axis; (3) *gliding* if the only movement produced is simple displacement between articulating surfaces; and (4) *special* if the movement produced is so unique that it must be described individually.

Angular movements. Angular movements are illustrated in Figure 4-9. **Flexion** decreases the size of the angle between the anterior or posterior surfaces of articulated bones. An exception to this definition is the shoulder joint. Shoulder flexion occurs as the arm is elevated forward in the sagittal plane. Flexing movements are bending or folding movements. Bending the head forward on the chest, for example, is flexion of the joint between the occipital bone at the base of the skull and the atlas, or first cervical vertebra. Bending the elbow, as when the forearm bends back on the arm, is another example of flexion.

Extension is the return from the flexed position and generally results in an increase of a joint angle. Whereas bending movements are flexion, straightening or stretching movements are extension. Most major joints are in extension when a person restores an extremity or body part from a flexed position to the anatomic position. Continuation of extension beyond the anatomic position is called **hyperextension.**

Extension of the head, for example, means to return it to the upright anatomic position from the flexed position; hyperextension of the head would result in its being stretched backward from the upright position.

Flexion and extension of the ankle joint are termed *plantar* and *dorsal* flexion. **Plantar flexion** is movement of the sole of the foot downward, such as standing on your toes. **Dorsiflexion** is movement of the top (dorsum) of the foot upward. **Abduction** is movement of a body part or extremity away from the midline, or center, of the body. An example of abduction is movement of the arm away from the body in the frontal plane. **Horizonal abduction** is movement of the upper limb through the transverse plane at shoulder level away from the midline of the body.

Adduction is the opposite of abduction. It moves the body part toward the midline, or center, of the body. An example would be bringing the arms back to the sides of the body from the abducted position. **Horizonal adduction** is movement of the upper limb through the transverse plane at shoulder level toward the midline of the body.

In discussing abduction and adduction of the fingers and toes the plane of reference is not the midline of the body but an imaginary line drawn through the middle finger or second toe. Movement of the fingers or toes away from these imaginary reference lines results in "spreading" movements or abduction. Movement of the fingers or toes toward these imaginary reference lines results in adduction.

Rotation and circumduction. Figure 4-10 illustrates the movements of rotation and circumduction. **Rotation** is the pivoting of a bone on its own central or longitudinal axis, somewhat as a top turns on its axis. An example is holding your head in an upright position and turning it from one side to the other, as in saying no. To accurately describe the type of rotation, a qualifying word is normally used in conjunction with rotation. Directional words such as upward, downward, inward, outward, medial, or lateral help to explain the type of rotation.

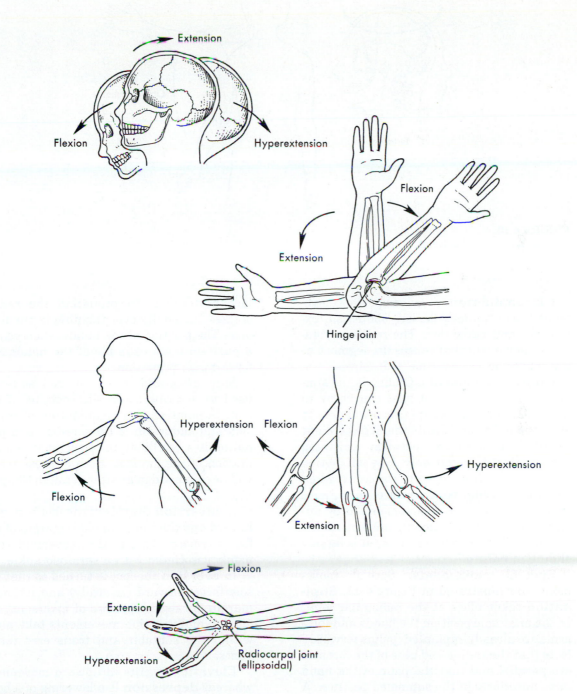

FIGURE 4-9
Examples of angular movements at synovial joints.

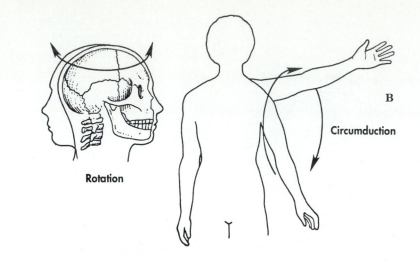

FIGURE 4-10
Rotation and circumduction. **A**, Rotation at the atlantoaxial joint; **B**, circumduction at the shoulder.

Circumduction is a composite movement that combines flexion, abduction, extension, and adduction. The result is rotational movement that causes the segment as a whole to describe a cone as it moves.

Gliding movements. Gliding is the simplest type of movement that can occur in movable joints and occurs to some degree in all of them. In some joints this type of slight relative displacement between adjoining bone surfaces is the only type of motion available. Gliding movements occur when one articulating bone surface in a joint moves over another, unaccompanied by angular or rotary movement. Movement between the carpal bones of the wrist is largely gliding in nature.

Special movements. Special movements are illustrated in Figure 4-11. **Supination** takes place at the radioulnar joint. In the anatomic position the hands and forearms are already supinated (palms forward). Note that the radius and ulna of the forearm are parallel and that the palm of the hand faces anteriorly in the supinated position. A handball serve involves supinating the hand.

Pronation describes the inward rotation or movement of the supinated forearm and hand, which causes the palm of the hand to face posteriorly. In pronation the radius crosses diagonally over the ulna in the forearm. The position of the hands when you do a push-up is an example of the hands and forearms in pronation.

Supination and *pronation* are also terms used to describe composite motions of the foot. Supination is a combination of inversion and adduction of the forefoot, and pronation is a combination of eversion and abduction of the forefoot. Both of these terms will be discussed in greater detail in Chapter 17.

In **inversion** the sole of the foot is turned inward and the inner (medial) margin of the foot is raised. This is the movement commonly associated with a sprained ankle.

In **eversion** the foot is turned so that the sole faces outward (laterally) and its outer margin is raised (opposite of inversion). Inversion and eversion movements take place within the subtalar and transverse tarsal joints.

Elevation results in upward movement, whereas **depression** is a lowering of a body part or return from an elevated position. These terms are commonly used to describe movements of the mandible and shoulder girdle.

Protraction refers to motion that moves

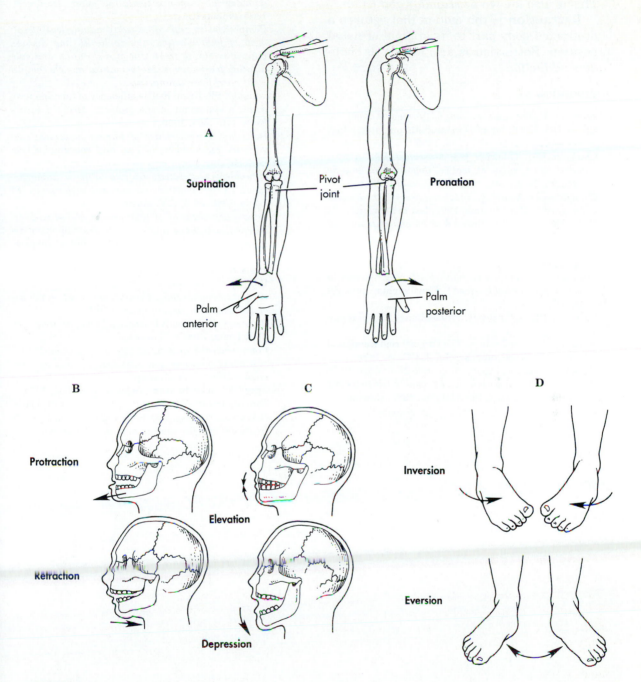

FIGURE 4-11
Examples of special movements at synovial joints. **A**, Pronation and supination; **B**, protraction and retraction; **C**, elevation and depression; **D**, inversion and eversion.

a part forward. Reaching for an object involves a protraction of the shoulder girdle. This is also known as *scapular abduction*.

Retraction is the motion that returns a protracted body part to its original or usual position. Retraction is also known as *scapular adduction*.

REFERENCES

Allman WF: The knee, *Science 83* November, 1983.

Clarke DH: Sex differences in strength and fatigability, *Res Q Exerc Sport* 57(2):144, 1986.

Clarkson HM, Gilewich BG: *Musculoskeletal assessment; joint range of motion and manual muscle strength,* Baltimore, 1989, Williams & Wilkins.

Clemente CD: *Anatomy: a regional atlas of the human body,* ed 3, Philadelphia, 1981, Lea & Febiger.

Hamilton WJ, editor: *Textbook of human anatomy,* ed 2, St. Louis, 1976, C.V. Mosby Co.

Hencke HR: *Arthroscopy of the knee joint,* Berlin, 1979, Springer-Verlag.

Norkin CC, Levangie PK: *Joint structure & function; a comprehensive analysis,* ed 2, Philadelphia, 1992, FA Davis.

O'Connor RL: *Arthroscopy,* Philadelphia, 1977, Lippincott.

Sonstegard DA and others: The surgical replacement of the human knee joint, *Sci Am* 238(1):44, 1978.

Walker PS: Joints to spare, *Science 85* November, 1985.

Wilson FC: *The musculoskeletal system: basic processes and disorders,* ed 2, Philadelphia, 1983, Lippincott.

SUGGESTED READINGS

Berme N and others: *Biomechanics of normal and pathological human articulating joints,* Dordrecht, 1985, Nijhoff Press.
Comprehensive and advanced (graduate level) treatment of joint biomechanics in health and disease. Especially strong treatment of dislocation and subluxation mechanisms. Mathematical models complement narrative explanations.

Cavanaugh PR, Kram R: The efficiency of human movement: a statement of the problem, *Med Sci Sports Exerc* 17(3):304, 1985.
Describes characteristics of human movement and adaptive mechanisms of gait and coordinated motion. An interesting and well-written reexamination of problems associated with locomotion in humans.

Johnson LL: *Diagnostic and surgical arthroscopy,* St Louis, 1985, ed 2, C.V. Mosby.
Advanced treatment of arthroscopy. Filled with excellent illustrations and accurate descriptions of arthroscopic surgical instrumentation and techniques.

Norkin CC, White DJ: *Measurement of joint motion: a guide to goniometry,* Philadelphia, 1985, FA Davis Co.
A comprehensive and well-illustrated text on the use of goniometer to measure joint ROM.

Thibodeau GA, Patton KT: *Anatomy and physiology,* ed 3, St Louis, 1993, C.V. Mosby.
Comprehensive undergraduate text covering the essentials of anatomy and physiology, including thorough coverage of arthrology.

Walker PS: Joints to spare, *Science 85* 6(9):56, 1985.
Popular treatment of joint replacement and repair. Interesting reading, easy to understand, and accurate treatment of a fascinating area in orthopedics.

CHAPTER 5
Myology

After you have completed this chapter, you should be able to:

- Define the term *myology* and describe the generalized functions of muscle tissue.
- Explain the relationship between strength of muscle contraction and range of motion (ROM) at joints.
- Identify the four component parts of a basic lever system and give examples of first-, second-, and third-class levers in the body.
- Describe the gross and microscopic anatomy of skeletal muscle.
- Discuss the types of muscle contraction.
- List the primary function of the major muscle groups of the body.
- Compare and contrast the origin and insertion points of muscle attachment.
- Discuss how skeletal muscles are named.
- Explain how muscle strength is estimated and how it can relate to athletic injury.
- Define: optimum angle of pull, motor unit, neuromuscular junction, sarcomeres, prime mover, holding strength.

We have already reviewed the basic architectural plan of the body as a whole (Chapter 2), the skeletal system (Chapter 3), and the system of joints or articulations that make the potential for movement possible (Chapter 4). Regardless of body type, bones and joints cannot move themselves. They must be moved by the contraction of muscle tissue. This chapter discusses the 40% to 50% of our body weight that is skeletal muscle—those muscle masses that attach to bones and make movement possible. We will cover only muscles of particular functional significance, with emphasis on those that can be located externally either by palpation or by sight. If appropriate, additional details of individual muscle attachment and function will accompany actual assessment procedures in subsequent chapters.

The study of skeletal muscles is termed **myology.** Each of the over 600 skeletal muscles in the body can be thought of as a separate organ. Ordinarily, however, muscles act in coordinated groups and not as single units. They tend to occur and function in pairs, or in sets of three, four, or more muscles. Kinesiologists, for example, identify over 215 functional pairs of skeletal muscles. Each pair performs a unique and essential muscular action. Muscles vary significantly in size and shape. In addition, their individual fibers are arranged differently and attach in differing ways to the bones they move. They all have the same function, however, and behave in the same way; that is, they shorten. As muscles fibers shorten, their ends are pulled toward the center and contractile force, or tension, is developed in the muscle. The result is the basic ingredient of all physical activity—movement.

GENERAL FUNCTIONS

The essential functions of skeletal muscle include the following.

Movement

Skeletal muscle contractions produce movements of the body as a whole (locomotion) or of its parts. Muscle tissue, because of its irritability, contractility, extensibility, and elasticity, is admirably suited to this function. The force of pull generated by the contraction of muscle tissue is generally applied through a leverage system of bones and joints. Whereas most of the systems of the body play some role in accomplishing movement, it is the skeletal, muscular, and nervous systems acting together that actually produce movement.

Heat production

Muscle cells, like all cells, produce heat as a by-product during the catabolism of nutrients for energy. Because skeletal muscle cells are highly active and numerous, they produce a major portion of total body heat. As a result, heat-related problems in athletes frequently occur as a result of muscular exertion in a hot and humid environment. In mild or cold environmental conditions, skeletal muscle contractions constitute one of the most important parts of the mechanism for maintaining homeostasis of temperature.

Posture, protection, and support

The continued partial contraction of many skeletal muscles makes possible standing, sitting, and other maintained positions of the body. In addition, skeletal muscle mass gives shape to the body and provides protection and support.

MUSCLES AND BONY LEVERS

Knowledge of the mechanics of lever systems and the points of muscle attachment to bones gives the athletic trainer a basis for understanding not only body movements but also muscle strength and range of motion (ROM) at specific joints. Maximal muscle strength and maximal ROM at the same joint are mutually exclusive. This inverse relationship between strength of muscle contraction and range of motion at a given joint is a basic principle of leverage, or mechanical advantage, and is of practical importance. As a general rule, if two muscles of equal length cross and act on the same joint, the muscle that inserts (attaches) farther from the fulcrum (joint) will produce the more powerful contraction, and the muscle inserting closer to the joint will produce the greater range of movement.

Another basic of muscle action in a lever system is called the **optimum angle of pull.** Generally, the optimum angle of pull for any muscle is a right angle to the long axis of the bone to which it is attached. When the angle of pull departs from a right angle and becomes more parallel to the long axis, the strength of contraction decreases dramatically. Contraction of the brachialis muscle demonstrates this principle very well. The brachialis crosses the elbow from humerus to ulna. In the anatomic position, the elbow is extended and the angle of pull of the brachialis is parallel to the long axis of the ulna. Contraction of the brachialis at this angle is very inefficient. As the elbow is flexed and the angle of pull approaches a right angle, the contraction strength of the muscle is greatly increased. If asked to assess brachialis muscle strength, how would you position the forearm? It is this type of information that makes a rational approach to the correct assessment of many joint and muscle injuries possible.

Lever Systems

A lever system is a simple mechanical device composed of four component parts: (1) a rigid rod or bar (bone); (2) a fixed pivot, or fulcrum, around which the rod moves (joint); (3) a weight, or resistance, that is moved; and (4) a force, or effort, that produces movement (muscle contraction). In Figure 5-1 the fulcrum is symbolized as a circle, the resistance as a square, and the effort as *E*. Figure 5-1 shows the three different types of lever arrangements that are categorized according to placement of the fulcrum, resistance

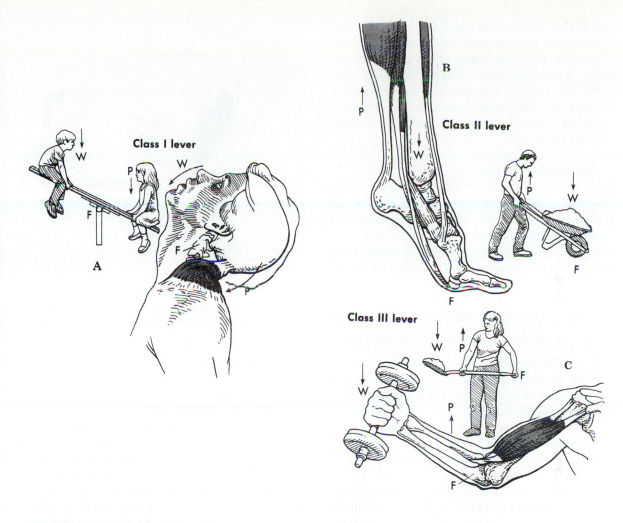

FIGURE 5-1
Classes of levers. Each class of lever is determined by the placement of fulcrum, effort, and resistance. **A**, First class lever; **B**, second class lever, and, **C**, third class lever.

and effort. All three types are found in the human body.

First-class levers

As you can see in Figure 5-1, the placement of the fulcrum in a first-class lever lies between the effort and the resistance, as in a set of scales, a pair of scissors, or a child's seesaw. In the body, the head raised or tipped backward on the atlas is an example of a first-class lever in action. The facial portion of the skull is the resistance, the joint between the skull and atlas the fulcrum, and the muscles of the back, such as the splenius

capitis, produce the effort. In the human body, first-class levers are not abundant. They generally serve as levers of stability.

Second-class levers

In the second-class levers the weight, or resistance, lies between the fulcrum and the joint at which the pull, or effort, is exerted. The wheelbarrow is often used as an example. The presence of second-class levers in the human body is a controversial issue. Some authorities interpret the raising of the body on the toes as an example of this type of lever (Figure 5-1). In this example the point of contact between the toes and the ground is the fulcrum, the resistance is located at the ankle, and effort is exerted by the gastrocnemius muscle through the Achilles tendon. Opening the mouth against resistance (depression of the mandible) is also considered to be an example of a second-class lever.

Third-class levers

In a third-class lever the effort is exerted between the fulcrum and resistance or weight to be moved. Flexing of the forearm at the elbow joint is a frequently used example of this type of lever. Third-class levers permit rapid and extensive movement and are the commonest type found in the body. They allow insertion of a muscle very close to the joint that it moves.

ANATOMY OF SKELETAL MUSCLES

Size and Shape

Each skeletal muscle is a separate organ consisting of skeletal muscle fibers plus important connective, nervous, and vascular tissue components. Individual skeletal muscles vary considerably in size and shape. They range from extremely tiny strands such as the stapedius muscle of the middle ear to large masses such as the quadriceps femoris muscles of the thigh. Some skeletal muscles are broad in shape and some narrow. Some are long and tapering and some short and blunt. Some are triangular, some quadrilateral, and some irregular. Some form flat sheets and others form bulky masses.

A typical muscle is often described as having a central fleshy, or meaty, contractile portion called the belly, or **gaster,** and two tendinous extremities by which the muscle is attached to bone. One attachment is called the **origin** and the other the **insertion.** The origin is the end that remains fixed or stationary when the muscle contracts. It is usually proximal to the joint. The insertion is the extremity that moves when the muscle contracts. It is distal to the joint and moves toward the origin when the muscle contracts (Figure 5-2).

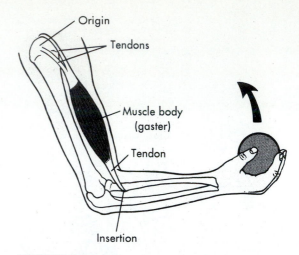

FIGURE 5-2
Attachments of a skeletal muscle. A muscle originates at a relatively stable part of the skeleton (origin) and inserts at the skeletal part that is moved when the muscle contracts (insertion).

Fiber Arrangement

Arrangement of fibers varies among different muscles (Figure 5-3). In some muscles, such as the rectus abdominis, the fibers are *parallel* to the long axis of the muscle. In the pectoralis major the fibers are said to be *radiate* in arrangement and converge from a broad area or origin to a narrow insertion. The deltoid exhibits a complex *multipennate* fiber arrangement that recalls from the convergence of fibers in several muscular components. The long sartorius muscle has longitudinally arranged fibers, and the rectus femoris has a *bipennate* arrangement, with fibers directed obliquely from both sides of a central tendon. A *unipennate* arrangement exhibits fibers inserting diagonally on only one side of a similar tendon that runs the entire length of the muscle, much like the feathers in an old-fashioned plume pen. *Circular* fiber bundles are curved to encircle an opening and are typical in sphincter muscles such as the orbicularis oris. The direction of the fibers composing a muscle is significant because of its relationship to function. Bipennate and unipennate fiber arrange-

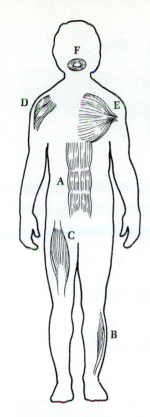

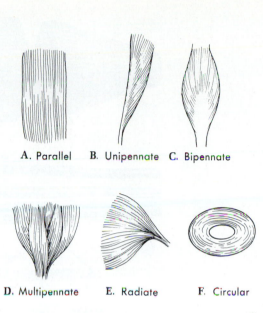

A. Parallel   B. Unipennate   C. Bipennate

D. Multipennate   E. Radiate   F. Circular

FIGURE 5-3
Types of muscle fiber arrangement.

ments, for example, produce the strongest contractions.

Connective Tissue Components

Every skeletal muscle contains a number of extremely important connective tissue elements (Figure 5-4). It is interesting to note that most muscular injuries in athletics occur in the connective tissue elements of the muscle. These noncontractile structures are intimately associated with muscle fibers, both anatomically and functionally. The contraction (shortening) of skeletal muscle cells cannot produce actual movement unless the cells are effectively attached to the structure to be moved. The connective tissue elements of skeletal muscle serve to "harness" the muscle to the structures they pull on during contraction.

A fine meshwork of loose connective tissue fibers, the **endomysium,** surrounds each muscle fiber. Groups of 15 to 40 fibers are bound into bundles called **fasciculi.** Each fascicle is covered by a coarser and more fibrous connective tissue sheath called the **perimysium.** The perimysium partitions between fasciculi merge with the endomysium and ultimately extend to the surface of the muscle, where they become continuous with a thicker, outer connective tissue sheath, the **epimysium,** which covers the entire muscle.

The epimysium, perimysium, and endomysium of a muscle become continuous with fibrous tissue that extends from the muscles as a **tendon,** a strong, tough cord continuous at its other end with the fibrous covering of bone (periosteum). The fibrous wrapping of a muscle may also extend as a broad, flat sheet of connective tissue (aponeurosis) attaching it to adjacent structures, usually the fibrous wrappings of another muscle.

Tubular structures of fibrous connective tissue, called *tendon sheaths,* enclose certain tendons, notably those of the wrist, hand, ankle, and foot. Like the bursae, tendon sheaths have a lining of synovial membrane. Its moist, smooth surface enables the tendon to move easily, almost frictionlessly, in the tendon sheath.

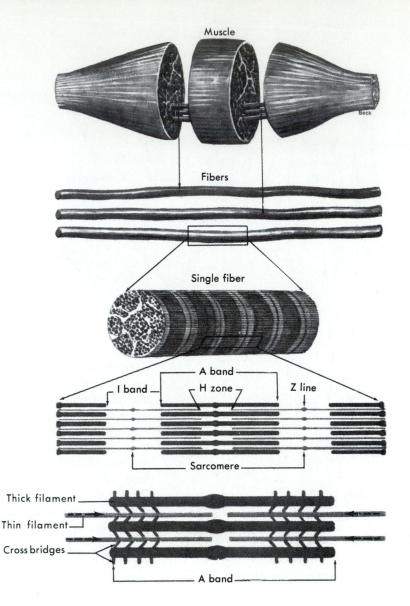

FIGURE 5-4
Connective tissue and contractile components of skeletal muscle. Illustration shows the increasingly more detailed submicroscopic structure of a muscle fiber.

You may recall that a continuous sheet of loose connective tissue known as the **superficial fascia** lies directly under the skin. Under this lies a layer of dense fibrous connective tissue, the **deep fascia.** Extensions of the deep fascia form the epimysium, perimysium, and endomysium of muscles and their attachments to bones and other structures and also enclose viscera, glands, blood vessels, and nerves.

Nerve Tissue

Nerves containing both sensory and motor components enter skeletal muscles through the covering epimysium and course between the fasciculi in the perimysium. Ultimately

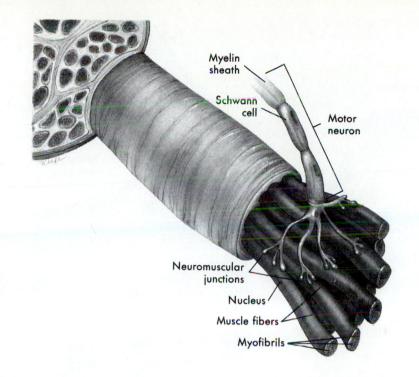

Myelin
sheath

Schwann
cell

Motor
neuron

Neuromuscular
junctions

Nucleus

Muscle fibers

Myofibrils

FIGURE 5-5
Motor unit. A motor unit consists of one somatic motor neuron and the muscle fibers supplied
by its branches.

each muscle fiber is innervated by a somatic **motor neuron.** One neuron plus the muscle fibers it innervates constitute a **motor unit** (Figure 5-5). The single axon fiber of a motor unit, on entering the skeletal muscle, divides into a variable number of branches. Those of some motor units terminate in only a few muscle fibers, whereas others terminate in numerous fibers. Thus, impulse conduction by one motor unit may stimulate only a half dozen or so muscle fibers to contract at one time, whereas conduction by another motor unit may activate a hundred or more fibers simultaneously. This fact bears a relationship to the function of the muscle as a whole. As a general rule, the fewer number of fibers supplied by a skeletal muscle's individual motor units, the more precise the movements that muscle can produce. For example, in certain small muscles of the hand, each motor unit includes only a few muscle fibers, and these muscles produce precise finger movements. In contrast, motor units in large abdominal or thigh muscles that do

not produce precise movements are reported to include more than a hundred muscle fibers each.

The area of contact between a nerve and a muscle fiber is known as the **motor endplate,** or **neuromuscular junction** (Figure 5-6). When nerve impulses reach the ends of the axon fibers in a skeletal muscle, small vesicles in the axon terminals release a chemical called acetylcholine into the neuromuscular junction. Diffusing swiftly across this microscopic trough, acetylcholine contacts the sarcolemma of the adjacent muscle fibers, stimulating the fiber to contract. In addition to motor nerve ends, there are also many sensory nerve endings in skeletal muscles. The purpose of the sensory nerves is to transmit impulses to the central nervous system to convey information concerning body position, pain, and other types of sensation. Examples of sensory components include muscle spindles and Golgi tendon organs.

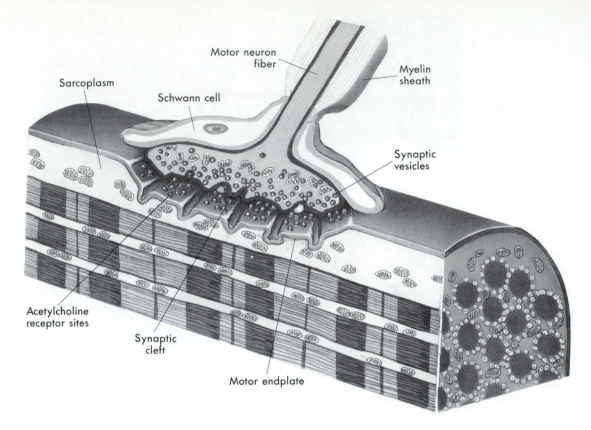

FIGURE 5-6
Neuromuscular junction. This figure shows how the distal end of a motor neuron forms a "chemical junction" with an adjacent muscle fiber. Neurotransmitters (acetylcholine) are released and diffuse across the synaptic cleft.

MICROSCOPIC ANATOMY

It is suggested that you review the basic microscopic anatomy of skeletal muscle in a textbook of anatomy and physiology or histology. Detailed information of this type lies beyond the scope of an assessment text but is useful in understanding cellular repair in muscle tissue after injury. In general, individual skeletal muscle cells (fibers) are multinucleated, elongated, and cylindric (Figure 5-7). When viewed under the microscope they show very distinct cross-striations of alternating light, or striped appearance. The cross-striations are produced by the repetitive or periodic arrangement and overlapping of interdigitating filaments. Individual contractile units are called **sarcomeres.** When adjacent sarcomeres contract simul-taneously the entire fiber shortens, and a measurable pulling force (contraction) is generated.

Types of Skeletal Muscle Contraction

Tonic contraction, or muscle tone, refers to the continual, partial contraction of muscles of normal individuals when they are awake. It is particularly important for maintaining posture. Loss of muscle tone occurs when a person loses consciousness, causing the individual to collapse. Muscles with less tone than normal are described as *flaccid muscles,* and those with more than normal tone are called *spastic.*

In addition to tonic contractions that maintain muscle tone and posture, other types of contractions also occur. Additional

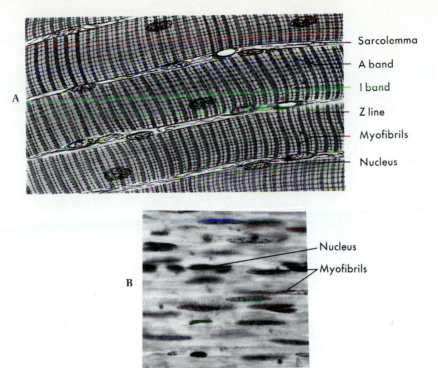

A ———

Sarcolemma

A band

I band

Z line

Myofibrils

Nucleus

B ———

Nucleus

Myofibrils

FIGURE 5-7
A, Skeletal or striated voluntary muscle tissue and, **B,** a higher magnification.

types of muscle contractions include:
1. Twitch contraction
2. Tetanic contraction
3. Isotonic contraction
4. Isometric contraction

Twitch and tetanic contractions

A **twitch** is a quick, jerky response to a stimulus. Twitch contractions can be seen in isolated muscles during research, but they play a minimal role in normal muscle activity. To accomplish the coordinated and fluid muscular movements needed for most activity, muscles must contract not in a jerky but in a smooth and sustained way.

A **tetanic contraction** is a more sustained and steady response than a twitch. It is produced by a series of stimuli bombarding the muscle in rapid succession. Contractions "melt" together to produce a sustained normal contraction called *tetanus*. Tetanic contraction is not necessarily a maximal

contraction in which each muscle fiber responds at the same time. In most cases, only a few areas of the muscle undergo contractions at any time. Tetanus is the kind of contraction exhibited by normal skeletal muscles most of the time.

Isotonic contraction

In most cases, **isotonic contraction** of muscle produces movement at a joint. With this type of contraction the muscle either shortens or lengthens. When the muscle shortens and the insertion moves toward the point of origin, it is called a **concentric contraction** (Figure 5-8, *A*). When a muscle is exerting tension but is being *lengthened* by some outside force or by gravity, it is known as an **eccentric contraction.** This is also called *negative work*. Most muscular contractions producing movement typical of athletic activity are examples of isotonic contractions.

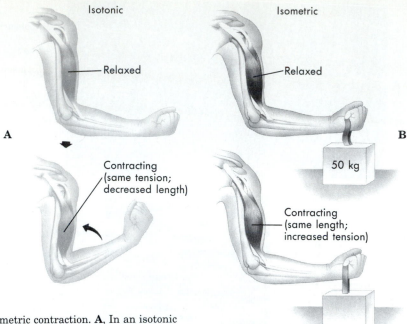

FIGURE 5-8
Isotonic and isometric contraction. **A**, In an isotonic contraction the muscle shortens, producing movement. **B**, In an isometric contraction the muscle pulls forcefully against a load but does not shorten.

Isometric contraction

Contraction of a skeletal muscle does not always produce movement. Sometimes, it increases the tension within a muscle but does not shorten the muscle. When the muscle does not shorten and no movement results, it is called an **isometric contraction.** Although muscles do not shorten (and thus produce no movement) during isometric contractions, tension within them increases (Figure 5-8, *B*). Because of this, repeated isometric contractions increase muscle mass and are important components in conditioning exercises.

MUSCLE ACTION

It is the voluntary contraction of specific skeletal muscles that produces the types of diarthrotic joint movements described in Chapter 4. Some muscles abduct a joint, whereas others may be positioned to adduct or flex it. Generally, muscles span the joint at which movement occurs and attach to both articulating bones. In most cases the body of the muscle lies proximal to the part moved. Thus muscles that move the forearm lie proximal to it, in the upper arm.

In understanding muscle actions it is important to realize that skeletal muscles almost always act in groups rather than singly. In other words, most movements are produced by the coordinated action of several muscles. Some of the muscles in the group contract while others relax. To identify each muscle's special function in the group, the following classification is used:

Prime movers, or agonists: Muscle or muscles whose contraction actually produces movement

Antagonists: One or more muscles that oppose the action of another group of muscles or the pull of gravity*

Synergists: Muscles that contract at the same time as the prime mover, assisting or supplementing a prime mover in producing a particular movement

---

*Antagonistic muscles have opposite actions and opposite locations. If the flexor lies anterior to the part, the extensor will be found posterior to it. For example, the pectoralis major, the flexor of the upper arm, is located on the anterior aspect of the chest, whereas the latissimus dorsi, the extensor of the upper arm, is located on the posterior aspect of the chest. The antagonist of a flexor muscle is obviously an extensor muscle and that of an abductor muscle, an adductor muscle.

Fixators: Muscles that serve to fix or stabilize a joint to augment the effectiveness of a prime mover

HOW SKELETAL MUSCLES ARE NAMED

Muscle names seem more logical and therefore easier to learn and remember when you understand the reasons for their use. Most muscles are named on the basis of one or more distinct features or characteristics. It is possible to learn much about a muscle just from its name. Characteristics used in naming muscles include the following:

Action of function: The name or part of the name indicates its function (such as flexor or extensor)

Direction of its fibers: For example, the external oblique muscle in the abdominal wall

Location: For example, the tibialis anterior muscle is located on the front of the leg

Number of diversions: Such as biceps, triceps, or quadriceps

Shape: Such as deltoid (triangular) or quadratus (square)

Size: Such as gluteus maximus and gluteus minimus

Points of attachment: The origin is the first part of the muscle's name and the insertion is last, as in brachioradialis—the brachium (arm or humerus) is the origin, and the radius is the insertion

A good way to start the study of a muscle is by trying to find out what its name means.

ORIGINS, INSERTIONS, FUNCTIONS, AND INNERVATIONS OF REPRESENTATIVE MUSCLES

The object of this chapter is to provide a generalized overview of myology. Rote memorization of many minute details will be counterproductive. Such facts only "make sense" when they help explain the rationale that undergirds actual assessment techniques. Necessary anatomic details will be a part of each assessment technique described in subsequent chapters of the text. Use the information and illustrations in this chapter as a reference source.

Basic information about many muscles is given in Tables 5-1 to 5-11 and Figures 5-9 to 5-16. Each table describes a group of mus-

Text continued on p. 80.

TABLE 5-1

Muscles That Move the Shoulder Girdle

Muscle	Origin	Insertion	Function	Innervation
■ Trapezius	**Occipital bone** (protuberance) Ligamentum nuchae	**Clavicle** (upper fibers)	Elevates shoulders Upward rotation of scapula	Spinal accessory, third and fourth cervical nerves
	Vertebrae (cervical and thoracic)	**Scapula** (spine and acromion) (lower fibers)	Depresses shoulder Upward rotation	
Pectoralis minor	Ribs, second to fifth	Scapula (coracoid)	Depresses shoulder Downward rotation	Medial pectoral nerve
■ Serratus anterior	**Ribs,** upper eight or nine	**Scapula** (anterior surface, vertebral border)	Protracts scapula; abducts and rotates it upward	Long thoracic nerve
Rhomboideus major	Vertebrae (upper thoracic)	Scapula (vertebral border)	Retract scapula Elevate shoulder Downward rotation	Dorsal scapular nerve
Levator scapulae	Vertebrae (upper cervical)	Scapula (superior angle)	Elevates shoulder Downward rotation	Third and fourth cervical nerves

TABLE 5-2

Muscles That Move the Vertebral Column

Muscle	Origin	Insertion	Function	Innervation
■ Sacrospinalis (erector spinae)	Three series of muscles: lateral, intermediate, and medial		Extend spine; maintain erect posture of trunk Acting singly, rotates trunk	Posterior rami of first cervical to fifth lumbar spinal nerves
Lateral portion: Iliocostalis lumborum	Iliac crest, sacrum (posterior surface), and lumbar vertebrae (spinous processes)	Ribs, lower six	Extends lumbar region	
Iliocostalis thoracis	Ribs, lower six	Ribs, upper six	Maintains erect position	
Iliocostalis cervicis	Ribs, upper six	Vertebrae, fourth to sixth cervical	Extends cervical region	
Intermediate portion: Longissimus thoracis	Same as iliocostalis lumborum	Vertebrae, thoracic ribs	Extends thoracic region	
Longissimus cervicis	Vertebrae, upper six thoracic	Vertebrae, second to sixth cervical	Extends cervical region	
Longissimus capitis	Vertebrae, upper six thoracic and last four cervical	Temporal bone, mastoid process	Extends head and rotates to opposite side	
Medial portion: Spinalis thoracis	Vertebrae, upper lumbar and lower thoracic	Upper thoracic spinous processes	Extends thoracic region	
Quadratus lumborum (forms part of posterior abdominal wall)	Illium (posterior part of crest) Vertebrae (lower three lumbar)	Rib (Twelfth) Vertebrae (transverse processes of first four lumbar)	Both muscles together extend spine	First three or four lumbar nerves One muscle alone, lateral flexor

TABLE 5-3

Muscles of the Anterior Abdominal Wall

Muscle	Origin	Insertion	Function	Innervation
■ External oblique	**Ribs,** lower eight	**Ossa coxae** (iliac crest and pubis by way of inguinal ligament) **Linea alba** by way of an aponeurosis	Compresses abdomen Important postural function of all abdominal muscles is to pull front of pelvis upward, thereby flattening lumbar curve of spine; when these muscles lose their tone, common postural faults of protruding abdomen and lordosis develop	Lower seven intercostal nerves and iliohypogastric nerves
■ Internal oblique	**Ossa coxae** (iliac crest and inguinal ligament) **Lumbodorsal fascia**	**Ribs,** lower three **Pubic bone** **Linea ulba**	Same as external oblique	Last three intercostal nerves; iliohypogastric and ilioinguinal nerves
■ Transversus abdominus	**Ribs,** lower six **Ossa coxae** (iliac crest, inguinal ligament) **Lumbodorsal fascia**	**Pubic bone** **Linea alba**	Same as external oblique	Last five intercostal nerves; iliohypogastric and ilioinguinal
■ Rectus abdominis	**Ossa coxae** (pubic bone and symphysis pubis)	**Ribs** (costal cartilage of fifth, sixth, and seventh ribs) **Sternum** (xiphoid process)	Same as external oblique; because abdominal muscles compress abdominal cavity, they aid in straining, defecation, forced expiration, childbirth, etc.; abdominal muscles are antagonists of diaphragm, relaxing as it contracts and vice versa Flexes trunk	Last six intercostal nerves

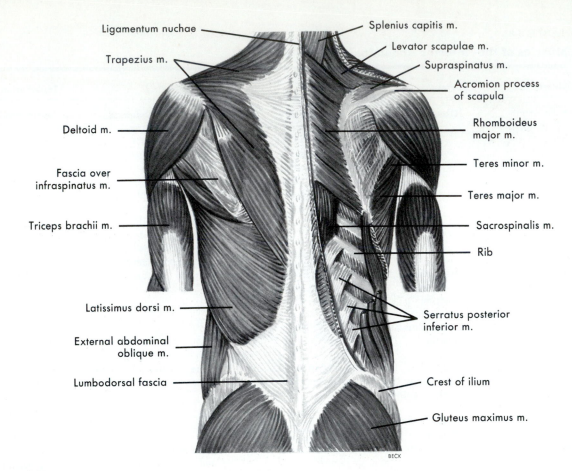

FIGURE 5-9
Superficial muscles of the posterior surface of the trunk.

TABLE 5-4

Muscles That Move the Head

Muscle	Origin	Insertion	Function	Innervation
■ Sternocleidomastoid	**Sternum Clavicle**	**Temporal bone** (mastoid process)	Flexes neck (prayer muscle) One muscle alone, rotates head toward opposite side	Accessory nerve
Semispinalis capitis	Vertebrae (transverse processes of upper six thoracic, articular processes of lower four cervical)	Occipital bone (between superior and inferior nuchal lines)	Extends neck One muscle alone, rotates head toward same side	First five cervical nerves
Splenius capitis	Ligamentum nuchae Vertebrae (spinous processses of upper three or four thoracic)	Temporal bone (mastoid process) Occipital bone	Extends neck One muscle alone, rotates head toward same side	Second, third, and fourth cervical nerves

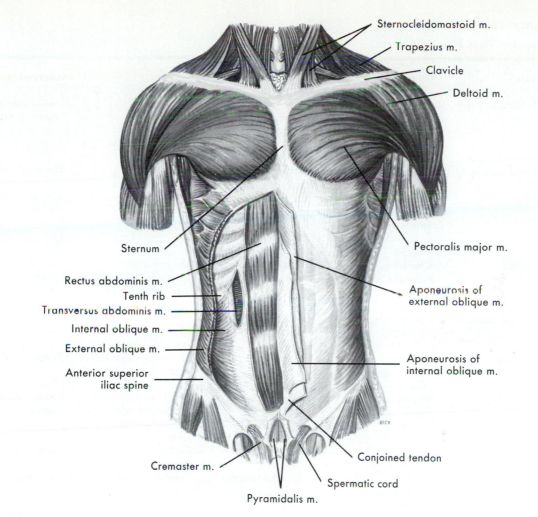

FIGURE 5-10
Superficial muscles of the anterior surface of the trunk.

TABLE 5-5

Muscles That Move the Chest Wall

Muscle	Origin	Insertion	Function	Innervation
External intercostals	Rib (lower border; forward fibers)	Rib (upper border of rib below origin)	Elevate ribs	Intercostal nerves
Internal intercostals	Rib (inner surface, lower border; backward fibers)	Rib (upper border of rib below origin)	Probably depress ribs	Intercostal nerves
■ Diaphragm	**Lower circumference of thorax** (of rib cage)	**Central tendon of diaphragm**	Enlarges thorax, causing inspiration	Phrenic nerve

TABLE 5-6

Muscles That Move the Arm

Muscle	Origin	Insertion	Function	Innervation
■ Pectoralis major	**Clavicle** (medial half) **Sternum** **Costal cartilages of true ribs**	**Humerus** (greater tubercle)	Flexes arm Adducts arm Rotates inward Horizontal flexion	Medial and lateral pectoral nerves
■ Latissimus dorsi	**Vertebrae** (spines of lower thoracic, lumbar, and sacral) **Ilium** (crest) **Lumbodorsal fascia**	**Humerus** (medial lip of intertubercular groove)	Extends arm Adducts arm Rotates inward	Thoracodorsal nerve
■ Deltoid	**Clavicle** **Scapula** (spine and acromion)	**Humerus** (lateral side about halfway down—deltoid tubercle)	Abducts arm Assists in flexion and extension of arm	Axillary nerve
Coracobrachialis	Scapula (coracoid process)	Humerus (middle third, medial surface)	Adduction; assists in flexion and inward rotation of arm	Musculocutaneous nerve
■ Supraspinatus	**Scapula** (supraspinous fossa)	**Humerus** (greater tubercle)	Assists in abducting arm	Suprascapular nerve
Teres major	Scapula (lower part, axillary border)	Humerus (upper part, anterior surface)	Assists in extension, adduction, and inward rotation of arm	Lower subscapular nerve
Teres minor	Scapula (axillary border)	Humerus (greater tubercle)	Rotates arm outward	Axillary nerve
Infraspinatus	Scapula (infraspinatus border)	Humerus (greater tubercle)	Rotates arm outward	Suprascapular nerve
Subscapularis	Scapula (subscapular fossa)	Humerus (lesser tubercle)	Rotates arm inward	Upper and lower subscapular nerves

cles that are located on, or move, one part of the body. Muscles that, in our judgment, are the most important for students of athletic injury assessment to know are preceded by a block, and the origins and insertions so judged are set in boldface type. The major actions are listed for each muscle, as well as the *innervations*. Remember that a single muscle contracting alone rarely accomplishes a given action. Instead, muscles act in groups as prime movers, fixators, synergists, and antagonists.

Start by familiarizing yourself with the names, shapes, functions, and general loca-

tions of the larger muscles. Refer often to illustrations and to a skeleton, if available, as you study individual muscles. Also, when possible, palpate each muscle on your own body. To understand muscle actions, you need first to know certain anatomic facts, such as (1) which bones muscles attach to and (2) which joints they pull across. If you relate these structural facts to functional assessment principles (for instance, those associated with lever systems), you will find the study of muscles more interesting and less difficult.

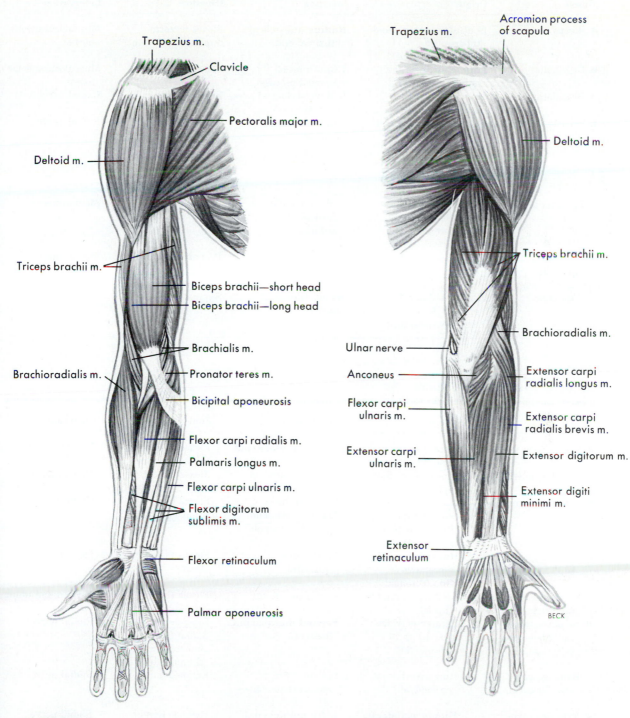

Trapezius m.

Clavicle

Pectoralis major m.

Deltoid m.

Triceps brachii m.

Biceps brachii—short head

Biceps brachii—long head

Brachialis m.

Pronator teres m.

Brachioradialis m.

Bicipital aponeurosis

Flexor carpi radialis m.

Palmaris longus m.

Flexor carpi ulnaris m.

Flexor digitorum
sublimis m.

Flexor retinaculum

Palmar aponeurosis

Trapezius m.

Acromion process
of scapula

Deltoid m.

Triceps brachii m.

Brachioradialis m.

Ulnar nerve

Anconeus

Extensor carpi
radialis longus m.

Flexor carpi
ulnaris m.

Extensor carpi
radialis brevis m.

Extensor carpi
ulnaris m.

Extensor digitorum m.

Extensor digiti
minimi m.

Extensor
retinaculum

BECK

FIGURE 5-11
Muscles of the flexor surface of the upper extremity.

FIGURE 5-12
Muscles of the extensor surface of the upper
extremity.

TABLE 5-7

Muscles That Move the Forearm

Muscle	Origin	Insertion	Function	Innervation
▪ Biceps brachii	**Scapula** (supraglenoid tuberosity) **Scapula** (coracoid)	**Radius** (tubercle at proximal end)	Flexes forearm Supinates forearm	Musculocutaneous nerve
▪ Brachialis	**Humerus** (distal half, anterior surface)	**Ulna** (front of coronoid process)	Flexes forearm	Musculocutaneous nerve
Brachioradialis	Humerus (above lateral epicondyle)	Radius (styloid process)	Flexes forearm	Radial nerve
▪ Triceps brachii	**Scapula** (infraglenoid tuberosity) **Humerus** (posterior surface—lateral head above radial groove; medial head, below)	**Ulna** (olecranon process)	Extends forearm	Radial nerve
Pronator teres	Humerus (medial epicondyle) Ulna (coronoid process)	Radius (middle third of lateral surface)	Pronates and flexes forearm	Median nerve
Pronator quadratus	Ulna (distal fourth, anterior surface)	Radius (distal fourth, anterior surface)	Pronates forearm	Median nerve
Supinator	Humerus (lateral epicondyle) Ulna (proximal fifth)	Radius (proximal third)	Supinates forearm	Radial nerve

TABLE 5-8

Muscles That Move the Hand

Muscle	Origin	Insertion	Function	Innervation
▪ Flexor carpi radialis	**Humerus** (medial epicondyle)	**Second metacarpal** (base of)	Flexes hand Flexes forearm	Median nerve
Palmaris longus	Humerus (medial epicondyle)	Fascia of palm	Flexes hand	Median nerve
▪ Flexor carpi ulnaris	**Humerus** (medial epicondyle) **Ulna** (proximal two thirds)	**Pisiform bone** Third, fourth, and fifth metacarpals	Flexes hand Ulnar flexion	Ulnar nerve
▪ Flexor digitorum superficialis	**Humerus** (medial) epicondyle **Ulna** (coronoid)	**Phalanges (middle)**	Flexes PIP of each finger	Median nerve
Flexor digitorum profundus	Ulna (proximal two thirds)	Phalanges (distal)	Flexes DIP of each finger	Median and ulnar nerves
▪ Extensor carpi radialis longus	**Humerus** (ridge above lateral epicondyle)	**Second metacarpal** (base of)	Extends hand Radial flexion (moves toward thumb side)	Radial nerve
Extensor carpi radialis brevis	Humerus (lateral epicondyle)	Second, third, metacarpals (bases of)	Extends hand	Radial nerve
▪ Extensor carpi ulnaris	**Humerus** (lateral epicondyle) Ulna (proximal three fourths)	**Fifth metacarpal** (base of)	Extends hand Ulnar flexion (moves toward little finger side)	Radial nerve
▪ Extensor digitorum	**Humerus** (lateral epicondyle)	**Phalanges** (middle and distal)	Extends fingers	Radial nerve

TABLE 5-9

Muscles That Move the Lower Leg

Muscle	Origin	Insertion	Function	Innervation
■ Quadriceps femoris group				
Rectus femoris	**Ilium** (anterior, inferior spine)	**Tibia** (by way of patellar tendon)	Flexes thigh Extends leg	Femoral nerve
Vastus lateralis	**Femur** (linea aspera)	**Tibia** (by way of patellar tendon)	Extends leg	Femoral nerve
Vastus medialis	**Femur** (linea aspera)	**Tibia** (by way of patellar tendon)	Extends leg	Femoral nerve
Vastus intermedius	**Femur** (anterior surface)	**Tibia** (by way of patellar tendon)	Extends leg	Femoral nerve
■ Sartorius	**Os innominatum** (anterior, superior iliac spine)	**Tibia** (medial surface of upper end of shaft)	Flexes thigh Flexes leg Rotates thigh outward	Femoral nerve
■ Hamstring group				
Biceps femoris	**Ischium** (tuberosity) **Femur** (linea aspera)	**Fibula** (head of) **Tibia** (lateral condyle)	Flexes leg Extends thigh	Tibial nerve from sciatic nerve
Semitendinosus	**Ischium** (tuberosity)	**Tibia** (proximal end, medial surface)	Extends thigh Flexes leg	Tibial nerve from sciatic nerve
Semimembranosus	**Ischium** (tuberosity)	**Tibia** (medial condyle)	Extends thigh Flexes leg	Tibial nerve from sciatic nerve

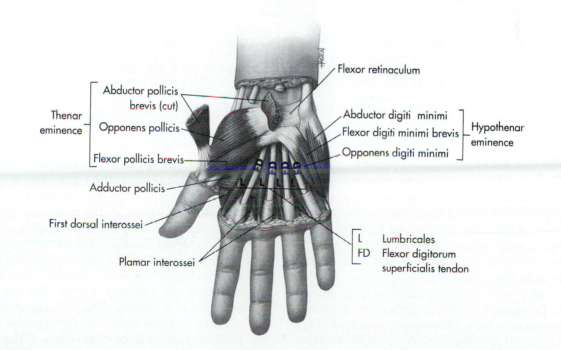

FIGURE 5-13

Palmer surface of the right hand. Abductor pollicis brevis has been cut. *L,* Lumbricales; *FD,* flexor digitorum superficialis tendons.

TABLE 5-10

Muscles That Move the Thigh

Muscle	Origin	Insertion	Function	Innervation
■ Iliopsoas (iliacus and psoas major)	**Ilium** (iliac fossa) **Vertebrae** (bodies of twelfth thoracic to fifth lumbar)	**Femur** (lesser trochanter)	Flexes thigh Flexes trunk (when femur acts as origin)	Femoral and second to fourth lumbar nerves
■ Rectus femoris	**Ilium** (anterior, inferior spine)	**Tibia** (by way of patellar tendon)	Flexes thigh Extends lower leg	Femoral nerve
■ Gluteal group Maximus	**Ilium** (crest and posterior surface) Sacrum and coccyx (posterior surface) Sacrotuberous ligament	**Femur** (gluteal tuberosity) **Iliotibial tract**	Extends and adducts thigh	Inferior gluteal nerve
Medius	**Ilium** (lateral surface)	**Femur** (greater trochanter)	Abducts thigh; rotates inward	Superior gluteal nerve
Minimus	**Ilium** (lateral surface)	**Femur** (greater trochanter)	Abducts thigh; stabilizes pelvis on femur Rotates inward	Superior gluteal nerve
■ Tensor fasciae latea	**Ilium** (anterior part of crest)	**Tibia** (by way of iliotibial tract)	Abducts thigh Tightens iliotibial tract	Superior gluteal nerve
Piriformis	Sacrum (anterior)	Femur (medial aspect of greater trochanter)	Rotates outward Abducts thigh	First or second sacral nerves
■ Adductor group Brevis	**Pubic bone**	**Femur** (linea aspera)	Adducts thigh	Obturator nerve
Longus	**Pubic bone**	**Femur** (linea aspera)	Adducts thigh	Obturator nerve
Magnus	**Pubic bone**	**Femur** (linea aspera)	Adducts thigh	Obturator enrve
Gracilis	**Pubic bone** (just below symphysis)	**Tibia** (medial surface behind sartorius)	Adducts thigh and flexes leg	Obturator nerve

Muscle Strength

Under optimal conditions, the strength of any muscle is dependent mainly on its size. Although different formulae can be used to calculate muscle strength as a unit of muscle mass, most values fall between 2.5 to 3.5 kg per cm² of an individual muscle or functional muscle group cross-sectional area.

In a well trained athlete a large muscle or functional muscle group such as the quadriceps may have a cross-sectional area of 125 cm² or larger. The quadriceps is the primary extensor of the knee and inserts on the patella and, by a common tendon, onto the tibial tuberosity. In this example, the 125 cm² cross-sectional area of the quadriceps would generate a contractile force of nearly 438 kg (964 lbs). However, if this muscle is already fully contracted during competition and some external force or trauma is applied to stretch it back out, a pull even greater than its shortening force is required. This characteristic is referred to as the *holding strength* of a muscle. The holding strength of most muscles is 30% to 40% greater than the contractile force. Therefore if the contracted quadriceps is stretched out, the resulting force applied could reach 613 kg

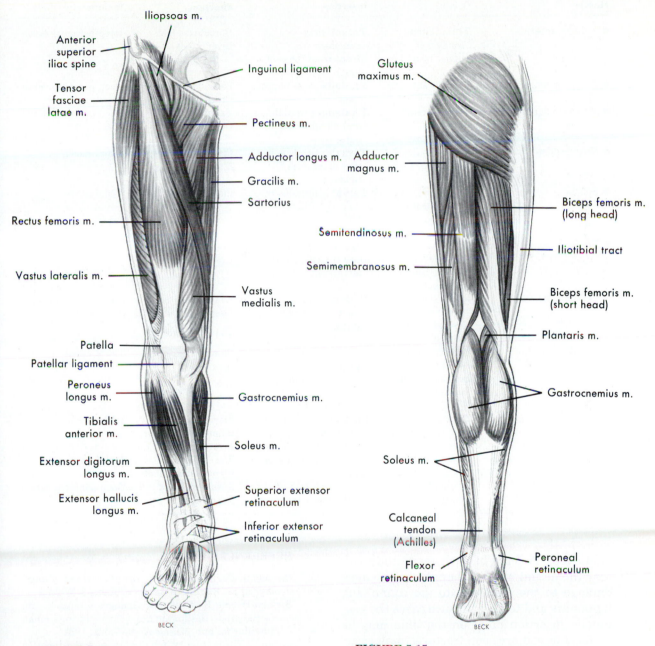

Iliopsoas m.

Anterior superior iliac spine

Tensor fasciae latae m.

Inguinal ligament

Pectineus m.

Adductor longus m.

Gracilis m.

Sartorius

Gluteus maximus m.

Adductor magnus m.

Rectus femoris m.

Biceps femoris m. (long head)

Semitendinosus m.

Iliotibial tract

Semimembranosus m.

Vastus lateralis m.

Vastus medialis m.

Biceps femoris m. (short head)

Plantaris m.

Patella

Patellar ligament

Peroneus longus m.

Gastrocnemius m.

Gastrocnemius m.

Tibialis anterior m.

Soleus m.

Extensor digitorum longus m.

Soleus m.

Extensor hallucis longus m.

Superior extensor retinaculum

Inferior extensor retinaculum

Calcaneal tendon (Achilles)

Flexor retinaculum

Peroneal retinaculum

BECK

BECK

FIGURE 5-14
Superficial muscles of the right thigh and leg—anterior view.

FIGURE 5-15
Superficial muscles of the right thigh and leg—posterior view.

TABLE 5-11

Muscles That Move the Foot

Muscle	Origin	Insertion	Function	Innervation
■ Tibialis anterior	**Tibia** (lateral condyle of upper body)	**Tarsal** (first cuneiform) **Metatarsal** (base of first)	Dorsiflexes foot Inverts foot	Deep peroneal nerve
■ Extensor hallucis longus	**Fibula** (anterior)	**Phalanx** (base of great toe)	Extends big toe Dorsiflexes foot	Deep peroneal nerve
■ Extensor digitorum longus	**Tibia** (lateral condyle) **Fibula** (anterior)	**Phalanges** (middle and distal of four outer toes)	Extends toes Dorsiflexes foot Everts foot	Deep peroneal nerve
■ Gastrocnemius	**Femur** (condyles)	**Tarsal** (calcaneus by way of Achilles tendon)	Plantar flexes foot Flexes lower leg	Tibial nerve
■ Soleus	**Tibia** (underneath gastrocnemius) **Fibula**	**Tarsal** (calcaneus by way of Achilles tendon)	Plantar flexes foot	Tibial nerve
■ Peroneus longus	**Tibia** (lateral condyle) **Fibula** (head and shaft)	**First cuneiform** Base of first metatarsal	Plantar flexes foot Everts foot	Superficial peroneal nerve
Peroneus brevis	Fibula (lower two thirds of lateral surface of shaft)	Fifth metatarsal (tubercle, dorsal surface)	Everts foot Plantar flexes foot	Superficial peroneal nerve
Tibialis posterior	Tibia (posterior surface) Fibula (posterior surface)	Navicular bone Cuboid bone All three cuneiforms Second and fourth metatarsals	Plantar flexes foot Inverts foot	Tibial nerve
Flexor digitorum longus	Tibia	Phalanges (distal four outer toes)	Flexes toes Plantar flexes foot Inverts foot	Tibial nerve
Flexor hallucis longus	Fibula (posterior)	Phalanx (base of great toe)	Flexes big toe Plantar flexes foot	Tibial nerve
Peroneus tertius	Fibula (distal third)	Fourth and fifth metatarsals (bases of)	Dorsiflexes foot Everts foot	Deep peroneal nerve

(1349 lbs). A force of such magnitude can tear the actual muscle fibers and also cause damage to the joint and to the connecting ligaments and tendon. In such cases the tendinous insertion point on the tibia may be avulsed or compression fractures may occur near the joint surface. In many cases, contractile forces applied to anatomic structures by shortening muscles, or by forces that attempt to stretch out already contracted muscles, are directly responsible for athletic injuries.

REFERENCES

Basmajian JV, Slonecker CE: *Grant's method of anatomy,* ed 11, Baltimore, 1989, Williams & Wilkins.

Bigland-Ritchie B, Woods JJ: Changes in muscle contractile properties and neural control during human muscular fatigue, *Muscle Nerve* 7:691, 1984.

Cohen C: The protein switch of muscle contraction, *Sci Am* 233(5):36, 1975.

Hardy L, Jones D: Dynamic flexibility and proprioceptive neuromuscular facilitation, *Res Q Exerc Sports* 57(2):150, 1986.

Hulton RS: Neuromuscular physiology. In Welsh RP, Shephard RJ, editors: *Curr Therap Sports Med,* Philadelphia, 1985, BC Decker.

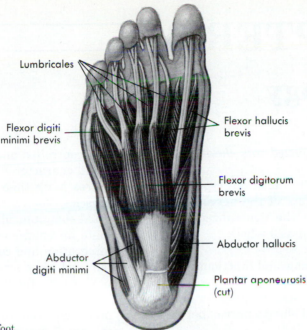

Lumbricales

Flexor digiti
minimi brevis

Flexor hallucis
brevis

Flexor digitorum
brevis

Abductor hallucis

Abductor
digiti minimi

Plantar aponeurosis
(cut)

FIGURE 5-16
Plantar surface of the right foot.

Huxley HE: The mechanism of muscular contraction, *Sci Am* 213(6):18, 1965. (Classic article)

Margaria R: The sources of muscular energy, *Sci Am* 226(3):84, 1972.

Murray JM, Weber A: The cooperative action of muscle proteins, *Sci Am* 230(2):59, 1974.

Noble BJ: *Physiology of exercise and sport,* ed 2, St. Louis, 1991, Mosby-Year Book.

Oster G: Muscle sounds, *Sci Am* 250(3):108, 1984.

Pavlou KN and others: Effects of dieting and exercise on lean body mass, oxygen uptake, and strength, *Med Sci Sports Exerc* 17(4):466, 1985.

Quiring DP: *The head, neck, and trunk,* Philadelphia, 1955, Lea & Febiger.

Quiring DP, and others: *The extremities,* Philadelphia, 1954, Lea & Febiger.

Snell RS: *Atlas of clinical anatomy,* Boston, 1978, Little, Brown.

Sobotta J, Figge FHJ: *Atlas of human anatomy,* ed 8, New York, 1963, Hafner Publishing.

Wilson FC: *The musculoskeletal system: basic processes and disorders,* ed 2, Philadelphia, 1983, Lippincott.

SUGGESTED READINGS

Jones NL, McCartney N, McComas AJ, editors: *Human muscle power,* Champaign, 1986, Illinois University Press.
Proceedings of the 1986 International Symposium on human muscle power. Excellent reviews of mechanics of muscle power, including theoretical implications for optimization of muscle contraction. Comprehensive coverage of morphology, energy metabolism, fatigue, and adaptation/maladaptation.

McMahon TA: *Muscles, reflexes and locomotion,* Princeton, 1984, Princeton University Press.
Well-written and comprehensive treatment of coordinated motion. Considerable emphasis on mathematical models.

McMinn RMH, Hutchings RT: *Color atlas of human anatomy,* ed 2. St. Louis, 1988, Mosby-Year Book.
An excellent supplemental text of color plates showing surface anatomy, bones, bony structures, various levels of cadaver dissections, and radiographs of all areas of the human body.

Netter FH: *Atlas of human anatomy,* Summit, NJ, 1989, CIBA-Geigy Corporation.
An excellent collection of color illustrations of the musculoskeletal system. A supplemental text for all athletic trainers.

Smith A: *The body,* New York, 1986, Viking Penguin.
Engagingly written and interesting presentation of factual material related to basic human anatomy and physiology.

Vidic B, Suarez F: *Photographic atlas of the human body,* St. Louis, 1984, Mosby-Year Book.
Outstanding photographic atlas of human anatomy. Surface anatomy, myology, and color plates of cadaver dissections are reinforced by exceptional line drawings.

Wickiewicz TL and others: Muscle architecture and force velocity relationships in humans, *J Appl Physiol* 57(2):435, 1984.
One of the first research reports to suggest that inhibition of muscle contraction by protective reflex mechanisms limits force production in human subjects. Hypothesis now advanced to explain inhibition at slow movement speeds with large forces.

CHAPTER 6

Neurology

After you have completed this chapter, you should be able to:

- List the organs, divisions, cell types, and specialized receptors of the nervous system and describe the generalized functions of the system as a whole.
- Discuss reflexes.
- Identify the anatomic and functional components of a three-neuron reflex arc.
- Compare and contrast the propagation of an action potential along a nerve fiber and across a synaptic cleft.
- Compare and contrast spinal and cranial nerves and discuss the formation of spinal nerves.
- Discuss the sensory system and the tests for primary, cortical, and discriminatory forms of sensation.
- Discuss the importance of understanding the relationship between myotomes, dermatomes, and specific reflex testing in the neurologic examination of an injured athlete.

The controlled and highly integrated movement characteristic of athletic activity requires more than intact bones, joints, and muscles. Such activity depends on sophisticated communication mechanisms that regulate an enormously complex function: the integration and control of diverse body systems, which must operate together to ensure proper body function.

The nervous system transmits, interprets, and coordinates the vast amount of information required for the fluid, powerful, and interdependent activity of athletic performance. It handles this information rapidly by means of nerve impulses conducted from one body area to another. These impulses are rapidly moving electrical signals generated by specialized nerve cells. It is the nerve impulse that communicates information to body structures—initiating, increasing, or decreasing their activities as needed for normal body movement and function. Although the nervous system serves a primary communication function, it also acts as a control and integrating system.

Most athletic-related injuries come to the attention of the athlete or athletic trainer through signs or symptoms associated with nervous system function or malfunction. In addition, direct injury to nervous system structures also occurs quite frequently as a result of athletic-related trauma. Such injuries have a profound impact on performance. Because athletic trainers are routinely involved in assessing injuries that involve some aspect of trauma to the nervous system, a review of the basics of neurology is important and necessary. Such information forms the basis for the neurologic examination component of the athletic injury assessment process. It is also important in implementing rational assessment sequences and in understanding many of the signs and symptoms of injury to the many structures of the nervous system. Additional neurologic information is incorporated in the discussion of individual assessment procedures in subsequent chapters of the text.

It is not the intent of this chapter to present in-depth information related directly to specific neurologic assessment techniques. Instead, in each chapter of the text there will be full discussion of the neurologic screening and assessment tests related to the types of athletic injury discussed in that chapter. Depending on the nature and extent of a particular injury you will learn to use numerous observation techniques and assessment tests to make an appropriate neurologic screen. The appearance of an athlete (grooming, body language, and emotional status); his or her cognitive abilities (conscious level, memory); emotional stability (mood); and speech and language status (coherence, comprehension of instructions, voice quality) will be a part of the evaluation. In addition, specific cranial or spinal nerve functions, proprioception and cerebellar functions (accuracy of movements, gait), and sensory function tests and evaluation of numerous reflexes will be discussed as appropriate for specific injuries. This chapter provides a review of the basic structure and function of the nervous system. The material was selected, organized, and presented in a way intended to help you build a rational basis for understanding information related to very specific neurologic tests as they are introduced later in the text.

The organizational plan for this chapter is to (1) name the organs and divisions of the nervous system, (2) relate basic information about the nervous system's special kinds of cells, (3) identify a typical reflex arc and the various types of reflexes, and then (4) discuss the mechanism of nerve impulse transmission and the various organs of the nervous system, including the cranial and spinal nerves. The importance of dermatomes and myotomes in assessment of athletic-related injury will also be discussed.

THE NERVOUS SYSTEM
Organs and Divisions

The organs of the nervous system include the brain and spinal cord, the numerous nerves of the body (Figure 6-1), the specialized sense organs such as the eyes and ears, and the microscopic sense organ receptors found in the skin. The system consists of two principal divisions: the central nervous system and the peripheral nervous system. Because the brain and spinal cord occupy a midline or central location in the body, together they are called the **central nervous system (CNS).** Similarly, the usual designation for the nerves of the body is the **peripheral nervous system (PNS).** The term *peripheral* is appropriate because nerves extend to outlying, or peripheral, parts of the body. A subdivision of the peripheral division of the nervous system is the **autonomic nervous system (ANS).**

The brain and spinal cord constitute the CNS, and the PNS includes all nervous structures that lie outside of the CNS: the (1) *nerves,* which connect receptors in outlying body parts to the brain or cord, and (2) *ganglia,* which are groups of nerve cell bodies found in close association to nerves. The most important groups of nerves in the PNS include 12 pairs of *cranial nerves,* which originate from the brain and exit from the cranial cavity through openings in the skull, and 31 pairs of *spinal nerves,* which originate in the spinal cord and pass through openings between the individual vertebrae of the spine. The spinal nerves include 8 cervical, 12 thoracic, 5 lumbar, 5 sacral, and 1 coccygeal nerve.

The PNS can be subdivided structurally into groups of nerves and ganglia and functionally into *sensory (afferent)* and *motor (efferent)* divisions. Sensory peripheral nerves carry impulses from receptors in the skin and from tissues surrounding the joints and other outlying body areas to the brain and spinal cord of the CNS. Motor peripheral nerves carry impulses to outlying body areas from the CNS and can be subdivided into *somatic* or *voluntary* nerves, which carry nervous impulses to skeletal muscles and

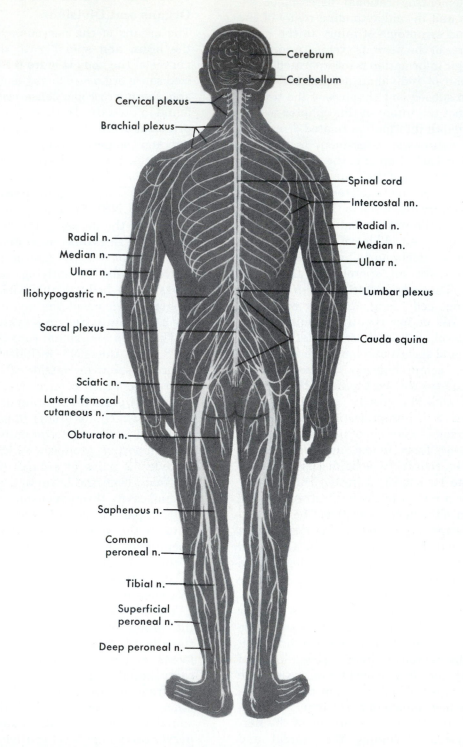

FIGURE 6-1
Central and peripheral divisions of the nervous systems. The central nervous system (CNS) consists of the brain and spinal cord. The peripheral nervous system (PNS) is composed of cranial and spinal nerves.

TABLE 6-1

Receptors Classified by Location

Type	Location	General senses
Superficial receptors (exteroceptors)	At or near surface of body; in skin and mucosa	Touch, pressure, heat, cold, and pain
Deep receptors (proprioceptors)	In muscles, tendons, and joints	Proprioception (sense of position and movement)
Internal receptors (visceroceptors)	In the viscera and in blood vessel walls	Usually no sensations result from stimulation of internal receptors; exceptions: hunger, nausea, and pain from certain stimuli (notably, distention and some chemicals)

are under conscious control, and the *visceral,* or *involuntary,* nerves, which transmit impulses to the heart, smooth muscles, and glands of the body. Components of the visceral, or involuntary, subdivision are referred to as the *autonomic nervous system* (ANS) and are classified as *sympathetic* or *parasympathetic* in nature. Sympathetic elements of the ANS are active during stress, and parasympathetic components dominate during periods of physical rest and emotional calm.

Receptors

Pain and other difficult to describe sensations called **paresthesias** are frequently associated with injury and may be the primary reason an athlete seeks assistance. A paresthesia is an abnormal or perverted sensation, which an athlete may describe as a burning, itching, "electric shock," or other type of unusual feeling located on the skin surface or deep within a muscle, joint, or body cavity. These sensations are caused by activation of nervous system structures called **receptors.** Receptors are specialized sensory components of the nervous system that generate nerve impulses. They are activated by *stimuli,* which may be internal or caused by external trauma or injury, temperature changes, or caustic chemicals. Receptor activity results in generation of nervous impulses that alert the brain to changes in the environment. When nervous impulses pass from a stimulated receptor to the brain, appropriate and often protective

responses can be initiated. Pain, for example, will often keep an athlete from aggravating an injury by discouraging movement of the affected body part.

Receptors are commonly classified according to location, structure, and types of stimuli activating them. Classified according to location, the three types of receptors are (1) superficial receptors, or *exteroceptors;* (2) deep receptors, or *proprioceptors;* and (3) internal receptors, or *visceroceptors.* For example, pain from a skin abrasion results from stimulation of superficial receptors on the body surface, whereas deep joint pain caused by a ligament rupture results from stimulation of proprioceptors located deep in the injured tissue. For the general senses resulting from stimulation of these receptors, see Table 6-1.

Classified according to structure, there are two general types of receptors, *free,* or naked, endings and *encapsulated nerve* endings. Free nerve endings are not enclosed by connective tissue, whereas encapsulated nerve endings are encased in some type of capsule (Figure 6-2). Most pain is mediated by free nerve endings, which are often referred to as **nociceptors.** Table 6-2 lists receptors classified by structure and gives examples of the general senses mediated by the differing types of receptors.

Cells

The two general types of cells in the nervous system are *neurons,* or nerve cells, and *neuroglia,* which are specialized connective tis-

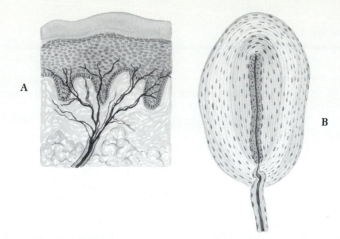

FIGURE 6-2

Receptors. **A**, Free nerve ending (pain receptor) and, **B**, encapsulated nerve ending—Pacinian corpuscle (pressure receptor).

TABLE 6-2

Receptors Classified by Structure

Type	Main location	General senses
Free nerve endings (naked nerve endings)	Skin, mucosa (epithelial layers)	Pain, crude touch, possibly temperature
Encapsulated nerve endings		
Meisnner's corpuscles	Skin (in papillae of dermis); numerous in fingertips and lips	Fine touch, vibration
Ruffini's corpuscles	Skin (dermal layer) and subcutaneous tissue of fingers	Touch, pressure
Pacinian corpuscles	Subcutaneous, submucous, and subserous tissues, around joints, in mammary glands and external genitals of both sexes	Pressure, vibration
Krause's end-bulbs	Skin (dermal layer), subcutaneous tissue, mucosa of lips and eyelids, external genitals	Touch
Golgi tendon receptors	Near junction of tendons and muscles	Subconscious muscle sense
Muscle spindles	Skeletal muscles	Subconscious muscle sense

sue cells. Neurons are the functioning units of the system responsible for generation and transmission of nerve impulses.

Neurons

Each neuron consists of three main parts: a *neuron cell body,* one or more branching projections called *dendrites,* and one elongated projection, an *axon* (Figure 6-3). Dendrites are the processes or projections that transmit impulses to the neuron cell bodies, and axons are the processes that transmit impulses away from the neuron cell bodies.

There are three types of neurons classified according to the direction in which they transmit impulses: *sensory neurons, motor neurons, and interneurons.* Sensory neurons transmit impulses to the spinal cord and brain from all parts of the body. Motor neurons transmit impulses in the opposite direction—away from the brain and cord. Motor neurons do not conduct impulses to

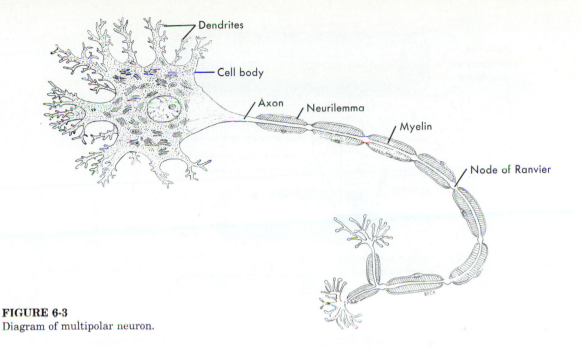

FIGURE 6-3
Diagram of multipolar neuron.

all parts of the body but only to two kinds of tissue—muscle and glandular. Interneurons conduct impulses from sensory neurons (afferent neurons) to motor neurons (efferent neurons). Interneurons are central, or connecting, neurons.

The axon in Figure 6-3 is surrounded by a segmented wrapping of a material called *myelin*. Myelin is a white, fatty substance that covers the axons of some nerve cells outside the CNS. Such fibers are *myelinated fibers,* and they make up the *white matter* of the nervous system. Note in Figure 6-3 that the membrane covering the myelin is the *neurilemma* and that indentations called *nodes of Ranvier* separate the myelin into distinct beadlike elevations along the axon. In a type of rapid nerve conduction along a myelinated axon, the impulse jumps from node to node by means of an impulse transmission called *saltatory conduction*. The transmission is rapid because the myelin acts as a good "insulator," covering the axon between nodes.

Axons in the brain and spinal cord have no neurilemma, which plays an essential part in the regeneration of cut and injured axons. Therefore axons in the brain and spi-

nal cord do not regenerate, but those in peripheral nerves do.

Nerve impulses

A nerve impulse may be defined as a self-propagating wave of electrical negativity that travels along the surface of a neuron's cytoplasmic membrane. Nerve impulses do not continually race along every nerve cell's surface. First they have to be initiated by a stimulus, a change in the neuron's environment. Pressure, temperature, physical trauma, and even chemical changes may serve as stimuli. When an adequate stimulus acts on a neuron, it greatly increases the permeability of the stimulated point of its membrane to sodium ions (Figure 6-4). In a resting or nonconducting neuron the membrane is characterized as "polarized" and exhibits a "resting potential" in which the inner surface of the neuron's membrane is slightly less positive—that is, slightly negative—to its outer surface. Following stimulation, positively charged sodium ions rush through the membrane into the interior of the neuron. The inward movement of positive ions leaves a slight excess of negative ions outside. A point of electrical negativity

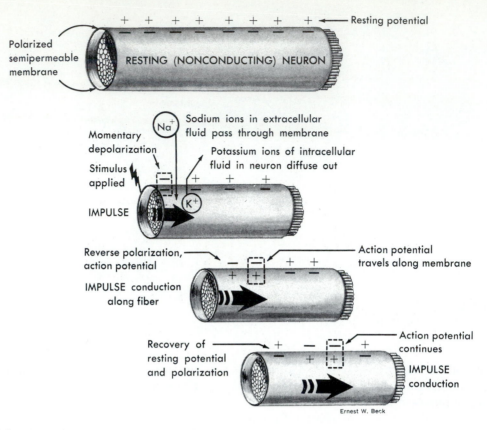

FIGURE 6-4
Upper diagram represents polarized state of the membrane of a nerve fiber when it is not conducting impulses. Other diagrams represent nerve impulse conduction followed by repolarization.

is created on the neuron's surface. A nerve impulse (a self-propagating wave of electrical negativity that speeds point by point along the entire length of the neuron's surface) begins. After passage of the impulse the membrane will return to its resting state. The process is "repolarization." To be effective a nerve impulse must not only progress along the surface of an individual neuron, it must pass from neuron to neuron and, in many cases, from neuron to effector cell. In doing so it must travel through a series of microscopic but "open" spaces between adjacent cells. This space is called a *synapse* and is discussed with the reflex arc.

Reflex arcs

Every moment of one's life, nerve impulses speed over neurons to and from the spinal cord and brain. If all impulse conduction ceases, life itself ceases. Only neurons can provide the rapid communication between the body's billions of cells that is necessary for maintaining life.

Nerve impulses can travel over literally trillions of routes made up of neurons because neurons are the cells that conduct impulses. Hence the routes traveled by nerve impulses are sometimes spoken of as neuron pathways. Their scientific name, is **reflex arcs.** The simplest kind of reflex arc is a *two-neuron arc,* because it consists of only two types of neurons: sensory neurons and motor neurons. *Three-neuron arcs* are the next simplest kind. They, of course, consist of all three kinds of neurons: sensory neurons, interneurons, and motor neurons. Reflex arcs are like one-way streets: they allow impulse

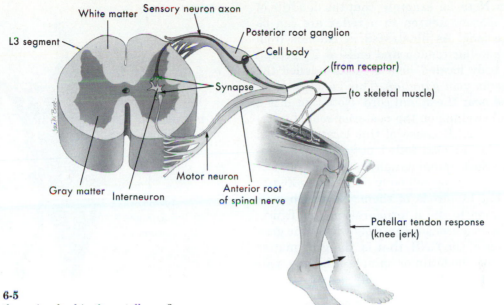

White matter   Sensory neuron axon
L3 segment   Posterior root ganglion
Cell body
(from receptor)
Synapse   (to skeletal muscle)
Gray matter   Motor neuron
Interneuron   Anterior root
of spinal nerve
Patellar tendon response
(knee jerk)

FIGURE 6-5
Neural pathway involved in the patellar reflex.

conduction in only one direction. Look frequently at Figure 6-5 as you read the next paragraph, which describes this direction in detail.

Impulse conduction normally starts in *receptors*. Receptors are the beginnings of dendrites of sensory neurons. In Figure 6-5 the sensory receptors are located in the patellar tendon of the knee joint. Receptors are often located at some distance from the spinal cord—for example, in other tendons, in skin, and in mucous membranes. In Figure 6-5, receptors in the patellar tendon are stimulated by a blow from a neurologic hammer. From receptors, impulses travel the full length of the sensory neuron's dendrite, through its cell body and axon, to the branching brushlike ends of the axon. The ends of the sensory neuron's axon contact interneurons. Actually, a microscopic space separates the axon endings of one neuron from the dendrites of another neuron. This space is called a **synapse.** After crossing the synapse the impulses continue along the dendrites, cell bodies, and axons of the interneurons. Then they cross another synapse. Finally, they travel over the dendrites, cell bodies, and axons of motor neurons to a

structure called an *effector* (because it "puts into effect" the message brought to it by nerve impulses). Effectors are either muscles or glands. When impulses reach skeletal muscle cells, they cause the cells to contract. This brings us to another definition. The response to impulse conduction over reflex arcs—in this instance muscle contraction—is called a **reflex.** In short, impulse conduction by a reflex arc causes a reflex to occur. Muscle contractions and gland secretion are the only two kinds of reflexes.

The term *reflex center* means the center of a reflex arc. The first part of a reflex arc consists of sensory neurons, and the last part consists of motor neurons. In spinal cord arcs the sensory neurons conduct impulses to the cord and the motor neurons conduct them away from the cord and out to muscles. The reflex centers of all spinal cord arcs, then, lie in spinal cord gray matter. In three-neuron arcs the reflex centers consist of interneurons. In two-neuron arcs they are simply the synapses between sensory and motor neurons. We might define a reflex center as the place in a reflex arc where incoming impulses become outgoing impulses.

Figure 6-5 reveals a number of important

facts. Note, for example, that the dendrite of the sensory neuron in a reflex arc can be quite long. As illustrated, it extends from the patellar tendon and ends at its neuron cell body located in a structure called the *posterior root ganglion*. This ganglion is located near the spinal cord. Note that it is a small swelling on the posterior root of a spinal nerve. (Because of this location, spinal ganglia are also called posterior root ganglia.) Each spinal ganglion contains not one sensory neuron cell body as shown in Figure 6-5 but hundreds of them. Now turn your attention to the interneuron in this figure. All interneurons lie entirely within the gray matter of the CNS, that is, the gray matter of either the brain or spinal cord. Gray matter forms the H-shaped inner core of the spinal cord.

Identify the motor neuron in Figure 6-5. Observe that its dendrites and cell body are located in the cord's gray matter. The axon of this motor neuron runs through the anterior root of the spinal nerve and terminates in the quadriceps muscle group of the thigh. Contraction of this muscle group following stimulation of receptors in the patellar tendon produces the familiar "knee jerk."

Look again at Figure 6-5 and note the two labels for synapse. The first synapse lies between the sensory neuron's axon terminals and the interneuron's dendrites. The second synapse lies between the interneuron's axon terminals and the motor neuron's dendrites. Conduction across synapses is an important part of the nerve conduction process. By definition, a synapse is the place where impulses are transmitted from one neuron, called the *presynaptic neuron,* to another neuron, called the *postsynaptic neuron.* Three structures make up a synapse: a synaptic knob, a synaptic cleft, and the plasma membrane of a postsynaptic neuron. A *synaptic knob* is a tiny bulge at the end of a terminal branch of a presynaptic neuron's axon (Figures 6-6 and 6-7). Each synaptic knob contains numerous small sacs or vesicles. Each vesicle contains a very small quantity of a chemical compound called a *neurotransmitter.* A *synaptic cleft* is the

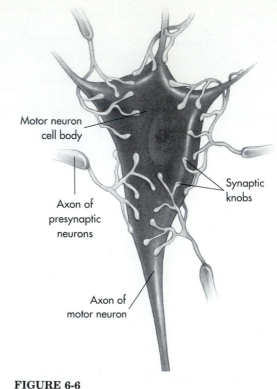

FIGURE 6-6
Synaptic knobs on motor neuron cell body.

space between a synaptic knob and the plasma membrane of a postsynaptic neuron; it is an incredibly narrow space—only about one millionth of an inch in width. Identify the synaptic cleft in Figure 6-7. The plasma membrane of a *postsynaptic neuron* has protein molecules embedded in it opposite each synaptic knob. These serve as receptors to which neurotransmitter molecules bind.

Once an impulse is generated and conduction by postsynaptic neurons is initiated, neurotransmitter activity is rapidly terminated. Either one or both of two mechanisms bring this about: (1) some neurotransmitter molecules diffuse out of the synaptic cleft back into synaptic knobs, and (2) other neurotransmitter molecules are metabolized into inactive compounds by specific enzymes.

Neurotransmitters are chemicals by which neurons talk to one another. As previously noted, at trillions of synapses in the CNS, presynaptic neurons release neuro-

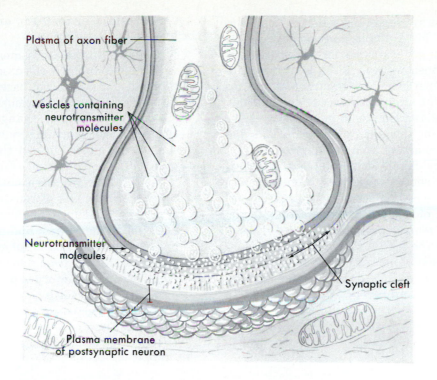

Plasma of axon fiber

Vesicles containing
neurotransmitter
molecules

Neurotransmitter
molecules

Synaptic cleft

Plasma membrane
of postsynaptic neuron

FIGURE 6-7

Diagram of a synapse showing its components: a synaptic knob (axon terminal) of a presynaptic neuron, the plasma membrane of a postsynaptic neuron, and a synaptic cleft (space about one millionth of an inch wide) between the two neurons. On the arrival of an action potential at a synaptic knob, neurotransmitter molecules are released from vesicles in the knob into the synaptic cleft. The combining of neurotransmitter molecules with receptor molecules in the plasma membrane of the postsynaptic neuron initiates impulse conduction by it.

transmitters that act to assist, stimulate, or inhibit postsynaptic neurons. At least 30 different compounds are established as neurotransmitters. They are not distributed diffusely or at random through the spinal cord and brain. Instead, specific neurotransmitters are localized in discrete groups of neurons and released in specific pathways.

For example, *acetylcholine* is released at some of the synapses in the spinal cord and at myoneural (muscle-nerve) junctions. Other well-known neurotransmitters include *norepinephrine, dopamine,* and *serotonin.* They belong to a group of compounds called *catecholamines,* which may play a role in sleep, motor function, mood, and pleasure recognition.

Two morphine-like neurotransmitters called *endorphins* and *enkephalins* are released at various spinal cord and brain syn-

apses in the pain conduction pathway. These neurotransmitters inhibit conduction of pain impulses. They serve the body as its own natural pain killers.

NEUROLOGIC ASSESSMENT

An understanding of nervous system structure and function permits the athletic trainer to incorporate elements of a basic neurologic examination into the assessment process. Direct injury may vary from minimal damage of free pain receptors in a skin abrasion to transection of an important nerve or serious brain or spinal cord injury. Because the nervous system is anatomically pervasive and functionally important, the athletic trainer must always be conscious of its potential for injury and must be skilled in recognizing the signs and symptoms of nervous system involvement.

Nervous system injury following a blow to the head, for example, may involve subtle changes in general behavior (eccentricities), level of consciousness (alert or drowsy), intellectual performance (retention of a series of numbers), orientation (recite date and day of the week), emotional status (excessive hostility), or thought content (illusions, delusions, or hallucinations). Other types of injuries may result in actual loss of reflex, motor, or sensory function to one or more areas of the body. Specific neurologic assessment techniques are incorporated into the total assessment processes covered in each chapter of the text. A review of the structure and function of nervous system components required to complete specific assessment procedures is presented in each chapter as required.

Cerebrum, Cerebellum, and Cranial Nerve Assessment

In Chapter 13 the assessment of an athlete with a head injury is discussed in detail. Establishing a neurologic baseline and monitoring the level of consciousness is emphasized. For example, changes in level of consciousness, general behavior, or intellectual performance suggest the possibility of injury to the cerebrum (Figure 6-8). This area of the brain is responsible for the integrative functions of consciousness, memory, use of language, and emotions. The **cerebrum** is the largest and most superficial area of the brain and is subject to traumatic injury resulting from blows to the head. Signs of cerebral injury to an athlete include difficulty in answering questions relevantly, carrying out instructions, identifying familiar sounds or objects, such as a wrist watch, or repeating one or two series learned in the

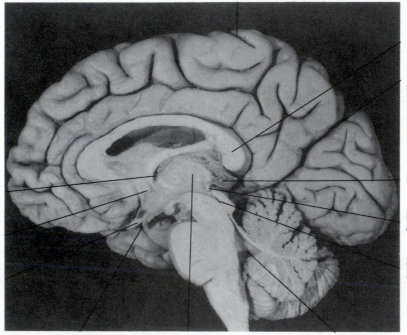

FIGURE 6-8
Right half of brain viewed from its medial aspect.

past such as days of the week or months of the year.

The thin covering of the cerebrum is the *cerebral cortex*. The highest levels of integration and abstract reasoning can occur only if the cortex is functioning properly. Injury to this critically important and superficial area of the brain can produce catastrophic but initially subtle and sometimes easily overlooked symptoms. Inability to understand or respond to abstractions suggests cortical trauma. This type of abstract reasoning is sometimes evaluated by asking the athlete to explain the meaning of a familiar proverb or slogan, for example "no pain—no gain."

The **cerebellum** is the second largest part of the brain (Figure 6-8), occupies the most inferior and posterior aspect of the cranial cavity, and is subject to injury following head trauma. In Chapter 12 the generalized functions of the cerebellum, which control balance and coordination of body movement, are explained. Assessment tests used to evaluate cerebellar function involve the ability of the athlete to produce skilled movements by coordinating the activities of groups of muscles. For example, the injured athlete might be asked to run each heel down the shin, to point to the examiner's hand with each big toe, or to make a "figure eight" in the air with each foot. Cerebellar injuries make it difficult to accomplish rapidly alternating coordinated movements such as patting the knees with the palms of the hands and backs of the hands, pronating and supinating the hands, or touching the fingers to the thumb in rapid succession.

In addition to cerebral or cerebellar injuries a blow to the head during athletic competition can also damage one or more of the 12 pairs of **cranial nerves,** which arise from the undersurface of the brain (Figure 6-9).

After leaving the cranial cavity through the small foramina in the skull, the cranial nerves extend to their respective destinations. Names and numbers identify the cranial nerves. Their names suggest their distribution or function. Their numbers indicate the order in which they emerge from front to back. Like all nerves, cranial nerves consist of bundles of axons. *Mixed cranial nerves* contain axons of sensory and motor neurons. *Sensory cranial nerves* consist of sensory axons only, and *motor cranial nerves* consist mainly of motor axons. Examine Table 6-3 to check the following summary:

Name	Number
Mixed cranial nerves	Fifth, seventh, ninth, and tenth
Sensory cranial nerves	First, second, eighth
Motor cranial nerves	Third, fourth, sixth, eleventh, and twelfth

Learn the names of the cranial nerves, using the memory aid given in the footnote to Table 6-3. Additional information, including assessment tests for each of the cranial nerves, can be found in Chapter 13.

By completing a basic neurologic assessment of cerebral, cerebellar, and cranial nerve function the athletic trainer can obtain information of nervous system functioning at the horizontal level above the spinal cord. Examination of the motor system, sensory system, and reflex activity of the body will add a vertical dimension to the assessment process. An understanding of myotomes, dermatomes, and reflex activity provides this additional information.

Spinal Nerves

Each of the 31 pairs of spinal nerves originates from the spinal cord within the spinal canal and is attached to the cord by two roots, a dorsal (posterior) or sensory root, and a ventral (anterior) or motor root (Figure 6-10). The two roots unite to form the spinal nerve, which then emerges through the small intervertebral foramen between the vertebrae. Table 6-4 lists the spinal nerves, the three major plexuses formed by elements of the spinal nerves, the specific spinal nerve branches, and the body areas supplied by each branch.

Text continued on p. 104.

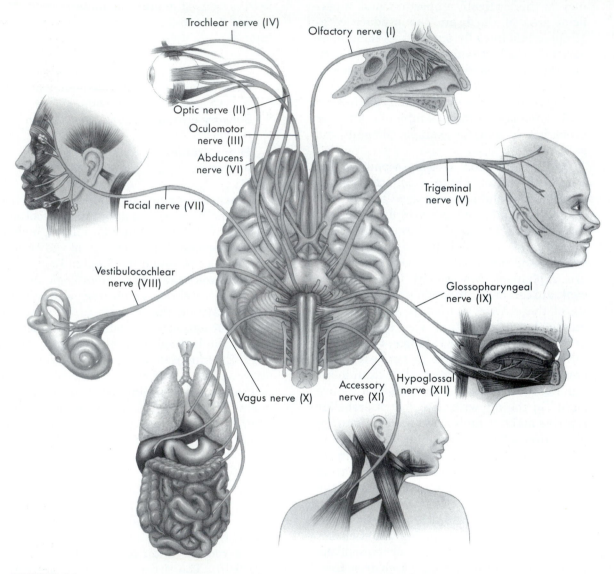

FIGURE 6-9
Cranial nerves. Ventral surface of the brain showing attachment of the cranial nerves.

TABLE 6-3

Cranial Nerves

Nerve*	Sensory fibers†			Motor fibers†		
	Receptors	Cell bodies	Termination	Cell bodies	Termination	Functions‡
I Olfactory	*Nasal mucosa*	*Nasal mucosa*	Olfactory bulbs (new relay of neurons to olfactory cortex)			*Sense of smell*
II Optic	*Retina*	*Retina*	*Nucleus in thalamus (lateral geniculate body); some fibers terminate in superior colliculus of midbrain*			*Vision*
III Oculomotor	*External eye muscles except superior oblique and lateral rectus*	?	?	**Midbrain (oculomotor nucleus and Edinger-Westphal nucleus)**	**External eye muscles except superior oblique and lateral rectus; fibers from Edinger-Westphal nucleus terminate in ciliary ganglion and then to ciliary and iris muscles**	**Eye movements, regulation of size of pupil, accommodation,** proprioception (muscle sense)
IV Trochlear	*Superior oblique*	?	?	**Midbrain**	**Superior oblique muscle of eye**	**Eye movements,** proprioception
V Trigeminal	*Skin and mucosa of head, teeth*	Gasserian ganglion	*Pons (sensory nucleus)*	**Pons (motor nucleus)**	**Muscles of mastication**	*Sensations of head and face,* **chewing movements,** *muscle sense*
VI Abducens	*Lateral rectus*	?	?	**Pons**	**Lateral rectus muscle of eye**	**Abduction of eye,** *proprioception*
VII Facial	*Taste buds of anterior two thirds of tongue*	Geniculate ganglion	*Medulla (nucleus solitarius)*	**Pons**	**Superficial muscles of face and scalp**	**Facial expressions, secretion of saliva,** *taste*
VIII Acoustic Vestibular branch	*Semicircular canals and vestibule (utricle and sacule)*	Vestibular ganglion	*Pons and medula (vestibular nuclei)*			*Balance or equilibrium*

Continued.

TABLE 6-3

Cranial Nerves—cont'd

Nerve*	Sensory fibers†			Motor fibers†		
	Receptors	Cell bodies	Termination	Cell bodies	Termination	Functions‡
Cochlear or auditory branch	*Organ of Corti in cochlear duct*	*Spiral ganglion*	*Pons and medulla (cochlear nuclei)*			*Hearing*
IX Glossopharyngeal	*Pharynx; taste buds and other receptors of posterior one third of tongue*	*Jugular and petrous ganglia*	*Medulla (nucleus solitarius)*	**Medulla (nucleus ambiguus)**	**Muscles of pharynx**	*Taste and other sensations of tongue,* **swallowing movements, secretion of saliva,** *aid in reflex control of blood pressure and respiration*
	Carotid sinus and carotid body	*Jugular and petrous ganglia*	*Medulla (respiratory and vasomotor centers)*	**Medulla at junction of pons (nucleus salivatorius)**	**Otic ganglion and then to parotid gland**	
X Vagus	*Pharynx, larynx, carotid body, and thoracic and abdominal viscera*	*Jugular and nodose ganglia*	*Medulla (nucleus solitarius), pons (nucleus of fifth cranial nerve)*	**Medulla (dorsal motor nucleus)**	**Ganglia of vagal plexus and then to muscles of pharynx, larynx, and thoracic and abdominal viscera**	*Sensations and* **movements** *of organs supplied; e.g.,* **slows heart, increases peristalsis, and contracts muscles for voice production**
XI Spinal accessory	?	?	?	**Medulla (dorsal motor nucleus of vagus and nucleus ambiguus)**	**Muscles of thoracic and abdominal viscera and pharynx and larynx**	**Shoulder movements, turning movements of head, movements of viscera, voice production,** *proprioception(?)*
				Anterior gray column of first five or six cervical segments of spinal cord	**Trapezius and sternocleidomastoid muscle**	
XII Hypoglossal	?	?	?	**Medulla (hypoglossal nucleus)**	**Muscles of tongue**	**Tongue movements,** *proprioception(?)*

*The first letters of the words in the following sentence are the first letters of the names of the cranial nerves. Many generations of anatomy students have used this sentence as an aid to memorizing these names. It is "On Old Olympus Tiny Tops, A Finn, and German Viewed Some Hops." (There are several slightly different versions of this mnemonic.)

†Italics indicate sensory fibers and functions. Boldface type indicates motor fibers and functions.

‡An aid for remembering the general function of each cranial nerve is the following 12-word saying: "Some say marry money but my brothers say bad business marry money." Words beginning with S indicate sensory function. Words beginning with M indicate motor function. Words beginning with B indicate both sensory and motor functions. For example, the first, second, and eighth words in the saying start with S, which indicates that the first, second, and eighth cranial nerves perform sensory functions.

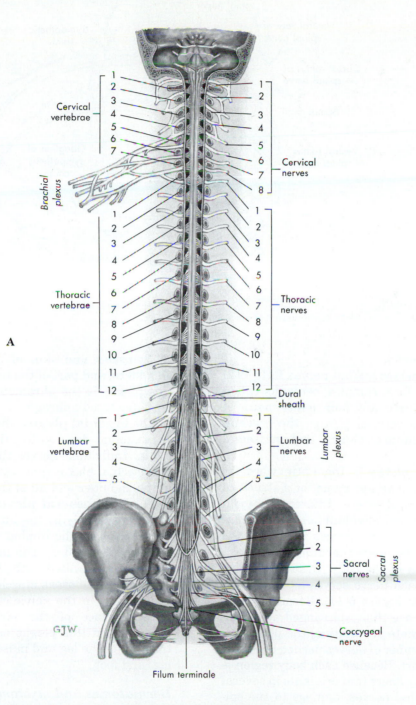

Cervical vertebrae

Brachial plexus

Thoracic vertebrae

A

Lumbar vertebrae

GJW

Cervical nerves

Thoracic nerves

Dural sheath

Lumbar nerves

Lumbar plexus

Sacral nerves

Sacral plexus

Coccygeal nerve

Filum terminale

FIGURE 6-10

Spinal nerves. **A**, Notice that after leaving the spinal cavity, many of the 31 pairs of spinal nerves interconnect to form networks called plexuses. The names of the vertebrae are given on the left and the names of the corresponding spinal nerves on the right.

Continued.

B

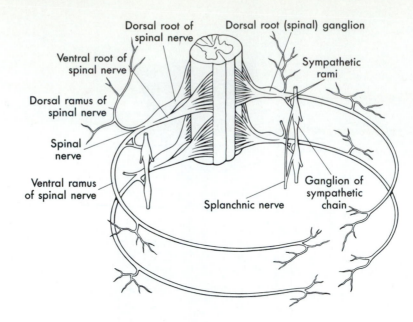

FIGURE 6-10, cont'd
B, The ventral and dorsal roots join to form a thoracic spinal nerve.

Nerve Plexuses

Most spinal nerves (all but nerves T2 to T12) subdivide to form complex networks called **plexuses.** There are four major pairs of plexuses: the cervical plexus, the brachial plexus, the lumbar plexus, and the sacral plexus.

The term *plexus* is the Latin word for "braid." This is an apt name for a structure in which fibers of several different rami join together to form individual nerves. Each individual nerve that emerges from a plexus contains all the fibers that innervate a particular region of the body. In fact, the destination of each nerve serves as a basis for its name (*see* Figure 6-11). Because spinal nerve fibers are thus rearranged according to their ultimate destination, the plexus reduces the number of nerves needed to supply each body part. Because each body region is innervated by fibers that originate in several different spinal nerves, damage to one spinal nerve does not usually mean complete loss of function in any one region.

The **cervical plexus,** shown in Figure 6-12, is found deep within the neck. Individual nerves emerging from this plexus innervate the muscles and skin of the neck, upper shoulders, and part of the head. Also exiting this plexus is the phrenic nerve, which innervates the diaphragm.

The **brachial plexus,** shown in Figure 6-13, is found deep within the shoulder and axilla. Individual nerves that emerge from the brachial plexus innervate the lower part of the shoulder and all of the arm.

The **lumbosacral plexus,** (Figure 6-14) is formed largely by the intermingling of fibers from both the lumbar and sacral plexuses (*see* Table 6-4). The lumbar portion of the plexus is located in the lumbar region of the back in the psoas muscle, and the sacral portion lies in the pelvic cavity on the anterior surface of the piriformis muscle. Nerves from this plexus emerge to supply the skin of the leg and muscles of the thigh, leg, and foot.

Dermatomes and myotomes

A **dermatome** is a defined area of skin supplied by the dorsal or sensory root fibers of a single spinal nerve, and a **myotome** is a muscle or group of muscles supplied by the ventral or motor root fibers from a specific

Text continued on p. 110.

TABLE 6-4

Spinal Nerves and Peripheral Branches

Spinal nerves	Plexuses formed from anterior rami	Spinal nerve branches from plexuses	Parts supplied
Cervical 1 2 3 4	Cervical plexus	Lesser occipital Great auricular Cutaneous nerve of neck Anterior supraclavicular Middle supraclavicular Posterior supraclavicular Branches to muscles Phrenic (branches from cervical nerves before formation of plexus; most of its fibers from fourth cervical nerve)	Sensory to back of head, front of neck, and upper part of shoulder; motor to numerous neck muscles Diaphragm
Cervical 5 6 7 8 Thoracic (or dorsal) 1	Brachial plexus	Suprascapular and dorsoscapular Thoracic nerves, medial and lateral branches Long thoracic nerve Thoracodorsal Subscapular Axillary (circumflex) Musculocutaneous Ulnar	Superficial muscles* of scapula Pectoralis major and minor Serratus anterior Latissimus dorsi Subscapular and teres major muscles Deltoid and teres minor muscles and skin over deltoid Muscles of front of arm (biceps brachii, coracobrachialis, and brachialis) and skin on outer side of forearm Flexor carpi ulnaris and part of flexor digitorum profundus; some of muscles of hand; sensory to medial side of hand, little finger, and medial half of fourth finger
2 3 4 5 6 7 8 9 10 11 12	No plexus formed; branches run directly to intercostal muscles and skin of thorax	Median Radial Medial Cutaneous	Rest of muscles of front of forearm and hand; sensory to skin of palmar surface of thumb, index, and middle fingers Triceps muscle and muscles of back of forearm; sensory to skin of back of forearm and hand Sensory to inner surface of arm and forearm

Continued.

*Although nerves to muscle are considered motor, they contain some sensory fibers that transmit proprioceptive impulses.
*Sensory fibers from the tibial and peroneal nerves unite to form the *medial cutaneous* (or *sural*) *nerve* that supplies the calf of the leg and the lateral surface of the foot. In the thigh the tibial and common peroneal nerves are usually enclosed in a single sheath to form the *sciatic nerve,* the largest nerve in the body with its width of approximately ¾ of an inch. About two thirds of the way down the posterior part of the thigh, it divides into its component parts. Branches of the sciatic nerve extend into the hamstring muscles.

TABLE 6-4

Spinal Nerves and Peripheral Branches—cont'd

Spinal nerves	Plexuses formed from anterior rami	Spinal nerve branches from plexuses	Parts supplied
Lumbar 1 2 3 4 5 Sacral 1 2 3 4 5 Coccygeal 1	Lumbosacral plexus	Iliohypogastric Ilioinguinal Sometimes fused	Sensory to anterior abdominal wall Sensory to anterior abdominal wall and external genitalia; motor to muscles of abdominal wall
		Genitofemoral	Sensory to skin of external genitalia and inguinal region
		Lateral cutaneous of thigh	Sensory to outer side of thigh
		Femoral	Motor to quadriceps, sartorius, and iliacus muscles; sensory to front of thigh and medial side of lower leg (saphenous nerve)
		Obturator	Motor to adductor muscles of thigh
		Tibial* (medial popliteal)	Motor to muscles of calf of leg; sensory to skin of calf of leg and sole of foot
		Common peroneal (lateral popliteal)	Motor to evertors and dorsiflexors of foot; sensory to lateral surface of leg and dorsal surface of foot
		Nerves to hamstring muscles	Motor to muscles of back of thigh
		Gluteal nerves, superior and inferior	Motor to buttock muscles and tensor fasciae latae
		Posterior cutaneous nerve	Sensory to skin of buttocks, posterior surface of thigh, and leg
		Pudendal nerve	Motor to perineal muscles; sensory to skin of perineum

ANTERIOR VIEW

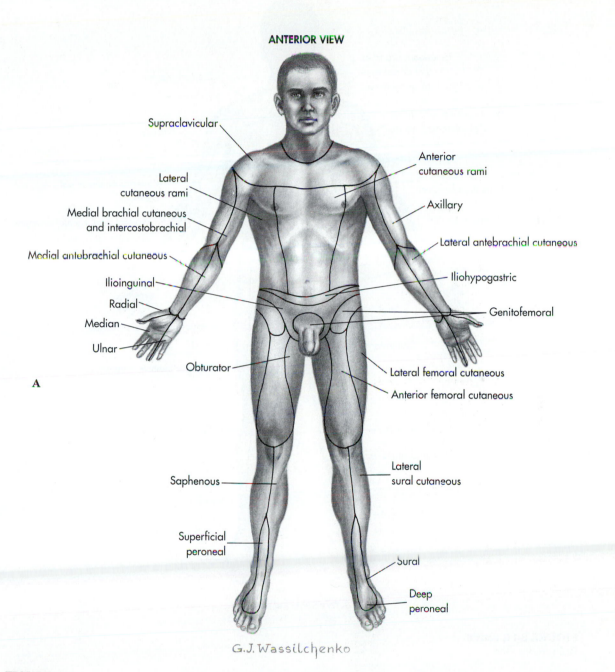

Supraclavicular

Lateral
cutaneous rami

Medial brachial cutaneous
and intercostobrachial

Medial antebrachial cutaneous

Ilioinguinal

Radial

Median

Ulnar

Obturator

Anterior
cutaneous rami

Axillary

Lateral antebrachial cutaneous

Iliohypogastric

Genitofemoral

Lateral femoral cutaneous

Anterior femoral cutaneous

Saphenous

Superficial
peroneal

Lateral
sural cutaneous

Sural

Deep
peroneal

A

G.J.Wassilchenko

FIGURE 6-11
Area of sensory innervation by certain peripheral nerves. **A,** Anterior view.
Continued.

POSTERIOR VIEW

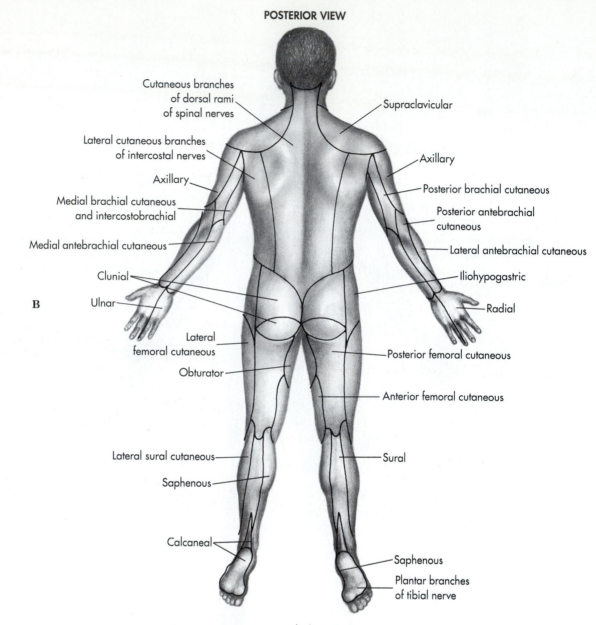

FIGURE 6-11, cont'd
B, Posterior view.

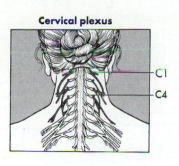

Cervical plexus

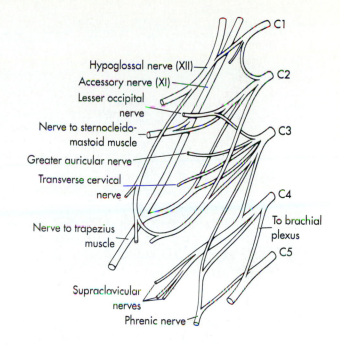

Hypoglossal nerve (XII)
Accessory nerve (XI)
Lesser occipital nerve
Nerve to sternocleido-mastoid muscle
Greater auricular nerve
Transverse cervical nerve
Nerve to trapezius muscle
Supraclavicular nerves
Phrenic nerve

C1
C2
C3
C4
To brachial plexus
C5

FIGURE 6-12
Cervical plexus. Ventral rami of the first four cervical spinal nerves (C1 through C4) exchange fibers in this plexus found deep within the neck. Notice that some fibers from C5 also enter this plexus to form a portion of the phrenic nerve.

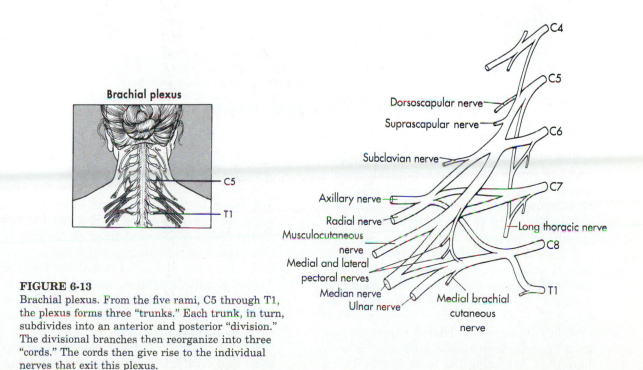

Brachial plexus

Dorsoscapular nerve
Suprascapular nerve
Subclavian nerve
Axillary nerve
Radial nerve
Musculocutaneous nerve
Medial and lateral pectoral nerves
Median nerve
Ulnar nerve
Medial brachial cutaneous nerve
Long thoracic nerve

C4
C5
C6
C7
C8
T1

FIGURE 6-13
Brachial plexus. From the five rami, C5 through T1, the plexus forms three "trunks." Each trunk, in turn, subdivides into an anterior and posterior "division." The divisional branches then reorganize into three "cords." The cords then give rise to the individual nerves that exit this plexus.

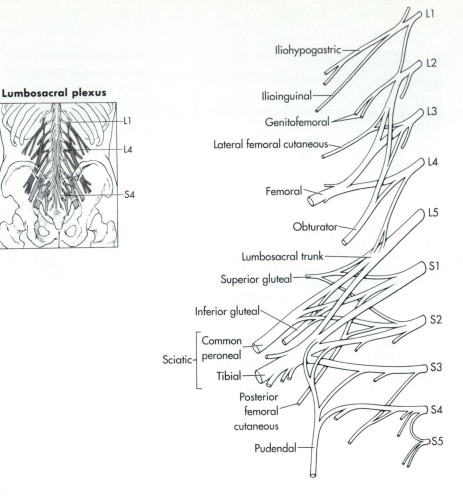

FIGURE 6-14
Lumbosacral plexus. This plexus is formed by the combination of the lumbar plexus with the
sacral plexus, as shown in the inset. Notice that the ventral rami split into anterior and
posterior "divisions" before reorganizing into the various individual nerves that exit this plexus.

spinal nerve. The ability to identify specific
areas of sensory loss (dermatomes), muscle
weakness and/or paralysis (myotomes) can
be extremely useful to the athletic trainer in
localizing injury to the spinal cord or to a
specific spinal nerve.

Figure 6-15 illustrates the segmental pattern of sensory innervation (dermatomes) of
the body surface. Sensations from each dermatome enter the spinal cord by way of afferent fibers in the dorsal or sensory roots of
specific spinal nerves. Therefore sensory loss
in a specific dermatome area can be very
helpful in assessing the level of spinal cord

damage following injury. For example, loss
of sensation in the skin covering the anterior
arm and lateral side of the lower forearm
and hand to the thumb and index fingers
suggests injury to spinal nerve root C6. Efferent fibers of the ventral or motor root of
this spinal nerve innervate the biceps brachii, supinator, and wrist extensors. Total or
partial paralysis of these muscles (C6 myotome) combined with sensory loss in the C6
dermatome confirms the area of injury in an
even more definitive way. In assessing injury to the spinal cord suggested by dermatome and myotome involvement, a physician

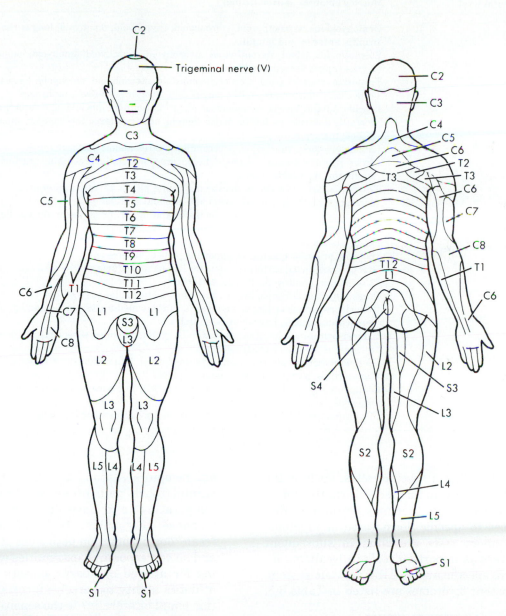

FIGURE 6-15

Segmental distribution of spinal nerves (dermatomes). There is often considerable overlap between adjacent dermatomes. Injury to a single spinal nerve will seldom result in complete loss of sensation in a discrete dermatome area.

TABLE 6-5

Important Myotomes

Segmental level	Muscles involved (partial listing)
C_1	Geniohyoideus, sternothyroid, sternohyoid, thyrohyoid, omohyoid, longus capitis, rectus capitis anterior and lateralis
C_2	Sternocleidomastoid, sternothyroid, sternohyoid, thyrohyoid, omohyoid, longus capitus, rectus capitis anterior and lateralis
C_3	Trapezius, sternothyroid, sternocleidomastoid, sternohyoid, omohyoid, longus capitis
C_4	Trapezius, semispinalis capitis, longus colli, levator scapulae, diaphragm
C_5	Brachioradialis, biceps, rhomboideus major and minor, subclavius, levator scapulae, serratus anterior, pectoralis major, deltoid, subscapularis, teres major, supraspinatus, biceps, infraspinatus, brachialis
C_6	Latissimus dorsi, subclavius, subscapularis, teres major, pectoralis major, serratus anterior, infraspinatus, biceps, deltoid, coracobrachialis, brachialis, brachioradialis, supinator, wrist extensors
C_7	Triceps, latissimus dorsi, pectoralis major and minor, serratus anterior, coracobrachialis, lumbricals, deep antebrachial muscles
C_8	Triceps, latissimus dorsi, pectoralis major and minor, flexor carpi ulnaris, flexor digitorum profundus, pronator quadratus, opponens pollicis, interossei
T_1	Pectoralis major and minor, flexor carpi ulnaris, flexor digitorum profundus, flexor pollicis, pronator quadratus, opponens pollicis, interossei
L_1	Gracilis, pectineus, sartorius, adductor longus and brevis
L_2	Psoas major, quadriceps, iliacus, sartorius
L_3	Psoas major, quadriceps, iliacus, sartorius, adductor longus and brevis
L_4	Quadriceps, adductor longus and brevis, gluteus medius, tensor fasciae latae, quadratus femoris, lateral crural muscles
L_5	Lateral crural muscles, gluteus maximus, gluteus medius, tensor fasciae latae, quadratus femoris, hamstrings
S_1	Gluteus maximus, gluteus medius, tensor fasciae latae, quadratus femoris, hamstrings, posterior crurals, lateral crurals
S_2	Gluteus maximus, hamstrings, posterior crurals, lumbricals and other intrinsic foot muscles
S_3	Flexor digitorum brevis, extensor digitorum brevis, intrinsic foot muscles

may also elicit a specific reflex, such as the brachial reflex, to further confirm the spinal segment or nerve that may be injured. References to specific dermatome or myotome assessment tests are cited in subsequent chapters as important tools in localizing injury to specific areas of the nervous system. Important myotomes are listed in Table 6-5.

THE SENSORY SYSTEM

Knowledge of receptor anatomy and physiology helps in the understanding of sensory phenomena. For example, in "mapping out" sensory loss using dermatomes, remember that sensory distribution varies from person to person and overlap between adjacent dermatomes is common. Also recall that differ-

ent receptors respond to different types of stimuli (touch, pain, pressure, vibration, and temperature) and have different stimulus-response thresholds. It is important to "scan" dermatomes on both sides of the body and on corresponding extremities when testing for altered or absent sensation. Is the athlete's ability to perceive a certain sensation equal bilaterally? Is the sensitivity level the same in distal and proximal parts of each extremity? A vibrating tuning fork, neurologic "pinwheel," cotton ball, camel's hair brush, your hand, or the blunt tip of an ordinary lead pencil can all be used in evaluating sensation.

There are different types of receptors classified according to location, structure, and the types of stimuli that activate them and various forms of sensation, which can be perceived at different levels of intensity. Sensations can also be abnormal or atypical, for example, a stimulus of normal but above threshold intensity that evokes an abnormally strong or weak response or no response at all. **Hypoesthesia** refers to diminished sensation, **hyperesthesia** is increased sensation, and **anesthesia** denotes total absence of sensation. As noted earlier, **paresthesia** refers to an abnormal or perverted sensation often described as "prickling."

When determining sensory responses an athlete should be tested with eyes closed. Sensory testing depends both on the subject's perception and interpretation of applied stimuli. Because sensory tests can be difficult to evaluate, the athlete's cooperation is essential. In most types of injury associated with athletics a diminution of sensation (hypoesthesia) occurs more frequently than total anesthesia.

Sensory System Tests

Tests for the sensory system include (1) *primary* and (2) *cortical and discriminatory forms* of sensation. The primary forms of sensation include superficial tactile sensation, superficial pain, sensitivity to temperature, sensitivity to vibration, deep pressure pain, and motion and position. The athletic trainer must be familiar with each type of primary sensation and skilled in appropriate assessment procedures. Abnormal reactions related to primary sensations suggest disturbances or injury along neural pathways between the receptors in the skin, joints, joint capsules, muscles and tendons, and the sensory cortex of the cerebrum.

Cortical and discriminatory forms of sensation are more complex in terms of evaluation and testing. The types of sensations usually included in this group are two-point discrimination, point localization, texture discrimination (can the athlete identify materials such as burlap or silk by feeling them with the fingers?), *stereognostic function* (ability to identify familiar objects such as a

ring when placed in each hand), and *graphesthesia* (the ability to recognize numbers or letters "written" on the body surface with a blunt instrument).

Abnormal cortical or discriminatory test results are most useful in localizing injury if the primary sensation tests are normal. In such cases neural involvement (injury) is most likely central and not in the peripheral pathways.

Reflex Status Tests

Refer to the earlier discussion of reflex arcs and the detailed examination of the neural pathway involved in the patellar reflex (Figure 6-5) for an understanding of tests for reflex status. Eliciting reflex responses is an important part of many assessment procedures explained in subsequent chapters of the text.

The reflex arc is the unit pattern or functional unit of the nervous system. Therefore the presence, strength, or absence of reflexes can provide valuable information in the athletic injury assessment process. Normally, reflexes are rapid, direct, stereotyped, and persistent. Further, in the absence of injury or disease most reflexes are modified or inhibited only with difficulty.

There are many reflex tests that can be performed. The reflexes listed in Table 6-6 are perhaps the most frequently elicited as part of an athletic injury assessment procedure. Others such as the "winking" or corneal reflex caused by an object striking the cornea, "swallowing reflexes" elicited by touching the back of the tongue or pharynx, or avoidance-type reflexes caused by pain are also useful to the athletic trainer in certain circumstances. If reflexes are hyperactive, a test for *clonus* (rapidly alternating involuntary contraction and relaxation of skeletal muscles) is often performed. In addition to reflexes mentioned here and listed in Table 6-6, other very specialized reflex testing procedures are sometimes employed to localize nervous system injuries and will be discussed as appropriate in subsequent chapters.

The reflexes listed in Table 6-6 are sub-

TABLE 6-6

Tests for Reflex Status

Reflex	Site of stimulus	Normal response	Segmental level involved
Deep Reflexes			
Biceps	Biceps tendon	Contraction of biceps	C_5, C_6
Brachioradialis	Styloid process of radius	Flexion of elbow and forearm	C_5, C_6
Triceps	Triceps tendon above olecranon	Extension of elbow	C_6, C_7, C_8
Patellar	Patellar tendon	Extension of the leg at the knee	L_2, L_3, L_4
Achilles	Achilles tendon	Plantar flexion of the foot	S_1, S_2
Superficial Reflexes			
Upper abdominal	Abdomen above umbilicus	Umbilicus moves up toward area being stroked	T_7, T_8, T_9
Lower abdominal	Abdomen below umbilicus	Umbilicus moves down	T_{11}, T_{12}, L_1
Cremasteric	Skin of inner thigh	Scrotum elevates	T_{12}, L_1, L_2, L_3
Plantar	Lateral surface of sole— heel to ball of foot	Flexion of toes	S_1, S_2
Gluteal	Skin of gluteal area	Skin tenses in gluteal area	L_4-S_3
Pathological Reflexes			
Babinski	Lateral surface of sole— heel to ball of foot	Fanning of toes and dorsiflexion of the big toe	Pathologic
Chaddock	Lateral aspect of foot below the lateral malleolus	Same as Babinski	Pathologic
Oppenheim	Anteromedial tibial surface	Same as Babinski	Pathologic
Gordon	Squeeze calf muscles	Same as Babinski	Pathologic

divided into (1) *deep reflexes,* (2) *superficial reflexes,* and (3) *pathologic reflexes.* Deep reflexes are elicited by tapping a tendon or bony prominence; superficial reflexes are obtained by stroking the skin with a noncutting but pointed object. Although pathologic reflexes are seldom encountered by the athletic trainer, they are listed for information purposes.

REFERENCES

Barr ML, Kiernan JA: *The human nervous system,* ed 6, New York: 1993, Lippincott.

Carson WG Jr and others: Physical examination, *Clin Orthop Relat Res* 185:165, 1984.

Cervical Spine Research Society: *The cervical spine,* Philadelphia, 1983, Lippincott.

Coen CW, editor: *Functions of the brain,* New York, 1985, Oxford University Press.

Collins K and others: Nerve injuries in athletes, *Phys Sportsmed* 16(1):92, 1988.

Hoppenfeld S: *Orthopaedic neurology; a diagnostic guide to neurologic levels,* Philadelphia, 1977, Lippincott.

Judge RD, Zuidema GD, Fitzgerald FT: *Clinical diagnosis: a physiologic approach,* ed 5, Boston, 1988, Little, Brown.

Malasanos L, Barkauskas V, Stoltenberg-Allen K: *Health assessment,* St. Louis, ed 4, 1990, Mosby-Year Book.

Nauta WJH, Feirtag M: *Fundamental neuroanatomy,* New York, 1985, WH Freeman.

Reilly BM: *Practical strategies in outpatient medicine,* ed 2, Philadelphia, 1990, WB Saunders.

SUGGESTED READINGS

Dunant Y, Israel M: The release of acetylcholine, *Sci Am* 252(4):58, 1985.
Clear and up-to-date review of the sequence of events that occurs at a synapse during impulse transmission.

Nathan P: *The nervous system,* ed 3, Oxford, 1988, Oxford University Press.
This account of the nervous system remains one of the best and most readable texts available.

National Geographic Society: *The incredible machine,* Washington DC, 1986, National Geographic Society.
Compilation of excellent articles describing the human body. Each article is accurate, up to date, and written in a very readable style. Good coverage of nervous system functions.

Snyder SH: The molecular basis of communication between cells, *Sci Am* 253(4):132, 1985.
Communication explained as a cellular phenomena. Reviews available research. Data helpful in understanding how cells exchange information. Well-written and filled with excellent illustrations.

Stevens CF: The neuron, *Sci Am* 241(3):54, 1979.
Generalized functions of the neuron are detailed in this frequently cited review article. Easy to read and historically accurate.

UNIT II

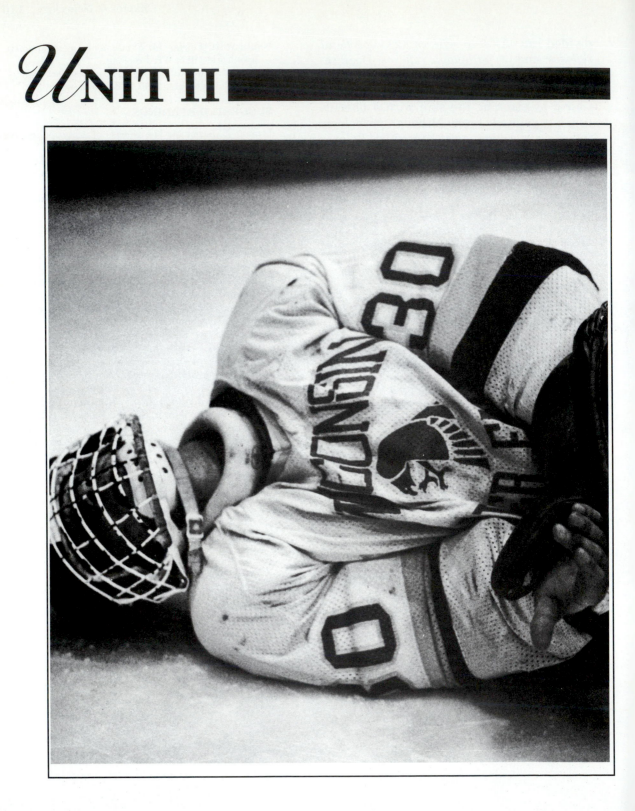

Athletic-related Trauma

To become competent and efficient in assessing athletic injuries, the athletic trainer must be familiar with the broad scope of athletic injuries or conditions and possess a fundamental knowledge of how the body responds to various types of traumas or stresses associated with athletic activity. Athletic injuries or conditions normally result from some type of physical trauma but can be caused by other circumstances such as infectious agents or exposure to hot or cold environments, as well as psychological trauma. The information in this unit will enable you to better understand the body's responses to athletic-related trauma and how the associated signs and symptoms can assist in the assessment process.

7 **The body's response to trauma and environmental stress**
8 **Athletic injuries and related skin conditions**
9 **Psychological aspects of injury**

CHAPTER 7

The body's response to trauma and environmental stress

After you have completed this chapter, you should be able to:
- Briefly describe the body's response to physical trauma, including the inflammatory process.
- Describe the immediate care of athletic injuries.
- Define shock and list its signs and symptoms.
- Explain the body's response to thermal exposure.
- List heat-related conditions and describe their treatment.
- Describe the body's response to cold exposure.
- List cold-related conditions and describe their treatment.

When the body is subjected to injurious trauma or stress, it will usually respond in a systematic and predictable manner. Fortunately, when changes in normal body functions occur, they are manifested by signs or symptoms that provide important clues to assist in identifying underlying medical conditions. To adequately and effectively care for athletic injuries, it is necessary for the athletic trainer to have a fundamental knowledge of the anatomic and physiologic responses to an injury and to understand how diagnostic signs and symptoms develop. The incorporation of this knowledge into athletic injury assessment and management strategies can provide for a rational approach to both the initial evaluation and the subsequent care of an injured athlete. Poor management of an athletic injury can contribute to such circumstances as delayed healing, an unsightly scar, or more serious, permanent disability or possibly death. This chapter discusses some of the body's basic responses to *trauma* resulting from athletic activity and adverse environmental conditions and the associated signs and symptoms. This chapter also briefly discusses procedures an athletic trainer can employ to positively affect and influence these body responses.

BODY'S RESPONSE TO PHYSICAL TRAUMA

The body's immediate and long-term responses to physical trauma are essentially the same for all types of athletic injuries; that is, the process of inflammation and healing. Although these phenomena are not completely or clearly understood, the phys-

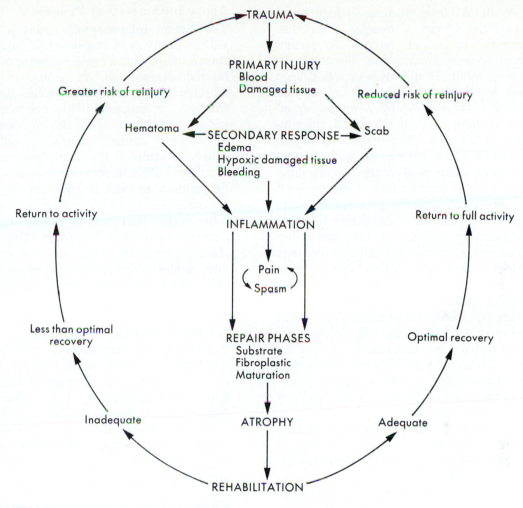

FIGURE 7-1
Cycle of an athletic injury.

iologic and anatomic changes that characterize each step are reliable and predictable indicators from which a trained observer can deduce a great deal of information about both the initial injury and the subsequent course of the recovery process. The body's basic response to a traumatic athletic injury is illustrated in Figure 7-1. This cycle outlines the sequence of events following an injury through the inflammatory and healing process. Ideally, the end result is optimal recovery. Of course, depending on the severity of the injury and the management procedures used, this cycle can vary greatly in its length and conclude in less-than-optimal re-

Trauma
Direct blow
Rotational stress
Abnormal motion
Overstretching

covery and possibly reinjury or permanent loss of function.

The majority of athletic injuries are caused by some type of trauma, such as direct blow, rotational stress, forced abnormal motion, and overstretching or tearing forces. When these forces are greater than the tissues can withstand, varying degrees of damage result. Athletic trauma frequently involves the skin, muscles, tendons, ligaments, bones, or nerves. A certain amount of *hemorrhaging,* or bleeding, will also be present if capillaries or other blood vessels are damaged. This bleeding may be external, if there is an open wound, or internal, if there is no disruption in the continuity of the skin. The body responds to hemorrhage by activating the clotting mechanism in an attempt to control the bleeding. In this type of injury there is also at least some direct cell damage as a result of the trauma. Cells that are damaged or torn lose their nutrition and, as a result, the ability to maintain the necessary cellular activities required for normal function. The result is often cell death or **necrosis.** These necrotic tissue cells and the **extravasated** blood remaining outside the blood vessels as a result of hemorrhage will eventually develop into a mass called a **hematoma.** With open injuries, the blood and necrotic debris may form a thin blood clot, fill the apposed margins of the wounds, and subsequently form a scab on the surface.

The damaged tissue and extravasated blood resulting primarily from direct trauma are termed the *initial insult,* or **primary injury.** Other than initiating procedures to bring bleeding under control as quickly as possible, athletic trainers have little if any effect on the extent of primary injury. Although it is considered the end of damage directly caused by initial trauma, swelling and tissue damage may not cease with the control of bleeding. Frequently, additional damage will occur that is secondary to the initial trauma or primary injury. This is called the secondary response, or **secondary injury** and is discussed along with the inflammatory process. Athletic trainers can greatly affect this phase of the athletic injury cycle.

Acute Inflammatory Process

The acute inflammatory process begins within minutes of the onset of injury. **Inflammation** is the basic response of vascularized tissues to an injurious agent, whether the source is physical, bacterial, thermal, or chemical. This nonspecific response is designed to be the body's defense mechanism against trauma, regardless of cause. In athletics the most frequent cause of inflammation is physical trauma. The inflammatory process is an evolving process characterized by vascular, chemical, and cellular events that lead to tissue repair, regeneration, or scar formation. The goal of the inflammatory process is threefold: (1) to localize the extent of the injured area, (2) to rid both the body as a whole and the injury site of waste products resulting from the initial trauma and secondary response, and (3) to enhance healing. There are three phases in the inflammatory process of athletic related injuries: (1) the acute vascular inflammatory response, or substrate phase, (2) repair and regeneration, or the fibroplastic phase, and (3) the remodeling and maturation phase. The exact duration of each phase is not definite because the phases overlap and there is much variability from one injury or individual to another.

Phase I: Acute vascular response

The initial phase of the acute inflammatory response is characterized by localized vascular changes and is also called the **substrate phase**. Immediate vasoconstriction occurs and is followed by vasodilation and increased vascular permeability. After the injury there is an immediate transient constriction of local blood vessels, resulting in a decreased blood flow to the injured area. The initial vasoconstriction may last from 5 to 10 minutes, providing sufficient time for initial evaluation of the injury and transportation

Primary Injury
Blood Damaged tissue

Substrate Phase
Vascular changes Phagocytosis

of the athlete off the field or court if necessary.

Transient vasoconstriction at the time of injury is followed by active vasodilation of local blood vessels and a rise in blood vessel hydrostatic pressure. These changes are attributed to chemical substances released at the injury site, the most significant being histamine. Histamine is released from mast cells and blood platelets at the injury site and causes vasodilation and increased vascular permeability. Concurrent to this increased blood flow and vascular permeability is congestion in the blood vessels that allows the white blood cells (leukocytes) to line up along the vessel walls (a process called **margination**) (Figure 7-2, *B*). Edema formation at this stage is primarily blood fluids and is known as **transudate**. As hydrostatic pressure and vascular permeability continue to increase, white blood cells, plasma proteins, and fluids leak out or escape the blood vessels to migrate toward the injury site (Figure 7-2, *C*). This ameboid type of movement of leukocytes and proteins from intact vessel walls into the tissue spaces is known as **diapedesis.** This protein-rich fluid is called **exudate** and contributes to the collection of blood fluids in the tissue spaces surrounding the blood vessels at the point of injury. This leakage into the interstitial tissues accounts for much of the swelling (**edema**) associated with an injury and may continue for 24 to 48 hours, causing the injury site to be more extensive than that caused by the initial trauma. In addition, this increased swelling and pressure in the area can result in a decreased blood flow and reduced amount of oxygen and nutrients being delivered to the injury site and may cause cells uninjured by the initial trauma to be damaged by **hypoxia.** Cells that undergo secondary hypoxic death add to the debris from the initial injury, increasing the size of the hematoma. As a re-

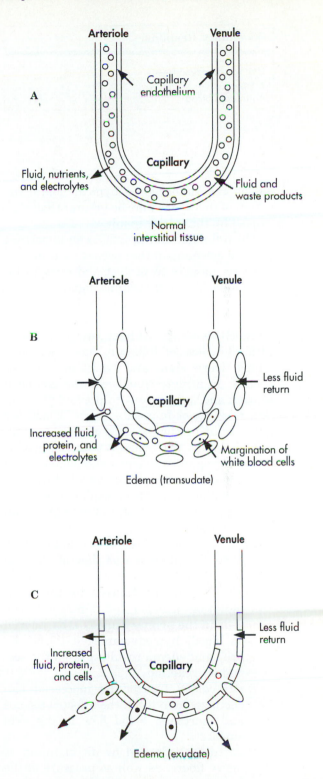

FIGURE 7-2
Formation of edema. **A,** Normal fluid, nutrient, and electrolyte exchange. **B,** Initial edema formation as hydrostatic pressure and vessel permeability continues to increase. **C,** Edema formation continues as white blood cells, plasma proteins, and fluids escape the vessel.

Secondary Response
Hypoxic-damaged tissue
Edema
Additional blood

Inflammation
Redness
Swelling
Heat
Pain
Loss of function

sult of cells undergoing hypoxic death, the extent of the injury may be greater than that caused by the initial insult.

The inflammatory process is an important defense mechanism that occurs for a specific purpose, namely to protect and heal an injured area. The four cardinal signs of inflammation, which were originally identified by Celsus in the first century AD, are (1) redness, (2) swelling, (3) heat, and (4) pain. A fifth sign, loss of function, has since been added. These signs and symptoms serve to remind an athlete that he or she has been injured and are present to prevent the athlete from exceeding safe limits of activity and reinjuring the area. To effectively manage an injury the athletic trainer must be able to recognize the signs and symptoms of inflammation and understand what they indicate. Following is a brief explanation of the signs and symptoms of inflammation and their causes:

Redness (rubor): Caused by dilation of arterioles and increased flow of blood to the injured area

Swelling (tumor): Caused by the accumulation of blood and damaged tissue cells in the primary injury area, as well as blood, hypoxic-damaged tissue debris, and edema resulting from the secondary reaction

Heat (calor): Caused by increased biochemical activity in the affected tissues and increased blood flow to the skin surface

Pain (dolor): Caused by direct injury to nerve fibers, as well as pressure of the hematoma or area of edema on nerve endings

Loss of function (functio laesa): Caused by

the resulting pain and swelling and/or the actual destruction of an anatomic structure, such as a fractured bone, ruptured ligament, or torn muscle

The primary function of the inflammatory process in the days following an injury is to rid the area of waste products resulting from the primary and secondary responses in preparation for the healing process. As the blood vessels become more permeable and allow blood cells to migrate into the tissues, leukocytes infiltrate the injured area and concentrate at the injury site. In the early stages of the acute inflammatory response, these leukocytes engage in **phagocytosis,** which is the ingesting and disposing of unwanted substances, such as elements of the hematoma. During the later phases of acute inflammation, the predominant phagocyte is a macrophage type of cell that emigrates to the injury site in large numbers. After the debris is ingested, these phagocytes reenter the blood stream or lymphatic system and are carried away from the injury site. The successful completion of this phagocytic activity usually marks the end of the acute inflammatory reaction. In most wounds not contaminated with bacteria or large amounts of foreign material, the acute inflammatory process subsides within several days, and the repair process continues to evolve.

Pain-spasm cycle. An additional response to trauma is the pain-spasm cycle. Generally, pain and muscle spasm of varying degrees accompany musculoskeletal injuries. Muscle spasm is a protective mechanism, designed to prevent further damage to an already injured area. The body attempts to splint the area surrounding the injured

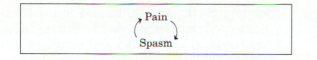

area through the involuntary contraction of muscles or groups of muscles. The resulting contraction is called muscle spasm. As the muscle spasm develops, there is increased pressure on the nerve endings, resulting in more pain. The body responds to increased pain with increased muscle spasms, resulting in more pain; hence the name pain-spasm cycle.

The process of wound healing begins with the acute inflammatory reaction and then accelerates when enough of the hematoma has been removed to permit the growth of new tissue. The formation of new tissue is required to replace tissues that were damaged by the injury. Most tissues involved in athletic injuries do not have the ability to regenerate their respective specialized cells and instead undergo a relatively nonspecific repair process—that of scar formation. Human epidermis and bones, however, do have the ability to regenerate, or heal, with the same type of tissue that was damaged. Unfortunately, most soft tissues in the body heal with the formation of scar tissue, which is less than an ideal replacement. Scar formation is virtually identical in all tissues of the body. However, the final appearance of a scar and its effect on function will vary, depending on the tissue involved and the treatment given. Treatment and rehabilitation procedures differ somewhat between various types of tissues injured. These procedures are briefly discussed later.

Phase II: Repair and regeneration

The removal of most of the necrotic debris from the injury site is followed by development of a dense network of capillaries early in the healing process. Along with the formation of this capillary network, **fibroblasts,** which are connective tissues in the body, proliferate in the damaged area. This phase of wound healing or scar formation is known as **fibroplasia.** These fibroblasts

Repair Phases
Fibroplastic
Collagen fibers
Maturation
Scar develops

manufacture **collagen,** which is the main supportive protein in skin, tendon, bone, cartilage, and connective tissue. Significant amounts of collagen are laid down by the fourth or fifth day after an injury, so that a loose mesh of fibrous connective tissue occupies the injured area. This newly formed connective tissue is vascular and fragile. It lacks cross-links between fibers. The phenomenon of fibroblast proliferation and collagen accumulation after injury usually continues for 2 to 4 weeks. During this time the vascularity of the new fibrous connective tissue continues to decrease, cross-linking becomes established, fibers acquire a more organized pattern, and the tensile strength increases. As a sufficient quantity of collagen is produced, the number of fibroblasts in the wound diminishes. The disappearance of these fibroblasts marks the end of the fibroplastic phase and the beginning of the **maturation phase.**

Phase III: Remodeling and maturation

During the remodeling and maturation phase of wound healing, pronounced changes occur in the newly formed fibrous connective tissue. The scar that is formed during fibroplasia is an enlarged and dense but unorganized structure of collagen. The fibers of collagen are initially randomly arranged but, in time, will line up along lines of stress. The union between the damaged tissues is still moderately fragile. During the next several months, the strength of the scar continues to increase and the collagen fibers and cross-links change to a more organized pattern. As the scar tissue matures, it shrinks and becomes avascular and acellular. This maturation process may continue for a year or longer.

It is important for athletic trainers to understand the basic fundamentals of wound repair and scar formation to gain optimum treatment results and achieve full recovery with injured athletes. It is the responsibility of the athletic trainer to localize the inflammatory response, promote the healing process, and ensure that athletes are not imposing undue stress on healing tissue that is not mature or ready for strenuous physical activity.

Open wounds, those involving a break in the continuity of the skin, should be thoroughly cleansed to remove any foreign material, obvious necrotic tissue, or bacterial contaminants. Wound edges must be restored as closely as possible to normal anatomic relationships to minimize the amount of fibroplasia required for healing to occur and the width of the resulting scar. Although this is primarily a physician's responsibility, the athletic trainer will be called on to protect the injured area when the athlete returns to activity and to inspect the wound periodically to ensure that it does not reopen or become infected. Remember, the epidermis is undergoing constant replacement by regeneration, and injuries involving only this outer layer of the skin will heal without scar formation. Epidermal wounds heal by migration and proliferation of epithelial cells originating in the margins of the wound.

Athletic injuries involving structures deep to the skin must be treated to heal in such a way that function of the involved anatomic part will be restored to an optimum level. In many instances, when a structure is ruptured or torn, it is desirable to repair it surgically. The goal of surgical repair is to bring the ruptured ends together so that a shorter distance has to be spanned by scar tissue. The injured area must be protected from abnormal stresses, which can interfere with the healing process and weaken, stretch, or tear the developing scar tissue and result in loss of function or instability. This protection or immobilization may be in the form of a cast, brace, splint, tape, or rest.

Rehabilitation procedures will differ, depending on the type of tissues injured. Injuries involving the contractile unit (muscles and tendons) are treated and managed differently than those involving noncontractile tissues such as ligaments. If muscles and tendons are allowed to heal without active early motion, it may be very difficult to restore full strength and range of motion. Range of motion exercises should be started as early as possible once swelling and tenderness have subsided to the point that exercises are not unduly painful. However, starting too early may impede the healing process, cause additional hemorrhage and swelling, and result in a bigger scar and possibly a limitation in function. Allowing the musculotendinous unit to heal in a shortened state will result in a loss of motion, requiring constant stretching and making the athlete more vulnerable to repeated strains. These contractile tissues may require a certain amount of support and protection when activity is resumed. Occasionally injuries to the contractile unit will result in the formations of fibrous **adhesions** that bind the tendon or muscle to surrounding tissues and interfere with normal movement.

Ligament injuries require a long period of time (possibly as long as 6 months) to heal to the point of regaining near normal tensile strength. The tensile strength of collagen is specific to the mechanical forces imposed during the remodeling phase. Forces applied to the ligament during rehabilitative exercises will develop strength specifically in the direction that force is applied. However, if ligaments are subjected to abnormal stresses too early in the healing process or at an excessive level, the healing process may be extended. The developing scar tissue may also elongate, resulting in some degree of permanent instability of the involved joint. Early mobilization can assist in producing a more viable injury result; too long a period of immobilization can delay healing. External means of protection or immobilization, such as a cast, brace, or taping, may be used until the healing ligament is moderately strong and the surrounding muscles can be rehabilitated to assist in the support of the joint. In many cases the injured joint will require continued support and protection when athletic activity is resumed.

Another result of the injury cycle of which an athletic trainer must be aware is **atrophy.** Atrophy is the wasting away or deterioration of a tissue, organ, or part. During the healing process, if the injured area has been immobilized or otherwise inactive, atrophy will occur. In most cases the degree of atrophy is directly proportional to the amount and length of time of immobilization. Occasionally, changes in vascularity and innervation of a body area will also result in atrophy. Regardless of the cause, an area of the body that has atrophied is more susceptible to reinjury, thus instigating repetition of the injury cycle. Therefore the injured athlete should not be returned to full athletic activity until the area has been rehabilitated to an optimum level.

The Immediate Care of Athletic Injuries

Standard procedures for the immediate care of athletic injuries are based on how the body responds to trauma and the acute inflammatory process. These initial treatment procedures are designed to control the swelling and minimize the magnitude of the hematoma, which allows the process of healing to begin earlier and proceed at a more rapid rate. The standard procedures for the initial care of an athletic injury are universally accepted and can be remembered by the acronym ICERS. These letters stand for the steps of *I*ce, *C*ompression, *E*levation, *R*est, and *S*upport. Each of these steps is important and should not be overlooked when caring for an acute athletic injury (Figure 7-3).

Initial Treatment

Ice
Compression
Elevation
Rest
Support

Ice

The first step is to put some form of cold application on the injured area, whether it is an ice pack or cold immersion. Cold applied promptly after an injury can slow down or minimize some of the acute inflammatory reactions previously discussed. In addition, cold diminishes local blood flow and helps constrict capillaries in the area of injury. The local application of cold also decreases clotting time because it increases the viscosity of the fluids and decreases the rate of flow in the injured area. This quicker clotting reduces hemorrhaging in the area of injury. Another important effect of cold is to lower tissue temperature, thus decreasing the metabolic demands and slowing the chemical actions in cells surrounding the injured area. This reduces the build up of waste products in the area and allows more tissue cells to survive the period of temporary hypoxia. To summarize, applying cold to an injured area reduces tissue damage and results in a smaller hematoma to be resolved. Cold applications are also beneficial in reducing the amount of muscle spasms that usually accompany athletic injuries. Therefore there is less discomfort associated with the pain-spasm cycle.

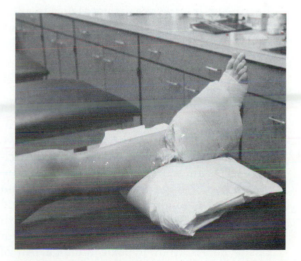

FIGURE 7-3
Standard procedure of initial care for an athletic injury: ice, compression, elevation, rest, and support.

Compression

The purpose of compression on an acute injury is to help control or reduce the amount of edema and provide mild support. Compression about an injured area is normally accomplished by the use of an elastic wrap or appropriate taping. Compression also increases the tissue pressure outside the blood vessels, thus helping to prevent edema caused by plasma seepage or extravasation. Normally, compression will also make an injured area feel more comfortable. Although an elastic wrap offers only mild support, the pressure appears to provide some relief of pain.

Elevation

Elevation of an injured area limits fluid pooling and encourages venous return. If possible, elevate the injured area above the level of the heart. Elevating an injured area also decreases the hydrostatic pressure within the blood vessels, which helps decrease the amount of edema by decreasing the volume of fluid filtered out of the blood vessels and into the tissue spaces. Controlling the edema associated with an injured area decreases tissue damage and results in a smaller area to be repaired.

Rest

Resting an injured area is necessary to allow the body time to get the effects of the trauma under control and to avoid additional stress and damage to injured tissue. The period of rest required will vary, depending on the athletic trainer's and physician's philosophy and on the severity of the injury. The length of rest may range from a 10-minute break in a practice to many months of postoperative recovery. Athletes who continue to participate with an acutely injured area may increase hemorrhage and the amount of initial tissue damage, as well as the amount and severity of secondary injury response such as edema formation and the accumulation of tissue debris from hypoxic damage. All of this can result in a larger hematoma, slower healing, and a longer recovery period.

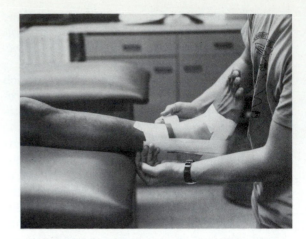

FIGURE 7-4
Injured ankle supported by adhesive tape.

Support

Another very important aspect of the initial treatment is that of support and protection. Often an injury requires stabilization or immobilization to prevent further injury. Athletic trainers employ the use of various materials, such as braces, splints, casts, tape, pads, or crutches, to protect and support injured areas (Figure 7-4). Varying degrees of support or protection often have to be provided throughout the healing phase and perhaps longer. Athletic trainers attempt to provide for optimum conditions for recovery during the healing phase.

The purpose of the initial treatment procedures of ice, compression, elevation, rest, and support is to minimize the effects of an injury at its onset and to create an optimum environment for healing, thereby reducing the loss of function and length of the recovery period. Normally these procedures are used for at least 2 to 3 days after a significant injury. Although athletic trainers can do little to speed up the actual healing process, they can have a tremendous effect on the total recovery time and on the quality of the repair.

Follow-up Treatment Procedures

Treatment procedures used after the immediate postinjury period are designed to

Rehabilitation
Heat or cold applications Exercise

rehabilitate the athlete toward full functional use of the injured area and return him or her to an optimum level of performance in a minimal period of time. Both heat and cold modalities are used after the initial treatment period; however, heat should not be used until you are relatively sure no further bleeding or swelling will occur. Heat is used primarily to increase the circulation to an area. Cold is used primarily to relieve pain, thereby allowing early and more extensive range of motion. Both of these modalities should always be used in conjunction with some type of exercise. Exercise is the primary modality used to rehabilitate an injured area, and it is the most effective method of increasing blood flow to an area. The increased blood flow helps resolve the hematoma and deliver oxygen and nutrients required in rebuilding injured tissues.

Athletic trainers must be familiar with rehabilitation procedures. He or she must assume a leadership role in convincing an injured athlete that the key to a good rehabilitation program is continued progressive exercise, not just an extension of passive treatment activity for a longer period of time. The type of exercises used to restore normal function depend on the nature and severity of the injury, as well as the athletic trainer's philosophy. Basically, exercises should be performed essentially pain free and progress as fast as possible from active range of motion to full participation. This may be completed in days or may take 3 to 4 weeks or longer. Pain is the primary governing force for all treatment procedures. As long as the exercise is pain free, the athlete should be encouraged to increase the level of activity. If the exercise is painful or if residual swelling and pain are present following treatment, the activity is too strenuous and should be modified.

Chronic Inflammation

Chronic is defined as long lasting. Although there is no sharp delineation of time between acute and chronic, **acute** generally refers to a matter of hours or days, whereas chronic refers to weeks, months, or years. Chronic inflammation may result from overuse, improper technique, continued stress, or repeated injury to a structure or area of the body. For whatever reason, the inflammatory response continues to repeat itself and can be detrimental to an athlete's performance. Such conditions as tennis elbow, jumper's knee, and shin splints are typical examples of chronic inflammations. They can progress to a point at which they disable an athlete. Although these seem to be different conditions, chronic inflammatory responses are basically alike and require the same treatment: rest, local heat, protection against reinjury, and often antiinflammatory medications prescribed by a physician. In chronic conditions, identification of possible causes and the initiation of corrective measures are very important.

The purpose of any training program is to build up the body's structures gradually so they can withstand progressively heavier workloads, thus increasing their strength, endurance, and ability to avoid injury. Once a chronic inflammatory condition occurs, it is up to the athletic trainer or physician to attempt to identify and eliminate the possible causes. These problems can be magnified by the fact that in many cases relief will require a sharp reversal of activity. A period of complete rest may be required, which must then be followed by a gradual increase in workload. This can be very frustrating and burdensome to the athlete, athletic trainer, or coach, especially if the injury occurs during the athletic season. The athlete's impatience to resume activity too soon or at too great an intensity level often results in recurrence of the condition and an even more frustrating period of disability.

Summary

The body's response to trauma is generally well established and programmed. When some type of trauma occurs, there is a certain amount of damaged tissue and blood that accumulates as the result of the primary injury. In addition to hematoma formation, there is frequently a secondary response that causes the injury site to become even more extensive. This secondary response includes edema and hypoxia and may continue for 24 to 48 hours. The body responds to this trauma with an inflammatory reaction designed to localize the extent of the injured area, rid the body of waste products, and enhance healing. The processes of inflammation and healing form a continuum that can be subdivided into three phases; substrate (vascular changes and phagocytosis), fibroplastic (laying down of collagen fibers), and maturation (scar development). However, portions of these phases can occur simultaneously. For example, fibroplasia begins during the substrate phase, and scar maturation begins while collagen production continues. Possessing a fundamental knowledge of what happens to the body as a result of trauma provides the athletic trainer with a more rational basis for the management of various athletic injuries.

One of the primary responsibilities of an athletic trainer is to positively affect and influence the healing process to gain optimum treatment results with the injured athlete. This is initially accomplished by reducing the effects of the initial injury or trauma. Bleeding and swelling must be controlled as quickly as possible to minimize the magnitude of the hematoma. Limiting the hematoma allows the healing process to commence earlier, reducing the length of inactivity caused by the injury. Follow-up treatment procedures using exercise in conjunction with various methods of heat or cold applications are designed to optimally rehabilitate the injured athlete in a minimal period of time. It is not the intent of this text to discuss the various modalities and treatment procedures used by athletic trainers. We recommend that you aggressively seek new information in this area and continue to improve and refine your treatment and rehabilitation techniques.

✤ SHOCK

Another of the body's responses to trauma is shock. **Shock** is a state of collapse or depression of the cardiovascular system. Although it does not occur often in athletics, any significant athletic injury can result in shock. The possibilities of shock developing are much greater with severe bleeding (external or internal), spinal injuries, major fractures, or significant intrathoracic or intraabdominal injuries. There are three main causes of shock: (1) the heart is damaged so that it fails to pump properly, (2) blood is lost so that there is an insufficient volume of fluid in the circulatory system, and (3) blood vessels dilate so that blood "pools" in the larger vessels, resulting in a diminished amount of fluid available to provide efficient circulation. Either of these last two causes are most often responsible for shock when it occurs because of athletic injuries.

Types of shock

Shock can be associated with many types of injuries or conditions. Following are the main types of shock.

Anaphylactic shock is a life-threatening reaction of the body to an allergen, something to which the athlete is extremely allergic. It is the most severe form of an allergic reaction.

Cardiogenic shock is caused by inadequate functioning of the heart.

Hypovolemic shock is caused by the loss of body fluids or blood. Dehydration due to diarrhea, vomiting, or heavy perspiration can lead to its development. When caused by blood loss, this type of shock is called *hemorrhagic shock*.

Metabolic shock may be associated with a profound fluid loss from uncontrolled diseases such as diabetes mellitus. Other possible causes could be diarrhea, vomiting, and excessive urination. Such conditions can cause loss of body fluids and changes in body chemistry.

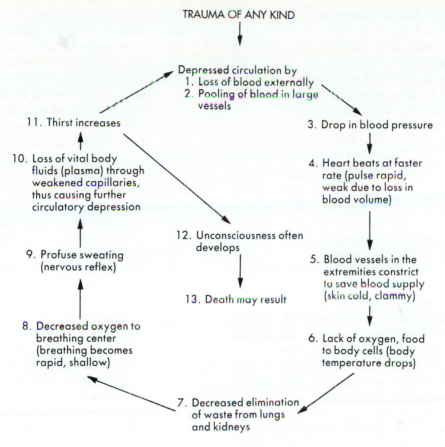

FIGURE 7-5
Continuous cycle of traumatic shock.

Neurogenic shock is caused by a failure of the nervous system to control the size and muscular tone of the blood vessels. This type of shock may be seen with spinal injuries.

Psychogenic shock is caused by a sudden, temporary dilation of the blood vessels to the brain, causing the individual to faint. This is also known as **syncope.**

Septic shock is almost always associated with some form of serious illness and is caused by severe infection. Toxins are released into the bloodstream and cause blood vessels to dilate.

The result of shock is the same no matter what the cause, that is, failure of the cardiovascular system, resulting in a diminished amount of blood available in the circulatory system. This results in an insufficient perfusion of blood providing oxygen and nutrients through the tissues and organs of the body. All bodily processes are affected. Body systems are depressed, and vital functions slow down. Shock is always serious; if this condition is not treated properly and promptly, death can result.

Shock develops in distinct stages. It can progress quite rapidly or develop over a period of hours. Figure 7-5 traces a continuous cycle of traumatic shock and outlines how each of the signs of shock develop. It is important for an athletic trainer to recognize these signs and to be prepared to properly care for an injured athlete. The important signs indicating possible shock are:

1. Rapid, weak pulse
2. Cool, clammy skin

3. Rapid, shallow breathing
4. Profuse sweating
5. Pale skin, and later, cyanotic mucous membranes
6. Nausea, possibly vomiting
7. Dull, lackluster eyes; pupils may dilate
8. Steadily falling blood pressure
9. Unconsciousness

As soon as the athletic trainer recognizes any of these signs, the athlete should be treated for shock. Shock is a serious condition, but if recognized quickly and treated effectively, it can be reversed. The general treatment for shock is as follows:

1. Establish and maintain a clear airway.
2. Control obvious bleeding.
3. Keep the athlete lying down, and elevate the lower extremities if the injury will not be aggravated. If there is a head, spinal, or abdominal injury or breathing difficulties, keep the athlete flat or in a comfortable position.
4. Loosen or remove any pieces of uniform or equipment that may hinder breathing or circulation.
5. Maintain body temperature as near normal as possible. In cold temperatures, keep the athlete warm and reduce the loss of body heat.
6. Do not give anything to eat or drink.
7. Give oxygen if available.
8. Transport the athlete to medical facilities or summon medical assistance.

BODY'S RESPONSE TO THERMAL EXPOSURE

It is extremely important for the athletic trainer to understand the body's response to thermal exposure, especially any abnormal responses such as heat exhaustion or heatstroke. Athletes participating in activities such as running, tennis, cycling, baseball, and softball regularly engage in vigorous exertion during hot and humid weather. The popularity of distance running, marathons, and triathlons has increased problems related to heat stress. Early season practices in fall sports such as football, cross country, soccer, or field hockey frequently necessitate participation in a hot, humid environment.

It is possible to find these same environmental conditions indoors, such as in wrestling rooms and gymnasiums. An elevated room temperature and a number of exercising, sweating bodies can create a hot, humid environment indoors even during the winter. The improper use of saunas, steam baths, rubberized sweat suits, and whirlpools can also increase the risk of heat-related problems.

Heat-related problems vary in severity from temporary heat cramps to fatal heatstrokes. Life-threatening situations in athletics are rare; however, they occasionally occur as the result of heat stress. The devastating effects of heat illness are needless and preventable. The athletic trainer can have a tremendous impact on prevention of heat-related illnesses by intelligently counseling coaches and athletes about the variables concerning activity in hot weather. Therefore it is extremely important for athletic trainers to understand the physiologic mechanisms active in thermoregulatory responses and how environmental conditions can significantly contribute to heat illness. The athletic trainer must also know how to acclimate athletes, initiate preventive measures to avoid potentially fatal heat-related incidents, recognize associated signs and symptoms indicating the development of heat-related conditions, and be proficient in the use of emergency procedures required to care for athletes suffering from heat-stress conditions.

Physiologic Basis of Heat Exposure

The human body is continually striving to maintain a constant internal (core) temperature of 98.6° F (37° C). The brain and the thoracic and abdominal visceral structures are considered core organs. To maintain constant temperature to these organs, heat lost must equal heat gained. If heat gain exceeds heat loss, the core temperature will rise; conversely, core temperature falls when heat loss exceeds heat production. The body has various mechanisms to gain, as well as lose, heat (Figure 7-6), and it is extremely important to maintain a balance between these mechanisms during athletic activity.

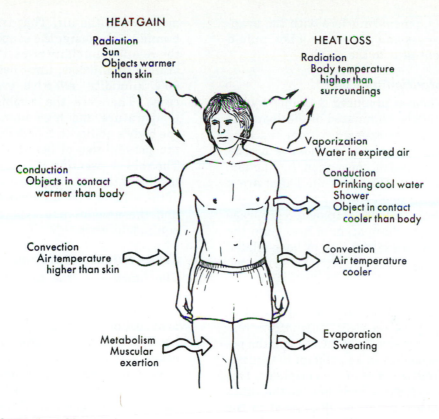

FIGURE 7-6
Mechanisms of heat gain and loss.

Heat production

The body produces heat and energy during **metabolism.** During exercise and muscular exertion accompanying athletic activity, the metabolic rate increases, as does the heat production. The greater the energy expenditure, the greater the heat production. This heat diffuses from the muscle cells to capillary blood, which passes through the lungs. A relatively small amount of heat is lost through **vaporization** of water in the air expired during respiration. However, most of the heat is carried by the blood into the circulatory system.

Heat gain

Heat can be gained by the body from the environment through radiation, convection, and conduction (Figure 7-6). We gain heat by **radiation** from the sun and surrounding objects. On an athletic field, a considerable amount of heat can be gained from the sun in this way. This is especially true when there is little or no cloud cover, or during the middle portion of the day when the sun is directly overhead and the radiation is more concentrated. Remember, the heat radiating from an artificial turf is usually higher than that radiating from a natural or grass playing field. We also gain heat by radiation from objects surrounding the body when they are warmer than the skin's temperature.

Convection is the transfer of heat from one place to another by motion or circulation. If the temperature of the air surrounding the athlete is higher than the athlete's temperature, he or she may gain heat through convection. An increase in the athlete's core temperature may also occur through **conduction** or contact with a solid or liquid that is warmer than the athlete's body. This is not usually a significant source of heat gain unless heavy clothing or equipment is worn close to the body. Heavy clothing and equipment interfere with the evaporation process and can create a hot, humid environment next to the skin.

Heat dissipation and loss

As excess heat is produced or gained by the body, it must be eliminated or dissipated to keep the body temperature from reaching detrimental extremes. Heat loss is accomplished by radiation, convection, conduction, and evaporation (Figure 7-6). There are a number of strategies and preventive measures athletic trainers employ to encourage or promote the dissipation of heat from the body and minimize the risk of heat-related illness during athletic activity; these are discussed on pp. 136 to 139.

The body eliminates heat primarily by cutaneous vasodilation and sweating. When the core temperature rises, for whatever reason, the body responds by increasing the peripheral blood flow in an attempt to transfer the heat from the core to the periphery. This brings an increase of body heat to the skin's surface, where it can be dissipated to the outside environment. When the body temperature is warmer than surrounding objects, heat is lost through radiation. When the air temperature is cooler than the body's, heat can be lost by convection. Athletes who are running can lose heat in this manner, as can those standing in a breeze. The amount of heat lost by convection depends on the temperature and speed of the air flow over the body. The body can also lose heat by conduction, providing the object in contact with the body is cooler. Examples of this are drinking cold water, wiping off with a cool, wet towel, or taking a cool shower.

The major portion of heat loss during athletics is through **evaporation** of sweat from the surface of the body. This is the body's major defense mechanism against overheating and serious heat illness. The body produces sweat that accumulates on the surface of the skin and cools the body as it evaporates. Our bodies are cooled only if the sweat evaporates. The effectiveness of this sweating and evaporation mechanism is strongly influenced by the relative humidity, or the moisture in the air. That is, the lower the humidity, the faster the evaporation rate. As the relative humidity rises, the rate of evaporation diminishes, until between 70% and 80% humidity, effective evaporation may cease. Therefore the combination of high temperature and high humidity decreases the body's ability to cool down and increases the possibilities of heat-related conditions. The rate of sweating also depends on the intensity of the activity, the physical condition of the athlete, how acclimated the athlete is, and the amount and type of clothing and equipment worn.

Temperature regulation

The function of the thermoregulatory system is to maintain a relatively constant internal body temperature, whether the body is at rest or participating in strenuous activity. This system is controlled by the temperature regulatory center in the hypothalamus, which receives its information from various thermal receptors located throughout the body. The role of this center in the brain is analogous to that of the thermostat in a house. As information comes in that heat is being gained, the thermoregulatory center automatically relays information to appropriate thermal effectors, and mechanisms of vasodilation or sweating are initiated.

Cutaneous vasodilation brings warm blood to the body's surface, where excess heat can be dissipated. This mechanism functions well, as long as heat levels are not excessively high and the outside temperature is lower than the skin's surface. It is possible for an athlete's rate of heat gain and storage to become excessive in a very short period of time. If this occurs, it may overwhelm the body's mechanisms of heat loss. Such a situation can quickly develop into a serious heat illness. In addition, as the external temperature approaches that of the skin's surface or actually becomes higher, the heat dissipated by cutaneous vasodilation diminishes and may eventually cease completely. Body heat must then be dissipated primarily by the evaporation of sweat.

If peripheral vasodilation is quite marked, the effective volume of the vascular system is decreased and the heart must increase its output to compensate and maintain adequate blood flow. This is accomplished by an increase in both heart rate and stroke volume. Unfortunately, at least some degree of vasomotor control of the cutaneous vessels may be lost during heat stress; the result is pooling of blood in the extremities. As blood is progressively shunted into the periphery, less and less blood flows to the internal organs and central nervous system. These effects may combine to cause symptoms of headache, dizziness, exhaustion, restlessness, and impaired thinking.

Another important physiologic consideration is the volume of sweat lost from the body. Profuse sweating can cause excessive losses of body water, which can result in decreased blood volume and dehydration and a decreased rate of sweating and cooling by evaporation. If this water is not replaced, circulatory collapse (shock) may result from the continuing decrease in blood volume. As sweating decreases there is also a decrease in evaporative cooling, which can cause an excessive rise in core temperature. As water loss becomes extremely excessive, the mechanism of sweating is shut off to maintain or conserve blood volume. When this happens, internal body temperature soars, giving way to a serious heat condition, heatstroke, which is discussed on p. 136.

Some athletes will use a sauna, steam bath, or whirlpool in an attempt to lose weight. This is accomplished by raising the skin's surface temperature, causing vasodilation and sweating to dissipate the increased heat. As the athlete sweats, he or she loses water weight. Body heat is more effectively dissipated in the sauna because sweat evaporates more readily in hot, dry air. Because sweat does not easily evaporate in a steam bath or whirlpool, this method can result in an increase in skin temperature and, in turn, in an increase in the body's core temperature. In addition, saunas, steam baths, and whirlpools contribute to an athlete's dehydration. To avoid the effects of heat-related conditions, athletes who are already dehydrated must be especially careful when using one of these methods of applying external heat.

Increased physical exertion during athletic activity, combined with varying degrees of increased air temperature and humidity, can place abnormal demands on the thermoregulatory system. When this system fails, or the heat gained exceeds that lost, athletes are subjected to the effect of heat-related conditions. This is especially prevalent during early season workouts. The athlete who is not acclimated to physical activity in hot, humid weather is particularly susceptible. Acclimation is an important preventive measure because most serious heat-related problems occur in the first few days of practice.

Heat acclimation
Heat acclimation is the process of becoming accustomed to athletic activity in hot weather. It improves the circulatory and sweating responses and facilitates the dissipation of heat. Heat acclimation helps minimize changes in body temperature. Acclimation renders the athlete more capable of adapting to or tolerating the stresses of heat and is the most efficient method of handling increased external temperatures. The acclimated athlete exhibits less heat stress during workouts in hot, humid weather than does the nonacclimated athlete. As an athlete becomes acclimated, several important body adjustments occur to allow the athlete to more effectively handle the stresses of heat. The body responds to heat acclimation by increasing cardiac output, circulating blood volume, and venous tone. The basal metabolic rate, core temperature, and pulse rate are reduced. In addition, the body is able to more precisely regulate sweat production, electrolyte concentrations, and peripheral blood flow and maintain a more stable blood pressure under varying conditions of stress.

For heat acclimation to occur, athletes must work out or exercise in hot weather. It is best for an athlete to acclimate gradually over a period of time before scheduled practices or an athletic season begins. Each athlete will acclimate at a different rate. Further, the athlete in good condition is capable of more work in the heat and will acclimate more rapidly than the nonconditioned athlete. It is believed that optimal acclimation requires an athlete to exercise with progressively increasing intensities between 1 to 2 hours daily. With this type of schedule, acclimation is usually well developed in 5 to 7 days and complete in 12 to 14 days. In addition, athletes should have adequate access to water during the acclimation period because withholding fluids significantly retards this process.

Some athletes use a sauna to acclimatize to warm weather conditions. This method of acclimation is more common for athletes exercising in moderate climates as they prepare for competition in a hot, humid climate. This process is generally believed to be safe if the athletes are monitored and rehydration is practiced. Another method used to acclimatize athletes for competition in hot, humid climates is to exercise while wearing excess clothing or a nylon sweat suit. These procedures stimulate the microenvironment around the body and increases the skin temperature. Although this method may be successful in improving an athlete's ability to tolerate exercise in warmer environments, caution must be used.

Heat-Related Conditions

Three specific heat illnesses or syndromes can result from thermal exposure: (1) heat cramps, (2) heat exhaustion, and (3) heatstroke. These three are listed in order from the least serious to the most serious. Each is normally caused by the same set of circumstances; that is, strenuous activity in a combination of hot and humid weather, resulting in a loss of body water and a derangement of the body's thermoregulatory system. Although the cause of these heat-related conditions is normally the same, each represents a different bodily reaction to excessive heat, with its own set of signs and symptoms and treatment procedures. It

is extremely important for athletic trainers to be familiar with signs and symptoms that indicate the development of heat illnesses, as well as emergency measures necessary to adequately care for athletes suffering from serious heat stress.

It is important to remember that heat cramps and heat exhaustion can lead to heatstroke. This is especially true when working with athletes. In most types of activity, a person will voluntarily stop working and seek relief from the heat when heat cramps or heat exhaustion appears to be developing. Athletes, on the other hand, especially highly competitive or motivated athletes, are more likely to continue working out or exercising even though symptoms may be developing. Athletes in a sport such as football are required to wear heavy protective equipment and uniforms that cover much of the body and add to the problem of heat dissipation. Athletes are also engaged in strenuous activity under the influence of the coaches' or trainers' philosophies concerning the number of breaks, availability of water, and the intensity of the exercise sessions. All of these factors are pertinent to the development of heat-related conditions.

✤ *Heat cramps*

Heat cramps are the least serious of the three heat illnesses. These cramps are painful spasms of skeletal muscles. Past training literature suggested that heat cramps are caused by salt or electrolyte loss. More recent literature, however, suggests that heat cramps result from a fluid volume problem and can normally be prevented by providing unlimited amounts of water to athletes throughout activity in hot weather.

When heat cramps occur, they normally accompany strenuous physical activity and profuse sweating in hot weather. The most common muscles involved are the calf muscles or abdominals, but any of the voluntary muscles can be affected by a sudden and painful spasm or cramp. Heat cramps may be mild, with slight cramping, or they may be quite severe and incapacitating, with intense pain. Athletes suffering heat cramps

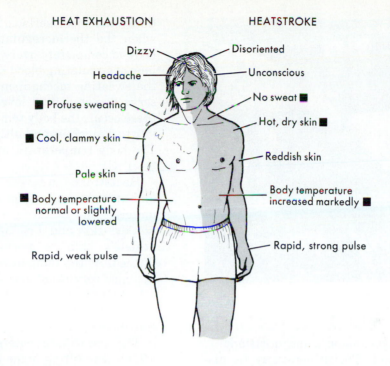

HEAT EXHAUSTION   HEATSTROKE

Dizzy —   — Disoriented

Headache —   — Unconscious

■ Profuse sweating —   — No sweat ■

■ Cool, clammy skin —   — Hot, dry skin ■

Pale skin —   — Reddish skin

■ Body temperature   — Body temperature
normal or slightly   increased markedly ■
lowered

Rapid, weak pulse —   — Rapid, strong pulse

FIGURE 7-7
Main signs and symptoms associated with heat
exhaustion and heatstroke.

are normally alert and oriented to their surroundings. The skin will be wet and warm
as a result of excessive sweating. The body
temperature, pulse, and respiratory rate
should be normal or slightly elevated.

In most cases heat cramps are not a serious problem and can be relieved by slowly
stretching the contracted muscle. The application of ice, firm pressure, or gentle mas-
sage to the area may facilitate relief. The
athlete should also be encouraged to drink
liquids. Many times the athlete will resume
activity after alleviation of the muscle
spasms; however, a severe episode of heat
cramps may require the athlete to avoid further exertion for a longer period of time, perhaps 12 to 24 hours. Should heat cramps frequently recur in the same athlete, additional
assessment of specific causes is warranted,
and medical referral may be necessary. Remember, athletes who suffer heat cramps
should be closely observed because this condition may precipitate heat exhaustion or
heatstroke.

Heat exhaustion

✤ **Heat exhaustion** is probably the most common condition caused by exertion in hot
weather. The physiologic basis for heat exhaustion has been previously described; that
is, peripheral vasodilation, loss of vasomotor
control, and vascular pooling. Because of
this peripheral vascular collapse, these athletes are suffering from an abnormally decreased volume of blood (hypovolemia) circulating in the body.

It is important for an athletic trainer to
recognize the signs and symptoms associated with heat exhaustion and be able to differentiate them from those associated with
heatstroke. Figure 7-7 illustrates the main
signs and symptoms associated with both
conditions, with a block representing those
most important.

Heat exhaustion is characterized by profuse sweating, which makes the skin wet,
cool, and clammy. The skin may also appear
pale or gray. The decrease in blood volume
normally results in headache, weakness,

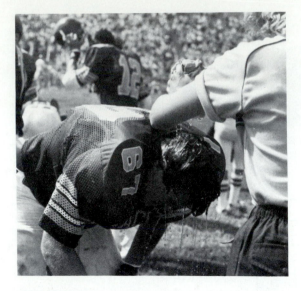

FIGURE 7-8
Assisting the cooling process.

dizziness, fatigue, nausea, and, occasionally, unconsciousness. The athlete may be disoriented, and heat cramps may accompany this condition. The body temperature is usually normal or slightly below normal, and the respiration is usually fast and shallow. Heat exhaustion may lead to complete collapse of the thermoregulatory system if not properly identified and treated.

Heat exhaustion is normally not life threatening, but proper medical care is required. The athlete should be treated as if in shock; that is, taken out of the hot environment and placed supine with the feet elevated. Remove as much equipment and uniform as possible. The cooling process can be assisted by sponging or toweling the athlete with cool water (Figure 7-8). If the athlete is conscious, allow him or her to drink cool fluids. The athlete will normally feel better in a short period of time; however, if symptoms persist, the athlete should be transported to a medical facility. Athletes suffering heat exhaustion should be withdrawn from further activity for the remainder of that day and closely observed. Fluids should be encouraged and monitored.

Heatstroke

✤ **Heatstroke** (sunstroke) is the least common of the heat-related conditions but certainly the most serious. Heatstroke occurs when the thermoregulatory system of the body is completely overwhelmed or the volume of circulating blood becomes so low that the sweating mechanism is shut off to conserve depleted fluid levels. When either of these occur, the body temperature rises rapidly to dangerous and ultimately fatal levels. The body temperature may go over 106° F (41.1° C).

Heatstroke is a severe medical emergency and must be recognized and treated immediately. This condition is characterized by hot, dry skin and a rising temperature. The athlete's skin is normally reddened or flushed. As the temperature rises, the pulse becomes very rapid and strong. Initially the athlete may experience headache, dizziness, and weakness, which are often followed by convulsions and unconsciousness.

The immediate emergency care for an athlete exhibiting signs of heatstroke is to reduce the body temperature as quickly as possible by any means available. This may include cooling the body by placing ice or cold towels around the body, immersing the athlete in cold water, directing a fan at the athlete, or sponging the body with cool water or alcohol. Remove clothing and equipment to prevent the retention of body heat. If the athlete is conscious, allow him to drink cool water. Athletes suffering from heatstroke are critically ill and must be taken to a medical facility as soon as possible. Aggressive efforts to lower the body temperature should continue during the referral and transfer process.

Preventive Measures

Although acclimation is probably the most important method of preventing problems related to heat stress, there are other measures an athletic trainer can take to prevent or reduce the impact of heat stress on the body.

Medical history. Obtain a complete medical history, including any previous heat illnesses or problems caused by the heat. Has the athlete ever fainted from excessive heat? Has the athlete ever had any sweating problems? Athletes who have suffered previous heat-related problems may have some permanent damage to the thermoregulatory center and are more prone to future heat disorders.

Physical condition. Evaluate the general physical condition of the athlete. Has he or she been working out in the heat? Inquire about the duration and intensity of work and training activities. In some sports, athletes may be required to complete a physical fitness test, such as a 12-minute run, before hot weather practice. Athletes in poor physical condition are candidates for heat illness. In addition, athletes who are overfat have an appreciably decreased ability to dissipate heat.

Recording temperature and humidity. It is important for the athletic trainer to measure the temperature and humidity during hot weather activity. The information an athletic trainer must have to make reasonable estimates of the severity of climatic conditions as they may affect athletes is minimal. Effective environmental guide-

lines can be constructed from easy-to-obtain temperature and humidity measurements taken on the practice or playing fields. These measurements should be made before and during training sessions, and adjustments or modifications in activity made if so indicated. These adjustments include decreasing intensity levels of activity, providing more breaks and fluids, eliminating unnecessary clothing, or delaying or postponing practices until conditions improve.

There are several methods of monitoring the temperature and humidity. These readings can be obtained from the local weather bureau and then charted on a graph such as Figure 7-9. This type of guide was developed from weather data gathered at the time of heatstroke fatalities occurring in football. Any combination of environmental conditions in zone 1 would be considered safe. Conditions in zone 2 would be a warning area, and athletes would need to be carefully observed for signs and symptoms of heat illness. Zone 3 would be the danger area. If

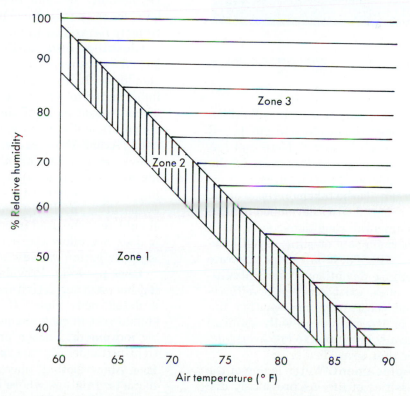

FIGURE 7-9
Weather guide for the prevention of heat stress.

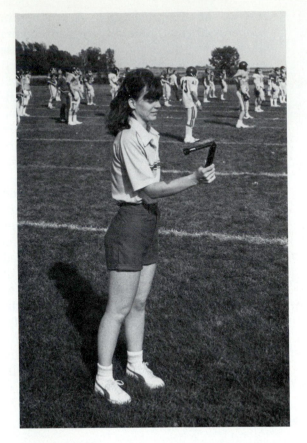

FIGURE 7-10
Using a sling psychrometer to monitor environmental conditions.

conditions in this zone were present, practices would have to be modified or postponed and athletes closely observed. Note that humidity is a significant factor, even in the presence of moderate temperatures.

Readings can also be taken on the athletic field using various devices developed to measure environmental conditions, such as a wet-bulb thermometer or sling psychrometer (Figure 7-10). These are more accurate methods because deviations of several critical degrees often exist between on-site recordings and those from the weather bureau. This is especially true with artificial surfaces because they tend to be several degrees hotter than grass fields.

Fluid replacement. Water is one of the major necessities of life. As previously discussed, decreased body fluids associated with profuse sweating diminishes the avail-

able blood volume and sweating necessary for body cooling. Dehydration can impair mental and physical performance and lead to severe heat-related conditions. **Fluids must be provided.** Ideally, for the body to remain in balance, water input must equal water output. Thirst alone is not an accurate indicator of body water needs. During intense exercise, more than 3 quarts of sweat can be lost in an hour, depending on weather conditions and the type of clothing worn. Athletes exercising in the heat never voluntarily drink as much water as they lose sweating. The fluid intake is usually about one half to two thirds of the water lost in sweat. Prevention of dehydration during work in hot weather requires scheduled fluid intakes and, perhaps, forcing fluids. Athletes should have unlimited and easy access to water during all athletic activity in hot weather (Figure 7-11). It is better for athletes to drink small amounts frequently than to schedule a break every hour or so, when they may gulp large amounts of water. Deliberately withholding water from athletes for purposes of weight loss may be extremely hazardous in hot weather.

Clothing and uniforms. In hot or humid weather, clothing and uniforms should be light-weight, loose fitting, and light colored to reflect the sun. Porous or net shirts expose more of the body surface for evaporation of sweat and dissipation of body heat. Avoid the use of long socks, long sleeves, excess clothing, and sweat suits during hot weather activity. This type of clothing can seriously limit heat loss by reducing evaporative cooling. Rubberized clothing should never be used in hot weather because it does not allow the evaporation of sweat and dissipation of body heat.

Rest periods. Provide rest periods during hot weather activities to dissipate accumulated body heat. If possible, athletes should rest in cool, shaded areas with some air movement. Loosen or remove heavy or tight-fitting jerseys to expose more skin surface. Allow football players to remove their helmets. In areas where hot weather conditions are especially severe, unique arrangements for moving air, such as placement of

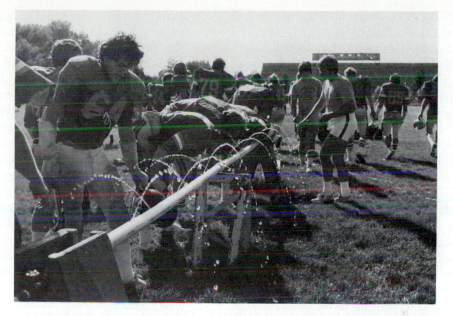

FIGURE 7-11
Athletes enjoying free access to water during practice.

large fans, may be required. Athletes also need to get adequate sleep at night.

Weight charts. Weight charts can facilitate the detection of an athlete who may be more susceptible to heat stress. Serious heat conditions usually occur in the individuals who lose the most body water. Athletes who have a large muscle mass or are overweight seem to be particularly susceptible. Daily measurements of weight loss, which mainly reflects water loss, should be taken and recorded. Athletes losing excessive amounts of weight each day, in excess of 3% of their body weight, which is not made up in a 24-hour period, should be observed carefully; they may be candidates for heat illness. Depending on the environmental conditions and the acclimation timetable, there are times when athletes should be weighed in and out of practice. Fluids can then be adjusted according to their weight loss.

Diet. A well-balanced diet is essential to athletic activity. A diet high in carbohydrates, 60% to 65% of caloric intake, will normally replenish electrolytes or body minerals lost during hot weather and provide the energy requirements necessary to help the body resist the effects of the heat. Suf-

ficient salt replacement will also occur with a balanced diet and it is not recommended that athletes ingest salt tablets.

Summary

The body's response to thermal exposure is basically one of maintaining heat balance; that is, the same amount of heat must be lost as produced or gained by the body during activity in hot weather. Heat is gained by the body mainly through metabolism but may also be gained through radiation, convection, and conduction. Heat is lost from the body by radiation, convection, conduction, and evaporation. The body functions to maintain a relatively constant temperature through the thermoregulatory system.

Our body eliminates heat gained during activity in hot weather, primarily by cutaneous vasodilation and sweating. Peripheral blood flow is increased to transfer heat from the core of the body to the periphery, where it can be dissipated. The evaporation of sweat from the skin's surface is the body's major defense mechanism against overheating. There are many factors, both internal and external, that influence or affect these two important heat-dissipating mechanisms. Whenever abnormal demands are placed on the thermoregulatory system and the heat gained exceeds that lost, athletes are subjected to the effects of heat-related conditions. These conditions can be significantly reduced by heat acclimation, adequate water replacement, and the awareness of various factors imposed on the athlete by the combinations of exercise, environment, and clothing.

Heat-related conditions include heat cramps, heat exhaustion, and heatstroke. Heat cramps are the least serious, heat exhaustion the most common, and heatstroke the most serious. Each of these is caused by basically the same set of circumstances, but each represents a different bodily reaction to excessive heat. It is extremely important for the athletic trainer to be familiar with signs and symptoms that indicate the development of these heat conditions, as well as emergency measures that should be immediately initiated if they occur.

BODY RESPONSE TO COLD EXPOSURE

Unlike heat-related conditions, injuries resulting from exposure to cold are not as big a problem in athletics. Of course, activities such as ice-skating and skiing are normally performed in cold weather. Athletes running or jogging outside during the winter months are subjected to cold environmental conditions. Occasionally other sports, due to a change in the weather, must be performed in a cold environment. Exposure to cold under these circumstances normally does not present a significant problem for two reasons: (1) exercise, as previously discussed, increases the heat production of the body, and (2) adequate clothing is usually worn by the athlete.

Humans possess much less capacity for adaptation to prolonged exposure to cold than to that of heat. However, it does appear that athletes can enhance their thermoregulatory defense to a certain extent against cold stress when exposed to regular and prolonged cold. This may be attributed to an elevated resting metabolism, some peripheral adaptations that increase blood flow

through areas subjected to repeated cold exposure, a more sensitive and larger shivering response, or an apparent psychological "toughness."

Just like evaluating the thermal quality of a warm environment, temperature alone is not always a valid indication of how cold it is. An important factor is the wind. On a windy day, air currents magnify heat loss as the warmer insulating air layer surrounding the body is continually replaced by cooler air. The cooling effect of wind is clearly shown in the Wind Chill Index presented in Figure 7-12. This figure illustrates the effects of wind velocity on bare skin for different temperatures and velocities. In addition, if an athlete runs, skates, or skis into the wind the effective cooling from the wind is increased in direct relation to the athlete's velocity. Conversely, performing athletic activity with the wind at the athlete's back creates less relative wind speed. The wind chill chart is divided into three areas or zones. In the zone on the left there is relatively little danger from cold exposure for a properly clothed athlete. In the middle zone there is increasing danger to exposed flesh, especially the ears, fingers, and nose. In the zone on the right there is serious danger to the freezing of exposed flesh within a matter of minutes.

Even though exposure to cold is seldom a problem, athletic trainers should possess a basic knowledge of how the body responds to cold, as well as the associated signs and symptoms and emergency measures necessary to care for athletes suffering from cold-related injuries.

Physiologic Basis of Cold Exposure

The physiologic basis required for regulation of a constant core temperature has been discussed. Just as the body has mechanisms to guard against overheating, there are thermoregulatory mechanisms designed to prevent abnormal cooling (hypothermia).

Heat production

As previously described, metabolism is the body's main source of heat. During cold weather, an athlete will normally increase his or her muscular activity in an effort to increase metabolism, thus producing more heat to stay warm. If the voluntary increase in muscular activity is not sufficient, the athlete normally begins to shiver, which also increases metabolism. If the core temperature continues to drop, the basal metabolic rate accelerates in an effort to increase heat production.

Heat preservation

During cold weather, the body attempts to conserve heat and maintain its core temperature. The skin and subcutaneous tissue, especially fat, form a natural insulation. As the body temperature decreases, cutaneous vasoconstriction occurs, shunting blood away from the skin and the cold environment to which it is exposed. This prevents excessive transfer of heat from warmer parts of the body to the areas being cooled by significantly reducing the amount of blood circulating in the extremities. This does not include the head, from which, on a cold day, a large amount of heat can be lost if it is uncovered. This vasoconstriction decreases surface temperature of the extremities, making them more susceptible to the injurious effects of exposure to cold. This is especially true of the fingers or toes because they provide a large surface area that is often poorly protected.

Athletes provide additional insulation to the cold weather by the clothing worn. The effectiveness of this insulation depends on thickness and layering more than the type or style of clothing.

Heat transmission

Heat is transmitted, or lost, from the body primarily by the mechanisms described earlier; that is, radiation, conduction, convection, and evaporation. Depending on the severity of exposure, athletes must attempt to reduce the transmission of heat from the body to prevent cold-related injuries. The amount of heat lost through radiation can be reduced by covering the exposed surface areas of the body, especially the head. Other body areas with a large surface/volume ratio, such as the ears, hands, and feet, are also particularly likely to lose heat by radiation. Reducing heat loss by conduction is accomplished mainly by avoiding contact with objects colder than the body. When the object is large and a good conductor of heat, such as water or metal, the heat loss can be considerable. Decreasing heat loss by convection can be achieved primarily by avoiding the cold wind and dressing appropriately. Persons exposed to a cold environment are normally not sweating. However, athletes who exercise or perform in cold weather usually sweat. Sweating dampens the clothing, which aids in the conduction of heat away from the body. Therefore, during cold weather, athletes should wear several layers of light, loose clothing that will trap air, a very effective insulator, and provide adequate ventilation to allow moisture to escape. Athletes should also change clothing, especially socks and gloves, when they become damp with perspiration. Clothing that becomes wet loses its ability to trap air and increases conductive heat loss by up to 20 times over dry clothing.

Cold-related Conditions

When heat regulating mechanisms fail or are insufficient to maintain the temperature of the core (brain, lungs, heart and abdominal organs) or shell (skin, muscles, and extremities), injury from cold can occur. There are two specific cold-related conditions that may result from cold exposure: (1) **frostbite** and (2) **hypothermia.** Although these conditions are seldom a problem in athletics, athletic trainers should be familiar with signs and symptoms that indicate their development, as well as emergency procedures necessary to adequately care for athletes suffering from exposure to cold. It is important to recognize the early stages of cold-related conditions and take preventive measures to avoid serious consequences.

❖ **Frostbite**

Frostbite is freezing of a part of the body and occurs when the heat supply to that part is insufficient to counteract the heat loss, causing the intracellular and interstitial water to crystallize. The resulting mechanical

Windchill Index

Cooling power of wind expressed as "eqivalent chill temperature"

Wind speed		Temperature (°F)																
Knots	Mph																	
Calm	Calm	40	35	30	25	20	15	10	5	0	-5	-10	-15	-20	-25	-30	-35	-40
3-6	5	35	30	25	20	15	10	5	0	-5	-10	-15	-20	-25	-30	-35	-40	-45
7-10	10	30	20	15	10	5	0	-10	-15	-20	-25	-35	-40	-45	-50	-60	-65	-70
11-15	15	25	15	10	0	-5	-10	-20	-25	-30	-40	-45	-50	-60	-65	-70	-80	-85
16-19	20	20	10	5	0	-10	-15	-25	-30	-35	-45	-50	-60	-65	-75	-80	-85	-95
20-23	25	15	10	0	-5	-15	-20	-30	-35	-45	-50	-60	-65	-75	-80	-90	-95	-105
24-28	30	10	5	0	-10	-20	-25	-30	-40	-50	-55	-65	-70	-80	-85	-95	-100	-110
29-32	35	10	5	-5	-10	-20	-30	-35	-40	-50	-60	-65	-75	-80	-90	-100	-105	-115
33-36	40	10	0	-5	-15	-20	-30	-35	-45	-55	-60	-70	-75	-85	-95	-100	-110	-115

Winds above 40 have little additional effect

Little danger

Increasing danger
(Flesh may freeze within 1 minute)

Great danger
(Flesh may freeze within 30 seconds)

Danger of freezing exposed flesh for properly clothed persons

Courtesy Director of Plans and Training, USARAL. In Alaska Med, March 1973.

FIGURE 7-12
Wind Chill Index

TABLE 7-1

Signs and Symptoms of Frostbite

Severity of frostbite	Skin color and appearance
Frostnip—1°	Initially red, then white—Painless Skin soft
Superficial—2°	White and waxy—Numb Skin firm but soft tissue beneath
Deep—3°	Blotchy, white to purplish tinge—Numb Skin solid the entire depth

damage caused by formation of ice particles can result in tissue injury or death. The frozen area is normally small and commonly occurs on exposed body areas such as the nose, ears, cheeks, or fingers. However, unexposed body areas such as the toes may also be affected. The penis is another commonly affected area of the body, especially in the northern climates. This condition occurs when an inadequately clothed but perspiring male athlete is running in extremely cold temperatures. With growing numbers of year-round runners and the common use of nylon shorts, the incidence of this condition is increasing. The extent of the injury from frostbite depends on such factors as temperature, wind velocity, duration of exposure, humidity, lack of protective clothing, or the presence of wet clothing.

There are various degrees of frostbite (Table 7-1). A minor case, or first-degree frostbite, often called **frostnip,** involves the skin's surface. The affected skin may at first become flushed or reddened because superficial blood vessels dilate in an attempt by the body to protect the area against frostbite. Burning and tingling sensations are common. With continued exposure, the skin may suddenly turn white and become painless. Because of this loss of sensation, the athlete may be unaware of the danger. This is the most common type of frostbite affecting athletes and, if identified early, can be reversed without any tissue damage. The treatment consists of rewarming by some means, such as covering the area, holding a warm hand over the area, blowing hot breath against the area, or holding the frost-nipped portion against the body. Rewarming usually produces burning and itching sensations accompanied by local redness and swelling.

Superficial frostbite involves the skin and subcutaneous tissue. The skin becomes firm, white, and waxy, although the tissue beneath it remains soft. Athletes with superficial frostbite should be removed from the cold, and the affected area should be carefully rewarmed as described for frostnip or in a warm water bath (100° F to 105° F). The area should not be rubbed. As the area is warmed, it may turn purple and swell. If superficial capillaries are damaged, edematous fluid will leak out into the tissue, causing superficial blisters to appear. Stinging, burning, or aching pain may follow and last several days to weeks. This area of the body is often extremely sensitive to further cold exposure and should be protected during additional activity in cold weather.

Deep frostbite involves freezing of the entire tissue depth, including muscles and bone. This type of frostbite occurs when someone is exposed to freezing weather for a prolonged period of time. This is a serious injury, and these persons should be transported to a medical facility immediately. There is often permanent damage associated with this type of injury.

✤ *Hypothermia*

Hypothermia is a condition in which the core temperature falls below 95° F (35° C). At temperatures below 95° F the body's thermoregulatory mechanism is overwhelmed, and the body is unable to rewarm itself without outside assistance. If the body temperature drops below 86° F (30° C), a life-threatening medical emergency exists. This condition will seldom affect an athlete, but if present, can result in a serious and potentially fatal injury. Participation in winter sports such as cross-country skiing can present opportunities that may result in a general cooling of the body to dangerous levels. In most cases of athletic-related hypothermia, exhaustion is a predisposing problem.

TABLE 7-2

Signs and Symptoms of Hypothermia

Core body temperature		Signs and symptoms
°C	°F	
37	98.6	Periperhal vasoconstriction; ↑ heart rate, ↑ respiratory rate
35	95	↑ Muscle tone, shivering ensues
32	89.6	Dilated pupils; muscular rigidity, shivering ceases, altered mental status, poor judgment
30	86	Basal metabolic rate depressed; ↓ heart rate, ↓ respiratory rate
28	82.4	Cardiac arrhythmias
27	80.6	Coma, no voluntary motion
25	77	Hypotension and shock; spontaneous ventricular fibrillation
24	75.2	Respiratory arrest
21	68	Cardiac standstill
18	64.4	Lowest accidental hypothermia recovery

In addition to cold temperatures, wind and wetness are major contributing environmental factors.

The degree of hypothermia present determines the signs and symptoms manifested. As can be seen in Table 7-2, as the core body temperature falls, drastic changes in respiration and cellular metabolism occur, and the associated signs and symptoms become progressively more severe. Early signs of hypothermia include shivering, depressed respiration, and a slow irregular pulse. The skin is cold and pale. As body temperature decreases, a person may show signs of an altered mental state, such as irritability, incoordination, stumbling, clumsiness, weakness, and difficulty in speaking. Continued temperature depression leads to muscular rigidity, collapse, coma, and failure of the respiratory and cardiovascular systems. The treatment of hypothermia is basically to prevent further heat loss, rewarm, and promptly transport to a medical facility. Rewarming techniques are usually grouped into passive rewarming, active external rewarming, or active core rewarming. Passive rewarming is removing the individual from exposure to the environment and using some type of insulating material, such as blankets. Passive rewarming is probably the only technique required of an athletic trainer in an athletic setting.

Summary

The body's response to cold exposure is primarily one of maintaining a constant core temperature. Just as the body has mechanisms to guard against overheating, there are thermoregulatory mechanisms designed to prevent abnormal cooling. Metabolism is the body's main source of heat. During cold weather, athletes normally increase muscular activity, which increases metabolism, producing more heat. If muscular activity is not sufficient, the athlete will begin to shiver, which also increases metabolism. The body also prevents an excessive transfer of heat from warmer parts of the body to the areas being cooled by cutaneous vasoconstriction, which reduces the amount of blood circulating in the extremities. Athletes can reduce the transmission of heat from the body by covering exposed surfaces, avoiding contact with colder objects or wind, and wearing several layers of light, dry, loose-fitting clothing.

Cold-related conditions include frostbite and hypothermia. Frostbite is freezing of a part of the body and can result in tissue damage or death. There are three degrees of frostbite. Frostnip involves only the skin's surface and can usually be easily reversed without any tissue damage by various means of rewarming. Superficial frostbite involves the skin and subcutaneous tissue, whereas deep frostbite involves the entire tissue depth, including muscles and bones. Superficial frostbite will often leave surface blisters after rewarming. There is often permanent damage associated with a deep frostbite.

Hypothermia is a condition in which the body temperature falls below 95° F (35° C), and the body is unable to warm itself without outside assistance. This condition seldom affects an athlete but can be a life-threatening emergency. The early signs of hypothermia include shivering, depressed respiration, and a slow, irregular pulse. The skin is cold and pale. As body temperature decreases, an athlete may show signs of an altered mental state and failure of the respiratory and cardiovascular systems. The treatment of hypothermia is to prevent further heat loss, rewarm the athlete by any means, and transport to a medical facility.

REFERENCES

American Academy of Pediatrics: Climatic heat stress and the exercising child, *Phys Sportsmed* 11(8):155, 1983.

Armstrong LE, Maresh CM: The induction and decay of heat acclimatization in trained athletes, *Sports Med* 12(5):302, 1991.

Bryant WM: Wound healing, *CIBA Clinical Symposia* 29:3, 1977.

Davidson M: Heat Illness in Athletes, *Ath Train* 20(2):96, 1985.

Doubt TJ: Physiology of exercise in the cold, *Sports Med* 11(6):367, 1991.

Duda M: The medical risks and benefits of sauna, steam bath, and whirlpool use, *Phys Sportsmed* 15(5):170, 1987.

Hafen BO, Karren KJ: *First aid for colleges and universities,* ed 4, Englewood Cliffs, 1993, Regents/Prentice Hall.

Hargarten D: Syncope in athletes: life threatening or benign, *Phys Sportsmed* 19(7):33, 1991.

Haynes EM: Physiological responses of female athletes to heat stress: review, *Phys Sportsmed* 12(3):45, 1984.

Hecker AL, Wheeler KB: Impact of hydration and energy intake on performance, *Ath Train* 19(4):260, 1984.

Heckman JD, editor: *Emergency care and transportation of the sick and injured,* ed 5, Park Ridge, 1992, American Academy of Orthopaedic Surgeons.

McArdle WD, Katch FI, Katch VL: *Exercise physiology: energy, nutrition, and human performance,* ed 3, Philadelphia, 1991, Lea & Febiger.

Murphy RJ: Heat Illness in the athlete, *Ath Train* 19(3):166, 1984.

Parcel GS: *Basic emergency care of the sick and injured,* ed 4, St Louis, 1990, Mosby-Year Book.

Nelson WE and others: Treatment and prevention of hypothermia and frostbite, *Ath Train* 18(4):330, 1983.

Vinger PF, Hoerner EF: *Sports injuries: the unthwarted epidemic,* Boston, 1982, John Wright—PSG.

SUGGESTED READINGS

American Academy of Orthopaedic Surgeons: *Athletic training and sports medicine,* ed 2, Park Ridge, IL, 1991, The Academy.
Chapter 8 does a good job of addressing the inflammatory process and the physiology of tissue repair.

Fox EL, Bowers RW, Foss ML: *The physiological basis of physical education and athletics,* ed 4, Philadelphia, 1988, WB Saunders.
One of the most highly respected texts for undergraduate exercise physiology courses.

Grant HD, Murray RH, Bergeron JD: *Emergency care,* ed 5, Englewood Cliffs, 1990, Prentice Hall.
A textbook often used in Emergency Medical Technician courses. Addresses all aspects of emergency medical care procedures.

Knight K: *Cryotherapy: theory, technique and physiology,* Chattanooga, 1985, Chattanooga Corporation.
An excellent guide to the physiological basis and clinical techniques involving the use of cold.

Reed B, Zarro V: In Michlovitz SL, editor: *Thermal agents in rehabilitation,* ed 2, Philadelphia, 1990, FA Davis.
Authors present a good chapter on inflammation and repair of body tissues.

Ryan GB, Majno G: *Inflammation: a scope publication,* Kalamazoo, 1977, Upjohn.
This monograph reviews the inflammatory process in an easily understandable format. The authors use numerous illustrations to help describe the mechanisms of the inflammatory reaction.

CHAPTER 8

Athletic injuries and related skin conditions

After you have completed this chapter, you should be able to:
- Briefly describe the structure and function of the epidermis, dermis, and accessory organs of the skin.
- Identify and describe the open wounds commonly found in athletic activity.
- List and describe the variety of skin lesions that can impair athletic performance.
- Identify and describe the unexposed injuries commonly occurring in athletic activity.

An **athletic injury** is defined as a disruption in tissue continuity that results from athletic or sports-related activity, causing a cessation of participation or restriction of usual activity. This definition implies that an athletic injury is more than the aches and pains that may accompany but not interfere with athletic participation. There is an almost infinite array of possibilities in the spectrum of athletic injuries, ranging from minor problems to severe and potentially lethal types of trauma. The care of athletic injuries also involves a wide range of treatment possibilities, from as little as the application of a Band-Aid to multiple operations and months of rehabilitation. Athletic injuries or illnesses that athletic trainers must often assess and manage are discussed in this chapter.

Athletic injuries result from the application of forces or stresses in excess of the body's or body part's ability to adapt. The manner and location by which these excess forces or stresses are applied to the body, better known as the **mechanism of injury,** determine the exact nature and extent of the injury and the tissues involved. These forces or stresses may be applied (1) instantaneously, resulting in an **acute traumatic injury,** or (2) over a considerable period of time, resulting in a **chronic overuse syndrome.** Traumatic injuries such as sprains, strains, and contusions are common to athletic activity, particularly during contact sports. Overuse syndromes such as tendinitis, bursitis, stress fractures, and shin splints are becoming much more common in athletic activity because of the increasing intensity of training and conditioning programs. As a group, overuse injuries occur more often in athletic activity requiring specific repetitive movements.

Athletic injuries are grouped into two main classifications, depending on the integrity of the skin: (1) **exposed** injuries, and (2) **unexposed** injuries. Exposed, or open, injuries disrupt the continuity of the skin. Unexposed, or closed, injuries are internal and do not break the skin. An athlete can suffer an injury in both classifications simultaneously; for example, an external blow resulting in a laceration and a contusion. This chapter deals with the skin, with athletic injuries in both classifications, and with the associated signs and symptoms that indicate presence of an injury. Guidelines for determining the severity of injury and when medical assistance should be sought are also present.

SKIN

The skin is the largest and one of the most important organs of the body, and when intact, serves as a barrier to protect us from many types of physical, chemical, and even biological attacks. In terms of surface area, the skin is as large as the body itself—probably 1.6 to 2.0 square meters (m²) in most adults. For the athletic trainer, the skin is often the window through which the physical assessment is performed. A large portion of the athletic injury assessment process takes place at the skin surface. Careful visual inspection of the skin, followed by palpation of structures beneath its surface, can provide valuable information when assessing athletic injuries. To gain this useful information, athletic trainers must possess a basic understanding of the anatomy, structure, and functions of the skin.

Visual Inspection

Unless a specific lesion is the chief complaint of the athlete, the initial visual examination of the skin during the secondary survey can be completed quickly. Look at the exposed skin surface in its entirety. Include in your examination the mucous membranes of the lips, mouth, and nasal openings. Assessment of specific skin lesions is covered later in this chapter.

Color, Temperature, and Texture

Skin color is influenced by a number of factors in addition to pigment distribution. For example, a bluish tint to the skin (cyanosis) may occur as a result of inadequate oxygenation of the blood, whereas a flushed or ruddy appearance may accompany fever or sunburn. Shock or exposure to cold temperatures will decrease blood flow to the skin and result in generalized pallor. Small, nonelevated patches of purplish or red discoloration may be the result of blood vessel trauma and localized hemorrhage into the layer of skin or mucous membranes. If very small or almost pinpoint in size, such localized lesions are called **petechiae** or petechial hemorrhages. Hemorrhagic spots larger than petechiae are called **ecchymoses.** Special attention should always be given to areas of increased or decreased pigmentation in skin that is otherwise normally pigmented.

In palpating the site of an injury, any detection of a localized increase in skin temperature suggests the presence of an inflammatory process or an increase in localized blood flow. A decrease in skin temperature is often noted in areas of inadequate circulation. In areas of swelling, the skin becomes stretched, and the texture feels tight and smooth. A highly skilled athletic trainer can detect edema in a body part by changes in skin texture long before obvious swelling occurs. Good assessment techniques and keen observational skills are especially important if the symptoms of a particular injury are insidious and gradual in their appearance. Remember, when involved in assessment of an injured extremity, always compare the skin and characteristics of the contralateral limb.

Anatomy and Structure

Two main layers compose the skin: an outer thinner layer, the **epidermis,** and an inner thicker layer, the **dermis** (Figure 8-1). The epidermis consists of stratified squamous epithelial tissue, the dermis consists of fibrous connective tissue. Underlying the dermis is *subcutaneous* tissue, or superficial fascia, made of areolar and, in many areas,

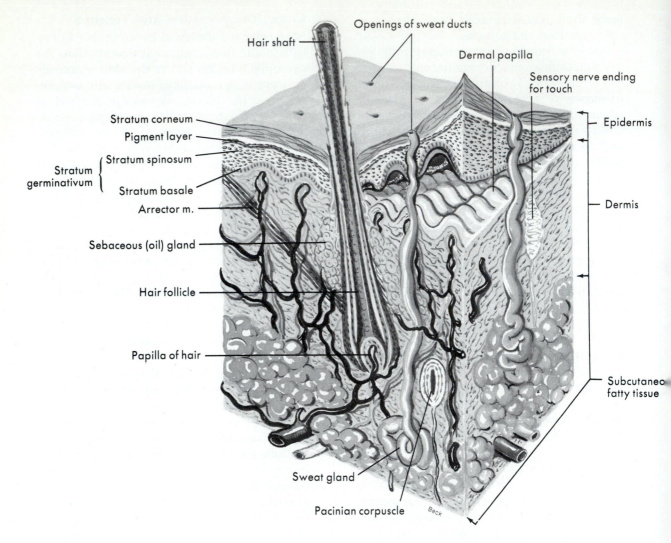

FIGURE 8-1
Microscopic view of the skin. The epidermis is shown raised at one corner to reveal the underlying dermis.

adipose tissue. The epidermis has four layers in all parts of the body except the palms of the hands and soles of the feet. In the skin of the palms and soles, there are five layers of epidermis. From the surface in, they are as follows:

1. *Stratum corneum* (horny layer): Dead cells converted to a water-repellent protein, called keratin, that continually flakes off (desquamates).

2. *Stratum lucidum* (Latin *lucidus,* clear): So named because of the presence of a translucent compound (elei-

din) from which keratin forms; present only in thick skin of palms and soles.

3. *Stratum granulosum* (granular cell layer): So named because of granules visible in the cytoplasm of cells (cells die in this layer).

4. *Stratum spinosum* (prickle-cell layer): Several layers of irregularly shaped cells.

5. *Stratum germinativum* (basal layer): Columnar-shaped cells, the only cells in the epidermis that undergo mitosis; new cells are produced in this deepest

stratum at the rate old keratinized cells are lost from the stratum corneum; new cells continually push surfaceward from the stratum germinativum into each successive layer, only to die, become keratinized, and eventually flake off, as did their predecessors. This fact illustrates nicely the physiologic principle that while life continues, the body's work is never done; even at rest it is producing new cells to replace millions of old ones.

An interesting characteristic of the dermis is its parallel ridges, suggestive on a miniature scale of the ridges of a contour-plowed field. Epidermal ridges, the ones made famous by the art of fingerprinting, exist because the epidermis conforms to the underlying dermal ridges.

Accessory Organs

The accessory organs of the skin consist of hair, nails, and microscopic glands.

Hair. Hair is distributed over the entire body except the palms and soles. The structure of a hair has several points of similarity to that of the epidermis. Just as the epidermis is formed by the cells of its deepest layer reproducing and forcing upward the daughter cells, which become horny in character, so a hair is formed by a group of cells at its base multiplying and pushing upward and in so doing becoming keratinized. The part of the hair that is visible is the shaft, whereas that which is embedded in the dermis is the root. The root, together with its coverings (an outer connective tissue sheath and an inner epithelial coating that is a continuation of the stratum germinativum), forms the hair follicle. At the bottom of the follicle is a loop of capillaries enclosed in a connective tissue covering called the hair papilla. The clusters of epithelial cells lying over the papilla are the ones that reproduce and eventually form the hair shaft. As long as these cells remain alive, hair will regenerate even though cut, plucked, or otherwise removed.

Each hair is kept soft and pliable by two or more sebaceous glands, which secrete varying amounts of oily sebum into the follicle near the surface of the skin. Attached to the follicle, too, are small bundles of involuntary muscle known as the arrector pili muscles. These muscles are of interest because when they contract, the hair stands on end, as it does in extreme fright or cold, for example. This mechanism is also responsible for gooseflesh. As the hair is pulled into an upright position, it raises the skin around it into the familiar little goose pimples.

Hair color results from different amounts of melanin pigments in the outer layer (cortex) of the hair. White hair contains little or no melanin.

Some hair, notably that around the eyes and in the nose and ears, performs a protective function in that it keeps out some dust, other types of particulate matter, and insects. For the hair on the bulk of the skin, however, no function seems apparent.

Nails. The nails are epidermal cells that have been converted to keratin. They grow from epithelial cells lying under the white crescent (lunula) at the proximal end of each nail.

Glands. The skin glands include three kinds of microscopic glands, namely, sebaceous, sweat, and ceruminous.

Sebaceous glands secrete oil for the hair. Wherever hairs grow from the skin, there are sebaceous glands, at least two for each hair. The oil, or sebum, secreted by these tiny glands has value not only because it keeps the hair supple but also because it keeps the skin soft and pliable. Moreover, it prevents excessive water evaporation from the skin and water absorption through the skin. And because fat is a poor conductor of heat, the sebum secreted into the skin lessens the amount of heat lost from this large surface. A **sebaceous cyst** may develop at this gland.

Sweat glands, although very small structures, are important and numerous—especially on the palms, soles, forehead, and axillae (armpits). Histologists estimate that a single square inch of skin on the palms of the hands contains about 3000 sweat glands. An athlete who sweats excessively is suffering from **hyperhidrosis.** An inflammation of noncontagious eruptions of red pimples

✦ with intense itching and tingling around the sweat ducts is called **prickly heat.**

Ceruminous glands are thought to be modified sweat glands. They are located in the external ear canal. Instead of watery sweat, they secrete a waxy, pigmented substance, the cerumen.

Functions

Vital, diverse, complex, extensive—these adjectives describe in part the function of the skin, its accessory organs, and related structures. Skin functions are crucial to survival and include protection from trauma (physical, chemical, biologic, and thermal), excretion, and sensation. In addition, the skin plays an extremely important role in maintaining fluid and electrolyte balance and normal body temperature. Sweat, in evaporating, cools the body surface. It also contains some nitrogenous wastes and therefore serves as a vehicle for both excretion and water loss.

In athletics, the function of the skin in temperature regulation is particularly important. The skin is very vascular and contains a large number of uniquely arranged blood vessels. The number of capillaries in the skin far exceeds what is required. Therefore, under resting conditions, a large quantity of blood is normally shunted around the excess capillary beds through direct connections (anastomoses) between small arteries and veins. These arteriovenous anastomoses can be closed if the internal body temperature increases, such as occurs in strenuous exercise. If these shunt vessels are closed, blood is forced into the many extra capillary beds near the skin surface, and excessive heat can be radiated into the environment.

EXPOSED ATHLETIC INJURIES

Exposed athletic injuries are those in which there is a disruption in the continuity of the skin. These injuries are common in athletics and include open wounds and various skin lesions that may or may not break the skin.

Open Wounds

Open wounds are normally caused by physical trauma and may range from a simple scratch to a large, deep, freely bleeding laceration. Table 8-1 outlines the five common types of open wounds. It is important for the athletic trainer to remember that an open wound may only be surface evidence of a more severe and often "hidden" athletic injury. Most open or exposed athletic injuries are minor in severity and do not result in significant hemorrhaging or loss of tissue. However, any bleeding must be controlled before a complete evaluation of the wound itself or of the possible involvement of deeper anatomic structures. The application of direct pressure over the site of bleeding, preferably with a sterile dressing (Figure 8-2), should be sufficient to control the hemorrhaging of most open wounds. The risk of infection is usually a greater concern for the athletic trainer treating an exposed wound than the amount of bleeding. Any open wound is susceptible to contamination with pathogenic bacteria or other harmful microorganisms. They may enter the body through even the smallest break in the skin. Contaminants may also be carried into the body by the object causing the wound. Although not all open wounds bleed freely, the flow of blood can aid in flushing out contaminants. Therefore minor wounds can be cleaned while they are bleeding in an attempt to clean out all dirty material and contaminants. The signs and symptoms of a wound infection generally appear 8 to 48 hours after the injury occurs. The typical signs and symptoms of a wound infection can be readily remembered by the acronym SHARP, which stands for *S*welling, *H*eat, *A*ching, *R*edness, and *P*us. Wound infections should be recognized and promptly managed or referred to a physician for definitive treatment.

Athletic trainers must also remember to protect themselves whenever working with open wounds or when any bodily fluids are present. The athlete may have a systemic infection or the open lesion may contain some type of pathogenic microorganism. Personal health demands attention to infection barriers and proper hygiene. Hands should be washed thoroughly before and after contact. Disposable gloves should be

TABLE 8-1

Types of Open Wounds

Type	Cause	Characteristics	Care
Abrasion	Fall Scraping or rubbing portion of skin away	Superficial Little bleeding, oozing, or weeping	Clean Remove debris Apply antiseptic treatment Apply sterile dressing Change dressing daily
Laceration	Wound made by tearing	Jagged edges May bleed freely Contusion and tearing Often leaves scar	Control bleeding Clean Suture if necessary Inspect daily
Incision	Cut by sharp object	Smooth edges Freely bleeding	Control bleeding Clean Suture if necessary Inspect daily
Puncture	Penetration by sharp object	Small opening Minimal bleeding	Clean Refer to medical assistance Inspect daily
Avulsion	Tearing loose flap of skin	Completely loose Hanging as a flap May bleed freely	Control bleeding Clean Save avulsed tissue Refer

worn anytime you are working with body flu-ids. Any equipment or instruments used in conjunction with an open wound should be thoroughly cleaned and disinfected before and after each use. An infection control pro-gram begins with one's own personal health.

❖ *Abrasions*

Abrasions occur when the epidermis and a portion of the dermis is scraped or rubbed away (Figure 8-3). This type of injury is very common in athletic activity and is usually caused by falling on a firm or rough surface. Athletes commonly refer to abrasions as "turf burns," "mat burns," "floor burns," or "cinder burns," depending on the surface that caused them. A reddish, irregular sur-face appearance gives rise to the descriptive name "strawberry." The bleeding associated with abrasions is usually limited to blood oozing from underlying injured capillaries. Although these injuries may be painful, the primary concern is that of infection. The abraded area will often contain contami-nants such as bits of dirt, debris, or bacteria embedded in the injured tissue.

An abrasion must be cleaned thoroughly.

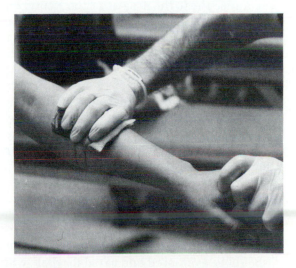

FIGURE 8-2
Application of direct pressure to control bleeding.

Soap and water will work well, but the area should be cleaned with an antibacterial scrub. Care must be taken to remove all for-eign material from the wound. Any dirt or debris left in an abrased area may cause in-fection or become incorporated into the heal-ing tissue and leave an unsightly "traumatic

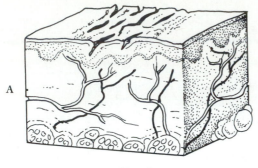

Abrasion

FIGURE 8-3
Abrasion. **A**, Schematic of typical abrasion injury.
Note that tissue damage is confined to epidermis. **B**,
Posterior forearm abrasion.

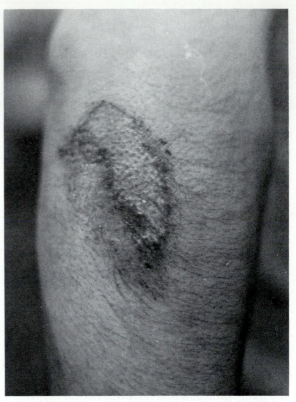

B

tattoo." Depending on the circumstances of
injury, you may have to use a soft brush to
clean the area thoroughly. A traditional
method of caring for an abrasion is to apply
an antiseptic to the area after the wound has
been cleaned and cover with a sterile, non-
adhesive dressing. An ointment dressing is
often applied when the abrasion is in the
vicinity of a joint so that a scab does not form
and be continually reopened during activity.

The contemporary treatment of abrasions
involves various self-adherent occlusive, hydrocolloid dressings. These dressings, applied after the abrasion has been thoroughly
cleaned, do not allow a scab to form by keeping the wound moist. This method has
shown to allow re-epithelialization to occur
faster than abrasions exposed to air. Occlusive dressings also assist in relieving the
pain associated with abrasions. Abrasions
should be evaluated and cared for daily with
either of these treatment routines. An abrasion should be referred to a physician for any
of the following reasons:

1. It is impossible to remove all the foreign material by washing the wound.
2. The area surrounding the abrasion becomes inflamed and infected a few
   days after the injury.
3. There is doubt about the status of the
   abrasion.

✤ Lacerations

Lacerations are wounds or cuts made by
tearing and are common in athletics (Figure
8-4). These injuries are usually the result of
some type of direct blow to the skin and are
especially common over bony prominences.
The skin may be stretched and actually torn
apart. Lacerations are often described as a
combination of contusion and tear. They
generally lack the clean appearance of a typical incised wound. The edges of a laceration
are usually jagged or irregular, and at least
some surrounding tissue damage occurs in
most laceration injuries. The severity of lacerations can range from a very small crack
in the skin to a large, deep wound with associated damage to surrounding and deeper
structures. The nature and severity of bleeding associated with lacerations is quite variable.

✤ Incisions

Incisions are wounds caused by cutting with
some type of sharp object such as a knife

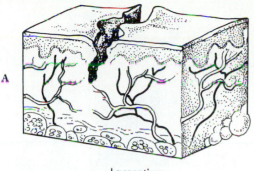

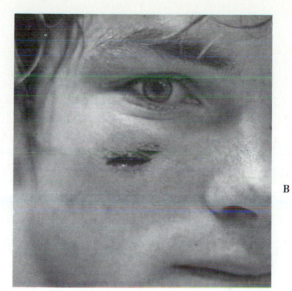

FIGURE 8-4
Laceration. **A,** Schematic of typical laceration injury. Note that injury extends into dermis. **B,** Facial laceration.

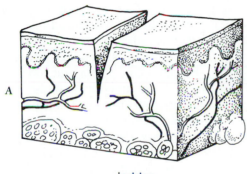

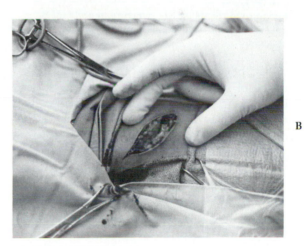

FIGURE 8-5
Incision. **A,** Schematic of incision injury and, **B,** an incision caused by glass fragment.

(Figure 8-5). The edges of an incision are smooth and cleanly cut, with little damage to surrounding tissue. Occasionally, an incised wound will be deep and there will be damage to blood vessels, muscles, tendons, or nerves well below the skin surface. Fortunately, severe incision wounds rarely occur as a result of athletic activity.

The initial care for incisions is essentially the same as for lacerations. Once bleeding has been controlled, carefully clean and inspect the wound. Is there any foreign material embedded in the wound? How deep is the wound? Was the mechanism of injury sufficient to cause other injuries in addition to the open wound? Remember, a laceration is caused by a crushing type of force, and there is probably an associated bruise. Athletic trainers must differentiate between lacerations and incisions that are "playable" and those that are not. Generally athletes will continue to play with smaller (less than 1 inch), superficial, and uncomplicated lacerations after the open wound has been sufficiently treated. After the game, the injured athlete can be referred to medical care. Occasionally, all that is necessary is to close the edges of the cut or tear with adhesive strips, such as butterfly closures or Steri-Strips, and apply a sterile dressing. In many

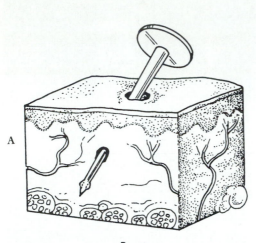

Puncture

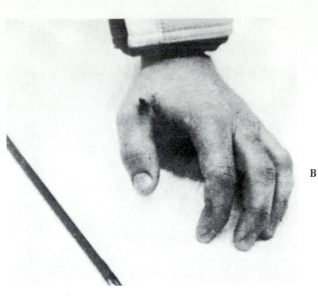

B

FIGURE 8-6
Puncture. **A**, Schematic of puncture injury and, **B**, puncture injury resulting from archery range accident.

cases, however, sutures are indicated. Because of activity required during athletics, sutures are more frequently recommended for athletes than nonathletes. Lacerations and incisions also need to be protected against additional trauma and stretching when the athlete returns to participation. The wound should be inspected daily for any signs of infection or further trauma. The athlete should be referred to a physician for any of the following reasons:

1. The wound may need sutures for adequate closure (more than ½-inch length and ⅛-inch depth).
2. There is foreign material embedded in the wound that cannot be removed.
3. Bleeding persists despite all efforts to control it.
4. The wound is on the face or another part of the body where scar tissue will be noticeable after healing.
5. The surrounding area becomes inflamed or infected.
6. There is doubt about how the laceration or incision should be treated.

✦ Puncture Wounds

Puncture wounds occur as a result of direct penetration of the skin by a pointed object (Figure 8-6). The opening may be quite small, with little or no bleeding. The penetrating object may, however, damage underlying structures and carry contaminants into the body. One of the first considerations in caring for a puncture is to determine the depth of penetration and the possibility of underlying damage. Only if the puncture is very minor and the penetrating object small, with little depth of penetration, is the athletic trainer justified in simply cleaning the wound and observing for signs of infection. The majority of puncture wounds should be cleansed and promptly referred to a physician. Large items that remain imbedded should be left in place until a physician can remove them. A tetanus toxoid booster is often indicated with puncture wounds. Punctures are not common in athletics but should be properly cared for when they occur. These wounds should be inspected frequently for signs of infection.

✦ Avulsions

An avulsion is the tearing away of part of a structure. When referring to an open wound, an avulsion is the tearing loose of a piece of skin, which may be torn completely free or remain partially attached, hanging as a flap (Figure 8-7). There may or may not be much bleeding. If an avulsed piece of skin or tissue of significant size is torn completely free of

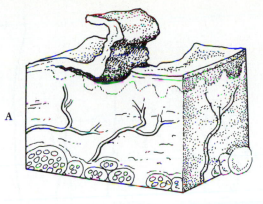

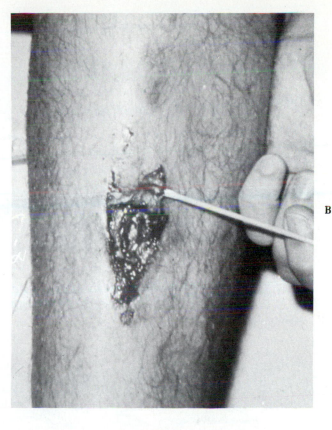

B

FIGURE 8-7
Avulsion. **A**, Schematic of avulsion injury and, **B**, avulsion injury to tibial area. Note avulsed skin flap.

the athlete, it should be saved and transported with the athlete to a medical facility. The avulsed portion should be wrapped in sterile gauze and kept moist and cool. Occasionally, significant portions of avulsed tissue may be successfully reattached. When the avulsed part remains attached, the flap of skin should be placed back in its normal position before bandaging and referral. Small flaps of skin, especially in highly vascular body areas such as the scalp and face, may remain viable and heal if replaced.

Common Skin Lesions

There are various skin lesions or disorders that can cause disability or impair athletic performance. These conditions may or may not break the surface of the skin, but they are discussed along with exposed athletic injuries because they involve the integrity of the skin. The integrity of the skin can be altered in many ways. Examples include physical trauma, infectious agents, and exposure to irritants in the environment, plant or insect poisons, and caustic chemicals. The skin problems and symptoms arising from these varied insults differ greatly among athletes. Prevention of skin problems, as well as the correct assessment and treatment of skin disorders when they occur, should be a major concern of the athletic trainer.

The assessment of any skin lesion should begin with a determination of the general characteristics of the eruption. This information is valuable in attempting to determine the nature and cause of the skin lesion and in describing the skin disorder when consulting a physician or dermatologist. The general characteristics of skin lesions include the (1) location, (2) configuration, and (3) structure of the eruptions. Location refers to the body areas affected. For example, contact dermatitis is sharply limited to the area of the body in contact with the causative agent. Configuration refers to the arrangement or position of several lesions in relation to each other (Figure 8-8). For example, ringworm is characterized by reddened circular areas. Structure refers to the physical signs used to classify skin lesions. A special vocabulary is used in describing the morphologic appearances or structure of skin lesions. These terms are defined later and illustrated in Figures 8-9 and 8-10.

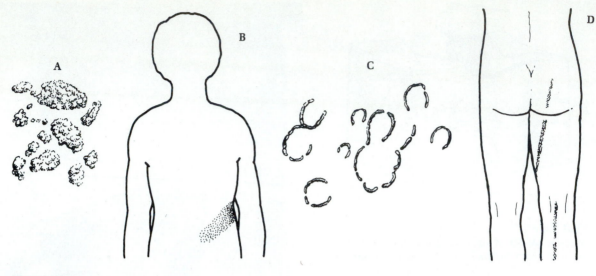

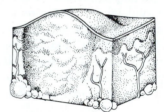

FIGURE 8-8
Configurations of skin lesions. **A**, Grouped (cluster); **B**, girdle (encircling pattern); **C**, ring-shaped (cyclic); **D**, linear.

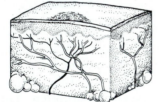

Macule or patch

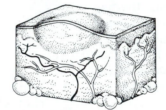

Papule or plaque

Nodule, tumor, or cyst

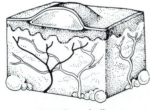

Vesicle or bulla

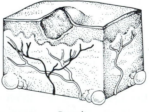

Pustule

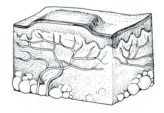

Wheal

FIGURE 8-9
Common primary skin lesions classified by structure.

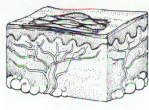

Crust

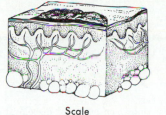
Scale

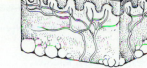
Erosion or ulcer

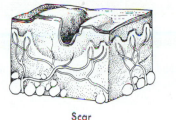
Scar

Fissure

FIGURE 8-10
Common secondary skin lesions classified by structure.

Lesions are classified as primary and secondary. **Primary lesions** are those that appear initially in response to some change in the internal or external environment of the skin. **Secondary lesions** do not appear initially but result from primary lesions. For example, a blister (primary lesion) may break and leave a small, moist area of skin, called an erosion (secondary lesion). When confronted with a diffuse skin eruption, it is important to examine the athlete closely to find primary lesions. These primary lesions may be obliterated by the secondary lesions of overtreatment, excessive scratching, or infection. By careful examination, it is usually possible to find some primary lesions at the edge of the skin eruption or on other less irritated areas of the body. A brief description of the common skin lesions under each classification is presented in Table 8-2.

Mechanically produced lesions

❖ **Blisters.** Blisters are normally caused by some type of skin friction or irritation. Many friction or shearing forces will cause the epidermis to separate from the dermis; the area between these layers then fills with fluid. This fluid is normally a clear exudate that has escaped from tiny blood vessels in the area. If the shearing force actually ruptures a blood vessel, such as might occur with a sharp pinching action, the blister may be filled with blood. Occasionally, a blister will become infected and the area between the two layers of skin will become purulent, that is, filled with pus.

Friction blisters can occur anywhere on the body, but are most common on the feet and hands (Figure 8-11). This is especially true early in an athletic season, when the skin of the feet and hands is soft and not accustomed to athletic activity. Over a period of time the skin will accommodate the friction, becoming tougher and much less likely to blister. The friction or shearing forces that cause blisters are enhanced by such things as poor-fitting or faulty equipment (especially shoes), participation on extremely hard surfaces, continued repetitive activity, or activity requiring frequent starting, stopping, and changing of direction. Athletes will normally feel a blister developing by detecting a "hot spot." This is an ideal time to care for the blister if at all possible. Blisters can often be contained if the "hot spot" is iced and/or the area is protected.

Blisters can be very handicapping to an athlete. Evaluating the severity of the blister and determining proper care depends on the cause, location, size, depth, and effect on performance. Identifying the cause, such as

TABLE 8-2

Types of Skin Lesions

Lesion	Description	Example
Primary skin lesions		
Macule	A small (less than 1 cm) circular discoloration of the skin without elevation or depression	Freckles
Patch	A macule larger than 1 cm	Senile freckles Measles rash
Papule	A small (less than 1 cm) solid, elevated area of the skin	Warts Closed comedo
Plaque	A papule larger than 1 cm, usually flat-topped, circumscribed elevation	Psoriasis Eczema
Nodule	A small, solid mass in subcutaneous tissue; deeper than a papule	Furuncle Epithelioma (skin cancer)
Cyst	A nodule filled with expressible material that is either liquid or semisolid	Sebaceous cyst
Tumor	Solid mass larger than 1 cm; may be above, level with, or beneath skin surface	Larger epithelioma
Vesicle	A circumscribed, elevated lesion containing serous fluid, up to 1 cm in size	Contact dermatitis Chicken pox
Bulla	A vesicle larger than 1 cm in diameter	Burn (2°) Friction blister
Pustule	A vesicle containing purulent fluid or pus	Acne Impetigo
Wheal	A papule or plaque resulting from edema in the skin	Hives Insect bites
Secondary skin lesions		
Crust	Dried exudate of serum, blood, or purulent material on skin; frequently results from breakage of vesicles, pustules, or bullae	Scab Impetigo Infected dermatitis
Scale	Dried, shedding, thin plates of epithelial cells; usually dry and whitish in color	Dandruff Chronic dermatitis
Erosion	A moist, circumscribed and often depressed area that reflects loss of epidermis; commonly implies a ruptured vesicle or bulla	Broken blister Scratches
Ulcer	Defect devoid of epidermis, as well as part or all of the dermis	Pressure sores
Scar	Formations of connective tissue replacing tissue lost through injury or disease; may be depressed or raised	Keloids
Fissure	A linear split or crack in the skin	Athlete's foot Chapping

poor-fitting shoes or a spike or cleat coming through the sole of a shoe, can help alleviate further complications. Many blisters can be drained and the skin protected, thus permitting the athlete to continue normal activity. In some cases the activity level will have to be modified for a few days so that the athlete does not continue to aggravate the blistered area. Infected blisters may require medical assistance.

❖ **Calluses.** Calluses are a thickening of the outer layer of skin (epidermis) normally present on the hands and feet. An excessive accumulation of callous tissue is usually found over a bony prominence and can develop from constant friction, pressure, or ir-

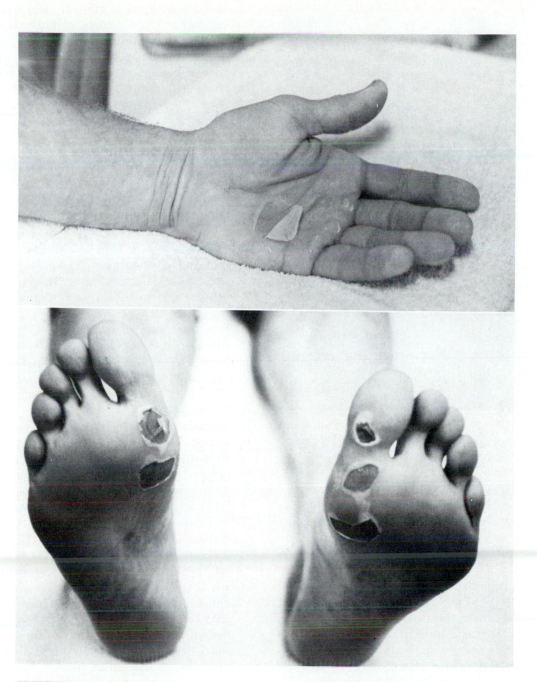

FIGURE 8-11
Examples of friction blisters.

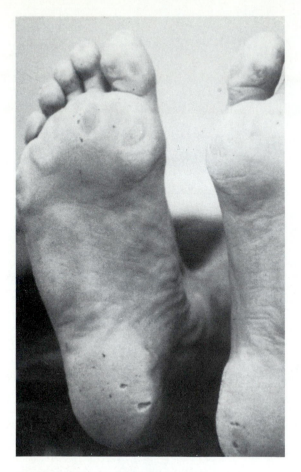

FIGURE 8-12
Calluses. Note development of calluses over the heads of the metatarsals.

ritation (Figure 8-12). This excess callus can become disabling and painful to an athlete as the mass becomes hard and inelastic. The most frequent sites for excessive callus formations are under the metatarsal bones at the ball of the foot, outer edge of the heel, inner edge of the big toe, or on the palm of the hand over the metacarpal heads. If left untreated, these hard masses are vulnerable to tearing and cracking and may cause painful bruising of the underlying tissues. Blisters may also develop under calluses.

Calluses can be differentiated from similar skin lesions, such as warts, by the skin lines, which will continue through to the surface. Treatment consists of preventing the excess callus accumulation and protecting the involved area. This may include re-

distribution of weight bearing in the shoe, proper foot hygiene, or the application of some type of pad or glove to reduce constant irritation. Once excess callous tissue has formed, it should be softened and trimmed periodically to prevent further problems and reduce the severity of symptoms. With callous formation the yellow epidermal layer should be trimmed until the epidermal layer just starts to turn pink. If too much of the epidermal layer is removed it leaves the area susceptible to blistering.

✤   **Contact dermatitis.** Contact dermatitis is an acute inflammatory reaction of the skin resulting from direct contact with a substance to which the skin is sensitive. The first apparent change in the skin is a redness (erythema) that is sharply limited to the area of contact with the causative agent (Figure A). Depending on the duration of contact and the intensity of the reaction, this initial irritation may develop quite rapidly into an intense inflammatory response. Along with the erythema, small itching papules (bumps) may form, and blisterlike elevations (vesicles) may develop. These vesicles may rupture and cause a crusty appearance.

Some of the possible causes of contact dermatitis in athletes are adhesive tape, dyes in leather or uniforms, elastic wraps, locally applied ointments, chemical powders, soaps, detergents, perfumes, deodorants, plants (such as poison ivy), and certain topical medications. When an athlete exhibits signs of contact dermatitis, the athletic trainer must attempt to identify the causative agent. This will require a complete and careful history. Investigate recent exposures to all possible causes, such as those listed previously. It may be possible to determine the cause and decrease the athlete's exposure to, or remove, the suspected irritants. If the problem persists or the inflammation becomes severe, oozing and spreading, the athlete should be referred to a physician specializing in skin care.

Bacterial lesions

Normal bacterial flora of the skin includes both pathogenic and nonpathogenic organisms, the major pathogenic type being the staphylococcus, followed closely by the streptococcus. The normal integrity of the skin, and the immune and cellular defenses, act as barriers to most bacterial organisms. Whenever the integrity of the skin is altered by any means, the potential for infection is increased. Skin trauma, friction, sweating, bruises, and warm, moist areas under equipment and protective pads, which are common in athletics, predispose to bacterial infections. Oily skin, exposure to another infected person, and poor hygiene can also facilitate or spread infections.

When dealing with bacterial infections, it is extremely important for the athletic trainer to prevent the infection from spreading over the body or to other athletes. Thorough cleansing of the area with soap and water will help prevent many bacterial infections, including impetigo, from spreading. An antibacterial ointment should be applied and covered with a thin dressing, which should be changed frequently. The athlete's towel, uniform, and clothing should be isolated until thoroughly laundered. The skin should be kept dry, with special attention given to the affected area because dryness inhibits the growth of bacteria. The affected athlete may have to be isolated from close contact with others, placed under a physician's care, and take antibiotic medication.

To prevent bacterial infection from spreading, it is important for the athletic trainer to aggressively care for *all* cutaneous lesions, no matter how small. This consists of cleansing the lesion and applying an antiseptic, and perhaps an antibacterial ointment dressing if the lesions are draining or moist. It is also important that the athlete carry out a sound personal hygiene program. The athletic trainer must constantly watch for bacterial infections to treat them effectively and prevent them from spreading. It is also important that facilities and equipment used by athletes, such as wrestling mats and shower rooms, be well cleaned each day. Bacterial infections are a constant area of concern for athletic trainers. A bacterial infection allowed to spread can sideline numerous athletes or an entire team in a short period of time and disrupt an entire athletic season.

❖   **Tetanus.** Tetanus is an acute infectious disease due to a toxin growing at the site of injury. It is characterized by severe uncontrolled skeletal muscle spasms. Tetanus normally begins with stiffness of the jaw, esophageal muscles, and some muscles of the neck. The jaws can become rigidly fixed *(lockjaw)*. It may involve the muscles of the back and extremities. The major risk to life is related to spasms of the muscles of respiration, which can lead to hypoxia and death. Individuals should have a tetanus toxoid booster every 10 years.

❖   **Boil (furuncle).** A boil is a common bacterial skin infection (Figure B). Boils are formed by staphylococci invading the skin through sebaceous glands or hair follicles. The follicles become inflamed, and the bacterial infection is localized in a painful red nodule and eventually a pustule. As a boil matures it becomes enlarged, hard, and tender. Most boils will eventually rupture spontaneously, releasing the contained pus. Occasionally, boils are lanced by a physician. Boils may occur anywhere but are more common on the upper extremities, buttocks, groin, axillae, neck, waist, and chest. Boils on the central face are of special concern because there is direct access to the veins of the brain from the superficial venous system. Athletes with boils should be under a physician's care, and their athletic activity may have to be limited until the infection is clear. Treatment includes systemic antibiotics.

❖   **Furunculosis.** Furunculosis is a self-limiting infection in which one or several furuncles are present.

❖   **Carbuncle.** A carbuncle is an extensive infection of several adjoining hair follicles that drains with multiple openings onto the skin's surface. A carbuncle is a cluster of boils that more commonly occur on the back of the neck, upper back, and lateral thighs. Therefore treatment is the same as that for a boil but with greater emphasis on systemic antibiotic therapy and rest from activity.

❖   **Folliculitis.** Folliculitis is a common infection of the hair follicles and can be caused by a staphylococci, chemical irritation, or physical injury (Figure C). The infection occurs most often in areas that have short, coarse hairs. Friction from protective pads or shaving may contribute to folliculitis. The lesions are frequently grouped together and can be recognized by finding a hair in the center of the pustule. Treatment includes eliminating friction and applying a medicated ointment.

❖ **Impetigo.** Impetigo is a highly contagious bacterial (streptococcal or staphylococcal) inflammation of the skin. It is characterized by the appearance of small vesicles, which form pustules and eventually honey-colored, weeping crustations (Figure D). Impetigo can be transmitted by direct contact with an infected athlete or contact with infected equipment or towels. Persons with impetigo should not engage in contact sports during the contagious period and should practice careful hygiene to protect other athletes. Treatment includes topical and systemic antibiotics.

❖ **Cellulitis.** Cellulitis is an inflammation of the dermis and subcutaneous tissue that is usually caused by a bacteria (group A streptococcus and *staphylococcus aureus*). The affected area is tender, deep reddish, swollen, and warm (Figure E).

❖ *Acne vulgaris*

Acne is the most common skin condition of adolescents and young adults. It is a chronic inflammatory disease of the sebaceous glands characterized by any combination of noninflamed comedones (blackheads and whiteheads) to inflammatory papules, pustules, and cysts (Figure F). Because there is often pus, it is easy to think of some type of infection. However, not all pustules are caused by pathogenic microorganisms. If infection is suspected, simple laboratory tests can confirm. In athletes, acne may be induced or aggravated by (1) traumatic physical contact with equipment and other competitors, (2) friction and occlusion from equipment and clothing, (3) skin hydration from excessive sweating or high humidity, and (4) psychologic stress from competition.

Treatment for acne is symptomatic and quite varied. The treatment routine often in-cludes gentle washing of the area and the application of various topical and/or systemic medications. Picking, scratching, and squeezing is harmful and should be avoided. Much of the skin damage is self-inflicted. Although the temptation to squeeze a fresh pustule is often overwhelming, it should be discouraged because it can produce more tissue damage, sometimes resulting in scars. The athletic trainer's role in the care of acne is to provide accurate information concerning this condition, to help the athlete comply with the physician's treatment program, and to assist in protecting the area from aggravation, such as from equipment and uniforms.

Fungal lesions

Fungal infections of skin, hair, and nails are common among athletes. Fungi are microscopic plants related to mushrooms and propagated by seeds called spores. Most fungal spores are highly resistant to drying or freezing and can survive for many years. These organisms thrive in dark, warm, and moist places, conditions often found in dressing rooms and lockers. There are many different fungi that grow in or on the human skin and can be transmitted from one athlete to another without bodily contact. This makes fungal infections an occupational hazard among athletes. Some athletes have a greater susceptibility to fungal infections than others.

The more common athletic fungal infections appear as an itching red rash consisting of small bumps or blisters and scales on the skin. Generally, a fungal infection tends to create more tissue reaction at the advancing borders of the infection than in the older center. This accounts for the ring-shaped lesions frequently seen, although not all fungal infections react in this manner. Sweating, heat, and physical activity contribute to the growth of fungi, commonly called ringworm (tinea) and classified according to the area of the body affected. The most common fungal infections among athletes are athlete's foot, jock itch, and ringworm.

❖ **Athlete's foot (tinea pedis).** Athlete's foot is a very common skin infection (Figure

G). This condition is characterized by redness, scaling, cracking, and itching of the skin of the feet. It is most common on the soles and between the toes.

✦ **Jock itch (tinea cruris).** Jock itch is a fungal infection that affects the groin area (Figure H). The infection usually begins near the crural folds and becomes fan-shaped as it spreads peripherally in the medial thighs. The infection usually exhibits an active advancing border with scaling, small papules, and varying degrees of itching. Jock itch may accompany athlete's foot, which can be spread by wiping the feet before drying the rest of the body.

✦ **Ringworm (tinea corporis).** Ringworm generally involves the upper extremities and trunk (Figure I). These lesions are characterized by reddened, ringlike areas that may be scaly or crusted.

✦ **Intertrigo.** Intertrigo is a red, macerated, half moon-shaped plaque occurring in skin folds. The most common area is in the groin area where moisture accumulates in the crural folds (Figure J). The borders touch where the opposed surfaces of the skin folds of the groin and thigh meet. Obesity contributes to this inflammatory condition, which may be infected with a mixed flora of fungi, bacteria, and yeast. In advanced cases, painful, longitudinal fissures occur in the crease of the crural fold.

The best management of fungal infections is, of course, prevention. Athletes must establish good daily personal hygiene habits such as washing and drying well, especially between the toes and in the groin, and wearing clean clothes. Natural material such as cotton is best. Synthetic materials such as nylon trap moisture and may cause additional irritation. It is also important to keep the shower and locker rooms clean. In treating mild cases of fungal infections, it is important to minimize heat and moisture in the affected areas. The athlete can accomplish this by drying thoroughly after a shower, applying a fungicide, and wearing clean clothing. Fungal infections will generally respond well to these routines. In moderate to severe cases of fungal infections, the athlete may also be under a phy-sician's care and possibly removed from activity until the condition improves. Remember, individual susceptibility varies from person to person.

Viral lesions

✦ **Herpesvirus.** The most common viral infection seen in athletics is **herpes simplex** (type 1) virus (Figure K). This is commonly called a fever blister or cold sore and is an acute infection of the mucous membranes and skin by this form of herpesvirus. The herpes simplex (type 1) virus is carried inactively by the majority of the population and does not erupt until a person's resistance is lowered by another condition such as sunburn, fever, stress, irritation, fatigue, or a dietary problem. The lesion is the result of recurrent infections that commonly affect the border of the lips, cheeks, mouth, and conjunctiva; however, it can occur on any skin surface. (Most genital lesions are caused by herpesvirus type 2 and are beyond the scope of discussion for this text. Athletes with genital herpes should always be referred to a physician for treatment.) Initially, groups of herpesvirus lesions appear as blisters, which rupture and form a crusted surface. The appearance of the vesicles is preceded by a burning and itching sensation. The condition is normally self-limiting and will disappear in 1 to 2 weeks. Some athletes are more susceptible to this condition, and lesions frequently recur at the same site. If an athlete develops this condition frequently, there may be an underlying causative factor that demands medical attention. The herpes simplex virus can be transmitted, largely through skin-to-skin contact, from one person to another during the vesicular phase. Contact with the infected area should be avoided until the crusted area is gone. The period of maximum contagious spread is 5 days after onset of eruptions. Herpes simplex can reach epidemic proportions among athletes in close-contact sports such as wrestling if it goes unrecognized and untreated. It is also possible to transmit the virus through shared equipment such as a wrestling mat.

There is no cure presently available for

herpes simplex. Treatment consists of keeping the area dry and clean to promote healing and prevent secondary infections. The athlete may have to be withheld from competition to avoid contaminating other athletes. A detailed history of foods, medications, and activities of the athlete may help in finding and eliminating the initiating trigger or stimulus, thus preventing recurrence.

✤ **Herpes zoster (shingles).** Herpes zoster is a unique viral infection that almost always affects the skin of a single dermatome (Figure L). It is caused by the varicella zoster virus of chicken pox. About 3% of the population will suffer from shingles at some time in their lives. In most cases the disease results from reactivation of the varicella virus. The virus most likely traveled through a cutaneous nerve and remained dormant in a dorsal root ganglion for years after an episode of chicken pox. Age, immunosuppressive drugs, fatigue, emotional upsets, and radiation therapy have been implicated in reactivating the virus. When this occurs, the virus will travel back down the sensory nerve to the skin of a single dermatome. The result is a painful eruption of red, swollen plaques or vesicles that eventually rupture and crust before clearing in 2 or 3 weeks. In severe cases, extensive inflammation, hemorrhagic blisters, and secondary bacterial infection may lead to permanent scarring. In most cases of shingles, the eruption of vesicles is preceded by 4 to 5 days of preeruptive pain, burning, and itching along the affected dermatome.

✤ **Warts (verruca vulgaris).** Warts are also caused by a virus. True warts are small tumors that may appear anywhere on the skin surface (Figure M). They are characterized by small dark spots in their center. The black central spot is actually a capillary or vascular bud in the center of the wart. Warts also have a distinct border at which all skin lines end. Normally, warts are treated only if they interfere with athletic activity. They frequently disappear with no treatment.

✤ **Plantar warts (verruca plantaris).** Plantar warts develop on the sole of the foot (Figure N). They may cause pain and dis-

ability, especially if they are located on a weight-bearing surface. During competition, plantar warts are protected with a donut-shaped pad to relieve pressure over the lesion. After the athletic season, the plantar wart can be removed by a physician or podiatrist.

✤ **Water warts (molluscum contagiosum).** Water warts are more contagious than warts, particularly in activities requiring direct body contact such as wrestling (Figure O). These viral infections appear as small, skin-colored, dome-shaped papules. When recognized, this condition should be referred to medical assistance for treatment.

✤ **Chicken pox (varicella).** Chicken pox is a mild, highly contagious viral infection marked by an eruption of vesicles on the skin and mucous membranes. It is characterized by a rash that begins on the trunk and spreads to the face and extremities. Symptoms in children are absent or consist of low fever, headache, and malaise, which appear directly before or with the onset of the eruptions. In adults, symptoms consisting of fever, chills, malaise, and backache are more severe and occur 2 or 3 days before the eruptions. Chicken pox passes through stages of macules, papules, vesicles, and crusts (Figure P). The disease is not infectious when the lesions have crusted.

✤ **Measles (rubeola).** Measles is a highly contagious viral disease transmitted by respiratory droplets. It typically has an incubation period of 10 to 14 days and lasts from 7 to 14 days. The onset of symptoms is much like the common cold with fever, malaise, cough, runny nose, and conjunctivitis. Three to 5 days after the symptoms begin, cutaneous eruptions appear as small, irregular, bright red spots with bluish-white centers on the forehead, cheeks, back of the neck, and spreading over the body. After 2 or 3 days the eruptions begin to fade and are gone in 1 to 2 weeks.

✤ *Acquired immune deficiency syndrome (AIDS)*

Although AIDS is not primarily a disease of the skin, it is discussed here because it is caused by a virus. AIDS is probably the most serious and frightening disease facing society today. AIDS is caused by a virus named human immunodeficiency virus (HIV). The signs of HIV infection initially surfaced in the United States as a general syndrome in 1978 and were described as a separate disease entity by 1981. HIV disrupts a complex T lymphocyte, crippling the immune system and leaving the body vulnerable to various viral, bacterial, and parasitic diseases. If the infection with HIV progresses, the onset of symptoms (the incubation period) ranges from about 6 months to 5 years or more. Symptoms may include fatigue, fever, loss of appetite, loss of weight, diarrhea, night sweats, and swollen glands. Some people infected with the virus develop less severe AIDS-related symptoms and may remain sick but stable for years. This condition is referred to as AIDS-related complex (ARC). ARC can but does not invariably lead to AIDS. To date there is no cure for AIDS.

All evidence indicates that AIDS is transmitted primarily through semen, vaginal secretions, and blood. AIDS is spread predominately through sexual contact with an infected partner, contaminated intravenous needle sharing, blood transfusion from an AIDS victim, or passage from mother to fetus through the placenta. Although low concentrations of HIV have been detected in the saliva and tears of some AIDS victims, there is no evidence that the disease can be transmitted through casual contact.

Of importance to athletic trainers is the fact that virtually all infected persons are able to transmit the infection. While the risk of acquiring the virus from an infected athlete may be slight, athletic trainers should always practice good hygienic techniques whenever working with open lesions. This is especially important if the athletic trainer has open skin breaks on the hands. Athletic trainers must remain informed about AIDS and continue to follow all established guidelines, including:

1. Every athletic training facility should have an infection control policy.
2. Disposable gloves should be worn whenever there is exposure to blood or body fluids.
3. Occlusive dressings should be used to bandage all wounds and breaks in the athlete's skin.
4. Hands should be washed with soap and water after every treatment.
5. All treatment areas should be cleaned in an appropriate manner.
6. Soiled laundry, pads, braces, mats, etc. should be cleaned and disinfected with bleach or other appropriate solution.
7. Materials used to dress wounds or clean up spills should be disposed of properly.

❖ *Environmentally produced lesions*
Sunburn. Sunburn is an injury to the skin caused by overexposure to ultraviolet rays of the sun or sunlamps. These lesions will vary in intensity from a first-degree **burn** characterized by a mild erythema (pink color) to a second-degree burn marked by the formation of large blisters. In addition to reddening of the skin, pain is normally present, and in severe cases the athlete may complain of headaches and even exhibit a fever. Persons with very light complexions are more susceptible to sunburn than are those with darker complexions. Athletes not accustomed to being in the sun are also more vulnerable to the effects of the sun's rays. Sunburns and their associated signs and symptoms occur between 4 and 12 hours after exposure to the ultraviolet rays, which makes it difficult to judge the optimum time necessary to prevent overexposure. The effects of a sunburn usually dissipate in 2 to 4 days.

Prevention of sunburn can be accomplished by asking athletes to follow several guidelines. Athletes should acclimate themselves to the sun's rays. The initial exposure should be brief and gradually increased each day until the athlete can tolerate being in the sun without ill effects. Avoiding exposure during midday, when the ultraviolet rays are at their peak, will help reduce burning of the skin. The use of some type of sunscreen designed to filter out the shorter ultraviolet rays, which are the burning rays, is also very helpful in avoiding a sunburn. Absorbent sunscreens containing paraaminobenzoic acid (PABA) affords the most effective protection against the harmful ultraviolet rays of the sun. Many sunscreens are labeled with a number between 1 and 15. This number is a sun protective factor (SPF) and helps indicate how long a person can remain in the sun. For example, a sunscreen with a number 4, indicates you can stay in the sun four times as long as you could without any protection. Remember that sunscreen must be applied frequently to ensure adequate protection if the person perspires heavily or goes swimming.

The treatment of sunburns is the same as for any thermal burn and depends on the degree of severity and extent of body area involved. Cool water immersion, cool compresses, or soothing lotions are helpful in milder cases. Aspirin is often administered to relieve pain and some of the inflammatory effects. In severe cases in which blistering and fluid loss is evident, a physician should be consulted for appropriate treatment.

✜ **Frostbite.** Frostbite was discussed in Chapter 7 but is presented again as an environmentally produced condition. Frostbite occurs when isolated areas of the body are exposed to severe cold. The ears, nose, cheeks, fingers, and toes are the body areas most frequently involved. As a result of exposure to cold, the superficial blood vessels constrict, decreasing the blood supply to the exposed areas. The extent of the injury depends on such factors as temperature, duration of exposure, wind velocity, humidity, and lack of protective clothing. The exposed area initially becomes red and inflamed, then, if frostbite continues the area will progressively turn grey. If freezing occurs, the affected area takes on a waxy white appearance. As these changes occur, the athlete will normally experience burning or stinging of the affected area, followed by pins-and-needles sensations and, finally, numbness. An athlete may be unaware of the development of severe frostbite because of the loss of sensations.

Frostbitten areas should be gently handled and rapidly rewarmed. In mild frostbite, rewarming will usually produce mild itching and burning sensations and some local redness and swelling. In severe frost-bite there may be some blister formation and possible tissue death and permanent damage to the area. Athletes with severe frostbite should be referred to a physician.

Infestation and bite lesions

✜ **Scabies.** Scabies is a contagious disease caused by a mite and is characterized by extreme nocturnal itching and elevated burrows (Figure Q). The female mite burrows into the stratum corneum and lays her eggs. The larvae hatch, reach maturity in 14 to 17 days, and repeat the cycle. In time, the number of mites reaching maturity can spread by migration or scratching and the patient has an acute dermatitis and intense, generalized itch. Diagnosis is made by scraping the burrow and examining the scrapings under a microscope.

✜ **Pediculosis.** Pediculosis is an infestation with lice. Lice are transmitted by close personal contact and contact with objects such as combs, clothing, hats, and bed linens. Lice feed by piercing the skin, injecting an irritating saliva, and sucking blood. The bite causes an itching dermatitis. Scratching can cause inflammation and secondary bacterial infections with pustules and crusting (Figure R). Diagnosis is made by visually identifying the louse or its eggs, which are attached to the shaft of a hair.

Additional skin lesions

✜ **Eczema.** Eczema is the most common inflammatory skin disease. The inflammation is caused by contact with an allergen and can vary from moderate to intense. Eczema will develop with a bright red swollen plaque with a pebbly surface and may develop into vesicles and blisters (Figure S). Often intense itching is associated with this condition.

✜ **Hives (Urticaria).** Hives are caused by some type of allergen such as foods, drugs, plants, or physical stimulation. Histamine release is induced by the allergens resulting in a localized capillary vasodilation. Hives are seen initially as a uniformly red edematous plaque (Figure T). The lesions tend to develop a pale center, or wheal, surrounded

TABLE 8-3

Types of Closed Wounds

Type	Cause	Characteristics	Care
Contusion (bruise)	Direct blow	Hematoma Ecchymosis Local tenderness	ICER Symptomatic care Protection
Strain	Overstretching Overstressing Violent contraction Strength imbalance to muscle tendon units	1°—Stretching Some discomfort No disability	ICER Symptomatic care Minimal support
		2°—Tearing of fibers Pain Disability 3°—Complete rupture Disability Deficit	ICER Symptomatic care Support during activity ICER Referral
Sprain	Joint forced in abnormal direction	1°—Stretching Some discomfort No instability 2°—Tearing of ligament Pain Swelling Instability 3°—Rupture of ligament Instability Swelling	ICER Symptomatic care Support during activity ICER Protection Support during activity ICER Referral
Dislocation	Joint forced beyond anatomic limits	Deformity Pain Loss of function	Cold Immobilization Referral
Fracture	Direct blow Indirect blow Twisting force Repetitive stress	Pain Crepitation Deformity Loss of function Guarding	Cold Immobilization Referral

by an erythematous edge. Hives resolve when the fluid is slowly reabsorbed.

❖ **Psoriasis.** Psoriasis is a chronic disease that fluctuates in intensity and occurs as sharply demarcated erythematous plaques with a dry, silvery scale (Figure U). Common sites are the elbows, knees, palms, soles, and scalp. Psoriasis is usually not itchy and vesicles are never formed, which distinguish it from dermatitis.

❖ **Pityriasis rosea.** Pityriasis rosea is a common, self-limiting skin eruption in young adults. It is of unknown etiology. It appears as round-to-oval patches most frequently on the trunk or proximal extremities. Within a few days to several weeks the disease enters the eruptive phase (Figure V). Smaller lesions appear and reach their max-

imum number in 1 to 2 weeks. There may be mild transient itching. The disease clears spontaneously in 6 to 8 weeks.

UNEXPOSED ATHLETIC INJURIES

Unexposed, or closed, athletic injuries are said to be internal, with no associated disruption or break in the continuity of the skin. Unexposed injuries can result in massive bleeding and significant damage to underlying structures, with little or no visible signs at the skin surface. Structures commonly involved in athletic injuries of this type include soft tissues such as muscles, tendons, blood vessels, and ligaments. Bones are also subject to unexposed injuries. Unexposed athletic injuries also involve such structures as nerves and internal (visceral)

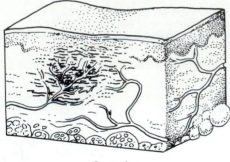

Contusion

FIGURE 8-13
Schematic and examples of contusion injuries.

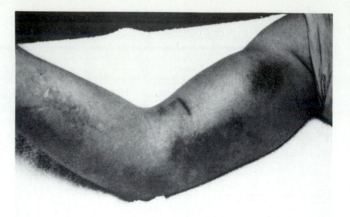

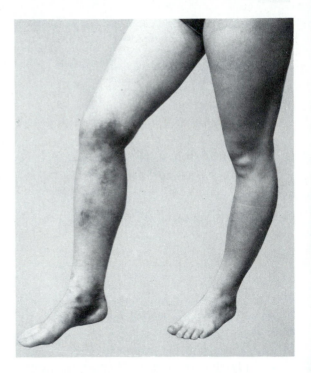

organs and their linings. The common unexposed athletic injuries are classified into contusions, strains, sprains, dislocations, and simple fractures (Table 8-3).

✤ **Contusions**

A contusion is a bruise and is among the most common type of injury that occurs in athletic activity. Contusions usually result from a direct blow or impact delivered to some part of the body, which causes damage to underlying blood vessels. The resulting bleeding into the skin or subcutaneous tissues may produce symptoms that range from very minor areas of discoloration to extremely large, debilitating masses (Figure 8-13). The collection of blood that forms at the site of a contusion is called a **hematoma.** As the blood leaks into the subcutaneous tissues, it often causes a black and blue discoloration known as **ecchymosis.** In addition to the swelling, a bruise usually results in an area of local tenderness.

The tissues involved in a contusion, as well as the extent of damage and bleeding, depends on the force of the impact, the size and shape of the object causing the bruise, and the part of the body receiving the blow. For example, a blow to a large muscular area such as the thigh will result in damage or bruising to the muscles. The involved mus-

cles respond by protective muscle spasms, causing a decreased excursion of the muscle fibers and a reduced ROM at the associated joints.

The objective of the initial treatment of contusions is to control the bleeding by means of ice, compression, and elevation. Heat and activity during this initial period may encourage or promote bleeding and should be avoided. After bleeding has stopped and the athlete exhibits a near nor-

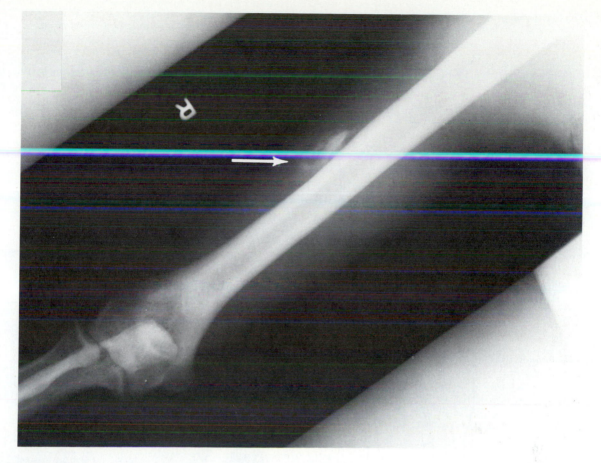

FIGURE 8-14
Myositis ossificans resulting from contusion injury to right biceps brachii.

mal ROM without a significant increase in pain, activity may be resumed. The level of activity is increased according to the athlete's tolerance until participation is at the level demanded by the sport. During recovery the athlete should be protected from reinjury by padding the bruised area and by avoiding excessive activity, which may aggravate injured tissues.

A complication to be aware of when dealing with contusions is (**myositis ossificans,** the formation of bone within or around a muscle, commonly called a **calcium deposit.** Myositis ossificans can result from a contusion injury and occurs when part of the hematoma is replaced with bone (Figure 8-14). It is believed that the bony deposits are caused by periosteal cells that invade the he-

matoma following the injury. The invasion of the hematoma by periosteal cells can occur when a severe bruise involves the bone as well as the muscle, causing a subperiosteal hematoma, or when the trauma causes a partial avulsion of muscle fibers from the periosteum. The bony deposit may be a separate piece of bone lying entirely within the muscle, or it may be attached to a bone (**exostosis**). This complication seldom occurs as a result of a single injury. It is more likely to occur after chronic irritation such as continued use of an injured part of repeated trauma to a body area. Whatever the reason, if the hematoma fails to resolve normally, myositis ossificans may result. The formation of myositis ossificans can be recognized by normal, plain, film radiographs about 3

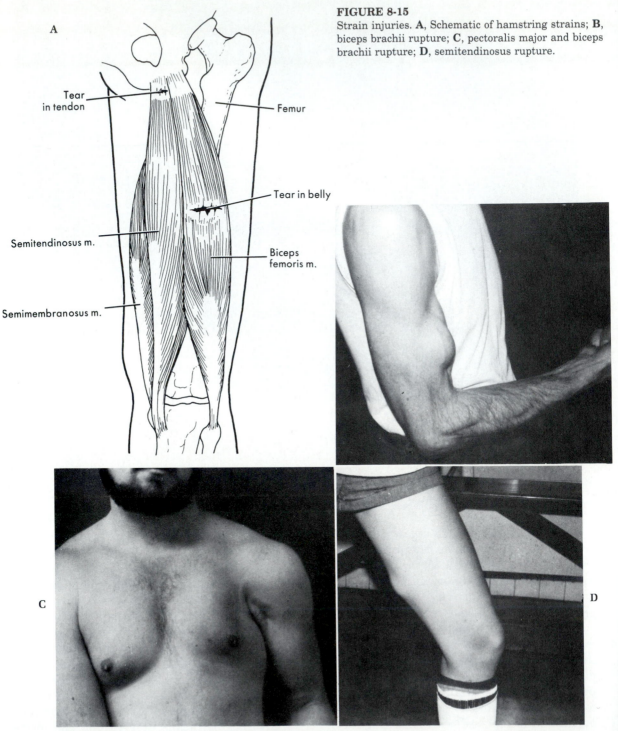

to 4 weeks after periosteal cell activity begins. It is important for the athletic trainer to recognize the possibility of myositis ossificans after a severe contusion or repeated bruising. Myositis ossificans can occur anywhere in the body but most frequently involves the quadriceps. This condition should always be suspected if hematoma formation does not promptly resolve and if pain, a palpable mass within the muscle, and loss of motion persist for 2 to 3 weeks. In this type of case the athlete should be withheld from activity until severe symptoms subside. It is important that athletes suffering from severe contusions should undergo frequent periodic evaluations.

✤ Strains

Strains are injuries involving the musculotendinous unit and may involve the muscle, tendon, and the junction between the two, as well as their attachments to bone (Figure 8-15). Strains or pulls can be caused by various mechanisms such as overstretching, overstressing, a violent contraction against heavy resistance, a strength imbalance between agonists and antagonists, or an abnormal muscle contraction. These injuries are generally dynamic; that is, there is no outside intervention and the athlete injures himself or herself. The portion of the musculotendinous unit that is damaged depends on which component is the weakest at the moment of injury. Generally, in younger athletes whose growth centers have not closed (ossified), the muscles and tendons are stronger. With these athletes, the attachment to the bone may fail and actually avulse a piece of bone with the tendon or separate at the epiphyseal, or growth, line (epiphyseal fracture) (Figure 8-16). In older athletes, the tendons and musculotendinous junctions become the weaker part and are more susceptible to injury.

Strains are graded into three groups by level of severity. Each is determined by the amount of damage to the fibers of the musculotendinous unit. The definitions, and the signs and symptoms delineating each grade of severity, are as follows.

A *mild strain (first degree)* involves

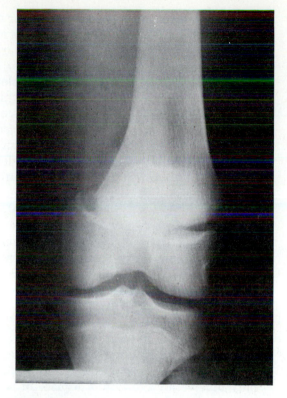

FIGURE 8-16
Epiphyseal fracture of the femur in a young athlete.

stretching and a minimal amount of tearing of the involved tissues. Although there is some discomfort during function after a mild strain, there is generally little or no disability. An athlete has normal or near-normal ROM and experiences only insignificant loss in strength. Athletes with these injuries require only minimal protection and support, such as an elastic wrap, to continue participation. Many times an athlete will continue activity and not report mild strains unless symptoms become more severe.

A *moderate strain (second degree)* involves a significant tearing of fibers, although at least some continuity of the musculotendinous unit remains. A few fibers may be torn, or the majority of the fibers in a given unit may be damaged. An athlete may complete a workout or activity in pain after suffering a moderate strain and then experience disability later that day or the next morning. The second-degree strain is the most common type of strain cared for by the athletic trainer. Signs and symptoms accompanying moderate strains include varying degrees of pain, swelling, loss of strength, and loss of flexibility. The athlete may hear or feel a snap at the time the tissue tears. An area of point tenderness is evident on palpation, as is local pain expressed during active, resistive, or stretching movements. Occasionally a palpable gap, or deficit, is evident immediately after the injury. The athlete should be treated symptomatically and returned to activity as tolerated. The time required for return to complete activity varies from a few days to several weeks after a moderate strain. Athletes normally require protection and support for the injured area when they return to activity.

A *severe strain* (*third degree*) involves complete destruction of the continuity of the musculotendinous unit, thus causing instant disability. The rupture may occur anywhere along the musculotendinous unit or may involve an avulsion of a piece of bone at its attachment. Frequently the athlete will hear or feel a snap as the tissue ruptures. Usually there will be an associated palpable, and many times visible, gap at the site of the injury. The muscle may bunch up because of spasmodic contractions. The athlete will experience a significant weakness and loss of function as a result of the injury. Severe strains should be treated initially with cold, compression, and elevation and then be referred to a physician for further diagnosis and treatment.

Strains should be referred to a physician for any of the following reasons:

1. A visible or palpable gap is noted.
2. Muscle fibers bunch as the result of spasmodic contractions and lack attachment of one extremity to a fixed point.
3. The athlete demonstrates a significant weakness and loss of function.
4. There is doubt about the status of the strain.

Acute musculotendinous strains resulting from athletic activity occur most frequently in the lower extremities. Treatment is aimed at restoring flexibility and strength. A period of complete inactivity will often result in a shortened, atrophied muscle that must be gradually stretched and strengthened to its normal state before full activity can be resumed. Severe strains therefore require repeated evaluations by the athletic trainer to return the athlete to full activity as quickly as possible.

Chronic strains can result from abuse or overuse of the musculotendinous unit. The most frequent mechanisms of injury involve workloads that are too stressful for the musculotendinous unit to withstand. Training and conditioning programs are designed to strengthen this contractile unit gradually, so that it is able to withstand progressively heavier work loads and thereby avoid strains. Chronic inflammation of a muscle may result if an athlete trains too intensely, performs specific repetitive movement over a considerable period of time, or continues to use an injured area. Any area of the musculotendinous unit can become irritated and inflamed, such as the muscle (**myositis**), the tendon (**tendinitis**), the musculotendinous junction, the tendon and its protective synovial sheath (**tenosynovitis**), or the tendinous attachment to bone. Although each of these chronic overuse syndromes involves a different area of the contractile unit, they require basically the same treatment. Treatment procedures normally include rest, local heat, antiinflammatory medication, and protection against continued aggravation. Most treatment programs require a modification of activity, or perhaps complete rest, which may be difficult and frustrating for both the athlete and the coach. After the cessation of symptoms, the athlete must resume activity gradually and progress within tolerable limits to avoid recurrence of the injury.

❖ Sprains

A sprain is an injury involving a ligament. Ligaments are basically inelastic and designed to prevent abnormal motion at a joint. Whenever a joint is forced to move in an abnormal direction, ligaments are stressed (Figure 8-17). If the ligament is forced beyond its limit, damage will occur at the weakest point in the ligament. The dam-

ATHLETIC INJURY ASSESSMENT

COLOR PLATES

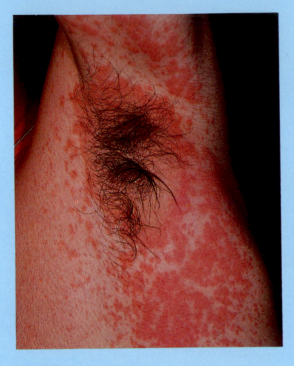

FIGURE A
Contact dermatitis.

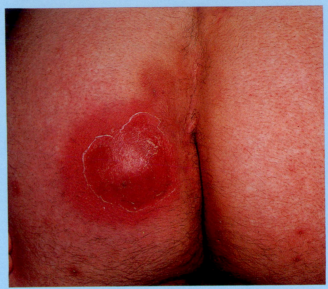

FIGURE B
Boil (furuncle).

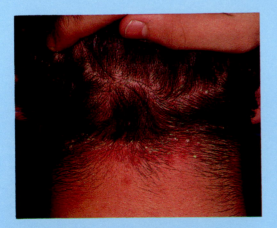

FIGURE C
Folliculitis.

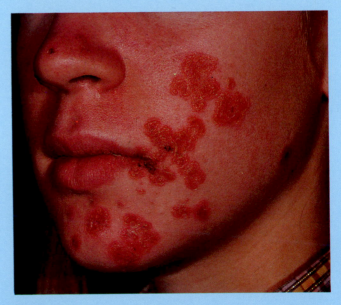

FIGURE D
Impetigo.

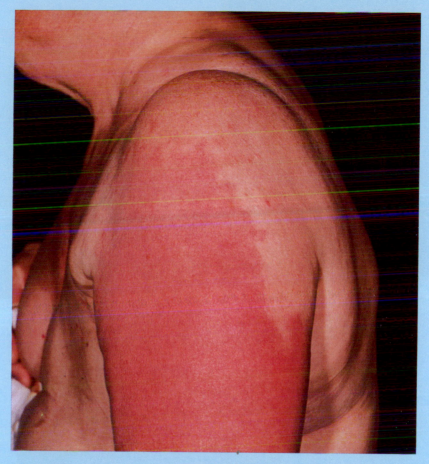

FIGURE E
Cellulitis.

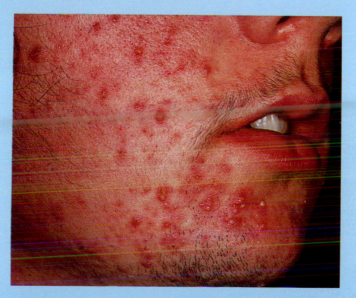

FIGURE F
Acne.

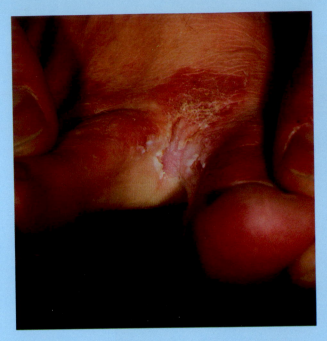

FIGURE G
Athlete's foot (tinea pedis).

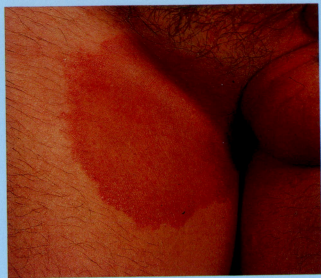

FIGURE H
Jock itch (tinea cruris).

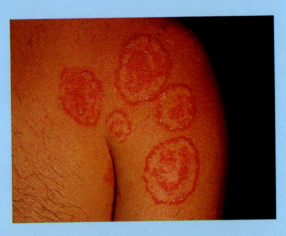

FIGURE I
Ringworm (tinea corporis).

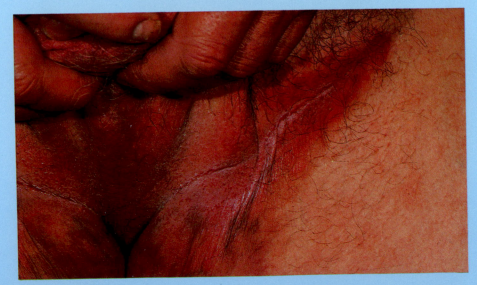

FIGURE J
Intertrigo.

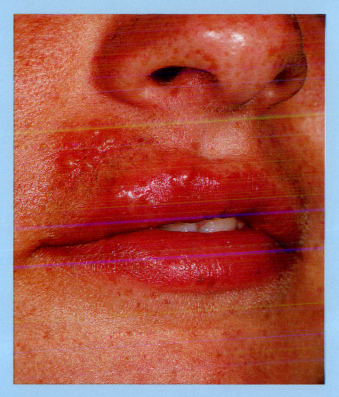

FIGURE K
Herpes simplex.

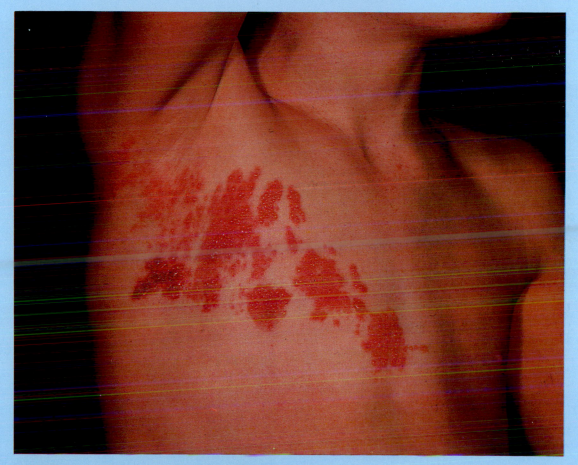

FIGURE L
Herpes zoster.

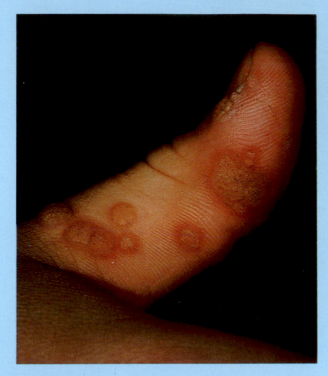

FIGURE M
Warts (verruca vulgaris).

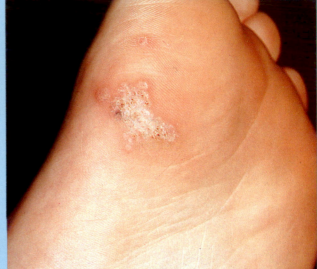

FIGURE N
Plantar wart (verruca plantaris).

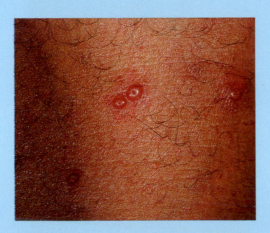

FIGURE O
Molluscum contagiosum.

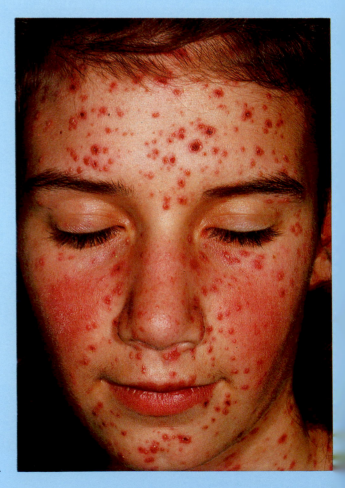

FIGURE P
Chicken pox (varicella).

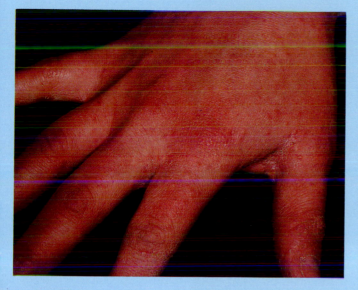

FIGURE Q
Scabies (mites).

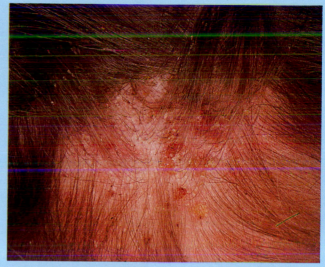

FIGURE R
Pediculosis (lice).

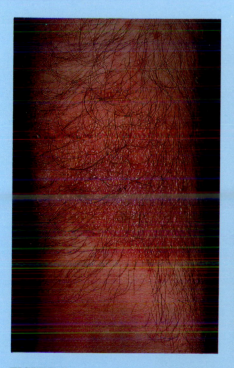

FIGURE S
Eczema.

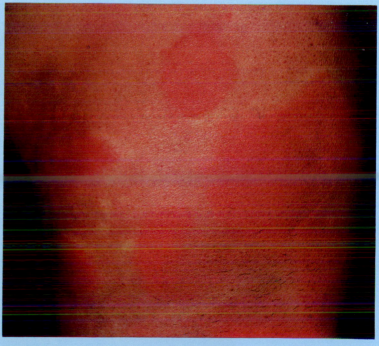

FIGURE T
Hives (urticaria).

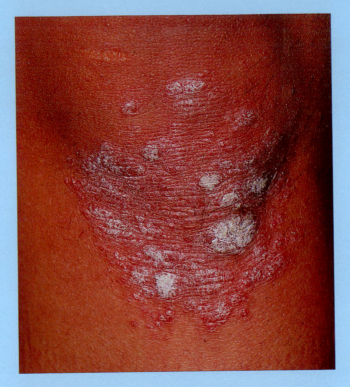

FIGURE U
Psoriasis.

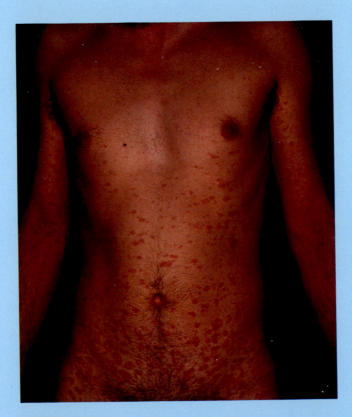

FIGURE V
Pityriasis rosea.

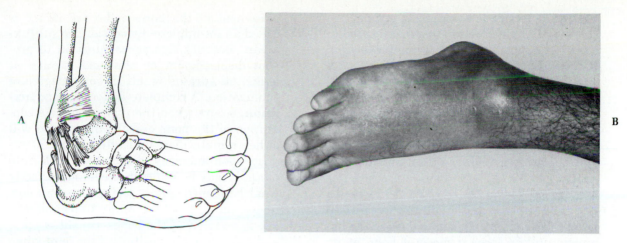

FIGURE 8-17

Sprain injuries. **A**, Ligament sprain resulting from inversion of the ankle during weight bearing and, **B**, second-degree sprain of anterior talofibular ligament 5 days after injury.

age may be within the ligament itself or at one of its attachments. The severity of damage depends on the amount and duration of the abnormal force. Hinge joints, those designed to function in only one direction or plane, are the most frequently sprained. Sprains may occur dynamically; for example, the injury may be self-inflicted during twisting or turning activity. Most sprains, however, involve some outside intervention, such as getting hit on the side of the leg or landing on someone or something in the wrong way.

Ligament sprains are among the more common injuries in athletics. They also are graded into three levels of severity, determined by the amount of ligament damaged.

A *mild sprain* (*first degree*) involves minor stretching or tearing, with minimal disruption in the continuity of the ligament. Although there may be some discomfort during function, there is little or no disability. The athlete will have no instability or abnormal motion of the joint during passive stress tests. The ligament is not weakened significantly, and the treatment is symptomatic. An athlete may continue activity and not even report a mild sprain.

A *moderate sprain* (*second degree*) involves a tearing of ligament fibers and a partial break in the continuity of this noncontractile structure. Like second-degree strains, moderate sprains include the widest range of severity and are the type most commonly reported to the athletic trainer. Moderate sprains are the most difficult to assess. Long experience and refined assessment skills are needed to determine with accuracy the amount of damage sustained by a ligament in a second-degree sprain.

Moderate sprains include varying degrees of pain, swelling, and instability. The athlete may hear or feel a snapping sensation and sense something giving way at the time of the injury. The torn fibers of the injured ligament will produce local pain and instability. The amount of instability will depend on the number of ligament fibers torn or ruptured. As long as some of the ligament remains intact, the passive stress test will normally have an end point, or a perceived limit to abnormal motion.

The goal when caring for moderate sprains is primarily to protect the injured ligament during the healing process. Protection is mandatory to keep damaged fibers immobile and close together to promote efficient repair. If injured ligaments are subjected to repeated stresses and reinjury during this healing process, they may heal in a lengthened and weakened state, resulting in an unstable joint. In most cases protection must be provided by external means, such as a cast, brace, splint, or tape. Once the healing ligament is moderately strong, the surrounding muscles can be rehabilitated to assist in support and to provide protection. Remember, ligaments heal by developing scar tissue, which takes a minimum of 6 weeks to develop and may take 6 months or longer to mature and provide maximum strength. Assessment, treatment, and rehabilitation of second-degree sprains provide the athletic trainer with a considerable challenge.

A *severe sprain* (*third degree*) involves a complete rupture and break in the continuity of the ligament. This may involve the ligament pulling loose a piece of bone at its point of attachment, causing an avulsion fracture. The athlete frequently hears or feels the ligament snap and has the sensation of the joint giving way in this type of injury. The athlete may or may not have pain initially with a completely torn or severed ligament. Passive stressing will produce significant instability and no end point of motion. Chapter 10 discusses some factors that may interfere with passive evaluation procedures.

Athletes suspected of having severe sprains should be treated with routine initial procedures, splinted, and referred to a physician for further diagnosis and surgical repair if necessary. Frequently surgical repair is required to reposition the ligament ends to ensure healing at or near normal length. Sprains should be referred to a physician for any of the following reasons:

1. Significant instability is demonstrated by passive stress tests.
2. Significant joint effusion occurs within a few hours after the injury.
3. There is doubt about the status of the sprain.

✛ Dislocations

A dislocation is the displacement of contiguous surfaces of bones composing a joint (Figures 8-18 to 8-20). This type of injury results from forces, usually external, that cause the joint to go beyond its normal anatomic limits. This may occur as a result of excessive force or from force in an abnormal direction. When there is an incomplete displacement of the bone ends, the injury is called an incomplete dislocation, or **subluxation.** Because ligaments function to prevent displacement or abnormal motion at joints, all sprains result in some degree of subluxation. A complete dislocation, or **luxation,** occurs when there is a complete separation of the bone ends. A dislocation will either remain displaced after injury or reduce spontaneously and move back into place. It may be difficult to evaluate exactly what happened unless the athlete can document the dislocation. Many times the athlete is aware that the bones are out of place and can relate the position of the joint when it was dislocated. Dislocations may be accompanied by avulsion fractures, which can be verified by radiographs, and by torn ligaments, resulting in moderate to severe sprains.

Joints that are designed to function in one direction or plane, such as hinge joints, are those more severely injured when dislocated. For example, when the ankle, knee, or elbow are dislocated, there is normally a significant amount of damage to surrounding structures. Damage to nerves and blood vessels is also more likely. On the other hand, when the shoulder, which has a great ROM and few restrictions, is dislocated, long-term complications and damage to nerves and blood vessels are not as common.

Dislocations that remain displaced are generally easy to recognize. Deformity is almost always apparent. Occasionally the athletic trainer may have to palpate and compare body contours with the uninjured extremity to reveal minimal deformity. Dislocations also cause a significant amount of pain, as well as loss of limb function. The objective of treatment is reduction of the dislocation by a physician. Initially, the athletic trainer should splint or support the injured joint to prevent any further damage. All dislocations and suspected dislocations should be referred to a physician for radiographs and further evaluation.

Treatment for dislocations, once they are reduced, depends on the joint involved, but essentially is the same as that for severe sprains. Surgical intervention is sometimes

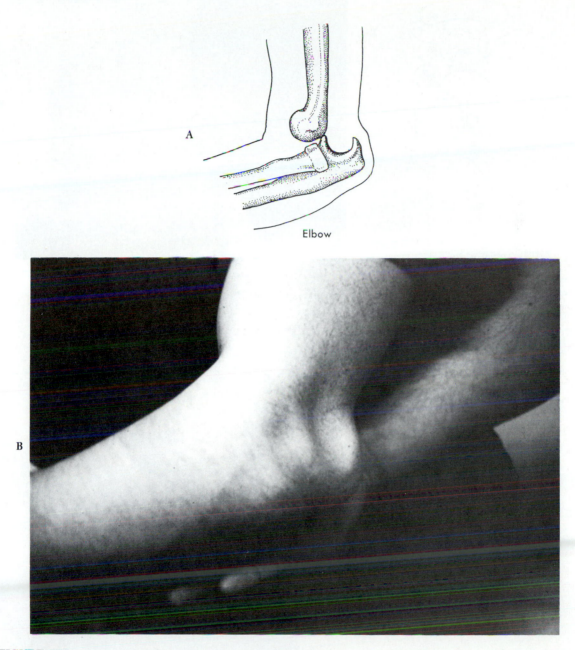

FIGURE 8-18
Elbow dislocation. **A**, Schematic of posterior displacement and, **B**, an actual posterior elbow dislocation.

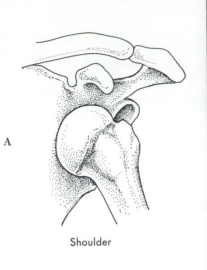

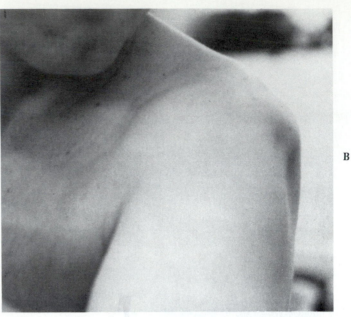

FIGURE 8-19
Shoulder dislocation. **A**, Schematic of anterior displacement and, **B**, an actual anterior shoulder dislocation.

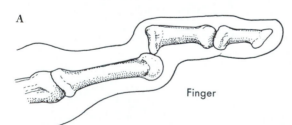

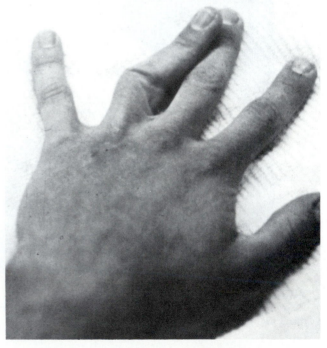

FIGURE 8-20
Finger dislocation. **A**, Schematic of proximal interphalangeal joint displacement and, **B**, an actual interphalangeal joint dislocation.

required, and the injured ligaments must be supported and protected throughout the healing process. Unprotected joints may heal with increased laxity in the ligaments, making the joints more vulnerable to subsequent subluxations and total dislocations.

✥ Fractures

A fracture is a disruption in the continuity of bone and can range in severity from a simple crack to the severe shattering of a bone with multiple fragments. Fractures are unique injuries in that they heal with the same type of tissue (bone) that was injured and can thus regain their preinjured strength. Bones can be fractured in several ways. A direct blow may cause a break at the point of impact, such as an athlete getting kicked in the lateral aspect of the leg, resulting in a fractured fibula. An indirect blow may cause a fracture away from the point of impact, such as an athlete landing on his or her hand and breaking one of the bones of the upper extremity. Severe twisting forces, such as turning and cutting maneuvers, may also cause a fracture. As previously described, severe sprains or strains may result in avulsion fractures.

Prolonged repetitive activity or chronic overuse can lead to another type of fracture,
✥ **stress fracture,** sometimes called fatigue fracture. This type of fracture occurs over a considerable period of time and without history of an acute traumatic episode. A stress fracture is generally an incomplete fracture and seldom results in separation of bone fragments. Many times the initial plain-film radiographs will be negative, and the stress fracture will not be confirmed until the appearance of new periosteal bone formation is recognized on follow-up radiographs 2 or 3 weeks later. The actual fracture line may never appear on radiographs. The athletic trainer should suspect a stress fracture when an athlete reports painful stress and tenderness over a bony area without any specific trauma but is involved in an activity with repetitive stress. If symptoms persist, repeated radiographs or a bone scan may be required to obtain a definitive diagnosis.

Fractures are divided into two major clas-

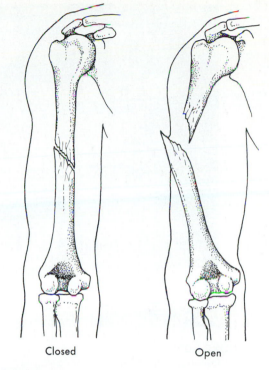

Closed   Open

FIGURE 8-21
Two major classifications of fractures: closed and open.

sifications according to involvement of the overlying skin. Fractures that do not break the skin are called **closed fractures,** whereas fractures that are associated with a tear of the skin are called **open fractures** (Figure 8-21). Open fractures may be caused by a broken bone end tearing the skin or by a direct blow that lacerates the skin at the time of fracture (Figure 8-22). These are generally the more serious type of fractures because of the additional possibilities of infection and external bleeding.

Fractures are also described by the manner in which the bone is broken. This classification is determined and confirmed only by radiographs. Although the athletic trainer is obviously not responsible for classifying fractures according to radiographic appearance, he or she should be familiar with the terminology. Various types of fractures are illustrated in Figure 8-23. Other terms an athletic trainer should be familiar with concerning fractures include:

Contrecoup: Fracture occurring at a dis-

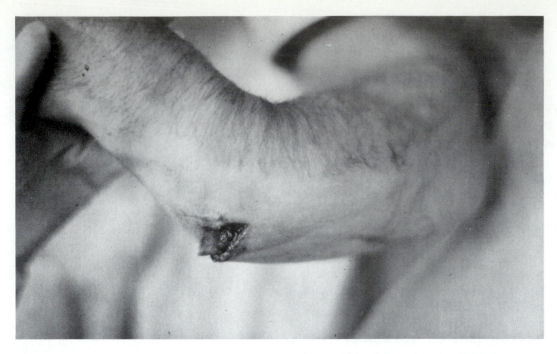

FIGURE 8-22
Open fracture of the ulna.

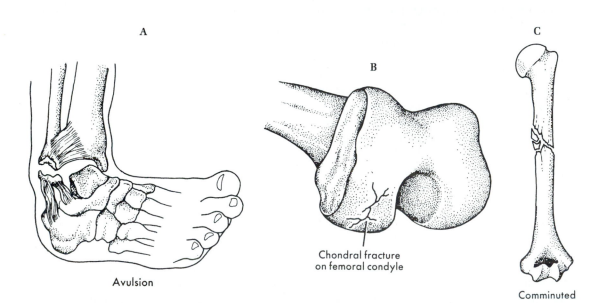

FIGURE 8-23
Various types of fractures. **A**, Avulsion, a fracture in which a piece of bone is pulled loose at the attachment of a tendon, ligament, or muscle, normally occurring with a sudden violent contraction or stress. **B**, Chondral, a fracture involving the articular cartilage. **C**, Comminuted, a fracture in which three or more fragments are produced.

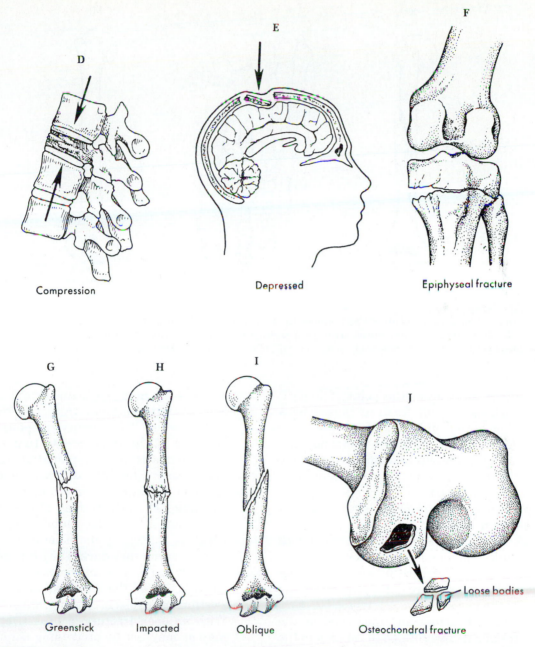

D   E   F

Compression   Depressed   Epiphyseal fracture

G   H   I

J

Greenstick   Impacted   Oblique   Osteochondral fracture

Loose bodies

FIGURE 8-23, cont'd

D, Compression, an impacted fracture characterized by crushed bone tissue, such as the body of a vertebra. **E,** Depressed, in which part of a flat bone is depressed inward or below the surface, such as the skull or cheek bone. **F,** Epiphyseal, a fracture at the growth plate of long bones. Occurs in growing children, as this is the weakest link along the bone. **G,** Greenstick, an incomplete fracture of a long bone that occurs in adolescent athletes whose bones are still pliable. A common example would be a greenstick fracture of the clavicle in children. **H,** Impacted, a fracture in which one fragment has been driven into and imbedded in another fragment. **I,** Oblique, a fracture that crosses the bone at an oblique angle to its long axis. **J,** Osteochondral, a fracture involving the articular cartilage and underlying bone.

Continued.

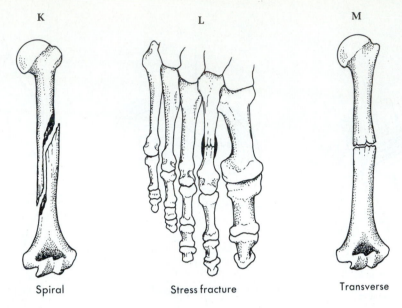

K   **L**   **M**

Spiral   Stress fracture   Transverse

FIGURE 8-23, cont'd
K, Spiral, a break that twists around and through the bone and is usually caused by a twisting injury. **L**, Stress (fatigue), a fracture occurring after prolonged repetitive activity. **M**, Transverse, a break across the bone at a right angle to its long axis, often caused by a direct blow.

tance away from the point of impact, such as a skull fracture caused by a blow to the opposite side.

Delayed union: Fracture that has not united successfully within expected period of time, although the healing process continues.

Nonunion: Failure of the ends of a fracture to unite.

Malunion: Fracture that has united with faulty alignment of fragments.

Overriding: Fracture in which the fragments overlap, resulting in shortening of the bone.

Rotated: Fracture in which one of the fragments has rotated in relation to the other.

Fracture-dislocation: Fracture near a joint that occurs simultaneously with a dislocation.

Displaced: Fracture in which the bone fragments are out of normal alignment.

Nondisplaced: The pieces of bone lie in relatively normal alignment. Occasionally this type of break may be difficult to see on a radiograph.

There are many signs and symptoms that may assist the athletic trainer in recognizing a fracture. The primary symptom is pain localized at the fracture site that remains consistent with motion, palpation, or stress maneuvers. The athlete may report the sound or sensation of something breaking or snapping. The athlete may also experience a grating or grinding sound (crepitation), which is caused by the bone ends rubbing against each other during any type of movement. There may be an obvious deformity or irregularity of the involved area such as swelling, protrusion, or shortening of a limb. With an open fracture, a broken bone end may or may not be protruding through the wound. There may be a loss of function or disability associated with a fracture. However, a loss of function does not always accompany a fracture, and it is a myth to believe, "If the injured part can be moved, it's not broken." The detection of any of these signs and symptoms deserves additional assessment procedures and referral to medical assistance for further diagnosis and radiographs. Forceful manipulation or stress procedures to evaluate bone integrity should be reserved as a final check of structural continuity, not as further proof of that which already clearly requires further diagnosis and radiographs. Athletes may demonstrate false motion or abnormal movement in an area, which is commonly called a false joint. However, in the presence of the above signs and symptoms there is little need to demonstrate false motion. In the absence of signs and symptoms indicating a fracture, more vigorous procedures should be applied to evaluate the bony integrity. A forceful levering both longitudinally and cross-wise to the bone should be performed before pronouncing any such injury free of fracture. Athletic trainers must maintain a high index of suspicion and never allow an athlete to return to activity with an injury that suggests a fracture. Similarly, athletic trainers must not decide any suspected fracture is safe from aggravation by continued athletic activity without further diagnosis.

The treatment for suspected fractures is that of protection for the injured area so that no further damage occurs because of improper handling or movement. This is normally accomplished by splinting the injured area. Remember to immobilize the joint above and below a fracture site to avoid movement to the bone fragments. If there is an open wound associated with the fracture, control the bleeding and apply a sterile dressing before splinting the area. Treat for shock if necessary. The athletic trainer should also feel for a pulse distal to major fractures to ensure circulation is adequate. Whenever circulation is jeopardized, a medical emergency exists and the injured athlete must be transported to a medical facility immediately.

REFERENCES

Comes JA: Myositis ossificans traumatica, pathogenesis and management, *Ath Train* 22(3):193, 1987.
Conklin RJ: Acne vulgaris in the athlete, *Phys Sportsmed,* 16(10):57, 1988.
Grant HD, Murray RH, Bergeron JD: *Emergency care,* ed 5, Englewood Cliffs, 1990, Brady.
Hamel R: AIDS; assessing the risk among athletes, *Phys Sportsmed* 20(2):139, 1992.
Lookingbill DP, Marks JG: *Principles of dermatology,* Philadelphia, 1986, WB Saunders.
Malasanos L, Barkauskas V, Stoltenberg-Allen: *Health assessment,* ed 4, St Louis, 1985, Mosby-Year Book.
Mellion MB and others: Hydrocolloid dressings in the treatment of turf burns and other athletic abrasions, *Ath Train* 23(4):341, 1988.
Nelson MA: Stopping the spread of herpes simplex; a focus on wrestlers, *Phys Sportsmed* 20(10):117, 1992.
O'Donoghue DH: *Treatment of injuries to athletes,* ed 4, Philadelphia, 1984, WB Saunders.
Reichel M, Laub DA: From acne to black heel: common skin injuries in sports, *Phys Sportsmed* 20(2):111, 1992.
Sauer GC: *Manual of skin diseases,* ed 5, Philadelphia, 1985, Lippincott.
Seltzer DG: Educating athletes on HIV disease and AIDS; the team physician's role, *Phys Sportsmed* 21(1):109, 1993.
Stauffer LW: How I manage athlete's foot, *Phys Sportsmed* 14(7):103, 1986.
Stauffer LW: Skin disorders in athletes: identification and management, *Phys Sportsmed* 11(3):101, 1983.
Stone MH: Muscle conditioning and muscle injuries, *Med Sci Sports Exerc* 22(4):457, 1990.
White WB, Grant-Wels JM: Transmission of herpes simplex type 1 infection in rugby players, *JAMA* 252(4):533, 1984.

SUGGESTED READINGS

American Academy of Orthopaedic Surgeons: *Emergency care and transportation of the sick and injured,* ed 5, Park Ridge, 1992, the Academy.
A textbook frequently used in Emergency Medical Technician courses that covers all aspects of emergency medical care.
Arnheim DD, Prentice WE: *Principles of athletic training,* ed 8, St Louis, 1993, Mosby-Year Book.
A comprehensive textbook covering all aspects of athletic injuries and athletic-related conditions.
Habif TP: *Clinical dermatology: a color guide to diagnosis and therapy,* ed 2, St Louis, 1990, Mosby-Year Book.
An excellent comprehensive text covering the etiology, diagnosis, and therapy of skin diseases. Contains numerous color photographs.
Maneval MW and others: The implication of acquired immunodeficiency syndrome for athletic trainers, *Sports Med Update* Summer, 1989.
An article intended to familiarize athletic trainers with AIDS information and outline preventive measures that will help control the spread of AIDS in the athletic environment.

CHAPTER 9

Psychological aspects of injury

After you have completed this chapter, you should be able to:

- Identify the factors that may predispose athletes to injury.
- Name some strategies that could be used to minimize the risk of injuries.
- Describe the psychological responses to injury.
- Explain the necessity of dealing with injured athletes as human beings to minimize the degree of psychological trauma.
- Identify psychological strategies and techniques that can be used to facilitate the rehabilitation process.

This chapter was contributed by Dr. Jim Lidstone. Dr. Lidstone is Professor and Coordinator of Graduate Studies in the Department of Health, Physical Education and Recreation at South Dakota State University. He has 10 years experience as a sport psychology consultant to athletes and has conducted research on the psychological impact of sports injuries in collegiate athlete populations.

This text is testimony to the fact that injuries occur as a result of participating in athletics. It has been documented through research that over one million injuries occurred in interscholastic athletics in a single year. Although it is inevitable that injuries will occur, one of the goals of the sports medicine professional is to reduce the number and severity of injuries and, for the injuries that do occur, to return the injured athlete to competition safely and successfully. A safe return means that the athlete returns to competition without an increased probability of reinjury. A successful return implies that the athlete not suffer a performance decrement as a result of his or her injury.

The field of sports medicine has advanced to such a stage that we are now able to return athletes to competition with unprecedented speed. Athletes are able to physically return to competition faster than at any time in history. However, what is forgotten is that athletes may suffer *psychological* trauma as well as *physical* trauma when injured, and if we are too efficient with our treatment methods and rehabilitation modalities, athletes may be ready to return to competition physically before they are ready to return psychologically (Figure 9-1).

The purpose of this chapter is to, first, identify athletes who may be psychologically and circumstantially at risk of injury so that this risk can be minimized, and secondly, in the event that injury does occur, to recognize that there are certain predictable and unpredictable psychological consequences of injury. Finally, some psychological rehabilitation strategies will be described that can be used by the sports medicine team to facilitate the athlete's safe and successful re-

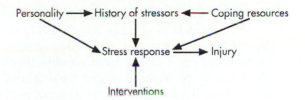

FIGURE 9-2
A model of stress and athletic injury.

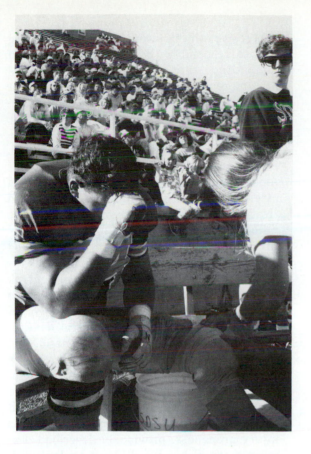

FIGURE 9-1
An athletic injury can be as traumatic psychologically as it is physically.

turn to competition, including both physical and psychological rehabilitation.

PRE-DISPOSITION TO INJURY

In addition to the assessment, treatment, and rehabilitation of athletic injuries, one of the athletic trainer's most valuable function is the prevention of athletic injuries. Taping, bracing, and orthotic devices are used to help deter injuries, but recently, research has shown that it may be possible to identify classifications of individuals who may be at a higher risk for injury to occur. This does not mean that we are able to predict with 100% certainty who will become injured; it simply means that certain groups of athletes may be *predisposed* to injury because of factors related to life stress, personality, attitude, and situational factors.

Life Stress Events

Intuitively it is tempting to believe that all injuries have certain physical mechanisms that cause them: a lateral blow to the knee; violent rotational movement while a foot is firmly planted on turf or the court surface; or a dramatic contraction of a muscle that produces a strain, tear, or rupture. Similarly, other readily observable factors such as equipment, environmental conditions, lack of training, lack of adequate warmup or stretching, and overtraining are cited as contributing factors to injury. However, a convincing body of research evidence has recently emerged that points to the fact that there is a fairly strong relationship between psychological factors and the occurrence of injuries. Variables such as personality factors, history of life stressors, and coping resources all contribute to whether or not an individual may be at increased risk of athletic injury. Based on this, a preliminary model has been proposed to explain the relationship among these variables (Figure 9-2). According to the model, numerous variables such as personality factors, coping resources, and whether or not the individual has been or is being schooled in intervention strategies, affect the magnitude and intensity of the stress response, which, in turn influences the occurrence of injury. A significant factor in the model is the concept of **life stress.**

Athletes who are, or have been, experiencing significant stressors in their lives are more likely to be injured, and the injuries are likely to be more severe. Stressors include, but are not limited to, such things as the death of family members, moving, change of occupation, and divorce in the family. As yet it is unclear why individuals experiencing excess life stress are predisposed to injury, but the most tenable theories have to do with muscular tension and attentional focus. Stress produces anxiety, which is accompanied by physiological **arousal.** One of the symptoms of excessive arousal is muscular tension, and muscles and limbs that are rigid and inflexible are more prone to injury. Additionally, it is well established that increased arousal results in a narrowing of **attentional focus,** as well as increased distractibility. Failure to attend appropriately to the task at hand in a volatile environment might result in individuals missing important cues and stimuli that might alert them to hazardous situations, particularly in contact sports.

Interacting with the concept of life stress are the individual's coping resources. Coping mechanisms such as relaxation techniques, mental imagery, and goal setting are invoked to help us overcome stressors in the environment. However, coping resources can be viewed as a reservoir that becomes depleted somewhat each time an individual encounters a stressful situation. Time replenishes the reservoir, but too many stressors in a short period of time can seriously deplete the individual's coping resources, thus making it more likely for injury to occur due to increased anxiety, physiological arousal, and narrowed attentional focus.

Personality Factors

Unfortunately, there is no clear pattern of personality traits that enables prediction of the individuals who are most likely to experience injury. However, several personality attributes consistently emerge in the psychological testing of injured athletes with established instruments such as the Cattell 16PF Questionnaire and the California Psychological Inventory. Factors such as anxiety, locus of control, and risk-taking behavior have proven to be significantly related to the incidence of injury.

Anxiety, and in particular, **competitive trait anxiety** is defined as a predisposition to perceive athletic situations as threatening and to respond with heightened levels of competitive state anxiety. Such individuals are more likely to approach games or matches with high levels of fear and apprehension (**cognitive state anxiety**) that are accompanied by increased levels of physiological arousal (**somatic state anxiety**). Excess arousal creates heightened muscular tension and a corresponding narrowing of attentional focus that may make the high trait–anxious individual more injury prone.

Related to the concept of anxiety is **locus of control.** Individuals can be classified along a continuum ranging from extreme *internal* to extreme *external* locus of control. Those who are classified as internals believe that they are responsible for their own actions and that they are in control of their destiny. Externals, on the other hand, feel "acted upon," in other words, that they have little control over what happens to them. They tend to approach situations with more caution and higher levels of anxiety, which carry with them the same consequences for injury proneness, previously described. Externals are also more difficult to deal with following an injury because they tend to progress more slowly through the stages of the grieving process, described later, and are reluctant to share in the responsibility for their rehabilitation.

Two final personality factors that may predispose an athlete to increased risk of injury are risk-taking behavior and a sense of invincibility. Although risk-taking behavior is to be expected and encouraged to a certain extent in achievement-oriented individuals, excessive risk-takers may push themselves into stressful situations that will tax their coping mechanisms. When coupled with the concept of invincibility found to exist particularly in college-age male populations, one has "an accident waiting to happen."

Situational Factors

If there is one thing learned through years of studying the relationship between personality and behavior, it is that one cannot consider personality factors without examining the environment or situational factors in which they exist. It is the interaction between personality, situational factors, and the individual's physical characteristics that dictate whether they are at increased risk of injury.

Certain situational factors, when combined with the personality characteristics mentioned previously, may alert the trainer to a potentially hazardous situation. Beware of, for example, the substitute or marginal player who aspires to a starting position. These individuals are more likely to engage in excessive risk-taking behavior and to mask pain and injury to gain the coaches' attention and favor. Similarly, the player who has just earned a starting role may be motivated to play through pain so as not to relinquish that which has been achieved. Another potentially problematic situation involves the marginal student whose primary sense of self-worth comes through participation in athletics. Such individuals have more to lose by not playing and therefore may be more inclined toward excessive risk taking. Similarly, the individual for whom an athletic scholarship is the only avenue to an education or who views success in sport

as a vehicle for launching a professional career may be more at risk of injury.

Attitudes

In a recent survey of coaches, the characteristic most admired and desired in their athletes is *mental toughness*. Athletes are socialized to believe that mental toughness, giving 110%, and sacrificing their bodies are essential for success in sports (Figure 9-3). Certainly it is important for athletes to strive to do their best and to persevere in the face of adversity, but it is important to realize that mental toughness and ignoring one's physical limitations can lead to injury and failure. Again, it may be the substitute or marginal player who is most at risk because he or she may disregard common sense to earn a starting position. Sports medicine professionals know that pain is a signal that something is wrong, yet among some coaches and athletes, it is considered to be a sign of mental toughness to ignore pain. Players are constantly lauded for "playing with pain," "playing hurt," or "toughing it out." In this sense, playing with an injury becomes a badge of courage and a

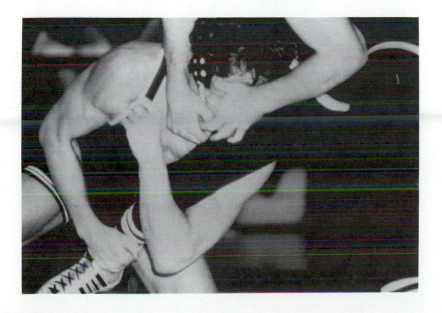

FIGURE 9-3
Coaches value athletes who exhibit mental toughness and may encourage them to take excessive risks for the "good of the team."

reinforcer. It is human nature to continue to seek rewards and reinforcement, and players learn to ignore pain to accrue the admiration of coaches, teammates, and spectators.

Self-Concept and Self-Esteem

The term **self-concept** is now accepted to mean the structure and organization of the self. Relatively stable and enduring, it is formed and shaped through interaction with significant others in the individual's environment. At the center of the self-concept is the "I," or essence of the self. The individual's identity, then, is comprised of all of the roles, characteristics, and attributes that the individual believes to be true about her or his existence (Figure 9-4). Roles such as student, spouse, son or daughter, athlete, or American define the individual's identity. Characteristics such as intelligent, personable, strong, lazy, fast, persistent, and industrious dictate the individual's acceptance of who or what he or she is. **Self-esteem** and self-concept are inextricably interrelated be-

cause one cannot contemplate the organization of the self without considering how one feels about those components.

It is also true that a hierarchy exists relative to these roles and attributes in the self-concept structure. Presumably, the closer these are to the center of the individual's existence (the "I"), the more important they are and, therefore, the more resistant they are to change. It is possible to conceive of four different individuals who each derive a positive sense of personal esteem through success in a different endeavor (academics, appearance, music, athletics). For individuals who have derived most of their reinforcement, identity, and esteem from athletic-related endeavors, the potential exists for severe psychological trauma to occur if they suddenly lose a role and the accompanying role-related characteristics that they hold in such high importance. The individual for whom the role of athlete is central in the self-concept hierarchy can be expected to exhibit more symptoms of psychological trauma in response to injury.

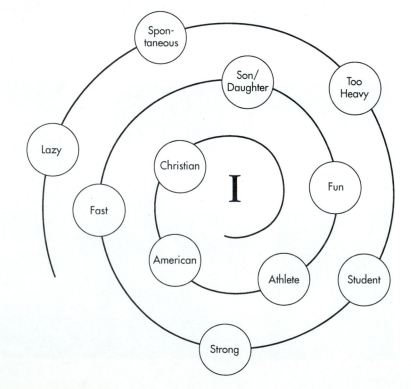

FIGURE 9-4
Structure and organization of the self.

Preventive Measures

Regardless of what precautionary measures are taken, injuries will occur. However, knowledge of a few simple strategies may help reduce the number of injuries for which psychological elements are contributing factors. For example, several excellent screening instruments are available that can alert the sports medicine professional to the individuals who are experiencing unusual amounts of life stress. The Athletic Life Event Scale (ALES), the Daily Hassles Scale (DHS), and the Stress Audit Questionnaire are a few examples. The latter instrument also has a coping resources (CR) scale to assess whether athletes have resources such as friends, family, and proper sleeping and eating habits to help them cope with stress.

Competitive trait anxiety can be easily assessed by administering Martens' Sport Competition Anxiety Test (SCAT). Individuals high in this construct who are experiencing excessive amounts of life stress, and who have low coping resources, are at high risk of injury. Referring these individuals to appropriate counseling services is a means of averting potentially dangerous situations through remediation of problems.

Techniques also exist to increase the coping strategies available to the athlete. A sports psychologist can be employed to teach the athlete appropriate relaxation techniques and concentration strategies to use when encountering stressful situations. As part of the pre-practice or pre-competition routine, athletes can be encouraged to "check their problems at the door," in other words to focus only on athletics while they are in the athletic venue. A useful strategy to help in this regard is the *focus stretch* employed during warmup exercises. During the first several minutes of stretching/warmup, athletes are permitted to engage their teammates in conversation regarding any subject whatsoever, including anything that is troubling them. During the middle portion of the warmup, conversation must be related to their sport. Finally, the last few minutes of the warmup must be spent in quiet, individual contemplation of the day's athletic activity.

PSYCHOLOGICAL CONSEQUENCES OF INJURY

Chapter 7 explained how the body responds to physical trauma. For all types of injuries the body can be expected to respond in the same way; that is, the process of inflammation and healing. In addition to these predictable physical responses of the body to trauma, there are certain psychological reactions that occur that have profound implications for how the sports medicine professional assesses, treats, and rehabilitates the injury.

The Grief Response

Although injuries are an inevitable consequence of participation in athletics, few athletes would acknowledge that a serious injury could ever happen to them. So, when an unexpected injury occurs, the impact is very sudden and severe, much like what one experiences during a loss due to separation, divorce, employment termination, or even the death of a loved one. Athletes are forced to deal with the injury as a loss. At the very least, they have lost physical function, but they also suffer a loss of a major aspect of their identity and a primary source of reward and reinforcement. The more severe the injury, the greater the sense of loss.

Some say that the psychological response of the athlete to injury is analogous to the five stages of grief outlined by Kubler-Ross in her epic work, *On Death and Dying*. The stages are denial, anger, bargaining, depression, and acceptance.

Denial. Initially, the athlete may refuse to acknowledge the fact that he or she has been injured. She or he may attempt to play through the pain, refusing to believe that it is serious. When the injury is diagnosed, the athlete may insist on a second and even third opinion before finally acknowledging the injury.

Anger. After acknowledging the injury, athletes may express anger with themselves and others. They may feel anger toward the individual or the situation that caused the injury, to themselves for not attending more rigidly to training and warmup regimens, or toward trainers and physicians who diag-

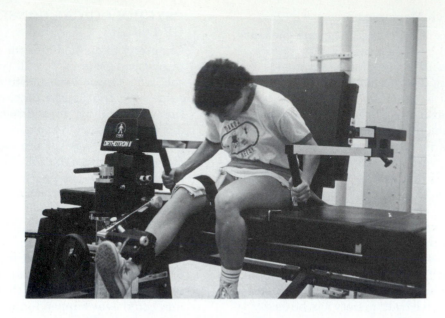

FIGURE 9-5
Once the injured athlete has accepted the injury, serious rehabilitation can begin.

nosed the injury. Obviously, the athlete can be a challenge to deal with during this phase.

Bargaining. At some point, the athlete may attempt to bargain his or her way out of the injury. "If I take the week off from practice, it will get better." "If I can just get through the remaining games, I'll have surgery in the off-season." It is not uncommon for athletes to risk more serious, long-term damage, to postpone radical treatment until season's end.

Depression. When athletes realize that the injury will cause them to miss extended amounts of practice and competition, they often respond with feelings of isolation, loneliness, and depression. This is to be expected since the athlete is experiencing a loss, and the length and severity of the depression will depend on the degree to which the player draws his or her identity from the role of athlete. Following a career-ending knee injury a college football player described his frustration at dealing with his new-found disability:

"For six days I didn't even get off my back. Then for another week and a half I didn't get off my back except to go to the bathroom. Then for three or four weeks I was in a wheelchair and relied on my friends to come and pick me up when it was time for class."

The sudden change from independence, health, and vitality to helplessness and dependence can have severe repercussions. Obviously it is critical to get the athlete into rehabilitation as quickly as feasible to help his or her transition through this stage.

Acceptance and Resignation. Once the athlete has entered this phase of the process, he or she has accepted the injury, and the process of healing and recovery can begin in earnest. It is important that the trainer adopt a positive approach to the recovery process and encourage the athlete to channel her or his energy into rehabilitation efforts (Figure 9-5).

Perceptions of Injury

Athletes vary in terms of their perceptions of an injury, and this has profound implications for the manner in which they progress through the stages of the grief process. Some may view the injury as a disaster, robbing them of playing time, physical function, future opportunities, and identity. It may also erode their sense of self-esteem. For others, the injury may be viewed as an op-

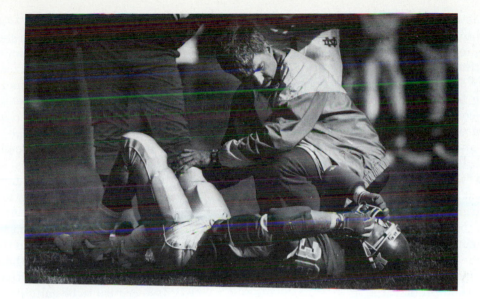

FIGURE 9-6
The pain that accompanies injury is a source of stress that can make the athlete fearful of returning to competition.

portunity for them to display their fortitude in the face of adversity. They embrace the challenge of returning to competition following a grueling period of rehabilitation. Still others wear their injury like a "badge of honor," a wound received in the line of duty. And, of course, other players may view an injury as an escape from a losing season, poor performance, or lack of playing time. The athletic trainer must be prepared for these varied reactions and be equipped to deal with each accordingly.

Fear

Fear is a very understandable and potentially damaging emotional response in the injury situation. First of all, the athlete probably experiences intense pain and accompanying anxiety, which will emerge again when the athlete contemplates returning to the competitive situation (Figure 9-6). In addition there are other fears that the individual may experience:

1. Fear of not recovering
2. Fear of losing one's job or position
3. Fear of losing income/scholarship
4. Fear of losing future opportunities
5. Fear of losing one's identity
6. Fear of reinjury on return to competition

It is important to realize that these are natural responses to a distressful situation that may be adequately dealt with using the athlete's coping mechanisms. However, it is equally likely that some individuals will benefit from psychological intervention to allay these fears and allow the rehabilitation process to proceed unabated.

Alienation

Athletes share a unique bond that can quickly dissipate when they lose that aspect of their identity through an injury. The injured athlete can no longer interact athletically with her or his teammates and can no longer contribute to the team effort; therefore the potential exists for them to become alienated from the situation. Attitudes of coaches, teammates, and allied personnel such as trainers, can contribute to this phenomenon when they "switch the injured player off" and don't include him or her to the same extent as before the injury.

Some coaches act as though they believe that the fastest way to recovery from an injury is to communicate to athletes in subtle ways that they are not contributing as long as they are injured. They isolate the injured athlete from the rest of the team and generally convey the attitude that injured athletes are malingerers, lack mental toughness, and are not fully committed to the organization. Coaches like this clearly exhibit a "winning first" as opposed to an "athlete first" mentality.

Attitudes and behaviors that convey the notion that a player is no longer part of the organization contribute to players becoming isolated and alienated, which may lead to quitting or pushing too hard to return to competition prematurely.

Depletion of Coping Resources

As mentioned earlier, a lack of coping resources is significantly related to the incidence of injury. Individuals with depleted coping resources as a result of dealing with inordinate amounts of life stress are more likely to experience anxiety and arousal in competitive situations, thereby placing them at increased risk of injury. It also bears mention that an injury is, in and of itself, a significant stressor that further taxes an individual's coping resources, leaving him or her less able to deal with other stressful events that may come along.

PSYCHOLOGICAL CONSIDERATIONS IN TREATMENT AND REHABILITATION

In keeping with the assessment theme of this text, the bulk of this chapter is devoted to the psychological antecedents and consequences of athletic injury. The remainder of this chapter will address psychological considerations that affect the treatment and rehabilitation process. The intent is not to address these issues in detail but merely to inform the reader of their existence. For more complete information, the reader is directed toward the suggested readings.

The Athlete as Human Being

By virtue of their exposure to sheer numbers of injuries, the sports medicine professional becomes somewhat desensitized to injuries. At all costs, the athletic trainer must avoid dehumanizing the assessment and rehabilitation process by treating *injuries* rather than *human beings*. Although a particular injury might be the ninety-eighth anterior cruciate tear you have encountered, chances are that, for the athlete and his or her family, it is the first. It is wise to apply "The Golden Rule" in assessment and treatment of injuries. Treat them as you would like to be treated. As the first one on the scene it is your responsibility to help them cope with the immediate crisis of the situation (Figure 9-7). It is critical to be calming and reassuring to minimize the fears and emotions that the athlete is experiencing. Following initial assessment and treatment a positive and upbeat approach to rehabilitation is critical to help the athlete progress swiftly through the grieving stages.

Social Support

To combat loneliness, isolation, and alienation, which may occur in response to injury, it is critical to establish a network of social support for the injured athlete. This is particularly true when athletic identity is strong and the athlete's interaction with family and friends is primarily through the role of athlete. Indeed, many close friendships are established solely because the individual encounters new friends as a result of the athletic experience. The bonds are suddenly weakened or severed with injury.

It is important that coaches and sports medicine professionals maintain normal contacts and relations with the injured athlete. Keep him or her involved as much as possible in practice and game situations, and encourage him or her to contribute in appropriate ways so that he or she continues to feel a part of the organization. At all times, it is essential to communicate a sense of optimism about the athlete's progress to-

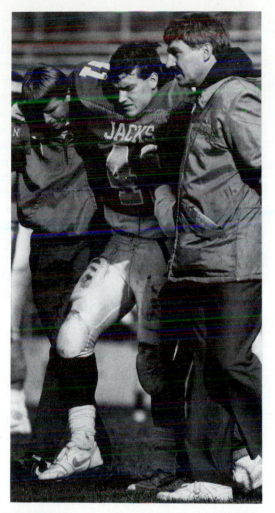

FIGURE 9-7
As first person on the scene the athletic trainer serves an important role in allaying the athlete's fears about the injury. This can minimize the amount of psychological trauma the athlete experiences.

evance to the sports medicine professional for the treatment and rehabilitation of athletic injuries. The purpose of this section is to briefly describe those techniques. In applying these strategies, the reader is encouraged to seek the help of a qualified professional.

Relaxation Techniques. Numerous relaxation strategies exist that can be taught to athletes. The ability to relax oneself on demand is an important coping strategy that can be employed whenever one encounters a stressful situation. Thus it has application beyond the athletic arena. Common relaxation strategies include progressive relaxation, passive relaxation, autogenic training, biofeedback, imagery, hypnosis, and controlled breathing. All are designed to elicit the relaxation response.

Imagery. Imagery is simply the experiencing of an event in the absence of the usual stimuli. It has been described as "making a movie in your mind," where you are the director and you control the outcome of your movie. Imagery has experienced widespread use for athletic performance enhancement but it is recently receiving attention in the sports medicine field for the rehabilitation of injuries. Following extensive patient education about the injury and the healing and rehabilitation process the athlete incorporates imagery of the healing process into his or her regular rehabilitation routine. Imagining oneself overcoming the adversity of injury and successfully recovering and returning to competition sets up positive expectations for the injured player. Effective imagery should include the following:

1. It should be done in a quiet place, free from distractions.
2. It should be preceded by relaxation.
3. It should incorporate all of the senses (visual, auditory, olfactory, tactile, and kinesthetic).
4. It should have a positive outcome.
5. It should be practiced daily for 15 to 20 minutes.

ward recovery. At the same time, injured players should be encouraged to broaden their horizons by seeking out and establishing new contacts, networks, interests, and identities so that they emerge from the injury experience even better than before.

Psychological Rehabilitation Strategies

The field of applied sport psychology uses many intervention strategies that have rel-

Cognitive Restructuring. Following injury and during the difficult treatment and rehabilitation phases, the athlete may exhibit a negative mindset, symptomized by a preponderance of negative self-talk. Statements such as "I can't do this" or "I'll never be able to play again" should alert the trainer to the need for intervention. Cognitive restructuring is a behavior modification technique that has, as its goal, the transformation of negative thought processes and negative self-talk into a positive mindset. The steps to cognitive restructuring are as follows:

1. Recognize and acknowledge the negative thoughts.
2. Stop the negative thoughts **(thought stoppage).**
3. Focus one's attention internally **(centering).**
4. Transform the negative thought into a positive thought.
5. Visualize yourself succeeding.

Statements such as "these exercises hurt too much to be beneficial" can be transformed to something like "this hurts, but the pain will decrease each day. The athletic trainer is knowledgeable and wouldn't be prescribing this if it wasn't helpful." With practice and improvement the frequency of negative thoughts should decrease.

Systematic Desensitization. In instances of severe trauma, the fear response may be so strongly conditioned in the individual as to warrant strong intervention. Systematic desensitization involves teaching the individual to substitute a newly learned response (relaxation) for the previously conditioned response (fear and anxiety). Systematic desensitization should only be implemented by a qualified professional such as a clinical psychologist. It involves the establishment of a *fear hierarchy* related to the feared situation (e.g., making a tackle similar to the one that resulted in injury). The client is then taught relaxation techniques. Once the client has learned to control his or her relaxation the individual is asked to imagine the fearful situations in the fear hierarchy from least fearful (e.g.,

walking past the football field) to most fearful (e.g., preparing to tackle the running back). At each step the client is told to relax in the presence of the feared stimuli. Once the individual is able to maintain a state of relaxation to the imagined stimuli, he or she is ready to transfer it to the real situation.

Goal Setting. Perhaps the single most effective motivational strategy that exists is goal setting. Goal setting has been proven to work in numerous situations and has obvious applications to the rehabilitation of athletic injuries. Goal setting is thought to be effective because goals (a) direct attention and action, (b) mobilize energy expenditure, (c) prolong effort (persistence), and (d) motivate strategy development. The following are principles of effective goal setting:

1. Goals should be specific.
2. Goals should be challenging.
3. Goals should be realistic.
4. Goals should be believable.
5. Goals should be measurable.
6. Goals should be short-term (30 to 60 days).
7. Goals should be written down and made public.

When helping an injured athlete set goals it is critical to remember that he or she is going to experience frustration at having difficulty doing things that once were easy. Be certain to maintain a positive approach and continually reinforce progress.

Building Self-Confidence. It has been proven repeatedly that a key ingredient to success is first believing that you can succeed. Self-confidence or self-efficacy is the belief that you can successfully perform a given task. For the injured athlete facing a long, difficult rehabilitation process, it may be necessary to enhance his or her self-confidence. Self-confidence is enhanced through (a) successful performance, (b) **vicarious experience,** (c) verbal persuasion, and (d) emotional arousal. For the athletic trainer this means paying particular attention to goal-setting and structuring the setting so that the athlete experiences only success (no matter how small) and never failure. Additionally, it is extremely effective if he or she is intentionally paired during rehabilitation with someone who has experienced a similar injury but is further along in the rehabilitation process. Seeing the progress of another (vicarious experience) raises the expectations of success of the newly injured player. Finally, it is essential that all who have contact with the injured player be upbeat, positive, enthusiastic, and encouraging about the individual's progress and prognosis for a timely return to competition.

REFERENCES

Anderson MB, Williams JM: A model of stress and athletic injury: prediction and prevention, *J Sport Exerc Psych* 10(3):294, 1988.

Bandura A: Self-efficacy: toward a unifying theory of behavioral change, *Psychol Rev* 84(2):191, 1977.

Blackwell B, McCullagh P: The relationship of athletic injury to life stress, competitive anxiety, and coping resources, *Ath Train* 25(1):23, 1990.

Deutsch RE: The psychological implications of sports related injuries, *Int J Sport Psych* 16(3):232, 1985.

Dunn R: Psychological factors in sports medicine, *Ath Train* 18(1):34, 1983.

Kraus JF, Conroy C: Mortality and morbidity from injuries in sports and recreation, *Ann Rev Public Health* 5:163, 1984.

Kubler-Ross E: *On death and dying,* New York, 1969, Macmillan.

Martens R: *Sport competition anxiety test,* Champaign, 1982, Human Kinetics.

Meggyesey D: *Out of their league,* New York, 1971, Paperback Library.

Miller LH, Smith AD: Stress audit questionnaire, *Bostonia: in-depth* Dec:39, 1982.

Nideffer RM: The injured athlete: psychological factors in treatment, *Orthop Clin North Am* 14(2):374, 1983.

Passer MW, Seese MD: Life stress and athletic injury: examination of positive versus negative events and three moderator variables, *J Human Stress* 9:11, 1983.

Purkey WW: *Self concept and school achievement,* Englewood Cliffs, 1970, Prentice-Hall.

Rotella RJ, Heyman SR: Stress, injury, and the psychological rehabilitation of athletes, In Williams JM: *Applied sport psychology: personal growth to peak performance,* Palo Alto, 1986, Mayfield.

Terkel S: *Working,* New York, 1974, Avon Books.

Weiss MR, Troxel RK: Psychology of the injured athlete, *Ath Train* 21(2):104, 1986.

SUGGESTED READINGS

Cox RH: *Sport psychology: concepts and applications,* Dubuque, 1990, WC Brown.
A comprehensive sport psychology text with an excellent chapter on intervention strategies.

Pederson P: The grief response and injury: a special challenge for athletes and athletic trainers, *Ath Train* 21(4):312, 1986.
An excellent article for helping the athletic trainer better understand the grief response and how to manage it.

Rotella RJ, Campbell MS: Systematic desensitization: psychological rehabilitation of injured athletes, *Ath Train* 18(2):140, 1983.
This piece thoroughly describes the process of systematic desensitization with specific applications to injury rehabilitation.

Samples P: Mind over muscle: returning the injured athlete to play, *Phys Sportsmed* 15(10):172, 1987.
An easily understood article that identifies psychological strategies for returning injured athletes to competition.

Singer RN, Johnson PJ: Strategies to cope with pain associated with sport-related injuries, *Ath Train* 22(2):100, 1987.
This article describes behavioral and cognitive intervention strategies that may be used to deal with pain as an alternative to drugs, surgery, and physical therapy.

Williams JM: *Applied sport psychology: personal growth to peak performance,* Palo Alto, 1986, Mayfield.
An edited volume of sport psychology topics of relevance to the sports medicine professional including goal setting, relaxation training, imagery training, confidence building, concentration training, self-hypnosis, psychological aspects of injury rehabilitation, and termination from athletics.

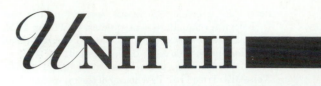UNIT III

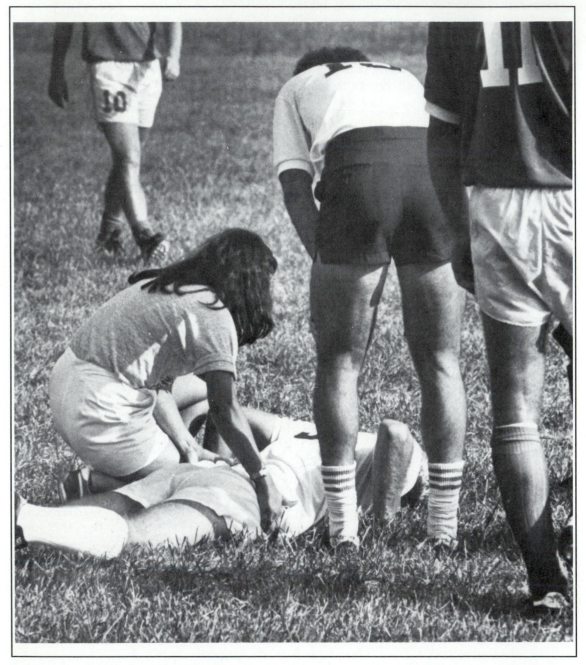

Athletic Injury Assessment Process

The athletic injury assessment process is a necessary and extremely important skill for anyone who shares responsibility for the medical care of athletes. A primary factor in the successful management of athletic injuries is the earliest possible determination of the type and extent of injury. To ensure a complete and effective evaluation, the athletic trainer must have meaningful and well-established assessment procedures to follow with every injury. In addition to the skilled execution of carefully organized steps in an assessment sequence, the athletic trainer must constantly sharpen and refine basic observation and communication skills essential for effective information gathering. This unit is designed to assist the athletic trainer in preparing his or her assessment techniques. The remainder of this text is concerned with evaluative techniques for injuries to specific areas of the body.

10 **Factors related to athletic injury assessment**
11 **Assessment procedures**

CHAPTER 10

Factors related to athletic injury assessment

After you have completed this chapter, you should be able to:
- Define athletic injury assessment and discuss some of the factors interrelated with this process.
- Discuss the various considerations and personal skills necessary for an individual to competently assess athletic-related injuries and conditions.
- Describe the difference between a sign and a symptom.
- Briefly describe the various diagnostic procedures that may be employed to assist in the evaluation of an athletic injury.

Athletic injury assessment is defined as the comprehensive evaluation of an athletic injury beginning when the injury occurs and continuing through the healing process until the injured area has been rehabilitated to its fullest extent. The initial evaluation involves accurately recognizing the nature, site, and severity of the athletic injury. This is the first step in properly caring for an injury and is accomplished by talking with and listening to the athlete and observing, touching (palpating), and perhaps stressing or manipulating the injured area. The knowledge gained during this initial evaluation will assist the athletic trainer in formulating the most effective and appropriate follow-up care and treatment procedures. This information will also provide the basis for decisions that may be required concerning referral to medical assistance. Without this knowledge, an injured area may not be cared for properly, which can result in further injury or delayed recovery. Thus effective treatment and recovery programs depend on the accuracy of the initial assessment of athletic injuries.

The athletic injury assessment process involves more than just the initial evaluation of an injury. Periodic reevaluations are necessary after the injury to give the physician, athletic trainer, coach, and athlete information about the current status of the injured area. The knowledge gained during these repeated evaluations is used to determine such things as how the injured athlete is progressing, whether or not the treatment or rehabilitation programs should be changed, and when the athlete can return safely to activity. The entire process of assessing an injured area ends only after the part has healed and been rehabilitated to its fullest extent.

Athletic injury assessment is not an easy task. The recognition and accurate identification of an injured area is often difficult and challenging. Knowledge, experience, practice, and acquired skills are all necessary prerequisites for competence in the assessment of athletic injuries. Of course, there is no substitute for experience and practice.

ATHLETIC INJURY ASSESSMENT CONSIDERATIONS

There are many considerations related to the total process of athletic injury assessment. Following is a brief discussion of several considerations you should be aware of as you prepare to develop proficiency in athletic injury assessment techniques.

When to Assess

The optimal time to begin assessing an athletic injury is as quickly as possible after it has occurred. As time passes, some of the signs and symptoms necessary for an accurate evaluation may be masked by pain, swelling, inflammation, and muscle spasms. If the evaluation is delayed for a period of time until the athlete is referred to medical assistance, an accurate diagnosis may be hindered by conditions that have developed since the onset of injury. In addition, the period of least discomfort for the athlete is usually right after the injury occurs. Hours or days later the injured area may be very painful and swollen, making an accurate evaluation very difficult. Of course, not all injuries are reported when they occur. There will be times when an athlete will not report an injury for days or even weeks. Such a delay in reporting an injury will make the evaluation more difficult and may require that you wait for the pain and swelling to subside to gain an accurate assessment.

Assessment is an ongoing process. Many athletic injuries will require reassessment or periodic evaluations to obtain an accurate and complete impression of the injury and all associated consequences. For example, after a head injury, what happens to the neurologic baseline? How soon did the swelling occur? How much pain, swelling, and muscle spasm is there the next day and days following? What are the functional abilities of the injured part? Depending on the signs and symptoms, how much can the athlete do? Once an athletic injury or condition is evaluated, an appropriate course of action is initiated. The athletic trainer must evaluate and reevaluate the results of this action. Is the athlete getting better or worse? What can be done to improve or enhance the athlete's recovery? Assessment of an athletic injury continues until the injured area has been rehabilitated to its fullest extent.

Where to Assess

Athletic injuries occur almost anywhere and at any time during athletic activity. Whenever possible, the ideal place to evaluate an injured athlete is right where the injury has occurred. If an injury occurs during a scheduled contest or game, the initial assessment may be limited to a cursory evaluation as to the nature and severity of the injury. After this evaluation, if indicated, the injured athlete can then be removed from the contest to a place where clothing and equipment can be removed and a more thorough examination conducted. If any serious injury is suspected, a thorough examination should be conducted on the playing field without moving the injured athlete and using all the time necessary.

Athletic injuries during practices should also be assessed where they occur if at all possible. It is easier to evaluate an injury without a cluster of players or fans around. If spectators are present, ask them to move elsewhere, or complete a limited examination to determine the nature and severity of the injury and then move the athlete to an area more suitable for a thorough assessment.

Personal Assessment Skills

Athletic injury assessment is not an easy task. The ability of one person to accurately interpret what is felt by another can be very difficult. Signs and symptoms may be masked and misleading, or there may be some abnormal preexisting conditions that complicate the evaluation. The athlete may feel excitement, panic, or concern about the injury, and facts may be distorted. Many factors may contribute to make the assessment difficult. However, if you are responsible for the injury evaluation, there are some personal skills you should be aware of and practice to help you make the injury assessment procedures less difficult and more informative.

Know the athletes

Knowing the athletes can be quite an asset when they become injured. All coaches and athletic trainers should make an attempt to get acquainted with each athlete. The more you know about an athlete, the better prepared you are to assess athletic injuries occurring to that person. This knowledge includes the medical history and the current medical status of the athlete. Does the athlete have any current injuries, diseases, allergies, or other medical problems? Is the athlete taking any medications or under psychologic stress? Does the athlete wear contact lenses or have dental appliances?

It is also important to know something about the various athletes' personalities. How do they react to emergencies or stressful situations? How do they react to pain? Some athletes complain about every little pain, whereas others never complain of pain even though it can be seen he or she is hurting. It is important to know and understand psychologic and personality traits for effective athletic injury care. You should observe each of the athletes and try to ascertain more about his or her personality.

Know the sport

Unlike a coach, who may work with only one sport, an athletic trainer works with all athletes in all sports. Therefore athletic trainers must understand the basic fundamentals and physical demands of each sport with which they may be working. This information can be an asset when deciding whether or not an athlete can return to activity after an injury. The physical skills demanded in one sport may prevent an injured athlete

from participating, whereas an athlete with a similar injury may be able to safely participate in another sport. In addition, knowing the types of injuries that are associated with a particular sport enables the athletic trainer to take appropriate preventive steps and thus lessen the incidence of particular injuries.

Remain calm

Try to remain calm. In many situations the first task is to calm the injured athlete. It is difficult to evaluate an injured area when the athlete is excited, scared, or anxious. If the athletic trainer is equally excited, the athlete may become more anxious about the severity of the injury than warranted by the circumstances. Action and words should not reflect panic. Do not hurry the assessment. Make it as thorough as possible under the circumstances.

Be alert

Be alert during athletic activity. Watch more than just the play or performance. Keep your eyes moving. Do not just watch the center of play. You are more than a fan. Attempt to observe all the athletes. Is anyone not getting up? Is anyone staggering, limping, or acting unusual? Observing an injury as it occurs allows the athletic trainer to have a better idea of the cause of the injury and what to expect when performing evaluation procedures. Keep a special eye on athletes who are known to have special conditions or problems. Depending on the environmental conditions, always be on the lookout for signs of heat illness. Also watch for safety problems, dangerous equipment, and improper teaching techniques or drills.

Use good judgment

There are many outside influences surrounding athletic injuries, thus making it important to always use sound judgment and common sense. Athletic trainers frequently work under a certain amount of pressure to quickly return the athlete to activity. The athlete is usually in good physical condition at the time of injury and strongly motivated to return to activity. The athlete expects the evaluation to be performed quickly and accurately and wants to know exactly what is wrong, as well as when a return to action can be expected. Athletic trainers may have additional pressure from the coach, parents, fans, or other athletes. Because of the nature of the sport, athletic trainers may even be under time restraints to hurry the evaluation. Remember, everyone makes mistakes, but it is better to err on the conservative side by being cautious, especially when you are unsure of the nature and severity of the injury. In athletic injury assessment, trainers must make rapid and accurate judgments, perhaps in front of many witnesses. Use sound judgment based on knowledge and experience.

Experience

There is no substitute for experience in assessing athletic injuries. Athletic trainers can gain the anatomic background, a knowledge of the specific signs and symptoms associated with various injuries, and the specific assessment techniques through study. However, the confidence developed in assessment skills will only increase through practice. It takes experience to refine assessment skills.

Patience

To become proficient at athletic injury assessment, athletic trainers must develop patience. There is an extremely wide range in the type and severity of athletic injuries. Some injuries may constitute an obvious evaluation and solution. Other injuries will constitute a grey area and will be very difficult to accurately assess. The injury may be masked by pain, swelling, or muscle spasm. The signs and symptoms may be insidious. These types of athletic injuries may require a long, meticulous evaluation to recognize the nature of the injury. A hurried evaluation may result in an inaccurate assessment.

Referral Skills

An area often neglected by those assessing athletic injuries is that of referral. Contacting a physician and scheduling the athlete

for an examination is not all there is to referring. Information gained at the initial evaluation must also be conveyed to the next link in the injury management chain. As previously discussed, by the time the physician evaluates the athlete, pain, swelling, muscle spasms, and inflammation may have developed, making the assessment more difficult. Therefore the information gained on the initial assessment should be recorded and passed along whenever an injured athlete is referred.

Do not hesitate to refer an athlete to a physician or other professional person if you feel uncomfortable or have questions about the assessment. It is better to be cautious initially than sorry later that you did not refer the athlete. There will be some athletic injuries that will also require consultation with a specialist. Again, these injuries should be referred at the earliest possible time so the specialist can take advantage of the optimal time for treatment.

Plan of Action

The athletic trainer or coach who has the responsibility for the medical care of athletes should have a plan of action worked out ahead of time should an injury occur. Plan emergency procedures and routine assessment techniques in advance so that these procedures may be carried out as easily and efficiently as possible. Any moving, lifting, or transporting should be thought out and practiced in advance so that these maneuvers will go smoothly. A well-practiced plan of action can reassure athletes that they are and will be handled in the best possible manner. Maintain a calm environment and initiate the preplanned steps of the emergency network. Plan for the worst and hope for the best. If you have not planned for a severe emergency and it occurs, there is a good chance it will be poorly handled.

Know how to obtain professional assistance. The ambulance, hospital, and physician's phone numbers should be readily accessible, as should a telephone with an outside line. Emergency equipment must be readily available and not locked up some distance away. This emergency equipment

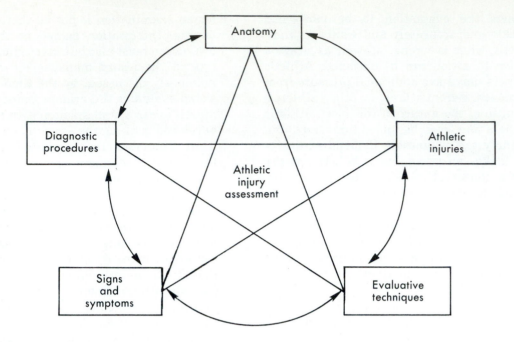

FIGURE 10-1
The five major areas of an athletic injury assessment process.

must also be operable, and the people handling it should be trained in its use. Athletic trainers should continually be updating their emergency care skills. Medical emergency plans should be well defined and detailed for each practice or game site, as well as the chain of command for notification of personnel in the event of a catastrophic type of injury.

Summary

As athletic training students develop procedures for assessing athletic injuries, many factors must be considered. These factors directly influence the effectiveness of the athletic injury assessment process and include knowledge and proficiency in the topics discussed. In addition, athletic trainers must continue to refine and improve these assessment skills in an attempt to provide their athletes with optimal medical care.

ATHLETIC INJURY ASSESSMENT PROCESS

Knowledge surrounding the athletic injury assessment process can be categorized into five main areas (Figure 10-1). Each of these areas is interrelated and important to the total process.

Anatomy

To accurately evaluate an injured area, the athletic trainer must understand the anatomy of the involved body part. A total assessment involves isolating and evaluating each anatomic structure suspected of being injured. This isolation process should be performed systematically to permit identification of the involved structures and to assess severity of involvement. Athletic trainers should be able to visualize the actual structures being evaluated. Without a good understanding of the underlying anatomic structures, it will be difficult or impossible to accurately evaluate the injury. A review of basic bone, joint, muscle, and nerve anatomy was presented in Unit I; more detailed regional anatomy is presented with each body area discussed throughout the remainder of this text. However, it is strongly recommended that courses in anatomy and kinesiology be taken by athletic trainers to strengthen their knowledge in these areas. Frequent review of this important information is encouraged.

Athletic Injuries

An overview of the body's response to trauma and the common athletic injuries was presented in Unit II. Everyone who has the responsibility for the medical care of athletes should be familiar with these processes and the various injuries that may result from athletic activities. To accurately assess these injuries, it is extremely important to understand how the body responds to trauma and how the associated signs and symptoms develop. Furthermore, it is important to have a general understanding of the mechanisms causing common injuries. All of this information can greatly assist the athletic trainer in the injury assessment process.

Evaluative Techniques

An important aspect of the athletic injury assessment process is the use of an organized examination sequence. Although each injury is unique, an evaluation of the injured area is easier to perform by using a systematic approach. Each athletic trainer must develop his or her own evaluative techniques within the limits of individual abilities and training. This text is intended to offer guidelines for development of athletic injury assessment skills, not to make medical diagnosticians out of athletic trainers. A properly trained person present at the time an injury occurs has the best opportunity to make an accurate initial evaluation, and most of the time this responsibility will fall on the athletic trainer. In the absence of trained personnel, the initial evaluation may be neglected and the injured athlete told to "wait and see" or "walk it off." In many cases an injured athlete is simply referred to a physician, and by the time the evaluation is performed, pain, swelling, and spasm make the assessment more difficult. Furthermore, initial evaluations performed by an athletic trainer immediately after a serious injury can be of great importance to the physician in establishing early treatment and planning of follow-up care.

Signs and Symptoms

Signs and symptoms exhibited by an injured athlete yield valuable information needed to make an accurate assessment (Figure 10-2). A **symptom** is subjective evidence of the injury or something the athlete relates. For example, pain that is associated with an injury is felt and can only be described by the athlete. A **sign** is objective evidence of the injury or something you as the examiner can see, hear, or feel. An example of a sign is swelling associated with an injury, which can be observed and felt by the athletic trainer. Interpretation of the signs and symptoms recognized during the assessment process provides information for the type of care the athlete should receive.

Diagnostic Procedures

Diagnostic procedures include all of the techniques a physician may employ to assist in the diagnosis of an athletic injury. Several tests or procedures are often required to pinpoint the location, extent, and seriousness of some injuries. An increase in the number, availability, and sophistication of these diagnostic procedures has made them extremely valuable tools in sports medicine. In many cases, complex laboratory tests or radiographic studies are required for a physician to complete the diagnosis of some athletic injuries. Because of their importance and frequency in use, several of these procedures will be discussed. It is often the responsibility of the athletic trainer to refer the injured athlete for additional diagnostic procedures indicated by the information gained during the assessment process.

It is not the intent of this text to discuss in any great depth the additional procedures a physician may use in diagnosing an injury. However, because they are important to the total assessment process, athletic trainers should possess some knowledge of these procedures. Such information is frequently useful in helping to prepare an athlete for referral or in explaining the rationale for specific procedures before or after they are performed. Following is a brief description of the more common diagnostic procedures a physician may use to assist in diagnosing an athletic injury.

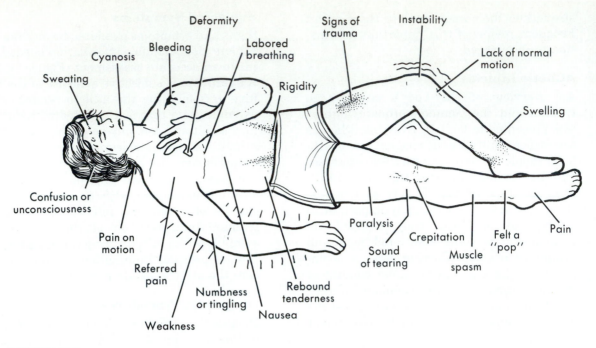

FIGURE 10-2
Signs and symptoms of athletic injuries. The left side indicates possible signs of an athletic injury, and the right side represents symptoms.

Radiology

Radiologic studies are very important and useful in diagnosing many athletic injuries or related conditions. Radiologic images or tests include a wide variety of techniques or procedures used individually or in combination to provide the physician with information necessary to assist in making a diagnosis. Radiologic techniques or procedures used most often in the diagnosis of athletic injuries are (1) plain film radiography, (2) contrast-enhanced radiography, (3) computed tomography (CT), (4) magnetic resonance imaging (MRI), and (5) nuclear imaging.

Plain film radiography

The term **plain film radiography** is used to describe radiologic procedures that use no special techniques or material to enhance the contrast of the various structures of the body. These procedures are adequate when natural radiographic contrast exists between body structures such as bone and ad-

jacent soft tissues. These are the most common types of radiologic procedures used in sports medicine. Plain film radiographs are used to clarify or confirm the clinical assessment in many types of athletic injuries. Plain film examinations are commonly used for bone and joint injuries, and the findings include information concerning bone integrity, atrophy, hypertrophy, erosion, contours, and density, as well as the relationships between articulating bones (Figure 10-3).

Stress radiograph. A stress radiograph is a procedure using radiographs taken while stress is being applied to the joint. These types of radiographs may have to be performed with the athlete under anesthesia to eliminate pain and accompanying muscular contractions. An unstable joint or one showing abnormal motion will be demonstrated on a stress film by a widening of the joint space as the stress is applied (Figure 10-4). This finding generally confirms a clinical impression of ligament instability. It

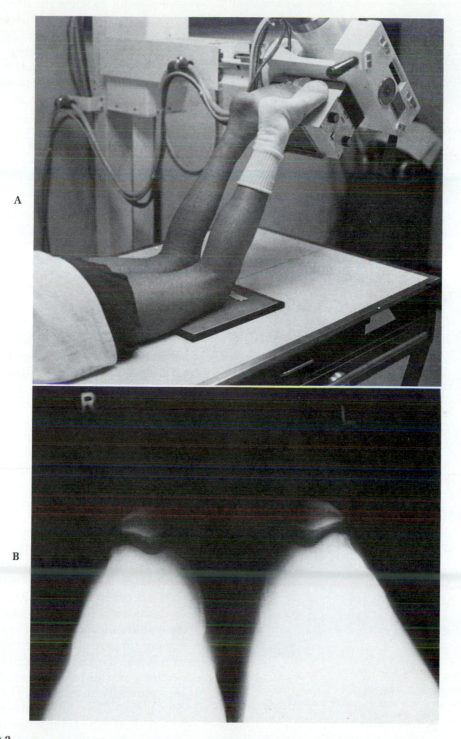

FIGURE 10-3
Plain film radiography. **A,** Procedure for taking sunrise view of patellae and **B,** the resulting radiograph.

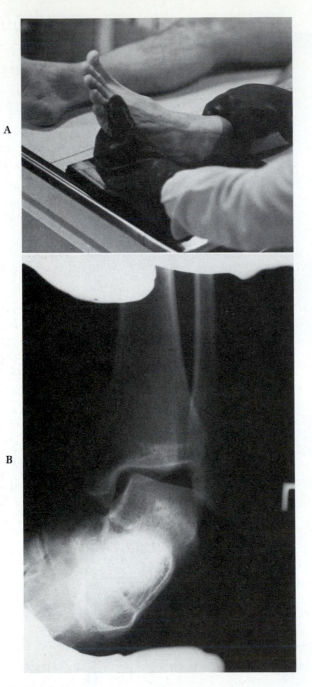

FIGURE 10-4
Stress radiography. **A**, Procedure for taking stress radiograph of an ankle and **B**, an ankle stress film.

is also possible to show the disruption of the growth plate in younger athletes by the use of stress radiographs.

Tomography. Tomography is a technique using radiographs taken with a specialized computer to give a two-dimensional view of one particular area of tissue at any depth (Figure 10-5). This is like taking a radiograph of one slice or section at any level of the extremity. As the X-ray is focused on a particular area, the X-ray tube and film are synchronized and move in opposite directions. This opposing movement blurs out unwanted structures while keeping the focal area in sharp contrast. Tomograms are helpful in delineating specific areas and are frequently used to evaluate bony structures. Tomography has been shown to significantly improve the diagnostic success in injuries involving the cervical spine.

Contrast-enhanced radiography

Contrast-enhanced radiographic procedures are those used to examine structures that do not have inherent contrast differences from surrounding tissues. With this type of radiologic technique, it is necessary to use one of various contrasting agents. These preparations can be administered orally, rectally, or by injection into the body. Some of the contrast-enhanced radiographic techniques that may be used with athletic injuries are as follows.

Arthrography. Arthrography is the study of joints using a contrast medium, with or without air, that is injected into the joint space. A radiograph is then taken, called an *arthrogram,* which outlines the soft tissue structures of a joint that otherwise would not show up on a plain film radiograph (Figure 10-6). The radiopaque dye outlines any irregularities in the soft tissue structures of the joint. After injection, the dye is generally absorbed by the body within a few hours. This procedure is frequently performed on athletic injuries involving the shoulder. As arthroscopy techniques improve, less arthrography is being done on the knee, but it still has its place in the diagnosis of certain conditions.

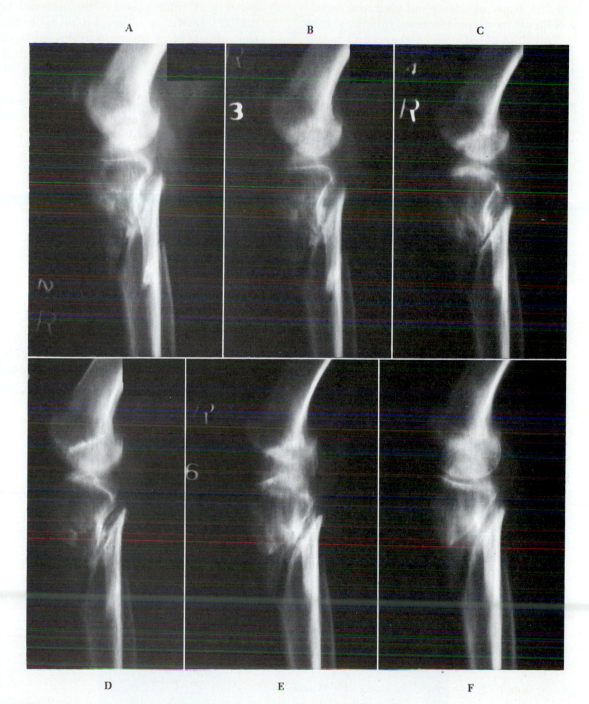

FIGURE 10-5
Tomograms of a fractured right proximal tibia, showing successive sections or slices of the fracture site from superficial (**A**) to deep (**F**).

Myelography. Myelography is the radiographic study of the spinal cord and canal. A contrast medium is injected into the spinal canal in the subarachnoid space, and radiographs are taken (Figure 10-7). Cerebrospinal fluid may also be removed for laboratory studies at this time. An abnormality on the resulting *myelogram* will show up in the dye column. The most common lesion evaluated by myelography is an intervertebral disc herniation with evidence of spinal cord or nerve root compression. The material normally injected is either an oil-type agent that must be withdrawn from the spinal canal later or a water-soluble agent that is absorbed by the body. Myelography is often enhanced with CT scanning.

Discography. Discography is the radiographic study of the spine for visualization of an intervertebral disc. Radiopaque dye is

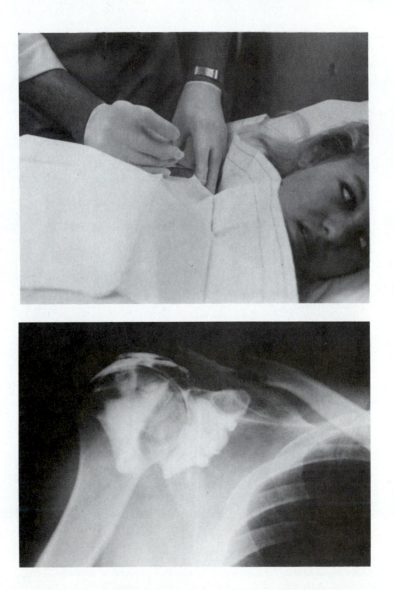

A

B

FIGURE 10-6
Arthrography of the shoulder joint. **A**, Preparing to inject radiopaque dye into the joint and **B**, an arthrogram showing a collection of dye outside the joint capsule indicating a rotator cuff tear. Note dye accumulating under the coracoid process.

introduced into the disc space between two vertebrae, and a radiograph, called a *discogram,* is taken (Figure 10-8). Ruptures of the intervertebral disc will be indicated by an abnormal dye pattern between the vertebrae.

Angiography. Angiography is the radiographic study of the vascular system. A water-soluble radiopaque dye is injected either intraarterially *(arteriogram)* or intravenously *(venogram),* and a rapid sequence of radiographs are taken to follow the course of the contrast material through the blood vessels (Figure 10-9). These tests are useful in diagnosing injury to or partial blockage of blood vessels.

Urography. Urography is the radiographic study of the urinary tract. A contrast medium is injected into the athlete intravenously and quickly passes into the urine. Radiographs are then taken of the kidneys, ureters, and urinary bladder (Figure 10-10). This is called an *intravenous pyelogram* (IVP); it is a common procedure when urinary tract injuries are suspected.

Computed tomography

Computed tomography (CT scan) is a sophisticated test that is performed with computerized radiographic equipment. The images give almost a three-dimensional view of the affected area. Images are displayed on a television monitor during the procedure, and permanent films are recorded at various levels or slices during the examination sequence (Figure 10-11). This is a representa-

FIGURE 10-7
Myelography. **A**, Injecting contrast medium into the spinal canal and, **B**, a myelogram.

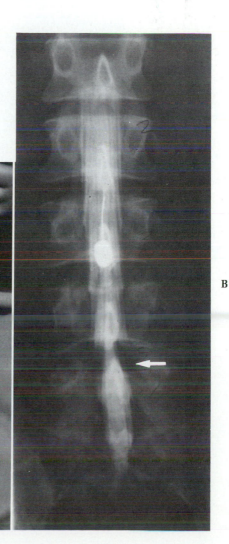

A

B

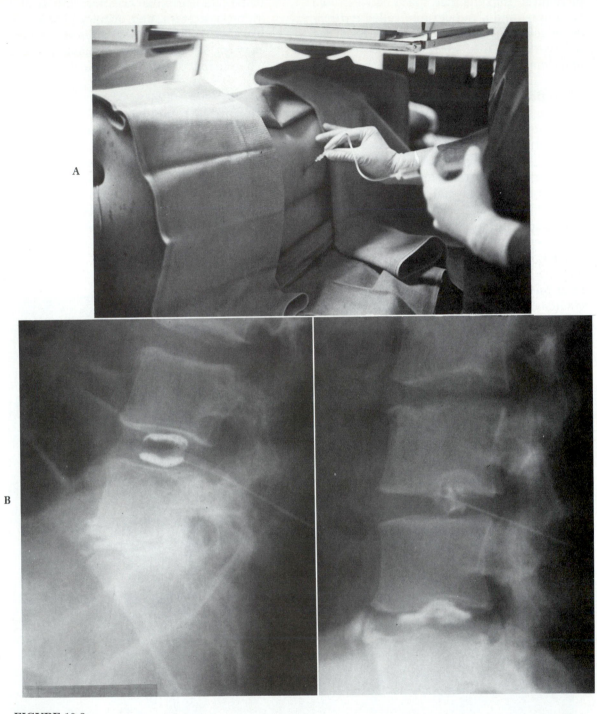

FIGURE 10-8
Discography. **A**, Injecting radiopaque dye into the disc space between vertebrae and, **B**, normal discogram (L4-S1) showing needle in place. Note that dye remains encapsulated at point of injection. **C**, Abnormal discogram (L5-S1). Note that dye has extravasated beyond injection site because of herniation.

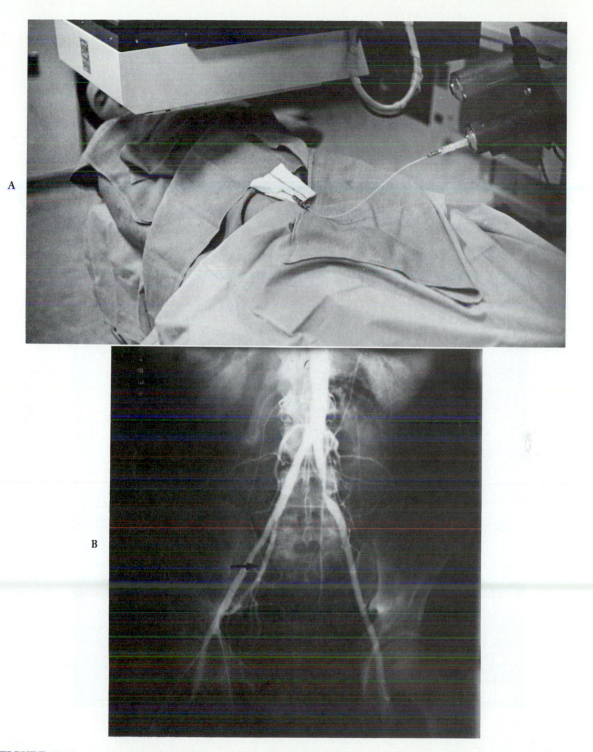

FIGURE 10-9
Angiography. **A**, Injecting radiopaque dye into the right femoral artery and, **B**, an arteriogram. Arrow points to right common iliac artery. Note absence of this artery on the left side.

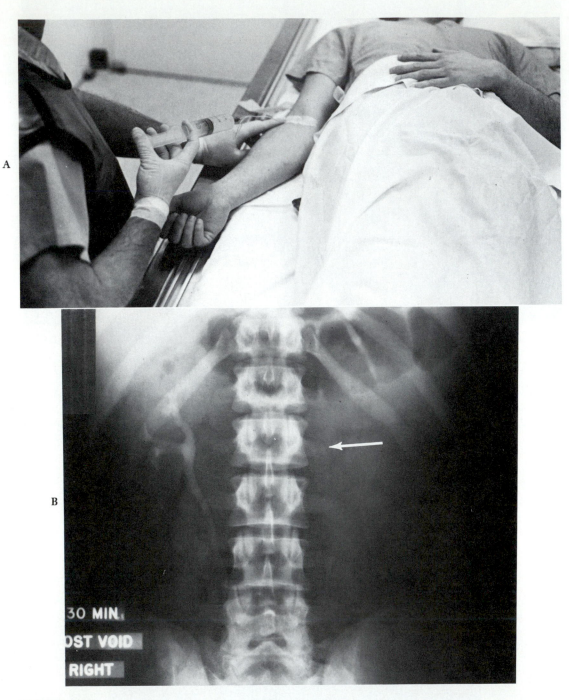

FIGURE 10-10
Urography. **A**, Injecting a contrast medium intravenously and, **B**, an intravenous pyelogram (IVP). Note the nonvisualization of the left ureter *(arrow)* following a contusion to the left kidney

tion of what would be seen with the athlete cut open on a transverse plane. The normal examination uses eight to ten slices of the head and twelve to fifteen slices of the body. CT scanning is the primary imaging procedure used in trauma involving the head because it shows both the contents of the skull and any injury that may have occurred. Small hematomas, localized swelling, and cerebral atrophy can be picked up by the CT scan almost unfailingly. This diagnostic procedure can also be used effectively on the trunk and extremities. In these cases, a contrasting agent is frequently injected intravenously to enhance the appearance of certain visceral structures.

Magnetic resonance imaging

Magnetic resonance imaging (MRI) has proven to be an important diagnostic tool in many musculoskeletal disorders. MRI is based on the way tissue protons, placed in a strong magnetic field, respond to a radio frequency signal. Protons spin about an axis, much like a top; when placed in a magnetic field, protons absorb energy, causing them to wobble (similar to a spinning top) at a higher rate. The magnetic field is created from radio waves equivalent to FM frequency. After the radio pulse is turned off, the protons emit energy as they gradually return to their equilibrium state. This constitutes the magnetic resonance signal. This process must be repeated many times before a significant number of signals are acquired to generate an image. By using different combinations of radio frequency pulses and "listening" to the returning relaxation signals, an infinite number of images can be created (Figure 10-12).

MRI produces highly detailed images of soft tissue, generally showing greater con-

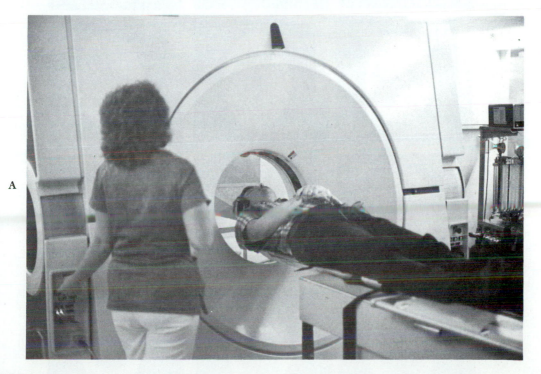

FIGURE 10-11
Computed tomography. **A**, Performing a (CT scan); **B**, an individual section of the CT scan; and, **C**, the resulting CT scan film series.   *Continued.*

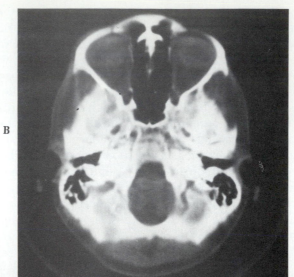

B

FIGURE 10-11, cont'd.

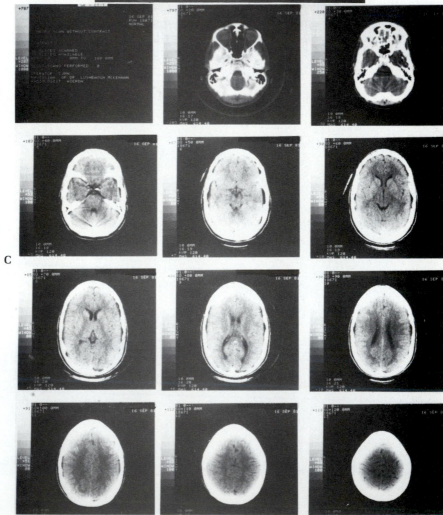

C

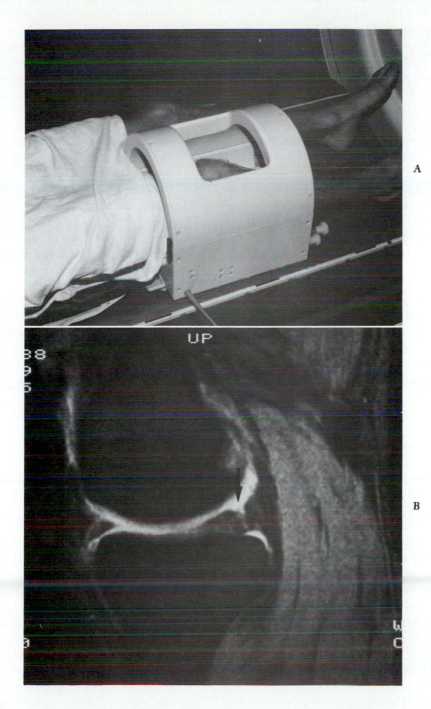

FIGURE 10-12
Magnetic resonance imaging (MRI). **A,** Preparing an athlete for MRI using a knee resonator or surface coil before being placed in the scanner and, **B,** one of the resulting MRI films. Note torn medial meniscus *(arrow)*.

trast between normal and abnormal tissue than CT. It also offers a clear view of the inner workings of joints, especially the knee. There are also no known risks or side effects. However, MRI costs far more than alternative diagnostic procedures. MRI may be warranted when the history and clinical findings suggest a primary, musculotendinous or soft tissue lesion that cannot be detected by conventional roentgenographic films.

Nuclear imaging

Nuclear imaging depends on the selective and unique absorption characteristics of certain radioactive compounds by different organs of the body. Typically, a radioactive isotope with a very short half-life is injected into the body, and the resultant radioactivity in a given area, organ, or tissue is calculated on a counter and recorded on a scanner. The most common nuclear imaging technique associated with athletic injuries is the **bone scan** (Figure 10-13). This test will detect particular areas of abnormal metabolic activity within a bone, which may indicate a tumor, infection, or recent fracture. Bone scans can detect sites of stress in a bone before a conventional radiograph shows any abnormality. Bone scans will often detect stress fractures before they are symptomatic. This can lead to an earlier diagnosis, earlier and more effective treatment, and less disability for the athlete. Bone scans can also be useful in determining if myositis ossificans or spondylolysis are still active or if they have matured. Nuclear imaging can also be used for examination of soft tissue areas. Examples include scans of the brain (largely replaced by CT scans), liver, lung, heart, or thyroid.

Laboratory Evaluations

There is a large and ever-increasing variety of laboratory evaluations or procedures that can be performed to supplement the assessment of athletic injuries. Laboratory tests make the basic sciences available to those who participate in the diagnosis and treatment of an injured athlete. In many cases, the professional athletic trainer needs to know, at least in general terms, the purpose of a particular test, how it is performed, and the significance of its results to serve effectively as a member of the sports medicine team. Biochemical data gained from laboratory studies of blood, urine, synovial fluid, cerebrospinal fluid, aspirates, or other materials can reveal information essential to diagnosis and treatment. For example, analysis of synovial fluid that is aspirated or removed from a joint will distinguish certain characteristics between infections, arthritides, acute injuries, and, occasionally, tumors or other unusual diseases. In acute injuries, blood is frequently present in the synovial fluid, which indicates that damage has occurred to a structure located within the joint capsule or to the joint capsule itself. An associated benefit of joint aspiration is the frequent relief of pain and an increased ROM.

Electroencephalography

Electroencephalography is the study of electrical currents emitted by the brain. This electrical activity is picked up by electrodes applied to the scalp and displayed on a monitor or printed on readout paper (Figure 10-14). The graphic recordings are called an *electroencephalogram* (EEG). The patterns and changes in electrical activity allow the neurosurgeon or neurologist to base a diagnosis on the activity of the brain rather than relying solely on neurologic assessments.

Electrocardiography

Electrocardiography is the study of electrical activity of the heart. This measure of electrical activity is picked up by electrodes placed on the chest and extremities and displayed on a monitor or recorded on paper (Figure 10-15). The graphic recordings are called an *electrocardiogram* (ECG or EKG) and are valuable in detecting suspected heart abnormalities. Although recordings are taken in resting and exercise conditions, the exercise ECG (stress test) is more discriminating in identifying abnormalities.

Echocardiography

Echocardiography is a technique that uses echoes or reflected high-frequency sound waves to locate and observe the activ-

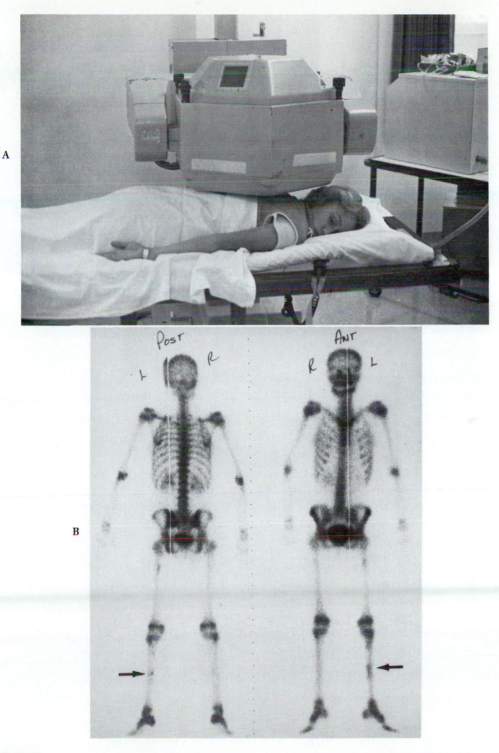

FIGURE 10-13
Nuclear imaging. **A**, Procedure for taking a bone scan and, **B**, a total body view bone scan. Note increased activity *(arrows)* in the midshaft of the left tibia, indicating a stress fracture.

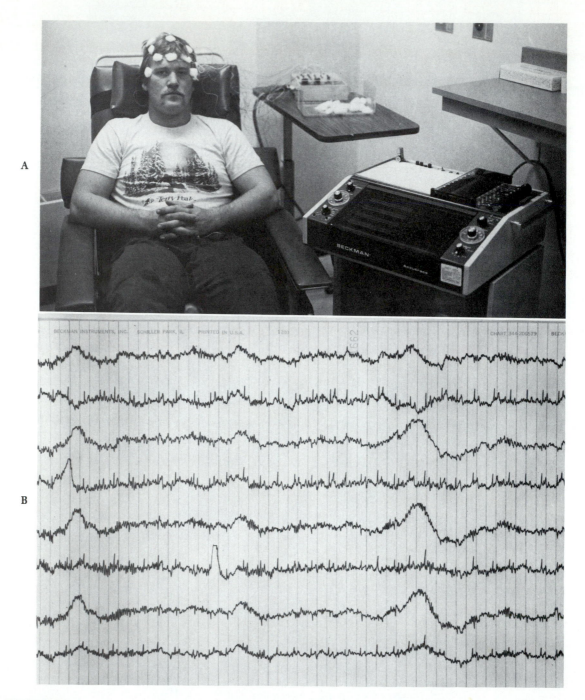

FIGURE 10-14
Electroencephalography. **A**, Electrodes are applied to the scalp and, **B**, a portion of the resulting electroencephalogram.

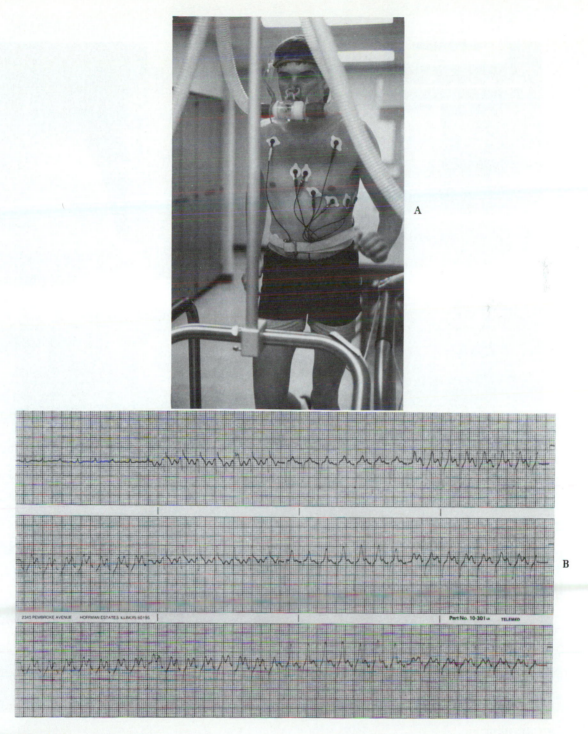

FIGURE 10-15
Electrocardiography. **A,** Athlete performing a graded exercise stress test (ECG). Note athlete is also being tested for maximal oxygen uptake, which can be administered during the stress test. **B,** Portion of the resulting electrocardiogram.

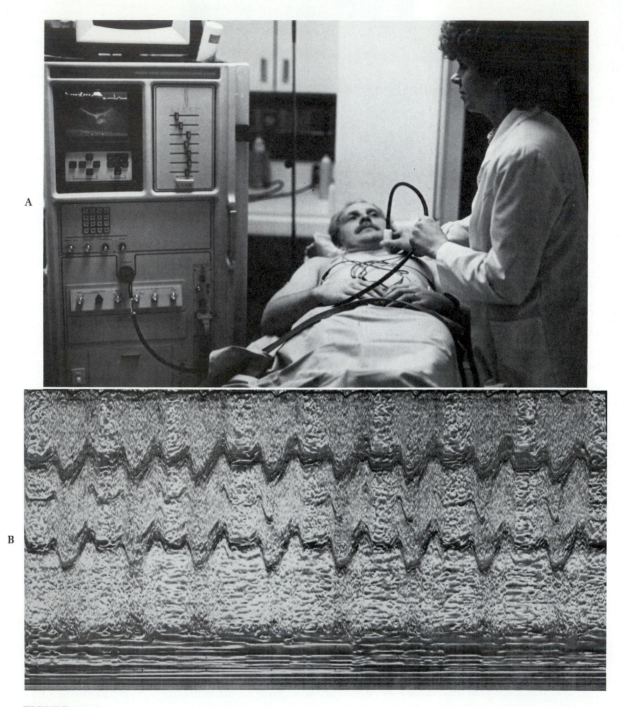

FIGURE 10-16
Echocardiography. **A**, Placement of the electrodes and sound head on athlete's chest and, **B**, a portion of the resulting echocardiogram.

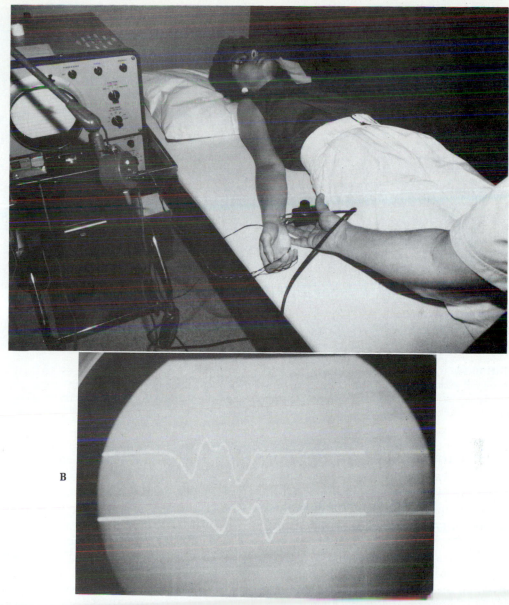

FIGURE 10-17
Electromyography. **A,** Conducting an ulnar nerve conduction test. The ulnar nerve is
stimulated above the elbow and at the wrist. Time difference is then calculated to determine if
there is an ulnar nerve entrapment at the elbow. **B,** Picture of oscilloscope display of test.

ity and integrity of cardiac structures. The
images are recorded on videotape and are
often processed by computer for quantita-
tion and enhancement of detail (Figure 10-
16). During the test, sound waves are generated by a transducer placed over the chest
wall. The technique is said to be noninvasive

because it does not break the skin or interfere in any way with the events that are
being observed. Echocardiography is often
used to measure the size of the cardiac
chambers to detect filling defects after injury. It is the most frequently used test in
the area of clinical cardiology after the electrocardiogram.

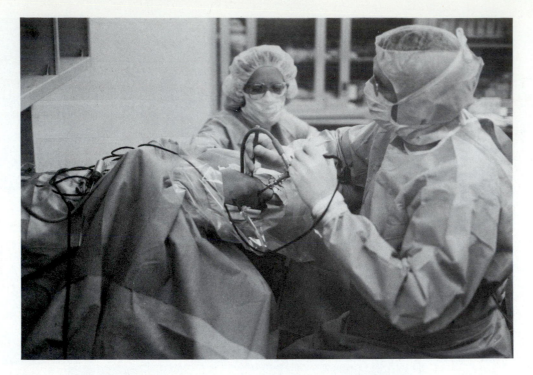

FIGURE 10-18
Arthroscopy of a knee joint. The arthroscope is inserted into the lateral side of the knee joint
and a probe is inserted into the medial side. Note surgeon is watching procedure on a television
monitor situated above the athlete.

Electromyography

Electromyography is the study of the electrical potentials generated in muscles. Electrodes placed on the surface of a muscle or sterile needle-type electrodes inserted into the muscle itself pick up the electrical potentials that are generated when the muscle contracts. These electrical signals are then displayed on an oscilloscope or printed on a paper strip recording (Figure 10-17). The graphic recordings are called an *electromyogram* (EMG). Interpretation of the electrical activity generated with slight and maximal-effort contractions is helpful in diagnosis of peripheral nerve injuries, muscle denervation, and intrinsic muscle disease.

Arthroscopy

Arthroscopy allows a surgeon to actually view the interior of a joint through a series of very small lenses with a fiberoptic light source. This diagnostic procedure is performed under sterile technique and local or general anesthesia. After the joint is distended with saline solution, a small incision (2 to 3 mm) is made, and the arthroscope is inserted into the joint space. A fiber bundle transmits light into the joint, and the surgeon, peering through an eyepiece, inspects the interior of the joint. The image can also be displayed simultaneously on a television screen (Figure 10-18).

The knee, because of its structure, easily lends itself to arthroscopy, although this procedure is now used to examine many joints of the body. Arthroscopy can contribute significantly to the preoperative diagnosis and has almost eliminated unnecessary exploratory surgery. This procedure frequently precedes more major and "open" surgical procedures. In certain conditions such as loose bodies or a torn cartilage in the knee the necessary surgery can be performed through or in conjunction with the

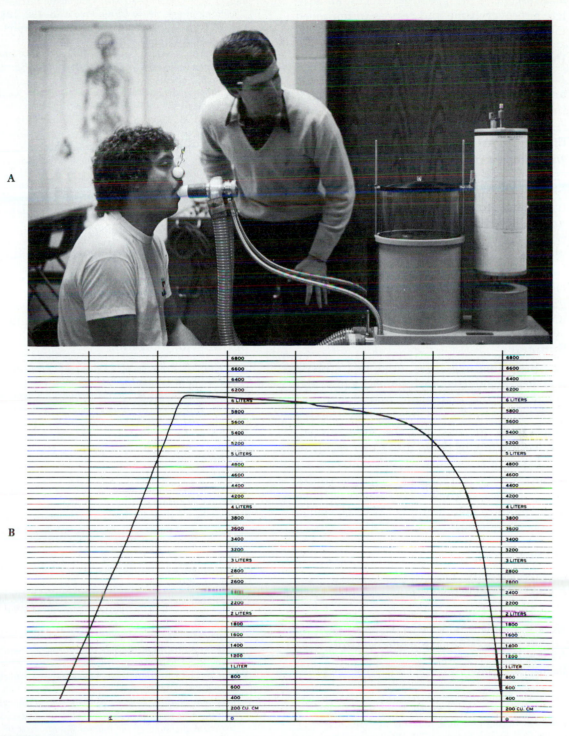

FIGURE 10-19
Pulmonary function test. **A**, Athlete performing a forced vital capacity test and, **B**, the resulting graph.

arthroscope. This greatly reduces an athlete's recovery time and results in improved medical care for athletes.

Pulmonary Function Tests

A large number of pulmonary function tests are available to measure the functioning of the respiratory system as a whole and the relationships of its various parts. As a group these tests are used to determine the presence of disease or injury, the type of disease or lesion that might be present and the extent of disability, and the proper course of treatment or therapy. Examples of pulmonary function tests include: (1) determination of lung volumes, such as vital capacity, (2) ventilation measurements, such as tidal volume and respiratory rate, and (3) pulmonary mechanics tests, such as forced expiratory volume and airway resistance (Figure 10-19).

Summary

The preceding five areas, anatomy, athletic injuries, evaluative techniques, signs and symptoms, and diagnostic procedures, are each important to the total athletic injury assessment process and are interrelated. Neglecting any of these areas can result in decreased effectiveness when evaluating an athletic injury. Accurate evaluations require that you possess knowledge in each of these areas and are able to apply that knowledge to specific injuries.

REFERENCES

Arger PH and others: Computed tomography in orthopedics, *Orthop Clin North Am* 14(1):217, 1983.

Baker BE, Lewinsohn EM: Radiologic diagnosis of pain in the athlete, *Clin Sports Med* 6(4), 1987.

Bosch E, Pathria M, Resnick D: Difficult-to-detect osseous injuries; MRI gives greater specificity, *Phys Sportsmed* 21(1):116, 1993.

Dalinka MK, editor: Radiographic imaging in orthopedics, *Orthop Clin North Am* 21(3), 1990.

Gartsman GM: Arthroscopic resection of the acromioclavicular joint, *Am J Sports Med* 21(1):71, 1993.

Hair JE: Intangibles in evaluating athletic injuries, *J Am Coll Health Assoc* 25:228, 1977

Hayes RG, Nagle CE: Diagnostic imaging of intracranial trauma, *Phys Sportsmed* 18(2):69, 1990.

James ME, Charboneau WJ: Diagnostic ultrasound—coming of age, *Mayo Clinic Proc* 57(3):198, 1982.

Lee BC: CT scans of the head: basic interpretation, *Hosp Med* 18(1):21, 1982.

Lee JK, Yao L, Wirth CR: Magnetic resonance imaging of major ligamentous knee injuries, *Phys Sportsmed* 18(4):97, 1990.

Levy RC, and others: *Radiology in emergency medicine,* St Louis, 1987, Mosby-Year Book.

Maywood RM, Jackson DW, Berger P: Athletic injuries to the knee: evaluation using magnetic resonance imaging, *Phys Sportsmed* 16(5):81, 1988.

Minkoff J, Sherman OH, editors: Arthroscopy, *Clin Sports Med* 6(3), 1987.

Radiology in sports medicine—a round table, *Phys Sportsmed* 9(5):61, 1981.

Speer KP, Lohnes J, Garrett WE: Radiographic imaging of muscle strain injury, *Am J Sports Med* 21(1):89, 1993.

Stark D, Bradley WG: *Magnetic resonance imaging,* St Louis, 1988, Mosby-Year Book.

Wichmann S, Martin DR: When to use MRI, *Phys Sportsmed* 20(8):116, 1992.

Zarins B: Arthroscopic surgery in a sports medicine practice, *Orthop Clin North Am* 13(2):415, 1982.

SUGGESTED READINGS

Arnheim DD, Prentice WE: *Principles of athletic training,* ed 8, St Louis, 1993, Mosby.
  Chapter 9 in this text addresses various aspects and techniques used in athletic injury assessment and evaluation.

Calkins D, Sartoris DJ: Imaging acute knee injuries; direct diagnostic approaches, *Phys Sportsmed* 20(6):91, 1992.
  Authors discuss different diagnostic procedures and their clinical applications to various pathologic conditions of knee injuries.

Nagle CE, Freitas JE: Radionuclide imaging of musculoskeletal injuries in athletes with negative radiographs, *Phys Sportsmed* 15(6):147, 1987.
  Authors discuss the use of bone scans and identify musculoskeletal injuries that are associated with specific sports.

Sartoris DJ, and others: MRI's role in assessing musculoskeletal disorders, *J Musculoskeletal Med* 4(12):12, 1987.
  Discusses the use of magnetic resonance imaging (MRI) and its importance in diagnosing a broad spectrum of musculoskeletal disorders.

Whipple TL, editor: Arthroscopy update, *Clin Sports Med* 10(3), 1987.
  With the help of several contributing authors, this volume addresses the rapidly evolving subspecialty of arthroscopic surgery for many common and troublesome athletic injuries.

CHAPTER 11

Assessment procedures

After you have completed this chapter, you should be able to:

- Describe the steps of a primary survey.
- List and briefly describe the basic steps of a secondary survey.
- Describe the factors for obtaining an accurate and thorough history of an athletic injury.
- Describe the factors for observing and inspecting an injured athlete.
- Discuss the four main areas of the physical examination.
- Discuss palpation procedures.
- List and explain the four types of movement procedures.
- Describe how to evaluate neurologic and circulatory status.

A comprehensive and accurate evaluation of athletic injuries or related conditions often requires a detailed and systematic assessment process. This chapter presents an approach to athletic injury assessment. It will discuss, in orderly sequence, the assessment procedures that should be performed by an athletic trainer when an athlete is injured. Everyone responsible for the medical care of athletes should develop an organized sequence of assessment procedures to perform a more accurate evaluation of athletic injuries. Mastery of complex assessment techniques requires a substantial personal commitment on the part of the athletic trainer in terms of the time and effort expended. In addition, it is essential that the student in an athletic training program have individualized professional supervision, guidance, and support. The procedures presented in this chapter will aid in the development of the skills that are essential to the successful assessment of athletic injuries.

A thorough athletic injury assessment can be broken down into two major parts: (1) primary survey and (2) secondary survey. Each survey is important and should be considered with each injury.

PRIMARY SURVEY

The **primary survey** is that portion of the assessment concerned with evaluation of the basic life support mechanisms: *A*irway, *B*reathing, and *C*irculation. These are usu-

Primary Survey
Airway
Breathing
Circulation

ally referred to as the ABCs of life support. The probability that life-threatening situations will arise as a result of athletic injuries is minimal; however, everyone involved in athletics must be aware that the potential for serious injury does exist. Critical injuries do occur, and death can result from an athletic injury. Life-threatening conditions must be recognized immediately and dealt with effectively to prevent needless loss of life. Persons responsible for the medical care of athletes must be trained to recognize and react appropriately to various life-threatening situations.

With most athletic injuries, the primary survey is completed easily and quickly. The experienced and observant athletic trainer will initiate a part of the primary survey even before reaching the injured player. Although a serious injury may exist that will only be revealed through a thorough examination, the critical life-support mechanisms (ABCs) can be evaluated almost immediately. For example, if an injured athlete is conscious and talking, one can assume that he or she is breathing and has a pulse. This type of basic observation is often completed while approaching the injured player. With this initial observation, the primary survey is begun.

Success in athletic injury assessment depends on the development of observational skills and the ability to remain calm and objective in times of stress and confusion. As you approach an injured athlete, be very observant. Survey the situation quickly and completely. As you conduct the primary survey, you should also note important details such as severe bleeding, level of consciousness, and body position. Completion of the primary survey can be accomplished quickly if you are disciplined in the use of an appropriate mental checklist.

Although athletic injuries are seldom life-threatening, it is important to consider and understand the aspects of basic life support. This section presents assessment techniques used to recognize possible life-threatening conditions. The purpose is not to present a discussion of specialized techniques, such as cardiopulmonary resuscitation (CPR), that are used to manage specific emergency situations. It should be emphasized, however, that a thorough understanding of basic life-support procedures is a necessary prerequisite to the study of assessment techniques.

Airway

Anything that blocks the passage of air through the *trachea,* or windpipe, into the lungs causes an airway obstruction. The most common cause of airway obstruction is blockage of the windpipe opening by the tongue and epiglottis. This may occur when an athlete is unconscious. In these cases the tongue may fall toward the back of the throat (pharynx) and block the airway opening into the trachea (Figure 11-1). This situation is life threatening and requires immediate action. Because the tongue is attached to the lower jaw directly and the epiglottis is attached indirectly, moving the lower jaw forward will usually lift the tongue and epiglottis away from the back of the pharynx and open the airway. This may be all that is required for breathing to resume spontaneously.

Head Tilt-Chin Lift

The currently recommended technique to open the airway is the head tilt-chin lift method. This maneuver is accomplished by tilting the head back with one hand and lifting the chin up gently with the other (Figure 11-2). With the athlete on his or her back, place the hand closest to the athlete's head on the forehead and apply firm backward pressure. At the same time, place the tips of your fingers under the lower jaw on the bony rim and lift the chin forward. You must be careful when compressing the soft tissues under the chin because this could obstruct the airway. The chin should be lifted so that the teeth are brought almost together. Avoid completely closing the mouth.

Jaw thrust without head tilt

When a neck injury is suspected, movement of the cervical spine must be avoided. The jaw thrust method can be used to open the airway. This is accomplished by grasping the angles of the athlete's lower jaw and lifting

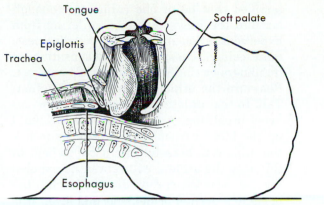

FIGURE 11-1
Tongue blocking the airway.

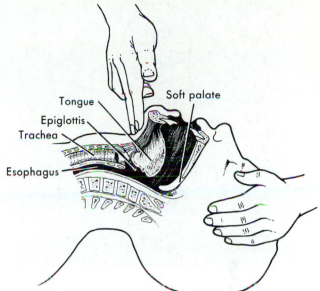

FIGURE 11-2
Opening the airway using the head tilt-chin lift procedure.

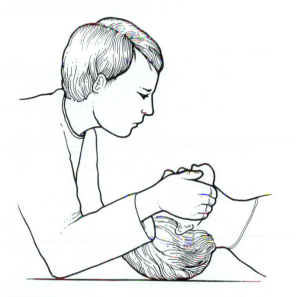

FIGURE 11-3
Jaw thrust procedure; the safest technique to open an airway when a neck injury is suspected because it usually can be accomplished without extending the neck.

with both hands to move the jaw forward (Figure 11-3). Your elbows should be on either side of the head and resting on the surface on which the athlete is lying. This is the safest technique to use when a neck injury is suspected because it can be accomplished in most cases without movement of the neck.

The airway can also become obstructed by various foreign objects, such as dental appliances, chewing tobacco, chewing gum, or

a mouth guard. An athlete should be advised to compete without substances other than a mouthpiece in his or her mouth. Take the time to explain the mechanism of airway obstruction. If an athlete understands how foreign objects in the mouth can easily block the trachea, such advice will more likely be followed. Any foreign object in the mouth should be removed immediately when assessing airway and breathing. If an object becomes lodged and occludes the airway, an effective method for removing it is the Heimlich maneuver. Although serious complications following use of the Heimlich maneuver are rare, the procedure involves some risk. Proper instruction in executing this emergency care procedure is essential.

Breathing

The term **apnea** refers to any temporary cessation of breathing. An athlete may stop breathing or be in respiratory arrest for various reasons, the most common being an obstructed airway. The airway may be obstructed by the tongue or foreign object, as previously discussed; swelling in the throat

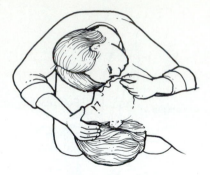

FIGURE 11-4
Opening the airway and assessing breathlessness using the head tilt-chin lift procedure.

caused by allergic reactions; or tissue damage caused by a severe blow to the neck. Respiratory arrest may also result from cardiac arrest, poisons, drugs, drowning, and intrathoracic injuries. Regardless of cause, it is extremely important that the person in charge recognize the condition immediately and initiate appropriate emergency care procedures. Assessment of breathing and adequacy of airway are closely coupled. The first priority in assessment and care of injuries involving an athlete's breathing is to establish an open airway. Remember, when the airway is opened, an athlete suffering from apnea may begin to breathe spontaneously. If it does not appear that the athlete is breathing, put your ear close to the athlete's mouth and nose as shown in Figure 11-4. Listen for an exchange of air. Feel for any breath against your cheek or ear and watch the chest for any breathing movements. If the athlete is not breathing after opening the airway, appropriate techniques of artificial ventilation must be initiated immediately.

A more common respiratory problem is difficult or labored breathing, called **dyspnea.** This can be a terrifying and serious condition for the athlete. In the absence of chest or lung injuries, dyspnea is often the result of **hyperventilation**, over-breathing to the extent that the carbon dioxide level in the blood is abnormally lowered. Hyperventilation can be a psychologic response to pain and trauma caused by an athlete breathing very rapidly and deeply. The athlete may be terrified that he or she cannot get enough air into the lungs. Athletes suffering from hyperventilation may experience dizziness, faint feelings, chest pains, and sensations of numbness or tingling of the hands and feet. Reassure the athlete with a calm manner. Talk to the athlete and encourage slow, relaxed breathing. A procedure used to build up the blood carbon dioxide level is to ask the athlete to breathe into a paper bag. In this way the athlete will rebreathe exhaled air and raise the carbon dioxide level in the blood to a normal or near-normal level. It is important to explain this technique to the athlete to gain his or her confidence. Once the athlete is calm and breathing normally, continue the assessment of any associated injuries.

Circulation

There are several reasons why an athlete's heart may stop beating, but should it occur, the exact cause is immaterial to the athletic trainer. Of utmost importance is the recognition of cardiac arrest and the immediate initiation of emergency measures. Circulation is assessed by palpating for a pulse. *Pulse* is defined as the alternate expansion and recoil of an artery caused by the intermittent ejection of blood from the heart. The carotid artery in the neck (Figure 11-5) is the most commonly used artery to check for a pulse during an emergency situation. This is the main artery in the neck, and it lies superficially in a groove between the sternocleidomastoid muscle and the trachea, or windpipe. The carotid artery is normally not obstructed by clothing or equipment and is easily accessible. Position yourself on one side of the athlete, place your index and middle fingers on the windpipe, and slide them toward you as shown in Figure 11-6. Press gently into the soft part of the neck next to the windpipe. The carotid pulse can be felt in the groove formed by the sternocleidomastoid muscle and the trachea. Always feel for the carotid pulse on the side of the neck closest to you.

If the athlete does not exhibit a pulse, appropriate emergency techniques of artificial circulation must be initiated immediately.

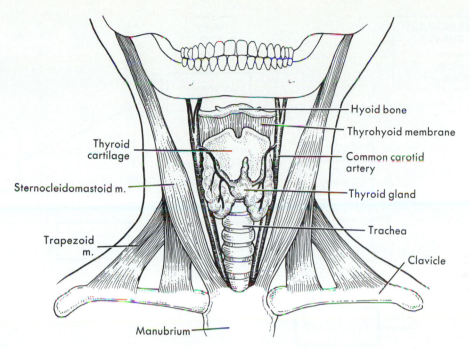

FIGURE 11-5
Anatomic illustration of neck showing the carotid arteries.

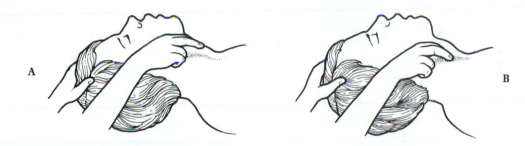

FIGURE 11-6
Assessing pulselessness by, **A**, placing index and middle fingers on the windpipe and, **B**, sliding them downward into the groove formed by the sternocleidomastoid muscle and the trachea.

Every athletic trainer must have a working knowledge of current cardiopulmonary resuscitation techniques. This knowledge can be gained only through supervised training and practice and should be reviewed at least annually.

Figure 11-7 is a flow chart illustrating the basic steps of the primary survey in sequential order.

Once the primary survey concerning the ABCs of life support has been completed and all life-threatening conditions have been brought under control, the secondary survey begins.

SECONDARY SURVEY

The **secondary survey** is the portion of the assessment that examines the athlete in an attempt to recognize and evaluate all injuries. In sports medicine, it is the secondary survey that usually comprises the largest portion of the total athletic injury assessment procedure. It consists of an ordered sequence of procedures used to assess the na-

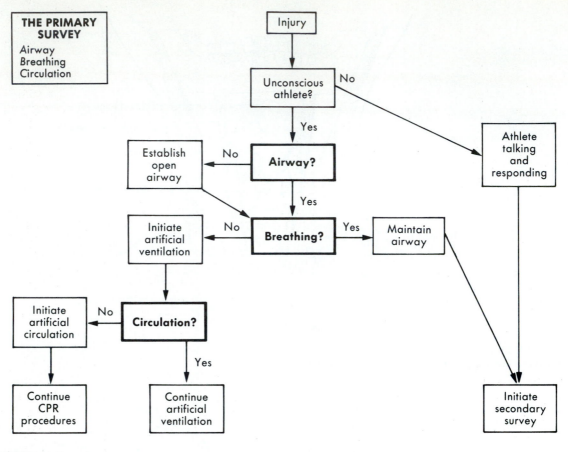

FIGURE 11-7
Basic steps of the primary survey.

ture, site, and severity of an athletic injury. When injury occurs, early, accurate assessment is essential in developing an effective treatment and rehabilitation program. In addition, the assessment can provide the athletic trainer with useful information for the development of programs to prevent similar injuries.

The importance of using a detailed and properly sequenced checklist in the assessment procedure cannot be overemphasized. By following a consistent pattern in your evaluation procedures, you are less likely to forget a procedure or miss an important detail. Pilots, for example, learn early in their flight training about the importance of using checklists. Sample checklists are provided for each body area discussed throughout the remainder of the text.

Secondary Survey
*H*istory
*O*bservation
*P*hysical Examination

The secondary survey can be divided into three main areas: History, Observation, and Physical Examination (Figure 11-8). An accurate assessment of an athletic injury often depends on a factual and reliable history, studious and diligent observations, and a careful and complete physical examination. The remainder of this chapter will discuss various concerns and procedures for each of these important segments of an athletic injury assessment. Of course, not all the procedures discussed in each area of the sec-

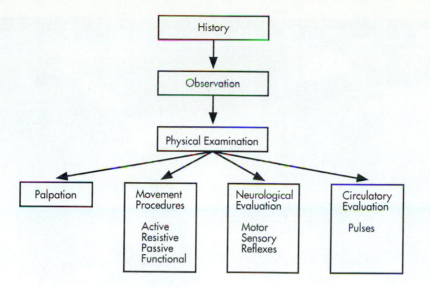

FIGURE 11-8
Basic steps of the secondary survey.

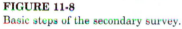

ondary survey will be carried out with each athletic injury. The nature, type, and severity of the injury will determine the evaluation techniques used. Every athletic trainer will at some time be faced with an athletic injury requiring very few assessment skills; for example, a fractured arm with the bone protruding through the skin. With this type of injury, immediate first aid and referral skills are the primary concern of the athletic trainer. Except in these types of obvious injuries, the athletic trainer should always initiate and conduct some type of a sequential assessment process. Shortcuts in evaluating athletic injuries should be avoided because they increase the risk of overlooking or missing important information. Athletic trainers must continue to improve and refine their assessment skills.

Another important aspect of the secondary survey is documentation of the results or findings. An athletic trainer should always document or record in writing the information gained during the evaluation process. This information becomes part of the athlete's permanent record, and it is important that it is recorded accurately and thoroughly. Documentation is also very helpful whenever referring an injured athlete, reevaluating the injured area, and following the

progress of treatment and rehabilitation programs. A common format for writing notes used for documentation is the **SOAP note.** SOAP is an acronym for *Subjective, Objective, Assessment,* and *Plan.* Each of these sections refers to the information gained during the evaluation and the resulting strategy for management of the injury. SOAP notes help establish an organized system of registering problem-oriented medical records and can assist an athletic trainer in organizing his or her thought process. SOAP notes form a method of communicating with other health professionals because this recording method, or some modification, is commonly used today.

The information gained during the assessment of an athletic injury can easily be adapted to the SOAP note format. Using the assessment techniques described in this text, the *subjective* segment of a SOAP note is the information gained during the history taking portion of the process. *Objective* information is gained during the observation portion of the athletic injury assessment process. The *assessment* segment refers to information gained during the physical examination portion of the athletic injury assessment process. The *plan* contains the strategies or approaches for management of the injury.

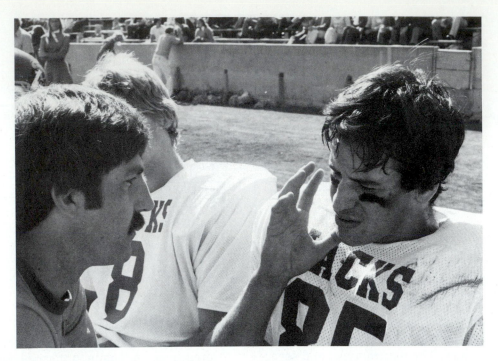

FIGURE 11-9
Obtaining a history from an injured athlete.

History

Obtaining an accurate history of an injury is one of the most important steps in the secondary survey portion of the total athletic injury assessment process (Figure 11-9). Taking a history involves finding out as much information as possible about the actual injury and the circumstances surrounding its occurrence. This is accomplished by talking with the injured athlete or others who have either witnessed or observed the injury. Information gained in a thorough history can provide important clues in determining which structures may be injured and which assessment techniques will be appropriate as you continue the examination.

Athletic injuries can happen almost anywhere and anytime during activity. They basically appear in two ways: (1) suddenly, such as those caused by trauma, and (2) gradually, such as the overuse syndromes that develop over a period of time. The direction taken when obtaining the history depends on the nature of the injury and how it occurred.

Injuries that appear suddenly

The history of a sudden traumatic injury (acute) is usually easy to obtain. This type of an athletic injury is frequently witnessed by persons who can provide useful information to help in completing the history. In many cases the athletic trainer will witness the injury and have an idea of the mechanisms involved before formal questioning begins. Sometimes, however, the athletic trainer does not witness the injury and must question the athlete and others who were present in an attempt to establish the facts. In some cases an athlete may not report the injury at the time it occurs or when the symptoms initially appear. In these cases, in addition to the history of the injury, you must find out what, if anything, has occurred since the injury happened. Specific questions required to elicit necessary information will vary, depending on the nature of the injury in question. Piecing together the complete history requires time, skill, patience, and thoroughness.

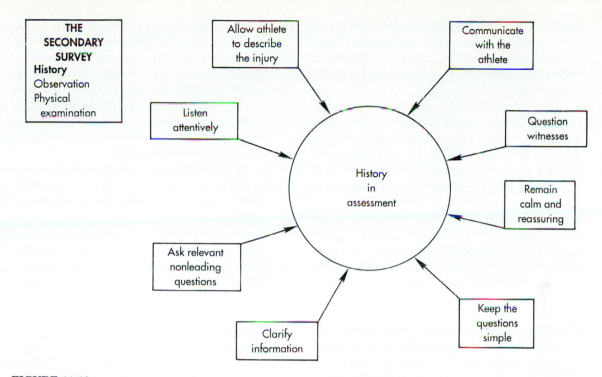

FIGURE 11-10
Factors related to obtaining an accurate and thorough history of an athletic injury.

Injuries that appear gradually

Accurate assessment of athletic injuries that develop over a period of time, such as chronic injuries and overuse syndromes, requires a very detailed history. If the athlete understands the importance of the history in assessing the extent of injury, he or she will more likely be patient and cooperative in answering questions. Sometimes the onset of the symptoms may be insidious, and the athlete will have few recollections of any injury or stress. The symptoms usually begin as a mild and sporadic ache and gradually become more painful and continuous. You must attempt to gain as much information as possible related to the injury. Did the symptoms appear suddenly or did they come on gradually? What has the athlete been able to do since the symptoms first appeared? Inquire about functional capabilities such as the ability to walk, climb stairs, twist, throw, or whatever activity is involved with the body area injured. What aggravates the injured area? Is it relieved by rest? In-

juries that appear gradually may be caused by any of a number of factors, such as errors in training, inappropriate or improperly fitted equipment, playing surfaces, structural abnormalities, poor flexibility, or poor conditioning. The history must take into consideration all of these factors. A meticulous history is required when attempting to assess injuries of this type.

There are several important factors to remember in attempting to gain a comprehensive history (Figure 11-10). Each of these factors involves the development and use of communication skills.

To gain an accurate history of the injury, you must communicate with the injured athlete if at all possible. The athlete is the only person who has experienced the injury and knows exactly how it feels. Of course, there will be times when it will be impossible to talk to the injured athlete, for example, if he or she is unconscious or unresponsive for any reason. When this occurs, you must question other athletes or persons who might have witnessed the injury. Attempt to gain as much information as possible from whomever observed the injury or has knowledge of important factors associated with its occurrence.

There are other factors to keep in mind as you attempt to talk with an injured athlete. Immediately after an injury, the athlete may not feel like talking. He or she may be in pain and frightened. Perhaps the last thing the athlete wants to do at that time is carry on a conversation about the injury. You should appreciate that every athlete responds differently to an injury. Some explain their injury in great detail; others volunteer little if any information. Some athletes try to minimize their injury; others try to maximize it. In addition, some persons become very emotional when in pain or under stress. These circumstances often complicate the assessment process and underscore the need to communicate with an injured athlete in a calm and reassuring manner. Make every attempt to relax the athlete so that he or she will be able to discuss the injury and respond to questions.

When speaking with the athlete, keep the questions simple. Most athletes are not interested in lengthy conversations after sustaining an injury. Ask only one question at a time, and get the answer before proceeding to the next. Attempt to follow an orderly or systematic format in taking an athlete's history, but allow for modifications on the basis of his or her responses.

One format used in the medical profession to elicit information during a history is to divide the information into five groups remembered by the acronym PQRST: (1) *Pro*vocative/*Palliative*, (2) *Quality*/*Quantity*, (3) *Region*/*Radiation*, (4) *Severity* scale, and (5) *Timing*. Examples of questions using the PQRST technique to elicit information are listed in the box.

So-called standard or canned questions are seldom useful. Each injury and each athlete is unique. The athletic trainer must develop interview or questioning skills that can be applied in a wide variety of situations. Clarify the information being gathered and ask questions that will elicit further essential information. Ask relevant,

---

Examples of Questions Using PQRST

Provocative/*Palliative*

What caused it?
What makes it better, or worse?
How did it start?

Quality/*Quantity*

How does it feel?
What sensations are associated with it?
Is it getting better or worse?
Can you compare this to a previous injury or condition?

Region/*Radiation*

Where is the injury located?
Are the resulting pain and abnormal sensations localized or radiating?

Severity scale

Does it interfere with activity?
How does it feel on a scale of 1 to 10?

Timing

When did it begin?
How often does it occur?
Was the onset sudden or gradual?
Have you had this before?

nonleading questions of an injured athlete. Examples of leading questions are "Did you turn your ankle under?" and "Does it hurt right here?" It is much easier for an athlete in pain to answer "yes" to such questions than to describe the injury in detail. If you lead the athlete with your questions, you may actually develop a false impression of the injury. Let the athlete describe the injury and tell you what happened.

As the athlete explains how the injury occurred, it is important to listen attentively to what he or she is saying. Many clues as to the structures injured, as well as severity of injury, can be gained by listening to the athlete's description of the injury. It is easy to make assumptions about an injury, especially if the injury was witnessed. If the athlete says he or she heard and felt a popping or cracking sensation and believes something is broken, it must be assumed correct until proved otherwise. Give the athlete the benefit of the doubt, even if it ap-

pears that he or she is overreacting to the injury. Do not begin the assessment with your mind made up about the injury. Each new injury must be evaluated separately. Begin with a complete history and allow the athlete to describe the injury and spell out in detail exactly what happened. The importance of being a good listener cannot be overemphasized. Obtaining a good history requires a high degree of proficiency in listening skills.

The importance of the history-taking process cannot be overemphasized; a vast amount of information can be gained by conducting an accurate and thorough history of all athletic injuries and related conditions (Figure 11-11). The history is of special significance because the physical findings associated with athletic injuries are often minimal.

In communicating with an injured athlete, determine the primary complaint early in the assessment process. Where does it

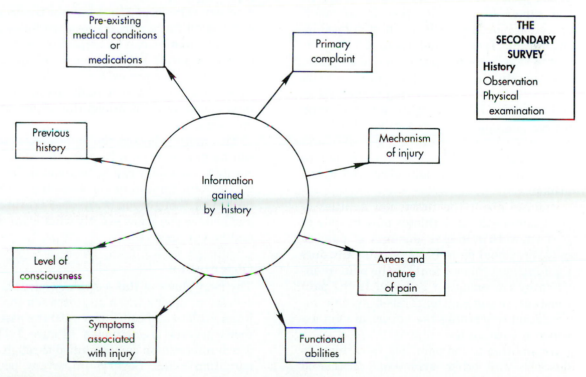

FIGURE 11-11
Information gained by taking the history of an athletic injury.

hurt? What type of injury has the athlete suffered? Attempt to find out the exact **mechanism of injury.** How and when did the injury occur? Did the athlete fall or was there a twist? Did the athlete receive a blow, and if so, from what direction? Did the athlete hear or feel anything? Attempt to recreate in your mind the mechanism of injury and visualize the position of the body when the injury occurred. It is important to have a clear conception of the mechanism of injury.

Attempt to locate the areas of pain. It is helpful if the athlete can point to the area of pain. Notice how he or she points to the painful area. Is the pain localized or is it spread over a large body area? Be as exact as possible in determining anatomic location. Is the pain around a joint, along a bone, or in a muscular area?

Inquire as to the type of pain the athlete is experiencing. Is the pain dull, sharp, constant, occasional, burning, deep, throbbing, etc? Is the pain changing? Has the intensity of the pain increased, decreased, or stayed the same? Has the location of the pain spread or moved since it was first noticed by the athlete? It can be helpful to ask the athlete to rate his or her perception of the pain. Ask the athlete to rate the pain on a scale of 1 to 10, with 1 representing almost insignificant pain and 10 being the worst pain the athlete can imagine or remember. There are also other various pain-rating scales and questionnaires that have been developed to gauge the amount of pain perceived by an athlete.

Inquire about the functional abilities of the injured athlete. Athletes may be able to perform with minimal amounts of pain or only occasional pain. Is there pain only during function or movement? Is the pain intensified by movement or activity? Is the pain constant or intermittent? Seek specific information concerning the nature of pain associated with athletic injuries.

In addition to the pain, ask the athlete to describe any other symptoms associated with the injury in as much detail as possible. Is the athlete experiencing any numbness, tingling, weakness, or burning sensations? Is reference made to any type of grinding or grating sensations (crepitation)? Did the athlete experience any abnormal sounds or sensations at the time of the injury? Does the athlete feel any tightness, tension, or swelling associated with the injury?

Talking with an athlete will also assist in assessing his or her level of consciousness. For example, is the athlete alert and responsive or confused and disoriented? It is important to evaluate the athlete's level of consciousness and establish a neurologic baseline early in the assessment process, especially when the injury involves the head. The importance of level(s) of consciousness will be discussed in greater detail in Chapters 12 and 13.

Knowledge of past injuries or problems can help in assessing the nature of current injuries. Inquire about any previous injuries to the affected part or surrounding body area. If there was a previous injury, probe for additional details. What type of injury? How long was the recovery period? Was the recovery complete? What kind of treatment and rehabilitation programs were followed? This information can be helpful in assessing current injuries. Also attempt to find out about any other pre-existing medical conditions that may have a relationship to the injury, or any medications the athlete may be taking.

The more relevant the information that can be gained from a history, the more accurately the injury can be evaluated. Do not overlook the importance of obtaining the history even though you witnessed the injury and believe you know exactly what is injured and how it occurred.

Observation

The next phase of the secondary survey, observation, begins when you first see the injured athlete and continues until the assessment process is completed (Figure 11-12). Much information can be gained through observation skills. Several important points should be remembered in observing an injured athlete (Figure 11-13). Begin by quickly

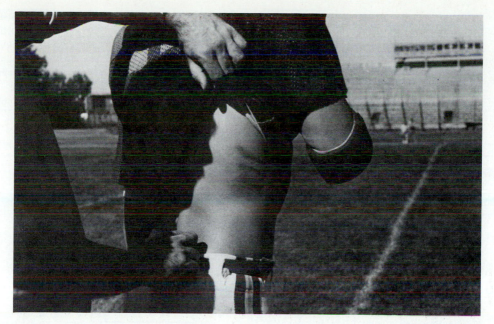

FIGURE 11-12
Observing and inspecting an injured area.

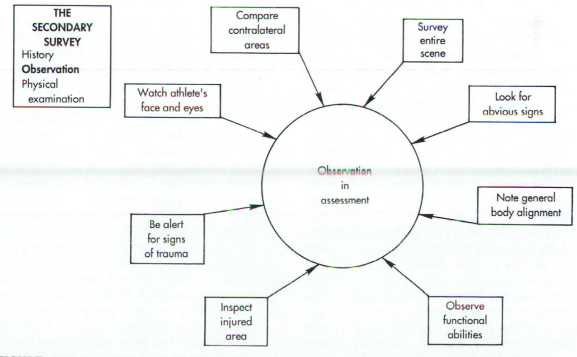

FIGURE 11-13
Factors related to observing an injured athlete.

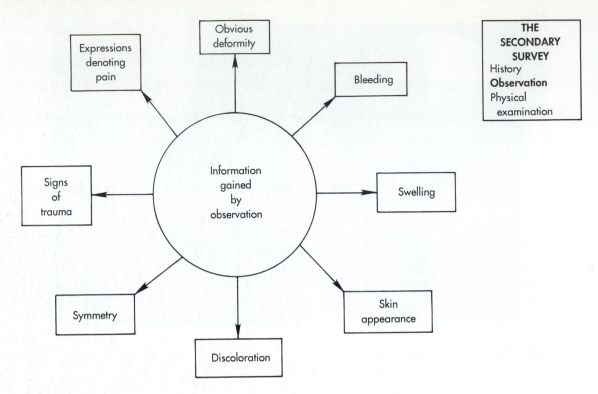

FIGURE 11-14
Information that can be gained during observation of an injured athlete.

surveying the entire scene. Notice the position of the athlete. Did you observe the mechanism of injury? Was there any apparatus or equipment associated with the injury? Look for any obvious bleeding, deformity, swelling, discoloration, or other signs of injury. Note general body alignment and posture of the athlete. Is the athlete holding a body part or grasping some body area? If the athlete is moving around, observe his or her functional abilities. Is the athlete using the injured part or protecting it? Is he or she limping?

After a general survey of the injury scene, carefully inspect the injured area and assess the results of the athletic injury. This is often accomplished in conjunction with the history-taking process. Watch closely as the athlete describes the injury. What is the position of the injured part? Be alert for any signs of trauma, such as abrasions or contusions, that may indicate the mechanism of injury. Some athletes try to disguise or min-

imize the extent of their injury. Observing the athlete's face and eyes as he or she describes the injury may give further clues as to the extent of pain. More pain may be reflected in the athlete's face than he or she is willing to admit.

When inspecting an injury, clothing and equipment that may obscure the area should be removed. Consider the athlete's modesty in removing clothing and equipment. If possible, adequate exposure should permit visualization of the area above and below the injury. Do not limit your examination solely to the area of injury. You should always compare the injured body part to the contralateral uninjured part and note any obvious differences. However, you must be aware of any abnormalities in the uninjured body part caused by such things as congenital conditions or previous injuries. If the athletic trainer has been involved with a preseason screening program of the uninjured athlete, this information will be readily

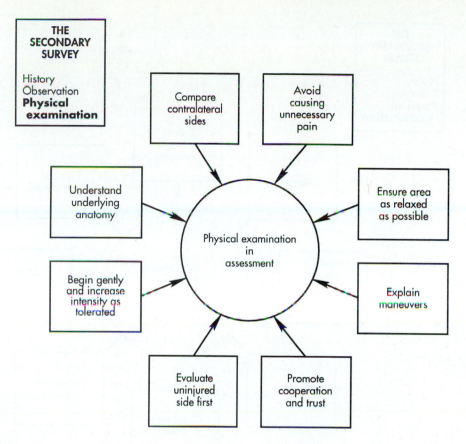

FIGURE 11-15
Factors associated with performing a physical examination on an injured area.

available. Attempt to gain as much information as possible by observation (Figure 11-14).

Physical Examination

The third phase of the secondary survey involves the selective use of various assessment procedures and maneuvers designed to further locate and evaluate the integrity of the structures involved in the injury. Figure 11-15 illustrates several important factors to remember when performing the various assessment techniques. Most of the physical examination procedures discussed in this text can be broken down into the following areas: palpation, movements procedures, neurological evaluations, and circulatory evaluations. Each area is important and informative (Figure 11-16). However, not all procedures are necessary with every athletic

injury and do not need to follow the sequence outlined in this text. Which evaluative procedures or maneuvers are used and in what sequence will depend on the athletic injury. For example, for an athlete with a suspected spine injury, the motor and sensory function evaluations are extremely important and should be performed very early in the assessment process. Following is a basic description of each area of the physical examination. Specific tests and procedures to evaluate the various body areas are explained in more detail throughout the remainder of this text.

Palpation

Palpation means to touch and feel the injured area. After the history and observation steps, you can gain additional physical information concerning the injury by carefully

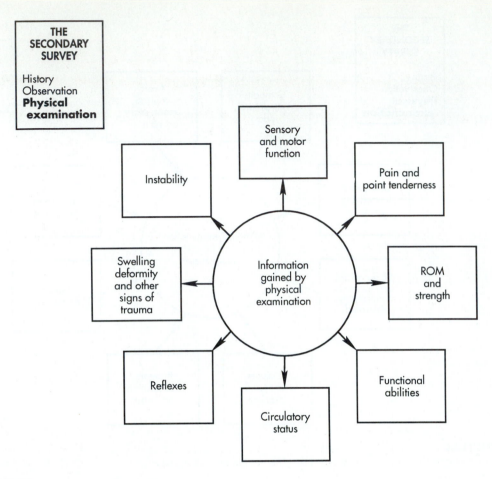

FIGURE 11-16
Information that can be gained during the physical examination of an injured athlete.

palpating the affected body area (Figure 11-17). There are several important points to remember as you prepare to palpate an injured athlete. Palpation procedures should begin in a tender manner to avoid unnecessary pain. If you cause the athlete unnecessary pain, he or she may become tense and uncooperative, making palpation assessment of the injury more difficult, if not impossible. To accurately palpate an injured area it should be as relaxed as possible. Treating the athlete gently helps demonstrate your concern and helps establish confidence and cooperation. The intensity or pressure used with each palpation maneuver can then be increased, depending on the athlete's tolerance and the severity of the injury. It is important that an athletic trainer develop a systematic approach to

palpating an area. A systematic approach can be beneficial in ensuring you evaluate all anatomical landmarks and structures that may be involved. It is a good practice to begin palpating distally and work toward the injury site to avoid unnecessary pain or apprehension and encourage the athlete's cooperation and confidence. In addition, by doing this you are not as likely to become so involved with the obvious injury that you overlook another, less apparent injury.

It is important that you visualize what structures are under your fingers. Are you feeling approximately where ligaments should be? Are you feeling an isolated tendon or a musculotendinous junction? Are you palpating predominately muscular tissue or bone? To visualize the structures that are being palpated, you must have an un-

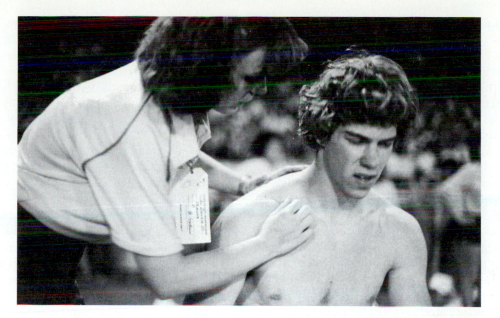

FIGURE 11-17
Palpating an injured area.

derstanding of the surface anatomy as well as the underlying anatomy. This text will illustrate surface anatomy with each body area discussed. It may be helpful to look at anatomic charts or drawings to verify underlying anatomy and show them to the injured athlete to help him or her understand the injury. Remember to also compare contralateral areas.

Important information can be gained by careful palpation procedures. Pain is one of the most obvious and consistent symptoms of injury. Use of palpation techniques to localize pain is extremely useful in assessing athletic injuries. It is especially important to locate areas that are most painful to touch. These are called areas of *point tenderness.* Regardless of the anatomic structures involved, point tenderness is usually found at the site of injury. This location of point tenderness, and knowledge of underlying anatomic structures, can provide important clues in evaluating the site and nature of an injury. It may be necessary to observe the athlete's face for wincing or grimacing if he or she cannot provide reliable verbal responses.

Another physical sign that can be recognized by palpation is swelling. Swelling, or edema, may be localized at the injury site or diffused over a larger area. Swelling may result from bleeding caused by trauma or by accumulation of pus or tissue fluid as a result of some inflammatory process (described in Chapter 7). As a rule, the amount of swelling is generally related to the severity of injury. There are cases, however, in which serious injuries produce very limited swelling and minor injuries cause severe and extensive swelling or edema. In areas of extensive swelling, the skin becomes stretched and feels tight and smooth.

Additional information gained during palpation may be related to the temperature and surface moisture of the skin. Normal skin is moderately warm and dry. In palpating the site of an injury, any indication of an increase in skin temperature suggests the occurrence of an inflammatory process. A decrease in skin temperature may be felt in areas of inadequate circulation. In addition, various combinations of skin color, temperature, texture, and moisture can assist in identification of generalized conditions such as shock and problems associated with body temperature regulation.

Muscle spasm may also be recognized while palpating an injured area. This is a body defense mechanism designed to protect an injured area from further trauma. When an injury occurs, the surrounding muscles often involuntarily contract, or become tight, as the body attempts to splint or brace the injured area. The area surrounding an injury may then feel tense or tight as you palpate the area. Remember to instruct the athlete to relax the injured area as much as possible before beginning palpation procedures.

Deformity may be caused by a fracture, dislocation, or the tearing of soft tissue such as ligament, muscle, or tendon. Deformity may be obvious and easily seen on observation, or it may be discreet and only recognized after careful palpation of the injured area. If there is any question regarding what the normal contour of the area should be, the corresponding uninjured side should be palpated as a basis for comparison.

Crepitation is a grating, grinding, or sticking sensation that may be produced by various conditions. When crepitation is associated with athletic injuries, it is commonly caused by the broken ends of a bone rubbing together or the thickening of synovial or bursal fluid and membranes. An athlete may describe a grinding sensation on movement of an injured part, and you may feel crepitus as you palpate the injured area.

Movement procedures

Up to this point in the assessment process, the injured athlete does not have to move or be moved. If necessary, history, observation, and palpation can be completed with the athlete remaining in the original position he or she is in immediately after injury. Movement procedures, however, do involve some movement of a body part or the athlete. However, should a serious injury be suspected, it is not necessary to perform this step of the assessment process, and appropriate emergency measures should be initiated.

Movement procedures involve selective use of some type of manipulation or stress to the injured body area. These procedures are employed in an attempt to locate and define the structures involved in the injury, as well as to evaluate the integrity of affected tissues. Information gained in this way is extremely valuable and usually cannot be obtained in any other manner. A complete and detailed evaluation of an athletic injury is often not possible unless the injury is subjected to some movement or stress. Unfortunately, this important step in athletic injury assessment may be neglected or even omitted completely.

There are several important factors to remember as you prepare to stress an injured area. Movement procedures should not be applied to an injured area until history, observation, and palpation have been completed. You must have an idea of the nature of the injury before you attempt to move the affected body part. For example, you would not attempt to stress an injured area when you suspect a dislocation or fracture. In addition to the information gained, completion of these three steps in the secondary survey serves another useful purpose. It provides the time necessary to calm and relax the athlete before manipulation and stress testing begins.

It is important that you explain what you are going to do and elicit cooperation from the athlete before beginning any stress tests. It is extremely difficult to use movement maneuvers effectively in assessment procedures if the injured athlete is tense and unable to relax. A mutual sense of trust between the athlete and the athletic trainer is essential to gain accurate information from the assessment. In addition to development of trust, the ability to communicate effectively is especially important during this step of the evaluation process.

Applying stress to an injured area will undoubtedly cause some additional pain. However, these procedures should not cause unnecessary pain, or you will most likely lose the cooperation of the injured player. Any stress applied to the athlete should begin slowly and gently to minimize pain and protective muscle spasms. In a painful injury, it is good practice to begin these maneuvers on the uninjured side. This will help lessen

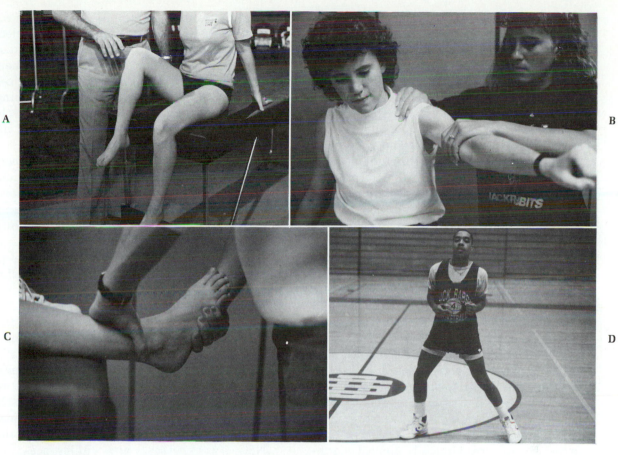

FIGURE 11-18
Applying stress procedures to an injured area. **A**, Active ROM; **B**, manual resistance applied against an injured body part; **C**, passive stress applied to a joint; and, **D**, functional activities performed by an athlete.

apprehensions and prepare the player for procedures that will be carried out on the injured side. This can also give you information necessary to compare the injured to the uninjured side.

Although there are many procedures for applying stress to an injured area, they can be divided into four basic types of maneuvers or movements: (1) active, (2) resistive, (3) passive, and (4) functional (Figure 11-18). Seldom is it necessary to subject an injury to tests from all four groups. Information gained during the first three steps in the assessment process will enable you to select the most appropriate procedures.

Active movements. Active movements are those that can be initiated and completed by the athlete without assistance of any kind. Such movements are usually the least stressful. To initiate this type of maneuver the athlete is asked to move the injured part as directed by the athletic trainer. Active motion is used to evaluate the athlete's willingness and ability to move the injured area. Active movements also assess the integrity of contractile and related tissues such as muscles and tendons and their junctions, attachments, integration, and control by the nervous system. Noncontractile tissues, such as joint capsules, ligaments, bursae, cartilage, and nerves, will also have some stress applied to them as the result of active motion. Note which movements, if any, cause pain and the amount and quality of pain that results. Does the movement increase the intensity of the pain? Where and when in the movement does the pain occur? Is there any restriction or limitation in the active motion?

Another important factor that can be evaluated with active motion is the range of motion (ROM) of surrounding joints. For example, an athlete may be asked to actively move an injured extremity through the pain-free ROM. Active motion will indicate the athlete's ability and willingness to perform the movements requested as well as the ROM possible. Pain will normally limit active motion so that additional injury to damaged structures does not occur as a result of the assessment process. Note the limits of active motion and, if necessary, compare it to the ROM of the uninjured side. You can accurately measure the ROM with a goniometer as described in Chapter 4.

Resistive movements. Resistance may be applied against active motion to further evaluate the integrity of the contractile tissues. Whenever a muscle or tendon injury is suspected or indicated, resistive movements can assist in identifying specific tender areas. Usually resistance is applied manually by the athletic trainer. Manual resistance can be applied throughout the ROM or isometrically in various positions in the range. Resistance applied *isometrically* (static contraction) helps rule out non-contractile tissue involvement and stresses primarily the contractile tissues. Low initial resistance against movement is gradually increased, depending on the athlete's tolerance. The ability of the athlete to tolerate increasing resistance loads can reveal a great deal about the extent of injury involving the contractile tissues. Note the site of pain at any specific point throughout the resisted ROM.

Resistive movements are also used to evaluate the strength of a body part. During the acute stages of an athletic injury, pain will normally limit an accurate evaluation of muscular strength. However, on repeated assessments used to determine when an injured athlete is ready to return to activity, **manual muscle testing** can be very bene-

ficial in evaluating muscular strength. In recent years, numerous mechanical and electronic devices have been developed to test muscular strength. Depending on their availability and applicability, these devices can provide valuable information concerning muscle function. However, manual muscle testing remains a readily available and inexpensive tool for the athletic trainer.

Manual muscle testing is normally performed throughout a full ROM for each muscle or group of muscles. The athlete is positioned in such a way that isolates the muscle or group of muscles being tested and allows movement through the full ROM. Substitution by muscles other than those being tested can usually be eliminated by careful positioning. Manual resistance is then applied throughout the movement by the athlete, or the athlete offers resistance to the movement performed by the athletic trainer. Those same resistive movements are usually performed on the contralateral or uninjured side for a comparison of strength. It is often necessary to carefully repeat manual muscle tests, comparing the strength to the normal side, because weaknesses can be subtle. Note weaknesses and differences in strength.

Manual muscle testing is graded subjectively, according to the athletic trainer's judgment of the athlete's responses. Various grading criteria and classifications have been used to record manual muscular strength. Table 11-1 indicates traditional systems frequently used. Other evaluators prefer descriptive words such as severe weakness, moderate weakness, minimal weakness, and normal. Whatever grading system is used, manual muscle tests should always be performed consistently, and movements should be coordinated and painless.

Passive movements. Passive movements are procedures performed completely by the athletic trainer and are the most difficult stress procedures to perform and evaluate. The athlete is asked to relax the injured area so that the effects of conscious control and muscular effort can be eliminated. Great care must be exercised in per-

TABLE 11-1

Grading for Manual Muscle Testing

Numeric grade	Percentage of normal	Muscular contraction	Functional level
5	100%	Normal	Complete ROM against gravity, with *full* manual resistance appropriate for age and sex
4	75%	Good	Complete ROM against gravity, with *some* manual resistance appropriate for age and sex
3	50%	Fair	Complete ROM against gravity and *no* manual resistance
2	25%	Poor	Complete ROM with gravity eliminated
1	10%	Trace	Evidence of slight contractility; no joint motion produced
0	0%	Zero	No evidence of muscular contraction by either palpated or visible means

forming passive movements because the potential to cause additional pain or injury is much greater than during active and resistive movements. Initially, these stress procedures must be performed very gently and slowly to avoid causing unnecessary pain and muscle spasms. The intensity of the procedures can then be increased, depending on the athlete's tolerance and the severity of injury.

Passive movements are used to evaluate the integrity of noncontractile tissues such as bones, joint capsules, ligaments, and bursae. There are numerous passive tests designed to analyze and locate any instability, pain, or crepitation present as the result of an injury. For example, each ligament around an injured joint should be stressed to check for pain and instability. The extent of instability or laxity must be recognized and noted to properly determine the severity of injury. These passive tests are often designed to reproduce the mechanism of injury. Specific passive procedures used to locate pain and instability in athletic injuries are described and illustrated throughout the remainder of this text.

Functional movements. Functional movements are a series of active movements or activities the athlete performs that simulate the type of activity required in a particular sport. These tests can be used during the initial assessment of an athletic injury but are most often used to determine if re-

covery is complete and if the athlete is ready to return to full participation or activity. The athlete is asked to perform specific movements necessary or required in his or her sport. In most cases the first functional movements are designed to generate relatively little stress. Stress intensity is then increased for subsequent movements until the extent of injury is determined or full recovery is apparent. For example, the athlete with an injured leg may be asked to begin jogging; if that does not cause any pain or problems, the athlete may progress to running and then jumping or cutting activities, depending on the sport.

Functional testing should always precede the return of the athlete to full activity. An athlete who has full strength and no pain or instability on active or passive stress tests must also demonstrate the ability to perform any activities required of his or her sport before returning to full participation.

Neurological evaluations

There are many neurological examinations that may accompany an assessment process. Athletic trainers should possess knowledge of neurological examinations of the cranial nerves (explained in Chapter 13), level of consciousness (explained in Chapters 12 and 13), and sensory functions, motor functions, and reflexes (Figure 11-19). This information was introduced in Chapter 6.

Sensory functions. Assessing the neu-

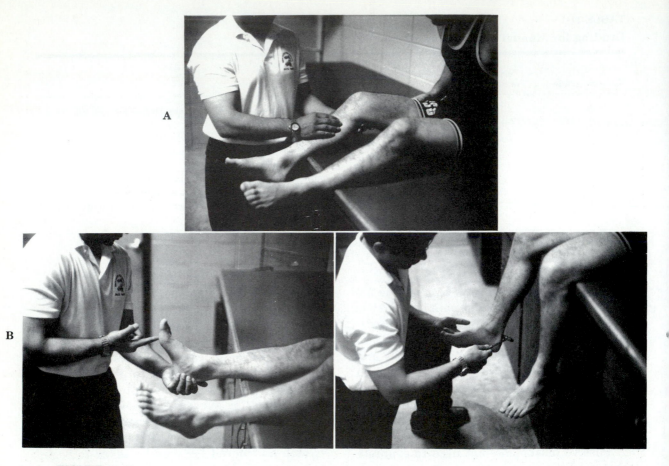

FIGURE 11-19
Using neurologic evaluations on an injured athlete. **A**, Sensory function; **B**, motor function; and
C, reflex testing.

rological status of sensory functions is accomplished by applying various stimuli to specific areas of the skin that are innervated by particular sensory nerves. The distribution of sensory nerves or *dermatomes* was discussed in Chapter 6. The athletic trainer should be familiar with the most likely areas of sensory loss associated with specific peripheral nerve and nerve root trauma.

Testing for altered sensations is usually completed quickly after an athletic injury. The athletic trainer should run a relaxed hand or fingers over the entire skin surface to be tested on the injured side, as well as the corresponding uninjured side. Does the athlete feel any difference in sensations between the two sides of the body? If an area of altered sensations is found, localize the

area or determine the boundaries. More specific tests can also be performed, such as testing for sensitivity to light touch or pain sensation. To assess touch, use a cotton swab, soft brush, or lightly scratch the skin's surface and note the athlete's response. To test for pain, apply the sharp and dull points of a pin or instrument to the skin and note whether the athlete correctly perceives the stimulus. Again, compare sensations on the uninjured side. Abnormal responses to sensory testing include tactile sensations that are decreased **(hypoesthesia),** absent **(anesthesia),** or increased **(hyperesthesia).** Testing for sensory function is especially important in assessing head and spinal injuries but should also be used after significant injuries involving the extremities. If distal

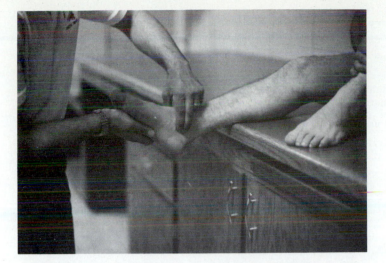

FIGURE 11-20
Evaluating the circulation of an injured extremity.

sensations are normal, it may be assumed the peripheral nerve is intact.

Motor function. Evaluation of motor function is carried out by asking the athlete to move the injured part as was previously discussed with active (ROM) and resistive movements (manual muscle testing). When a spinal injury is suspected, ask the athlete to carefully move his or her fingers or toes. Then proceed to the larger joints. If the athlete has normal motion in the extremities, proceed to check the speed and strength of movements. When a nerve injury is suspected, or to evaluate the integrity of a specific spinal nerve, check the muscle or group of muscles supplied by that nerve (myotome).

Reflexes. A **tendon reflex** is an involuntary contraction of a muscle in response to a brisk tap on its tendon. Testing a reflex can provide an indication of the state of the nerve or nerve root supplying that reflex. Reflexes can be altered by changes involving the sensory or motor nerve pathways. When evaluating reflexes, always test and compare each reflex bilaterally. Reflexes should be symmetrically equal. Do not be overly concerned if the reflexes are equally absent, diminished, or excessive on both sides, unless there is a suspected central lesion. Asymmetry between bilateral reflexes may

indicate a loss or abnormality of nerve conduction and can be diminished (**hyporeflexia**), lost (**areflexia**), or excessive (**hyperreflexia**). Common reflexes that an athletic trainer may evaluate are described in the remaining chapters.

Circulatory evaluations

We have already discussed the obvious importance of assessing if an athlete has adequate circulation. It is also important to evaluate the circulatory status in an extremity following an athletic injury to that area (Figure 11-20). After a fracture or dislocation it is especially important to palpate for a pulse distal to the injury to determine if the extremity has sufficient circulation. If no pulses are found distal to an injury, a medical emergency may exist, and appropriate care and referral measures should be initiated immediately.

EVALUATIONS OF FINDINGS

The remainder of this text includes various evaluative maneuvers and stress procedures that can be used to assist in the evaluation of athletic injuries. Obviously, not all athletic injuries require as complete and systematic a survey as outlined in this chapter. Athletic trainers must learn to select the appropriate evaluation procedures based on

Athletic Injury Assessment Checklist

Primary survey

_____ Airway
_____ Breathing
_____ Circulation

Secondary survey

_____ History
_____ Primary complaint
_____ Mechanism of injury
_____ Areas of pain
_____ Functional abilities
_____ Other associated symptoms
_____ Level of consciousness
_____ Previous injuries
_____ Pre-existing conditions
and medications
_____ Observation
_____ Bleeding
_____ Deformity
_____ Swelling
_____ Discoloration
_____ Signs of trauma
_____ Skin appearance
_____ Expressions denoting pain
symmetry
_____ Physical Examination

Palpation

_____ Point tenderness
_____ Pain
_____ Swelling
_____ Deformity
_____ Crepitation
_____ Muscle spasms
_____ Skin temperature

Movement Procedures

_____ Active movements
_____ ROM
_____ Resistive movements
_____ Pain
_____ Strength
_____ Passive movements
_____ Instability
_____ Pain
_____ Crepitation
_____ Functional movements
_____ Functional abilities

Neurological Evaluations

_____ Sensory functions
_____ Motor functions
_____ Reflexes

Circulatory Evaluations

_____ Pulses

the injured body part and the findings obtained throughout the assessment process. To become skilled in athletic injury assessment, a person must be well versed in both functional anatomy and the procedures used during the evaluation process.

REFERENCES

Arnheim DD, Prentice WE: *Principles of athletic training,* ed 8, St. Louis, 1993, Mosby.

Clarkson HM, Gilewich GB: *Musculoskeletal assessment: joint range of motion and manual muscle strength,* Baltimore, 1989, Williams & Wilkins.

Cyriax J: *Textbook of orthopaedic medicine,* vVol 1, ed 8, London, 1982, Bailliere Tindall.

Hoppenfeld S: *Physical examination of the spine and extremities,* New York, 1976, Appleton-Century-Crofts.

Kessler RM, Hertling D: *Management of common musculoskeletal disorders,* Philadelphia, 1983, Harper & Row.

Kettenbach G: Writing s.o.a.p. notes, Philadelphia, 1990, FA Davis.

Kinney B: Assessment: the key to quality patient care, *Emer Med Services* 18(4):30, 1989.

Malasanos L, Barkauskas V, Stoltenberg-Allen K: *Health assessment,* ed 4, St. Louis, 1990, Mosby.

O'Donoghue DH: *Treatment of injuries to athletes,* ed 4, Philadelphia, 1984, Saunders.

Rosen P, and others, editors: *Emergency medicine: concepts and clinical practice,* ed 3, St. Louis, 1992, Mosby.

SUGGESTED READINGS

Daniels L, Worthingham C: *Muscle testing, techniques of manual examination,* ed 5, Philadelphia, 1986, Saunders.

A highly illustrated manual that presents techniques used to perform manual muscle testing and grading.

Magee DJ: *Orthopedic physical assessment,* ed 2, Philadelphia, 1992, Saunders.

Developed to provide physical therapy students with a systematic approach to performing orthopedic assessments and an understanding of the reason for the various aspects of the assessment.

Post M: *Physical examination of the musculoskeletal system,* Chicago, 1987, Year Book Medical.

Reviews the principles of a history and physical examination for the basis of an effective medical evaluation.

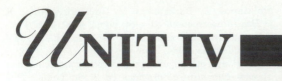# UNIT IV

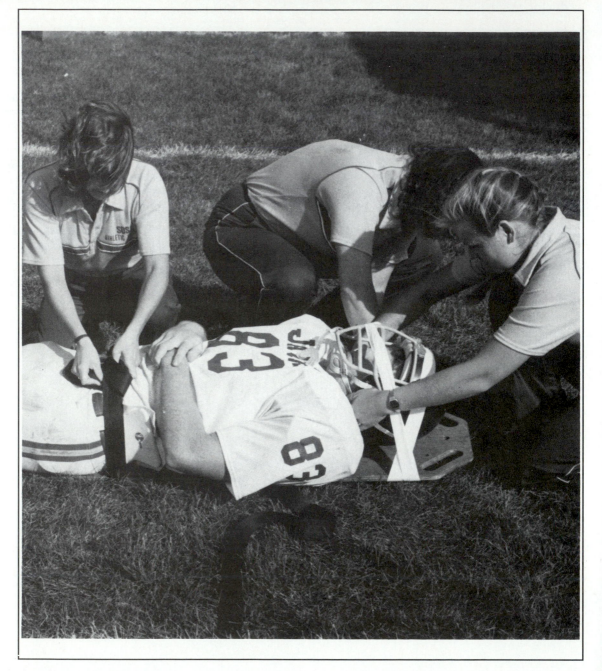

Athletic Injuries of the Axial Region

Athletic injuries to the axial region of the body are discussed first because of the vital organs within this region and the possibility that injuries involving these organs can be life threatening. The axial division of the body includes not only the head and spine but also the trunk, or torso, with its thoracic and abdominal subdivisions.

12 The unconscious athlete
13 Head injuries
14 Face injuries
15 Spine injuries
16 Throat, chest, abdomen, and pelvis injuries

CHAPTER 12

The unconscious athlete

After you have completed this chapter, you should be able to:

- Define unconsciousness and describe various levels of consciousness.
- Identify possible causes of unconsciousness in athletic activity.
- Explain the primary survey for an unconscious athlete.
- Explain the secondary survey for an unconscious athlete.
- List the vital signs that should be observed with an unconscious athlete.
- Describe briefly various abnormal breathing patterns that may indicate brain dysfunction.

One of the most difficult situations an athletic trainer may face is the assessment of an unconscious athlete. In most athletic injuries, the advantage of eliciting responses from the injured athlete greatly assists in making an accurate assessment. The unconscious athlete offers an unusual challenge in assessment, which again emphasizes the importance of having a prearranged sequence of evaluative techniques and a plan of action in the event you must care for an unconscious athlete.

UNCONSCIOUSNESS

Unconsciousness is defined as the inability to respond to any sensory stimuli, with the possible exception of those causing deep pain. The unconscious athlete is unaware of his or her surroundings and is unable to make purposeful voluntary movements. Consciousness is one of the highest functions of the brain, and evaluating the level of consciousness is one of the most reliable mechanisms for determining the neurological status of an athlete. An athlete is normally alert, oriented, and awake. Several terms are used to describe the various levels of consciousness. An athlete may be called **lethargic** when he or she seems drowsy but can be awakened easily by sound or a nudge, and when awake will answer questions. **Stuporous** describes an athlete who is partially or nearly unconscious. This condition is marked by reduced responsiveness. The stuporous athlete will fall asleep easily but can be awakened for short periods of time by verbal or physical stimuli and may be able to answer questions but rapidly falls asleep repeatedly. An **unconscious** athlete cannot be aroused to answer questions, but may pull away from or attempt to push away painful stimuli. **Coma** is a state of unconsciousness from which the athlete cannot be aroused, even by powerful stimuli. For the athletic trainer it is more practical to describe behavior than to label and define various levels of consciousness.

In most instances the unconscious athlete will regain consciousness in a short period of time. Should this occur, the assessment process takes on a different focus, which is discussed in Chapters 13 and 15. This chapter is concerned only with assessment of the unconscious and unresponsive athlete. It is extremely important that athletic trainers evaluate and monitor the level of consciousness of each injured athlete throughout the assessment process.

Causes of Unconsciousness in Athletic Activity

There are various reasons why an athlete may be rendered unconscious. Unconsciousness may result from derangement of the brain or from a problem in the body that interferes with the supply of oxygen and nutrients to the brain. The common cause of unconsciousness in athletics is traumatic head injury. Injuries of this type are discussed in more detail in Chapter 13. An athlete may also become unconscious from conditions such as heatstroke, diabetes, epilepsy, and cerebral or cardiac malfunctions. The fact that it may be difficult to determine the exact cause of unconsciousness underscores the importance of developing a systematic approach to managing an unconscious athlete.

Seizures

Seizures, or convulsions, are discussed at this time because they are periods of unconsciousness that must be managed before the assessment process can continue. Seizures occur suddenly and result from abnormal electrical discharges within the brain. The common cause of seizures during athletics is trauma to the head. However, any condition that irritates or damages brain cells may produce seizures or convulsions. A disorder of the brain that is characterized by a tendency for recurrent seizures is called **epilepsy.** There are several types of seizures, each characterized by disturbances of movement, unconsciousness, and altered sensa-

tions, behavior, mood, or perceptions. In a common type of seizure the person will fall down and display uncontrollable jerking or shaking movements of the extremities. This is known as a **grand mal seizure.** The teeth are often clenched and there may be excessive salivation and loss of bowel or bladder control. Breathing may be irregular because of spastic contractions of the diaphragm; as a result, a bluish color (cyanosis) is often noted in the lips and under the fingernails. Most seizures are self-limiting and cease after a few minutes. After a grand mal seizure, the individual is usually tired and will want to rest. Caring for an athlete who is having a seizure is primarily protective in nature. Protect the athlete's head, arms, and legs as they flail about so the athlete is not injured. The athlete must be protected but not restrained. Never place your fingers into the mouth of an athlete during a seizure. A return to normal respiration almost always follows a single convulsion or seizure, and breathing is not a problem unless successive seizures occur in a short period of time **(status epilepticus).** Should this occur, medical attention must be obtained immediately. An athlete who has experienced a seizure should also be referred to medical assistance. It is important to provide a careful description of the seizure on referral. This information can greatly assist in diagnosis and treatment by the physician.

ATHLETIC INJURY ASSESSMENT PROCESS

Primary survey

When approaching an injured athlete, always note if the person is alert and responsive. If the athlete appears unresponsive, try to communicate with him or her to evaluate level of consciousness. Call the athlete by name. It may be necessary to use loud and repeated verbal stimulation to evoke a response. An unconscious athlete will not respond to verbal or visual commands, and the status of the athlete's airway, breathing, and circulation requires immediate attention. Emergency care procedures of artificial respiration and circulation may have to be initiated before further assessment techniques can be considered. Remember, whenever an athlete is unconscious there is always the possibility that a severe injury has occurred and utmost care and caution should be used. Assume the unconscious athlete has a neck injury as well as a head injury, and treat accordingly. Whenever an unconscious athlete must be moved, extreme care must be taken to avoid causing additional injury.

Airway

Immediate attention must be given to the airway of any unresponsive athlete. As previously discussed, the parapharyngeal muscles may relax, allowing the tongue to fall backward and block the airway, especially if the athlete is lying on his or her back. As described in the previous chapter, tilt the head back and lift the chin (Figure 12-1). This moves the tongue away from the back of the throat. Remember, the unconscious athlete may have lost the normal protective reflex of coughing, which increases the danger of aspiration if blood or vomitus is present. Therefore an adequate airway must be maintained and constantly monitored in the unconscious athlete.

Breathing

In the majority of instances, the unconscious athlete will be breathing; however, always make sure the athlete is breathing before continuing the assessment process. Assessing breathlessness was discussed in Chapter 11. If an unconscious athlete is wearing protective headgear, such as a football helmet with a face guard, assessing breathlessness and initiating cardiopulmonary resuscitation (CPR) techniques may be difficult or impossible. If the protective headgear of an unconscious athlete must be removed, extreme caution must be used, because there may be an associated cervical spine injury. Removing the headgear can cause dangerous motion of the cervical spine and produce additional trauma, which may result in spinal cord transection, paralysis, and even death. Therefore your plan of action in this situation must include procedures for removing the headgear or cutting the face guard away

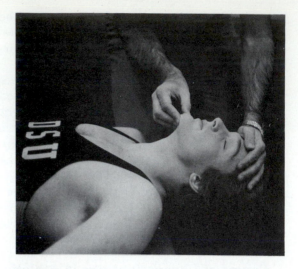

FIGURE 12-1
Positioning the airway in an unconscious athlete who is not breathing.

from the helmet without putting additional stress on the cervical spine. If the athlete is breathing sufficiently, leave the headgear in place because it can assist in stabilizing the head and neck.

Face guards can be removed by cutting them away from the headgear. If the face guard is attached by the type of supports that allow it to swing upward, cutting the side supports with a sharp knife or other appropriate tool will allow the face guard to swing up and away from the face during removal (Figure 12-2). Large bolt cutters can be used to cut the face guard at each point of attachment to the headgear. This procedure is difficult to perform without some movement of the head. You should be prepared to carry out one of the procedures to remove a face guard, depending on the style of face guards, supports used, and removal equipment available.

If a football helmet must be removed from an unconscious athlete, the easiest and safest method is shown in Figure 12-3. While one person holds the helmet firmly so there is no unnecessary movement, a second person removes the chinstrap and cheek pads. The cheek pads are removed with the help of a slender, flat object, such as a butter

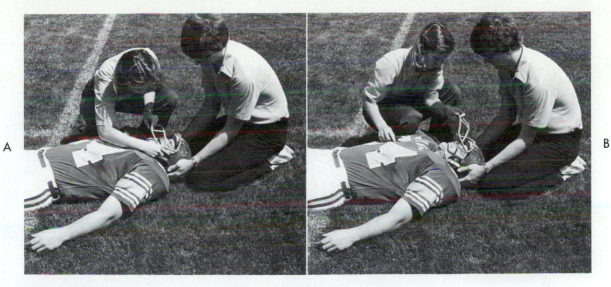

FIGURE 12-2
Removing the face guard. **A,** Cutting the side supports with a sharp knife and, **B,** swinging the face guard away from the face.

knife, spatula, tongue blade, screwdriver, or bandage scissors. It is a good practice to keep one of these objects (a butter knife is one of the best for this maneuver) readily available among your emergency supplies. The object is placed between the helmet and the cheek pad and twisted slightly to loosen the snaps holding the cheek pads in place. The cheek pads can then be carefully lifted out. The person holding the helmet then prepares to slide it off the athlete's head while the second person supports the head and neck. Putting the thumbs in the ear holes of the helmet will assist in spreading the helmet to clear the ears as it is slid off. Throughout the removal process, the second person applies longitudinal traction or stabilization to prevent movement of the head and maintain cervical alignment. After the helmet is removed the first person resumes responsibility for inline traction of the head and neck. This simple but critically important procedure should be practiced by anyone who has the responsibility of caring for injuries occurring in football. It should only be used when the helmet must be removed. Helmets and various types of headgear worn for protection in other sports can normally be removed much more easily than a football helmet. However, whatever type of headgear is being removed, use extreme caution to cause no unnecessary motion of the cervical spine and produce no additional trauma.

Circulation

In the majority of instances, the unconscious athlete will have a pulse. Assessing pulse-lessness is discussed in Chapter 11. If the unconscious athlete does not have a pulse and requires artificial circulation, uniforms and protective equipment may have to be removed. Remove a jersey by cutting up the middle with bandage scissors (Figure 12-4). To remove shoulder pads from the chest area, cut the laces in the front and pull laterally to expose the sternum enough to permit chest compressions (Figure 12-5).

When an unconscious athlete is not breathing and does not have a pulse, emergency cardiopulmonary resuscitation (CPR) techniques must be initiated. However, most of the time the unconscious athlete will be breathing, have a pulse, and recover consciousness rather quickly. For these persons, the secondary survey remains the largest portion of the assessment process.

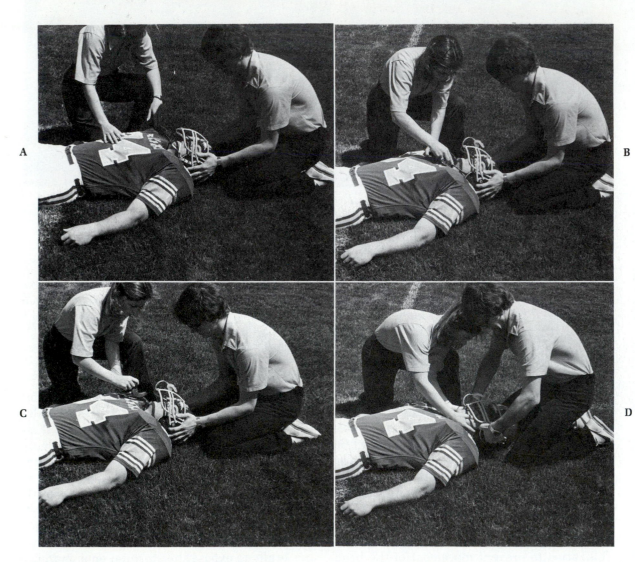

FIGURE 12-3
Removing a football helmet from an unconscious player. **A,** Supporting helmet so there is no unnecessary movement of neck; **B,** removing chin strap and loosening cheek pads with a slender flat object; **C,** lifting cheek pads out, and, **D,** sliding helmet carefully off while the head is supported.

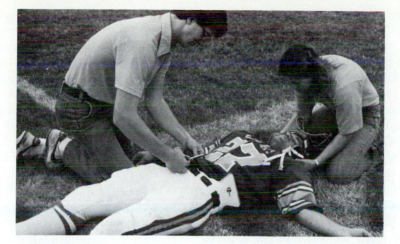

FIGURE 12-4
Cutting football jersey off using bandage scissors.

A   B

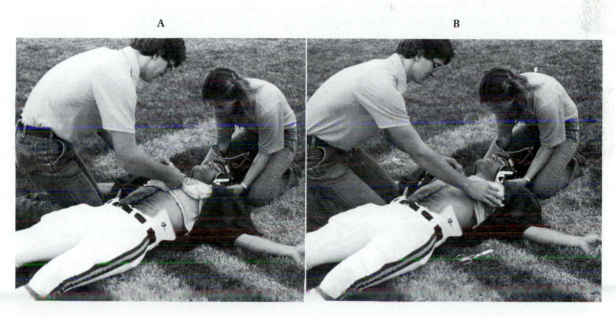

FIGURE 12-5
Removing shoulder pads from the chest area. **A**, Cutting laces in front and, **B**, pulling halves laterally, exposing the chest.

Secondary survey

The secondary survey becomes more difficult to complete on an unconscious athlete. When an athlete is unconscious, much of the secondary survey is concerned with evaluating and monitoring vital signs. Therefore, the remainder of this chapter is devoted to discussing these important health indicators. Information acquired on an unconscious athlete is very important and can be useful to the physician who will diagnose the extent of the injury after referral. The information gained should be written down and passed along to the physician whenever an athlete who was or is unconscious is referred. It can be a helpless feeling to care for an unconscious athlete who is breathing normally and has a good pulse. However, continue the assessment process to gain as much information as possible.

Vital signs. Vital signs are important indicators of the health status of the injured athlete, and they can change quickly. They are especially important for an unconscious athlete because the extent of injury is seldom known. Evaluate and continue to monitor the vital signs throughout the assessment of an unconscious athlete.

History

When the athlete is unconscious, the most important step in the athletic injury assessment process, the history, is not available from the usual source, the athlete. Nothing can narrow down the assessment more quickly than a good history. Even though the unconscious athlete is unable to communicate directly, proceed to obtain as complete and accurate a history as possible.

Find out as much information as possible from whomever is available. Question athletes, officials, or others who observed what happened. Perhaps you witnessed the injury. If so, immediately complete a mental list of possible causes. Did the athlete suffer some sort of blow to the head, or did he or she collapse unexpectedly in the absence of apparent trauma or injury? Remain constantly alert on the bench or sideline to witness any injury that may occur. Personal observation of circumstances surrounding an injury will make reliance on second-hand reports unnecessary and save considerable time. In addition, if you have a good working knowledge of the medical history of your athletes, you will be aware of possible conditions that may predispose them to unconsciousness, such as diabetes or epilepsy.

Level of consciousness. Evaluating the level of consciousness is a very important sign in assessing the status of the nervous system. Attempt to determine the level of consciousness of the injured athlete and then ascertain whether it is stable, improving, or deteriorating. All subsequent changes must be recognized and recorded. Your observations and documentation of the level of consciousness can play a major role in assisting physicians to determine the proper care for the athlete. The physician must know if the loss of consciousness was immediate or developed over a period of time. The athlete who loses consciousness rapidly or shows a lack of improvement with time suggests that medical care is needed. The athlete who progressively develops into a very deep state of unconsciousness or coma also requires immediate medical attention.

Questions that should be answered include: How long was the athlete unconscious? Could the athlete be aroused? Was there a response to pain? What was the depth of unconsciousness? Was the athlete aware of the correct time and oriented to the surroundings? Can he or she respond accurately to questions that require long and short-term memory? The level of consciousness has a direct relationship to intracranial involvement. The deeper the unconsciousness, the more intensive the possible damage. Remember, this information is important in establishing a neurological baseline and should be reported to the physician whenever the athlete is referred.

Observation

The unconscious athlete requires careful observation throughout the assessment process. Begin by observing the entire situation quickly. Note the alignment and position of the athlete. Look for any abnormal positions of the head or neck and unusual positions of any parts of the body. Note any apparatus or equipment that was in use at the time of injury. Look for any hemorrhaging and, if needed, initiate steps to control it. Measures to prevent or treat shock should also be initiated. Following are other vital signs that should be observed and carefully monitored.

Respirations. Determine the number of respirations per minute of an unconscious athlete. This can be accomplished by watching for movement of the chest and by listening and feeling for air exchange at the mouth

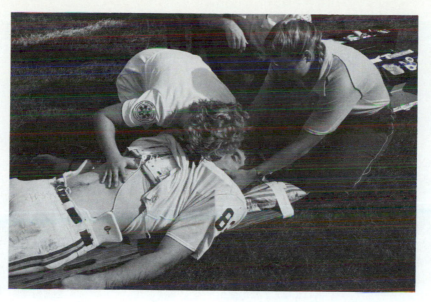

FIGURE 12-6
Counting respirations by placing hand on upper abdomen of unconscious athlete.

and nose. Another method is to place a hand on the chest or upper abdomen and count the number of breaths per minute (Figure 12-6). The normal adult respiratory rate will vary but is usually between 12 and 18 breaths per minute. In well-conditioned athletes the rate may be lower, and in younger athletes the rate may be slightly higher.

The character and pattern of the respirations should also be noted. Breathing should be quiet and effortless. Normal rate and rhythm of respirations in an unconscious athlete suggest that no severe brain damage has occurred up to that point. Abnormal breathing patterns suggest severe brain dysfunction and the need for immediate medical assistance. Table 12-1 briefly describes various abnormal breathing patterns that may indicate brain dysfunction. Any of these abnormal breathing patterns observed in an unconscious athlete, or in an athlete suffering from some sort of head injury, may indicate brain damage. The athletic trainer should be alert to recognize these patterns.

Pupils. The pupils should be examined for size, equality, and reactions in any unconscious athlete. Pupils are normally round, equal in size, and react to light very quickly. Changes in pupil size or their re-

TABLE 12-1

Abnormal Breathing Patterns

Term	Description
Hyperpnea	Abnormal increase in depth and rate of respiratory movements
Apnea	Periods of nonbreathing
Ataxic breathing	Irregular breathing pattern, with deep and shallow breaths occurring randomly
Hyperventilation	Prolonged, rapid hyperpnea, resulting in decreasing carbon dioxide blood levels
Cheyne-Stokes respirations	Periods of hyperpnea regularly alternating with periods of apnea, characterized by regular acceleration and deceleration in depth
Biot's respirations	Regular periods of hyperpnea and irregular periods of apnea
Cluster breathing	Breaths follow each other in disorderly sequence, with irregular pauses between them

action to light can give important information and must be noted. Check the size of the pupils of an unconscious athlete by gently raising the eyelids (Figure 12-7). Are both pupils the same size? Is one pupil larger than the other? Pupils of unequal size

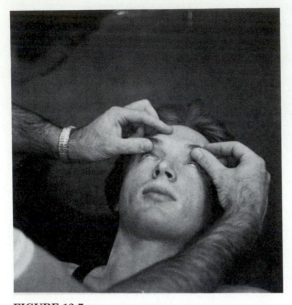

FIGURE 12-7
Checking size of pupils in an unconscious athlete.

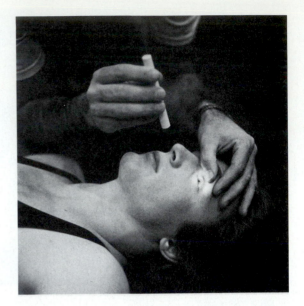

FIGURE 12-8
Using a flashlight to evaluate pupil response.

may indicate an expanding lesion within the skull. The larger, or dilated, pupil will usually be on the side of the lesion and is caused by pressure on the third cranial or oculomotor nerve. However, both pupils may be dilated slightly in an unconscious athlete. If the pupils appear to be dilated, check their response to light. Normally the pupils constrict promptly when light is directed at them. The rapidity with which the pupils respond to light can vary somewhat between persons. It is the presence of the constricting response, or **pupillary reflex,** and the equality of the response between the right and the left eye that is important to note. Pupillary response can be observed in two ways. You can use a flashlight to shine at the pupils to note the reaction (Figure 12-8). If you do not have a flashlight, shade the athlete's eyes with your hand (Figure 12-9) and then quickly take your hand away. When the sun or light hits the eyes, the reaction should be the same as using a flashlight. Failure of the pupils to react to light, or failure to react with equality, may indicate a serious situation. The athlete should be referred to medical assistance immediately.

Skin color. In assessing the unconscious athlete, changes in skin color can provide information useful in determining both adequacy of blood flow and blood oxygen concentration in a particular body part or area. In athletes with deeply pigmented skin, color changes related to blood flow or oxygenation are more apparent in the mucous membranes, the lips, the tongue, and the fingernail beds.

Areas of the body that are particularly susceptible to color changes include the face (cheeks), the bridge of the nose, the neck and upper chest, and the midline of the abdomen. The flexor surfaces of the extremities and the backs of the hands are also said to be **pigment labile** and should be observed carefully for changes in skin color.

Color changes to be aware of are red, white, and blue. Reddening of the skin, **rubor,** indicates the capillary vessels are dilated, resulting in an increased blood flow. This may be present in an athlete suffering from heatstroke or high blood pressure. A pale or white skin color, **pallor,** is caused by constriction of blood vessels in the skin, which results in decreased circulation. This

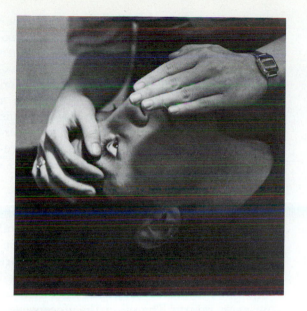

FIGURE 12-9
Checking pupillary response by shading an athlete's eye and quickly removing the hand, allowing light to reach the eye.

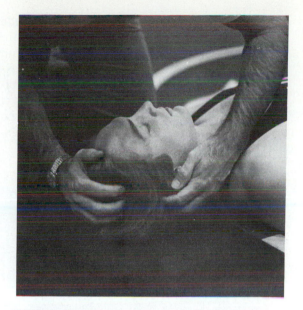

FIGURE 12-10
Examining scalp for signs of trauma.

may indicate severe hemorrhaging or shock. A bluish color, **cyanosis,** results from poor oxygenation of the circulating blood and may be the result of heart failure or airway obstruction. Observation of changes in skin color can help determine immediate care for the injured athlete.

Signs of trauma. Look for any obvious signs of trauma, especially about the head and neck. Examine the scalp for lacerations, bumps, or deformities (Figure 12-10). Is there blood in the hair? Check for any discharge coming from the ears **(otorrhea)** (Figure 12-11) or nose **(rhinorrhea)**. This discharge may be either blood or cerebrospinal fluid, or a combination of both. Cerebrospinal fluid is a clear fluid and indicates a probable skull fracture. Cerebrospinal fluid may be distinguished from blood when they are mixed together by collecting the discharge from the ears or nose on an absorbent pad, such as a gauze pad. The cerebrospinal fluid separates from the blood and forms a circle (halo) around the centrally located blood (Figure 12-12). Blood draining from an ear, even in the absence of cerebrospinal

fluid, may also be indicative of a skull fracture. Do not attempt to restrict the flow of cerebrospinal fluid or blood coming from the ear because this may increase the intracranial pressure.

Look for discoloration or ecchymosis about the head and face. Discoloration over the mastoid area just behind the ear may indicate a temporal bone or basilar skull fracture. This is called **Battle's sign** and may take up to 24 hours to develop. Discoloration of the eyelids and around the eyes, **racoon eyes,** may indicate an orbital or basilar skull fracture. This sign may take several hours to develop. Both of these areas on the head are at the base of the skull where blood may accumulate following a skull fracture.

Posturing. Neurological signs called *posturing of the extremities* may occur as a result of severe brain injuries, which are seldom seen as a result of athletic activity. Although it occurs only rarely, persons who deal with athletic injuries should be aware of what posturing is and be able to recognize it as a sign of severe brain malfunction. **De-**

cerebrate rigidity is a postural attitude resulting from involvement of the midbrain or brain stem. It has a poorer prognosis and is characterized by extension of all four extremities (Figure 12-13, *A*). **Decorticate rigidity** is a postural attitude resulting from involvement in the diencephalon area of the brain. It is characterized by the legs in extension and plantar flexion, while the upper extremities are adducted with marked flexion of the elbows, wrists, and fingers (Figure 12-13, *B*). Posturing can develop and be exhibited by an athlete during the observation phase or it may be a motor response to a painful stimulus. Whenever posturing is noted in an unconscious athlete, an emergency exists and the athlete must be referred to medical assistance immediately.

Physical Examination

Physical examination procedures for an injured athlete who remains unconscious will primarily be those involving palpation. Because the athlete cannot respond, you are unable to assess the severity of associated injuries. The athlete may have a severe head or neck injury. Therefore the unconscious athlete should not be subjected to movement or stress-type procedures until he or she regains consciousness and is responsive.

Palpation

Following are some additional physical signs that may be evaluated by palpation techniques. Remember, be gentle in palpating an unconscious athlete so as not to aggravate any existing injury or cause additional trauma.

Pulse. One of the first steps of the pri-

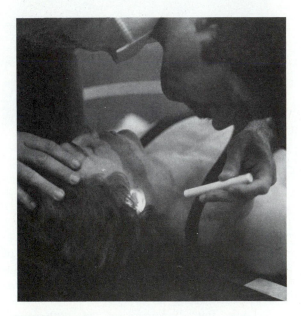

FIGURE 12-11
Checking for discharge (otorrhea) from the ear.

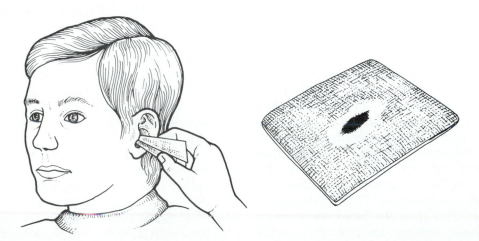

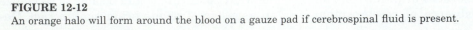

FIGURE 12-12
An orange halo will form around the blood on a gauze pad if cerebrospinal fluid is present.

mary survey is to determine whether or not an unconscious athlete has a pulse. Continue to monitor the pulse to note any changes in rate or character, such as a change in rhythm or strength. The normal pulse rate for an athlete at rest will vary greatly but is usually between 50 and 80 beats per minute, depending on conditioning. Pulse readings can be taken at any area where an artery lies close to the surface of the skin. The most common pulse is taken at the wrist by palpating the superficial radial artery (Figure 12-14). If circumstances make the radial pulse difficult to locate, the carotid pulse in the neck should be used. As intracranial pressure increases, an athlete's pulse rate slows down below normal.

Characteristics of the pulse indicate if the heartbeat is strong or weak, regular or irregular. These sensations are noted as you feel the pulse. Normally the pulse is strong and easily felt, indicating a full volume of circulating blood. Noting the rate, strength, and rhythm of the pulse can give important clues as to the health status of the athlete.

A weak, rapid pulse is an indication of shock. A strong, rapid pulse may indicate fright or hypertension. The pulse rate and character should be noted immediately and then checked throughout the assessment process to detect any changes.

Remember, when evaluating an obvious deformity, such as a fracture or dislocation, you must also feel for a pulse distal to the injury. The absence of a pulse below an injury, when the athlete has a heartbeat, suggests severe arterial damage, such as transection or occlusion. Absence of a pulse distal to an injury should be regarded as an emergency requiring immediate referral to a physician.

Blood pressure. Another vital sign is blood pressure. Monitoring blood pressure in conjunction with pulse rates can be helpful in evaluating the status of an unconscious athlete. Blood pressure is the pressure that circulating blood exerts against the arterial walls. It is measured with a sphygmomanometer (blood pressure cuff) used in conjunction with a stethoscope (Figure 12-15).

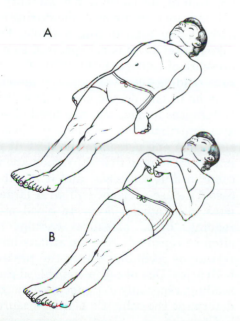

FIGURE 12-13
Posturing of the extremities. **A,** Decerebrate rigidity and, **B,** decorticate rigidity.

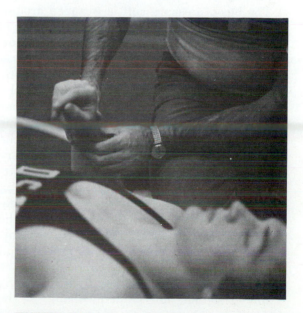

FIGURE 12-14
Monitoring the pulse of an unconscious athlete.

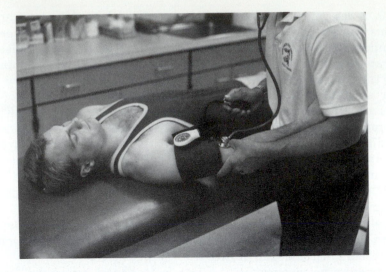

FIGURE 12-15
Taking the blood pressure of an unconscious athlete.

As the heart pumps blood into the closed circulatory system, a pressure wave is created, which keeps blood circulating throughout the body. The high and low points of this pressure wave are measured with the aid of the sphygmomanometer, which makes it possible to measure the amount of air pressure equal to the blood pressure in an artery. The blood pressure cuff is wrapped around the arm over the brachial artery, and air is pumped into the cuff by means of a compressible bulb. In this way, air pressure is exerted against the outside of the artery. Air is added until the air pressure exceeds the blood pressure within the artery or, in other words, until it compresses the artery. At this time no pulse can be heard through the stethoscope placed over the brachial artery at the bend of the elbow along the inner margin of the biceps muscle. By slowly releasing the air in the cuff, the air pressure is decreased until it approximately equals the blood pressure within the artery. At this point the vessel opens slightly and a small spurt of blood comes through, producing the first sound. This is followed by increasingly louder sounds that suddenly change as the air pressure decreases. They become more muffled, then disappear altogether. The first

sound represents the **systolic blood pressure.** The lowest point at which the sounds can be heard, just before they disappear, is approximately equal to the **diastolic blood pressure.** Blood in the arteries of the average adult exerts a pressure equal to that required to raise a column of mercury about 120 mm high in a glass tube during systole and 80 mm high during diastole. For the sake of brevity, this is expressed as a blood pressure of 120 over 80 (120/80). Blood pressure readings can vary greatly among persons or in one person throughout the day. Differences in age, sex, and level of activity also contribute to variations in blood pressure from one person to the next. It is also important to note that sphygmomanometers come in different sizes, and it may be necessary to use a bigger cuff with larger athletes to obtain an accurate blood pressure reading. Blood pressure readings should often be repeated after the athlete has been resting or reclining. Check the pressure in both arms. Do not rely on one blood pressure reading, especially if it appears abnormal, to determine the athlete's blood pressure.

Changes in blood pressure indicate changes in (1) blood volume, (2) integrity of the blood vessels, or (3) ability of the heart to pump blood. The loss of normal blood pressure indicates insufficient circulation. Whatever the cause of the decreased blood pressure in the cardiovascular system, the result will be insufficient perfusion of blood providing oxygen and nutrients to the tissues of the body. This is discussed in more detail under shock in Chapter 7. As shock develops, there is usually a reciprocal relationship between blood pressure and pulse; that is, blood pressure decreases and the heart pumps more rapidly to circulate the blood more efficiently.

Rising blood pressure in an unconscious athlete may indicate cerebral hemorrhage (*see* Chapter 13). This is especially true if the pulse rate is going down. Remember, athletes have increased blood pressure and pulse rates during activity, which should return to normal as they rest. Blood pressure can change rapidly and should be monitored frequently in athletes remaining unconscious or suffering head trauma.

❖ High blood pressure (**hypertension**) is one of the major health problems of today. As previously discussed, blood pressure varies widely and is affected by multiple factors. There is no clear-cut break between levels of blood pressure that defines hypertension. Therefore various definitions and arbitrary values are used to designate hypertension. One method considers systolic pressure less than 140 mm Hg and diastolic pressure less than 90 mm Hg as being normal. Systolic pressure between 140 and 160 mm Hg, or diastolic pressure between 90 and 96 mm Hg, is termed *borderline hypertension*. A systolic pressure of 160 mm Hg or greater, or a diastolic pressure over 96 mm Hg, is considered to be hypertension. These levels are somewhat higher for older individuals and lower for young individuals. Athletes with borderline or hypertensive blood pressures should be evaluated by a physician. The Joint Committee on Detection, Evaluation, and Treatment of High Blood Pressure more recently classified blood pressure as described in Table 12-2.

Skin temperature. Body temperature is normally taken with a thermometer. Be-

TABLE 12-2

Classification of Blood Pressure for Adults Age 18 and Older

Category	Systolic (mm Hg)	Diastolic (mm Hg)
Normal	<130	<85
High normal	130–139	85–89
Hypertension		
Stage 1 (mild)	140–159	90–99
Stage 2 (moderate)	160–179	100–109
Stage 3 (severe)	180–209	110–119
Stage 4 (very severe)	>210	>120

cause the skin is largely responsible for the regulation of body temperature, you can evaluate gross changes in body temperature by feeling the skin. Feel the athlete's skin at several locations using the back of your hand (Figure 12-16). The back of your hand is more sensitive to temperature change than roughened fingers. The athlete in shock or suffering from heat exhaustion will have cool, clammy skin. Hot, dry skin is indicative of excessive body heat such as that associated with heatstroke or high fever.

Signs of trauma. Along with observing the head and neck for signs of trauma, you can also palpate the area. Run your fingers gently over the scalp, through the hair, and along the neck if this area is accessible and not covered by headgear (Figure 12-17). Check for any depressions, lumps, or blood. You can also palpate for deformities and swelling in other areas of the body suspected of being injured.

Reaction to pain. Of course, the unconscious athlete is unable to respond and voluntarily move his or her extremities. However, it is normally possible to check the condition of the spinal cord of an unconscious athlete by providing a painful stimulus. A few methods of providing a painful stimulus include pricking the skin of the hands or feet lightly with a sharp object, pinching the skin, sternal compression, nipple pressure, calf pressure, squeezing the soft tissue between the thumb and first finger, and/or pinching the trapezius area (Fig-

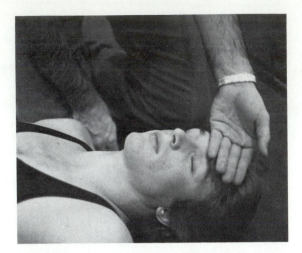

FIGURE 12-16
Feeling the athlete's skin for changes in skin temperature.

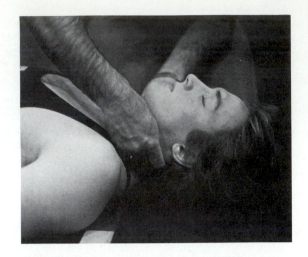

FIGURE 12-17
Palpating cervical spine for any obvious signs of trauma.

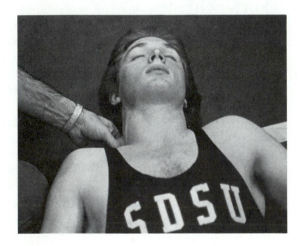

FIGURE 12-18
Providing a painful stimulus to note reaction of unconscious athlete.

ure 12-18). If there is no spinal cord damage, the athlete may involuntarily pull away from the painful stimulus or attempt to push it away. If there is no reaction to the painful stimulus, it may indicate that the spinal cord is damaged or the athlete is in a coma. If the unconscious athlete responds to the painful stimulus by posturing of the extremities, severe brain malfunctioning is indicated.

Evaluation of Findings

Fortunately, in most cases in which an athlete is rendered unconscious it is not a serious situation. Usually the athlete will breathe normally, have a strong pulse, and regain consciousness in a short period of time. The assessment of the unconscious athlete may be limited to the primary survey and determination of the vital signs. In these persons the majority of the assessment process will take place after the athlete begins to regain consciousness. However, serious injuries resulting in extended unconsciousness can and do occur, and the athletic trainer must be prepared for these situations. Much important information can be gained during the evaluation of an unconscious athlete. This information will indicate what emergency care should be provided for the athlete and provide important clues to the nature and severity of the conditions surrounding the unconsciousness. It cannot be overemphasized that this information must be documented and passed along whenever the athlete is referred to medical assistance. Information gained during these evaluation procedures can provide an important baseline for the physician's diagnosis and treatment.

Athletic Injury Assessment Checklist: Unconscious Athlete

Primary survey

———— Airway
———— Breathing
———— Circulation

Secondary survey

———— History
              ———— Question witnesses
              ———— Level of consciousness
———— Observation
              ———— Alignment and position
              ———— Bleeding
              ———— Respirations
              ———— Pupils
              ———— Skin color
              ———— Signs of trauma
              ———— Posturing
———— Physical Examination

Palpation
              ———— Pulse
              ———— Skin temperature
              ———— Signs of trauma
              ———— Reaction to pain

No movement or manipulative procedures applied as long as the athlete remains unconscious

---

When to Refer the Athlete . . .

Unconsciousness for an extended period of time (longer than 1 minute)
Unconsciousness that progressively develops into a coma
Rapid loss of consciousness
Dilated and unresponsive pupils
Pupils that are unequal in size
Signs about the head indicating possible skull fracture (clear fluid or blood coming from the ears, Battle's sign, racoon eyes, skull depressions)
Posturing of the extremities (decorticate or decerebrate rigidity)
Periodic or irregular breathing
Obvious deformities about the head and neck
No response to painful stimulus
Seizure following a head injury
Pulse that slows down below normal
Rising blood pressure
Unconscious situation in which there is doubt about what should be done with the athlete

---

When to refer the athlete

The unconscious athlete who regains consciousness in a matter of seconds and whose physical signs and symptoms appear normal may be treated by the athletic trainer. This is discussed further in Chapter 13. However, there are important physical signs that indicate the unconscious athlete should be referred to a physician for additional assessment and treatment.

The athletic trainer should be able to recognize these signs. Conditions that warrant referral to medical assistance are listed in the box above right.

REFERENCES

American Academy of Orthopaedic Surgeons: *Emergency care and transportation of the sick and injured,* ed 5, Chicago, 1992, The Academy.

American Red Cross: *First aid: responding to emergencies,* St. Louis, 1991, Mosby.

Grant HD, Murray RH, Bergeron JD: *Emergency care,* ed 5, Englewood Cliffs, 1990, Prentice Hall.

Parcel GS: *Basic emergency care of the sick and injured,* ed 3., St. Louis, 1986, Mosby.

Rosen P, and others, editors: *Emergency medicine: concepts and clinical practice,* ed 3, St. Louis, 1992, Mosby.

Stenger A: New guidelines for hypertension, *Phys Sportsmed* 21(2):55, 1993.

SUGGESTED READINGS

American Academy of Orthopaedic Surgeons: *Athletic training and sports medicine,* ed 2, Chicago, 1991, The Academy.
The sudden loss of consciousness is discussed. In addition to emergency care procedures, the authors present an extensive list of causes of unconsciousness in the athlete.

Caroline NL: *Emergency medical treatment,* ed 3, Boston, 1991, Little.
Includes chapter devoted to the general principles that apply to caring for any unconscious patient, regardless of the cause.

Smith RW, Sipe JC: The unconscious patient, seizures, and headache. In Warner CG: *Emergency care, assessment, and intervention,* ed 3, St. Louis, 1983, Mosby.
Discusses various causes of unconsciousness, as well as assessment, diagnoses, and intervention procedures.

Torg JS: *Athletic injuries to the head, neck, and face,* ed 2, St. Louis, 1991, Mosby.
Many experts contributed to this text on the problem, prevention, diagnosis, treatment, and rehabilitation of athletic injuries to the head, neck, and face.

CHAPTER 13

Head injuries

After you have completed this chapter, you should be able to:

- Describe the common head injuries involving the scalp, skull, and brain that can occur in athletic activity.
- Define cerebral concussion and list the signs and symptoms that are used to classify concussions by severity.
- Describe how to establish and monitor the level of consciousness of an athlete after a head injury.
- Describe the assessment process for an athlete suffering a head injury.
- Explain how to perform a basic cranial nerve assessment.
- List all conditions or findings that indicate an athlete with a head injury should be referred for medical attention.

Injuries involving the head and cervical spine constitute the most potentially serious of all athletic injuries. Correct assessment procedures, followed by proper emergency treatment and timely referral, may mean the difference between rapid, complete recovery or paralysis or death. Because head and neck injuries can occur together and result from the same mechanisms of injury, it is important to always consider these areas together when assessing athletic injuries. This chapter is concerned with injuries occurring to the head and face and includes signs and symptoms that indicate the athlete should be referred for medical attention. Spinal injuries are discussed in Chapter 15.

HEAD INJURIES

The term *head injury* may be used to describe damage to the scalp, skull, or brain. It is important to realize, however, that all three of these structures may not be damaged in any one injury. For example, it is possible for a skull fracture to occur with little or no injury to the scalp or the brain. As a matter of fact, most head injuries occurring in athletics are not associated with a skull fracture.

Head injuries can occur in any sport and in various ways. However, most head injuries are caused by the application of some type of sudden force to the head. This sudden force is usually the result of a direct blow. Trauma of this type may be caused by the athlete colliding with another athlete or object such as a goalpost, wall, bleacher, or the floor or ground. It may also occur if the athlete is struck by some sort of athletic equipment, such as a baseball bat or hockey stick. In addition, the head may be injured by a blow from a projectile such as a baseball, golf ball, discus, or hockey puck. The

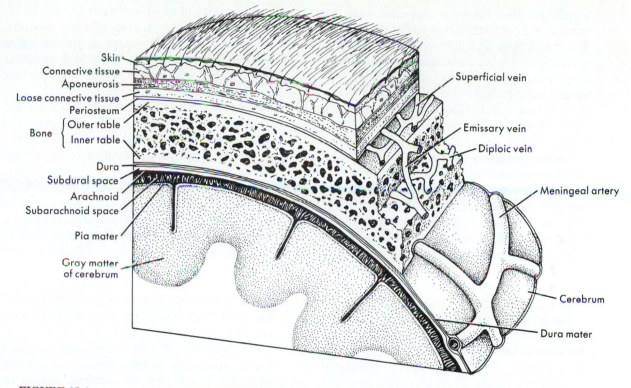

FIGURE 13-1
Layers of the scalp: skull, meninges, brain, and connecting blood vessels.

face or cervical spine may also be injured as a result of such sudden force.

Scalp

The scalp offers considerable protection for the skull. Without this protection, the skull could be fractured or the brain injured by much less force. It is important to understand the anatomy of the scalp because injury or infection to the scalp can also involve the skull or brain. The scalp consists of five layers (Figure 13-1):

S—Skin
C—Connective tissue (dense)
A—Aponeurosis of epicranius muscle
L—Loose connective tissue
P—Periosteum (pericranium)

The scalp is very vascular and has a profuse blood supply. Because of this, avulsed portions of the scalp can usually be saved and should never be cut away, even if points of attachment are minimal. In most instances, sufficient blood will reach the avulsed portion of the flap through remaining connections to permit healing if it can be sutured in place.

Skin. The skin of the scalp is denser than the skin anywhere else on the body and is similar in some ways to the thick skin on the soles of the feet and the palms of the hands. It is characterized by great numbers of hairs and sebaceous glands. The sebaceous glands may become infected, making the scalp the common site for sebaceous cysts, or **wens.**

Connective tissue (dense). The dense connective tissue layer acts to bind the skin above to the aponeurosis of the epicranius muscle below. This layer of the scalp, if cut, tends to bleed profusely because the blood vessels are firmly anchored by connective tissue and cannot retract. Because of the dense, unyielding nature of this layer of the scalp, inflammation here will generally result in only minimal swelling but much pain.

Aponeurosis. The aponeurosis (galea aponeurotica) is a very dense and strong membrane that becomes muscular over the frontal and occipital areas of the skull. It is this membrane that connects the muscular portions of the epicranius, or occipitofrontalis, muscle. This freely moveable, dense fibrous tissue helps absorb the force of external trauma, particularly that of glancing blows. Scalp wounds do not gape unless this layer is cut or split.

Loose connective tissue. The loose connective tissue component of the scalp lies between the dense aponeurotic layer above and the pericranium, or periosteal covering, of the skull below. It forms a potential space called the *subaponeurotic space,* in which large quantities of blood or pus can accumulate under the scalp and extend over the entire dome of the skull without undue stretching.

Important emissary veins connect the large venous sinuses inside the skull with the superficial scalp veins that traverse this area. These veins may carry infections through the skull. Therefore whenever the galea has been lacerated and the wound is wide open, the athlete should be referred to a physician for careful debridement, irrigation, and closure of the wound. There is a surgical axiom that states, "If it were not for emissary veins, wounds and infections of the scalp would lose half their significance."

Periosteum (pericranium). This fifth and deepest layer of the scalp is only loosely attached to the surface of the skull except at the suture lines. If this layer is torn as a result of a skull fracture, intracranial hemorrhage can leak into and collect in the subaponeurotic space of the scalp. Accumulation of blood in this space, instead of inside the skull, may for a time prevent compression of the brain and is aptly termed a *safety-valve* hematoma.

Scalp injuries

Injuries to the scalp may or may not involve the skull or brain. An athlete may suffer a severe brain injury without any observable trauma to the scalp; on the other hand, an athlete may have a dramatic-looking scalp injury with little or no brain damage. The true severity of head injuries may not be reflected by the appearance of scalp wounds. However, any scalp injury is indicative of forceful trauma to the head and suggests that further evaluation of the head should continue.

Common athletic injuries to the scalp are contusions and lacerations. Because the scalp is highly vascularized and may bleed profusely if cut, scalp wounds often appear worse than they actually are. Contusions about the scalp are marked by local tenderness and swelling. Bleeding between the skin and underlying tissue may result in a hematoma, which is commonly referred to as a "goose egg." If small blood vessels beneath the skin have been disrupted, there will be an ecchymosis in the area. Ecchymosis located in certain areas may indicate a possible skull fracture, as was discussed in Chapter 12.

Lacerations of the scalp usually bleed freely and have a frightening appearance initially. The source of bleeding should be located and the bleeding controlled by direct pressure before continuing the evaluation of the head. Remember, scalp wounds are indicative of trauma to the head and are secondary considerations to neurological assessment of the brain and spinal cord.

Skull

The skull consists of two major divisions: the cranium, or brain case, and the face. This section is concerned with the cranial portion of the skull; injuries to the face are discussed in Chapter 14. Review the anatomy of the cranial bones and landmarks in Figure 13-2. Table 3-4 lists and gives a brief description of the eight bones of the cranium.

The cranium is a rigid, bony cavity encasing the brain. The rounded vault is composed of an inner table and an outer table of bone, between which lies cancellous bone (Figure 13-1). Between these two layers of bone is the *diploic venous system,* which is connected to the superficial venous system of the scalp by emissary veins. The inner table of the skull also contains grooves in which the meningeal arteries lie.

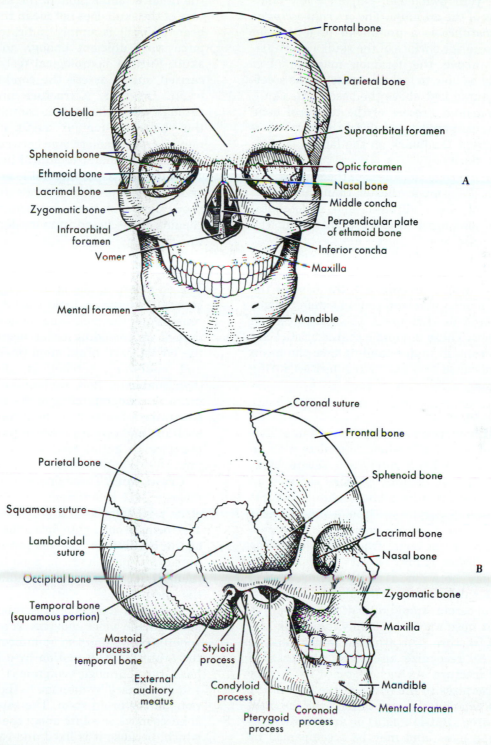

Frontal bone

Parietal bone

Glabella

Supraorbital foramen

Sphenoid bone

Optic foramen

Ethmoid bone

Nasal bone

Lacrimal bone

Middle concha

Zygomatic bone

Perpendicular plate
of ethmoid bone

Infraorbital
foramen

Inferior concha

Vomer

Maxilla

Mental foramen

Mandible

A

Coronal suture

Frontal bone

Parietal bone

Sphenoid bone

Squamous suture

Lacrimal bone

Lambdoidal
suture

Nasal bone

Occipital bone

B

Temporal bone
(squamous portion)

Zygomatic bone

Maxilla

Mastoid
process of
temporal bone

Styloid
process

External
auditory
meatus

Condyloid
process

Mandible

Pterygoid
process

Coronoid
process

Mental foramen

FIGURE 13-2
Skull views. **A**, Anterior and, **B**, lateral.

On your own head, palpate a few landmarks of the cranium. The *external occipital protuberance* is a prominent projection on the posterior surface of the skull a short distance above the foramen magnum. You should be able to feel this structure as a definite bump just above the base of the skull. The *mastoid process* of the temporal bone can be palpated just behind the ear. It is a prominent landmark on the lateral surface of the skull.

The average thickness of the skull is 2 to 6 mm. It is much thicker than this in the areas of the midfrontal and midoccipital bones and much thinner than this in the temporal fossa.

The inner surface of the skull, which covers the hemispheres of the brain, is relatively smooth. In contrast, the base of the skull is irregular and contains many ridges and grooves that make this surface much rougher. These anatomic characteristics are important in understanding how the brain can be raked over bony irregularities during trauma.

Skull injuries

✤ **Skull fractures** are not common in athletics but may occur when an athlete with an unprotected head receives a severe blow. This type of trauma is more common in sports that require a bat or club. Fractures of the skull may range from a simple linear fracture to a severe compound depressed fracture with bone fragments lacerating brain tissue. It may be very difficult to distinguish between a skull fracture and a subgaleal hematoma. Bleeding or the presence of cerebrospinal fluid draining from the ear or nose may be the only indication of a skull fracture. The athletic trainer must be alert to recognize any signs of a possible skull fracture. As was described in Chapter 12, fractures to the bones at the base of the skull can cause discoloration over the mastoid area (Battle's sign) or around the eyes (racoon eyes) and may be accompanied by leakage of cerebrospinal fluid from the ear (otorrhea) or nose (rhinorrhea).

It is possible for a fracture to involve only the inner or outer table of the skull. A fracture of the skull does not mean the brain has been injured; it simply indicates that the force was sufficient enough to crack the skull. Further neurological tests should be carried out to assess the condition of the brain. However, a fracture line running through one of the grooves containing either the venous system or meningeal arteries may result in hemorrhage between the skull and the dura mater (epidural hemorrhage). This bleeding, especially if it is arterial hemorrhage, can produce serious results in a short period of time. Intracranial hemorrhaging is discussed in more detail later in this chapter.

Brain

The adult brain, one of our largest organs, generally weighs a little over 3 pounds. It consists of the following major divisions, named in ascending order beginning with the lowest part: brain stem (medulla, pons, and midbrain), cerebellum, diencephalon (hypothalamus and thalamus), and cerebrum. An understanding of the anatomy and generalized function of the brain stem, cerebellum, and cerebrum are of particular importance in initial assessment of head injury.

Brain stem. Three divisions of the brain make up the brain stem, so called because of its resemblance to a stem (Figure 13-3). The medulla oblongata forms the lowest part of the brain stem, the midbrain forms the uppermost part, and the pons lies between them, that is, above the medulla and below the midbrain.

The brain stem is a fixed functional area between the more movable cerebral hemispheres above and the spinal cord below. If the brain is set in motion by a blow to the head, the neurologic symptoms that often result are caused by damage to the upper portions of the brain stem. The cerebral hemispheres move or rotate about the brain stem, which, because it is fixed and cannot move, tends to compress or buckle under the stress. The result is a brain stem concussion or a much more severe brain stem contusion.

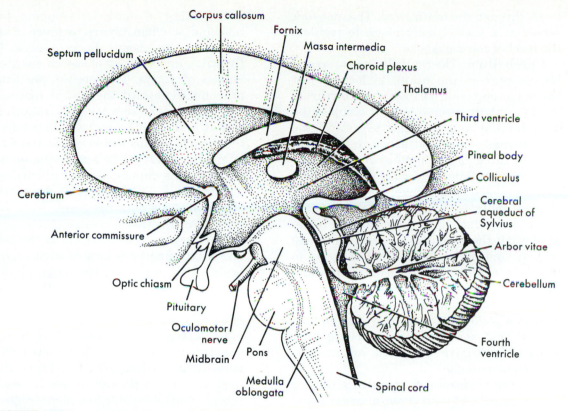

FIGURE 13-3
Sagittal section through midline of the brain. Note the components of the brain stem: medulla oblongata, pons, and midbrain.

The brain stem, like the spinal cord, performs sensory, motor, and reflex functions. Nuclei in the medulla contain a number of reflex centers. (The term *nucleus* used in reference to the nervous system means a cluster of neural cell bodies located in the gray matter of the central nervous system). Of first importance among reflex centers in the medulla are the cardiac, vasomotor, and respiratory centers. Because their functioning is essential for survival, they are called the vital centers. They serve as the centers for various reflexes that control heart action, blood vessel diameter, and respiration. Because the medulla contains these centers, it is the most vital part of the entire brain—so vital, in fact, that severe contusions that result in actual tissue damage and hemorrhage in this area often prove fatal. Severe blows at the base of the skull result in death if they interrupt impulse conduction by the vital respiratory centers. Other centers in the medulla are for various nonvital reflexes such as vomiting, coughing, sneezing, hiccuping, and swallowing.

The pons contains centers for reflexes mediated by the fifth, sixth, seventh, and eighth cranial nerves. In addition, the pons contains the pneumotaxic centers that help regulate respiration.

The midbrain, like the pons, contains reflex centers for certain cranial nerve reflexes, for example, pupillary reflexes and eye movements, which are mediated by the third and fourth cranial nerves, respectively.

An important network of nerve fibers, called the *reticular activating system,* extends through the brain stem. This network serves as a control mechanism to regulate the level of consciousness.

Cerebellum. The cerebellum, the second largest part of the brain, is located just below the posterior portion of the cerebrum and is partially covered by it. It occupies the most inferior and posterior aspects of the cranial cavity and is attached to the brain stem by three paired bundles of fibers.

The cerebellum performs three general functions, all of which involve the control of skeletal muscles. It acts with the cerebral cortex to produce skilled movements by coordinating the activities of groups of muscles. It controls skeletal muscles so as to maintain equilibrium and control posture. The cerebellum functions below the level of consciousness to make movements smooth instead of jerky, steady instead of trembling, and efficient and coordinated (synergic) instead of ineffective, awkward, and uncoordinated (asynergic).

Synergic control of muscle action is closely associated with cerebral motor activity. Normal muscle action involves groups of muscles, the various members of which function together as a unit. For example, in any given action the prime mover contracts and the antagonist relaxes, then contracts weakly at the proper moment to act as a brake, checking the action of the prime mover; the fixation muscles of the neighboring joint then contract. Through such harmonious, coordinated group action, normal movements are smooth, steady, and precise in force, rate, and extent.

Achievement of such movements results from cerebellar activity added to cerebral activity. Impulses from the cerebrum may start the action, but those from the cerebellum synergize, or coordinate, the contractions and relaxations of the various muscles once they have begun.

Injury to the cerebellum caused by hemorrhage or trauma produces certain characteristic symptoms, among which **ataxia** (muscle incoordination), **hypotonia,** tremors, and disturbances of gait and equilibrium predominate. One example of ataxia is overshooting a mark or stopping before reaching it when trying to touch a given point on the body (finger-to-nose test). Drawling and slurring of speech are also examples of ataxia. Tremors are particularly pronounced toward the end of movements and with the exertion of effort. Disturbances of gait and equilibrium vary, depending on the muscle groups involved, but the walk is often characterized by staggering or lurching and by a clumsy manner of raising the foot too high and bringing it down with a slap. Paralysis does not result from loss of cerebellar function.

Cerebrum. The cerebrum is the largest and most superiorly located division of the brain. A deep groove, the longitudinal fissure, divides the cerebrum into the right and left cerebral hemispheres. These halves, however, are not completely separate organs. A structure composed of white matter (tracts) and known as the corpus callosum joins them medially (Figure 13-3). Prominent grooves, or *fissures,* subdivide each cerebral hemisphere into four lobes (Figure 13-4). Each lobe bears the name of the bone that lies over it: frontal lobe, parietal lobe, temporal lobe, and occipital lobe.

Each hemisphere of the cerebrum consists of external gray matter, internal white matter, and islands of internal gray matter. The cerebral cortex is the thin surface layer of the cerebrum, composed of gray matter only 2 to 4 mm (roughly ½ to ⅙ inch) thick. Presumably, when early anatomists observed the outer darker layer of the cerebrum, it reminded them of tree bark—hence their choice of the name "cortex" (Latin for "bark").

The cerebrum performs three kinds of functions: sensory functions, motor functions, and a group of activities less easily named and even less easily defined or explained. "Integrative functions" is one name for them. What most of us think of as mental activities are part, but not all, of the cerebrum's integrative functions. Consciousness, memory, use of language, and emotions are important integrative cerebral functions. Very little is known about the neural mech-

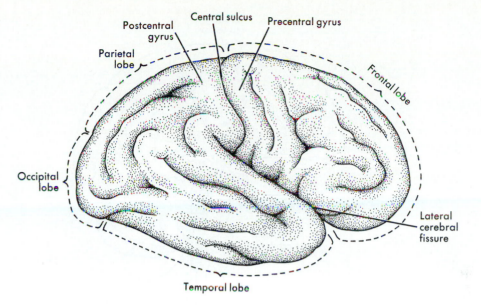

FIGURE 13-4
Right hemisphere of cerebrum, lateral surface. Note the subdivision of the hemisphere into four lobes, each bearing the name of the bone that lies over it.

anisms that produce consciousness. One known fact, however, is that consciousness depends on excitation of the cerebral cortex by impulses conducted to it through the brain stem reticular activating system. Without continual excitation of cortical neurons by reticular activating impulses, a person is unconscious and cannot be aroused (Figure 13-5).

Cranial nerves. The cranial nerves consist of twelve pairs of nerves that arise from various portions of the brain. These nerves are discussed in Chapter 6 and listed in Table 6-3. Athletic trainers should be familiar with the cranial nerves and know how to conduct a basic evaluation for each nerve. Testing of cranial nerves is discussed later in this chapter.

Meninges. Because the brain and spinal cord are both delicate and vital, nature has provided them with two protective coverings. The outer covering consists of bone: cranial bones encase the brain and vertebrae encase the spinal cord. The inner covering consists of membranes known as meninges. Three distinct layers compose the meninges: the *dura mater,* the *arachnoid membrane,* and the *pia mater.* Observe their respective locations in Figure 13-6. The dura mater, made of strong white fibrous tissue, serves as the outer layer of the meninges and also as the inner periosteum of the cranial bones. The arachnoid membrane, a delicate, cobweblike layer, lies between the dura mater and the pia mater, or innermost layer of the meninges. The transparent pia mater adheres to the outer surface of the brain and contains blood vessels.

Between the dura mater and the arachnoid membrane is a small area called the subdural space, and between the arachnoid and the pia mater is the subarachnoid space, which contains cerebrospinal fluid. This fluid serves as a protective cushion around and within the brain and spinal cord.

Brain injuries

Injuries to the brain constitute by far the most serious threat to an athlete. These injuries usually result from movement of the brain within the skull. The semisolid brain, surrounded by cerebrospinal fluid, has limited freedom to move about within the skull and is vulnerable to accelerative forces in a

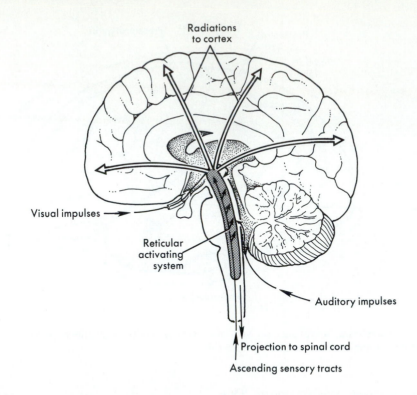

FIGURE 13-5
Reticular activating system, consisting of centers in the brain stem reticular formation and fibers that conduct from the centers to widespread areas of the cerebral cortex. Functioning of the reticular activating system is essential for consciousness.

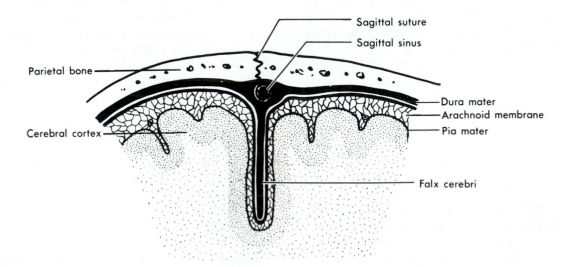

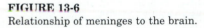

FIGURE 13-6
Relationship of meninges to the brain.

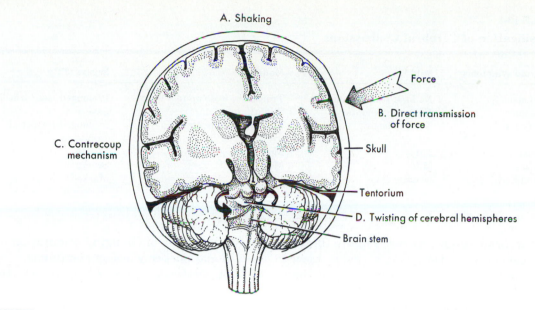

FIGURE 13-7
Common mechanisms resulting in brain injury. A sudden impact to the head can cause: *A*, shaking of the brain; *B*, direct transmission of force to the underlying brain tissue; *C*, contrecoup mechanism; or, *D*, twisting or swirling of the cerebral hemispheres on the brain stem.

variety of contact and collision sports. Whenever a sudden force or impact is applied to the head, there can be an abrupt change of momentum for the brain, resulting in significant movement of the brain within the skull. This gives rise to the common mechanisms resulting in brain injury (Figure 13-7).

A sudden forceful impact to the head can cause agitation of the brain, resulting in transient dysfunction (cerebral concussion). The brain may also be injured by direct transmission of force from the skull to the underlying brain tissue. This can result in the brain being contused (cerebral contusion) or lacerated as it collides with the skull. The brain can also be injured when it rebounds against the opposite side of the skull. This mechanism is called a **contrecoup** injury and is possible due to the movement of the brain within the skull. The extent of the injury to the brain depends on the magnitude and direction of impact, the structural features of the inner skull, and the response of the brain to the force. Any

blow to the head may be injurious to the brain. However, a brain injury is not necessarily the result of a single blow; it may be the cumulative effect of a series of blows.

In addition, injuries to the brain can occur as the result of a sudden force that causes tremendous twisting or swirling of the cerebral hemispheres within the skull. This can also result in cerebral contusions and lacerations as the moving hemispheres are raked over bony irregularities inside the skull. The twisting or swirling motion of the cerebral hemispheres can also cause a temporary malfunction of the brain stem. Consciousness depends on the interaction between the cerebral hemispheres and the upper brain stem. The brain stem is not as free to move as the hemispheres, and the twisting motion can cause an interruption of neural functions of the reticular activating system (center of consciousness). This can result in a loss of consciousness from a brief moment to an extended period of time, depending on the severity of injury. Normally this does not result in permanent damage,

TABLE 13-1

Classification of Cerebral Concussions

Signs and symptoms	Mild (1°)	Moderate (2°)	Severe (3°)
Consciousness	No loss, stunned, dazed	Transitory loss (up to 5 min)	Prolonged loss (over 5 min)
Confusion	None to momentary	Slight	Severe
Memory loss	None to slight	Mild retrograde amnesia	Prolonged retrograde amnesia
Tinnitus	Mild	Moderate	Severe
Dizziness	Mild	Moderate	Severe
Unsteadiness	Usually none	Varied	Marked

and the brain stem recovers rapidly (brain stem concussion). However, a severe blow that results in remarkable twisting of the brain stem may cause prolonged unconsciousness and tissue disruption (brain stem contusion) and hemorrhage from which the brain stem may not completely recover. The important signs to recognize during evaluation of injuries to the head will be discussed in more detail with each injury.

Concussion. There is no general agreement as to the exact definition of a concussion. A **concussion** appears to be a syndrome involving an immediate and transient impairment in the ability of the brain to function properly. It is usually caused by a direct blow to the head, as previously described. There have been various attempts to classify concussions by severity according to their accompanying signs and symptoms. A subcommittee of the American Medical Association Committee on the Medical Aspects of Sports classified concussions into the following three degrees of severity (Table 13-1).

A *mild cerebral concussion* (first degree) is caused by a mild blow to the head, resulting in an agitation of the brain. The symptoms include no loss of consciousness. There may be momentary mental confusion, possible memory loss, a mild ringing in the ears **(tinnitus),** mild dizziness, and headache. There is usually no lack of coordination or unsteadiness. The athlete normally recovers quickly, with no residual symptoms. However, the athlete should be watched closely

for any signs of changing orientation or additional post-concussion symptoms.

A *moderate cerebral concussion* (second degree) is caused by a blow of moderate intensity that results in a loss of consciousness lasting less than 5 minutes. This is usually followed by slight mental confusion and a temporary loss of memory (amnesia). Amnesia may take the form of **retrograde amnesia,** in which there is a loss of memory for events that occurred before the injury, or **anterograde amnesia,** in which there is a loss of memory for events occurring immediately after awakening. Dizziness, tinnitus, unsteadiness, blurred vision, double vision, nausea, and headache are also common symptoms and may be experienced in varying combinations.

The athlete usually recovers consciousness within 5 minutes but may have symptoms lasting several weeks. Athletes suffering moderate concussions should be referred to a physician for further evaluation and follow-up care. It is important that these athletes are closely observed for 24 hours for any changes or complications.

A *severe cerebral concussion* (third degree) is caused by a blow of severe intensity that results in a prolonged loss of consciousness (over 5 minutes). This is usually followed by prolonged retrograde amnesia, mental confusion, severe tinnitus, dizziness, headache, and marked unsteadiness. The recovery rate is slow and characterized by the presence of symptoms. An athlete exhibiting these symptoms must be referred to a physician.

Normally an athlete who has suffered a concussion will improve rapidly to an alert state of consciousness. The greatest concern for anyone who is responsible for caring for the athlete with a head injury is the possible development of an expanding intracranial or intracerebral lesion. The signs and symptoms of an athlete suffering from a concussion are reversible and will appear to be worse on the initial evaluation and then improve. If the signs and symptoms become progressively worse, it suggests that there is an expanding lesion within the cranium. For example, a neurologic assessment of an athlete who has a concussion should not reveal abnormalities in pupil size, movements, reflexes, sensations, strength, or respirations. Any deterioration in these neurologic signs indicate additional intracranial involvement, such as hemorrhaging or swelling. The neurologic evaluations are discussed in more detail later in this chapter as part of the assessment procedures.

❖ **Post-concussion syndrome.** Post-concussion syndrome consists of headache (especially with exertion), dizziness, fatigue, irritability, and impaired memory and concentration. These symptoms may persist for days or weeks and indicate altered brain functioning. These symptoms must be monitored periodically and the athlete withheld from activity as long as they persist.

Contusion. Contusions, or bruising of the brain, result when the brain collides against the skull or is raked over bony irregularities, especially on the floor of the skull. Contusions to the hemispheres may result in a lack of nerve function of the bruised portion of the brain but usually will not result in a loss of consciousness. Signs that suggest an athlete may have a cerebral contusion are any numbness, weakness, loss of memory, **aphasia** (loss of speech or comprehension), or general misbehavior when he or she is alert. An athlete with a cerebral contusion also remains stable or begins improving. Any deterioration suggests additional intracranial involvement.

Hemorrhage. Intracranial hemorrhaging is a potential life-threatening consequence of a head injury. Hemorrhaging can lead to rapid deterioration of the athlete's condition and must be recognized if death or disability is to be averted. The same sudden forces that may result in concussion or contusion (to any area) of the brain may also cause blood vessel damage and hemorrhaging. The hemorrhaging forms a hematoma, which may continue to enlarge after the injury. Hematomas are classified by their location within the skull.

❖ A **subdural hematoma** develops when bridging cerebral vessels that travel from the brain to the overlying dura are torn. This condition is the most frequent cause of death from trauma in athletics. Rupturing of cerebral vessels can occur as a result of the twisting motion of the cerebral hemispheres or the stretching of these vessels on the side opposite the point of impact. Hemorrhaging can result in low-pressure venous bleeding or rapid arterial bleeding into the subdural space. The signs and symptoms of a subdural hematoma will vary, depending on the type of hemorrhaging. They may occur in rapid progression or may not be evident for hours or days after the injury.

❖ An **epidural hematoma** develops when a dural artery is ruptured. Usually this hematoma is associated with a skull fracture, and it is commonly caused by a tear of the middle meningeal artery. The bleeding is between the dura mater and the skull. The clot formation is usually rapid, and signs and symptoms may occur in a matter of minutes

❖ to hours. An **intracerebral hematoma** develops when blood vessels within the brain are damaged. This may occur when a cerebral contusion is accompanied by significant bleeding.

Each of these hematomas can cause an increase in intracranial pressure and shifting of the hemispheres away from the hematoma (Figure 13-8). This accounts for the deteriorating neurologic signs and symptoms, such as a decreasing level of consciousness, loss of movements, slowing of pupil reactions, or a dilating pupil. It cannot be overemphasized how important it is for an athletic trainer to continue to evaluate an

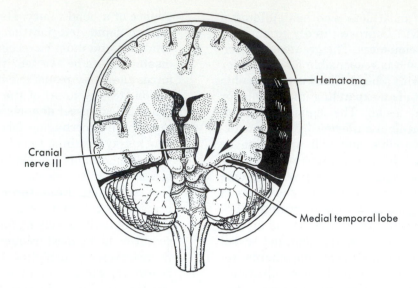

FIGURE 13-8
Hematoma causing increased intracranial pressure and shifting of the cerebral hemispheres away from the bleeding. Note the expanding pressure on the third cranial (oculomotor) nerve. This can result in a dilated pupil on that side of the head.

athlete who suffers a head injury for neurologic signs that may indicate hemorrhaging and an expanding lesion within the cranium. Failure to do so can result in death or disability for the athlete.

Second impact syndrome. Second impact syndrome occurs occasionally when an athlete sustains a second head injury before symptoms associated with a previous injury have cleared. Repeated closed head injuries can predispose the brain to vascular congestion due to loss of autoregulation of the brain's blood supply. This can lead to vascular engorgement within the cranium, increased intracranial pressure, and possibly death. Second impact syndrome can occur as a result of repeated trauma that may appear to be minor compared to the original episode. Prevention is the only sure cure. It is essential that an athlete who is symptomatic from a head injury not be allowed to participate in contact or collision activities until all cerebral symptoms have subsided.

ATHLETIC INJURY ASSESSMENT PROCESS

As previously stated, head injuries are potentially the most serious athletic injuries. Although fatalities in sports are relatively rare, injuries to the head account for more fatalities than injuries to any other area of the body. Permanently disabling brain damage resulting from athletic activity is also rare. However, injuries to the brain do occur, and no head injury should be treated lightly. Anyone who has the responsibility of caring for athletic injuries should plan and prepare for devastating injuries. Head injuries can produce an array of complex symptoms, and correct assessment procedures by the athletic trainer are extremely important.

Primary survey

The importance of maintaining airway, breathing, and circulation has been discussed previously. These important steps of basic life support can never be neglected with any athletic injury. Always check and continue to monitor an athlete's airway, breathing, and circulation throughout the assessment process to recognize and correct any life-threatening problems. Whenever an injured athlete is responsive, the primary survey can be completed quickly and with little difficulty.

Secondary survey

In evaluating an athlete with a head injury, it is extremely important to establish a neurologic baseline. This baseline gives the athletic trainer and the physician a point of reference. If the athlete improves from this baseline, there is a good chance that there is no additional intracranial involvement. Remember that intracranial involvement may take a period of time to develop. An athlete may appear to be doing fine immediately after an injury and then develop signs and symptoms hours later. An important aspect of the assessment of a head-injured athlete is the manner in which physical signs and symptoms progress. This is why it is important to repeat evaluations over a period of time with an athlete who suffers an injury to the head. Physical changes are only appreciated if the athlete's initial status is evaluated and documented. When an athlete's condition deteriorates from the original neurologic baseline, it suggests additional intracranial involvement; he or she must be referred for medical assistance. This baseline information is extremely important to the physician, who must diagnose the severity of injury after referral. It is, unfortunately, often neglected in the rush to get an injured athlete to medical assistance. Neurologic information should always be written down and reported to the physician.

Whenever the trauma is sufficient enough to cause a head injury, remember that there may be an associated neck injury. Always handle the athlete with a head injury as though he or she has a cervical spine injury, until proved otherwise. This includes protecting the injured athlete from any unnecessary movement during the assessment process. If movement of the athlete is necessary for any reason, absolute control of the head is essential.

Much information can be gained by performing a secondary survey on an athlete who has suffered a head injury. Throughout the evaluation process, look for signs and symptoms that may indicate the athlete has an expanding intracranial lesion or cervical spine involvement. Whenever any of these signs are recognized, it is not necessary to continue the assessment. It is time to seek medical assistance for the athlete. This point must be remembered and cannot be overemphasized.

History

It is vital to get a precise history for injuries involving the head. Gain as much information surrounding the circumstances of the injury as possible. Attempt to determine the mechanism of injury and direction of force. Was there a loss of consciousness? Did the athlete have a seizure? Does the athlete have any medical problems that may be associated with the injury? Has the athlete suffered any previous head injuries? Details of the injury, as well as specific time intervals between any changing clinical signs, should be recorded because this information is invaluable for diagnosis. Obtain as much information as possible from the injured athlete. Many symptoms may not be volunteered by the injured athlete but must be actively sought through questioning. If the athlete cannot remember or is stuporous or uncooperative, attempt to obtain information from anyone who witnessed the injury.

Level of consciousness. Establishing and monitoring the level of consciousness is the most important neurological sign to be gained during the assessment of a head injury. Question the athlete in an attempt to evaluate the level of alertness, responsiveness, awareness, and orientation. Begin by checking the athlete's awareness to person, place, and time. Can the athlete answer simple questions such as "What is your name?", "Where are you?", "How old are you?", and

"Do you know who I am?". Then ask the athlete questions that require more thought, such as "What do you do on a certain play?". Such questioning may require the assistance of a coach or another player who is aware of the correct answers. Also evaluate the athlete's memory. Can the athlete remember the events leading up to the injury? What was the first recollection after the injury? The severity of the injury is many times proportional to the lack of memory; that is, the longer the period of amnesia, the greater the injury to the brain.

When describing or reporting the level of consciousness, many examiners use terms such as alert, lethargic, stuporous, semicomatose, and comatose. These terms can be accurate in describing status of consciousness when they are accompanied by explanations and descriptions. *Alert* describes an athlete who is awake and responds immediately and appropriately to all verbal stimuli. A *lethargic* athlete is drowsy and frequently falls asleep but is easily aroused and oriented to person, place, and time. *Stuporous* describes an athlete who is asleep most of the time. This person is difficult to arouse and responds inappropriately to verbal commands. The athlete who is categorized as *semicomatose* has lost the ability to respond to verbal stimuli. This athlete has some response to painful stimuli, and this response is generally nonpurposeful reflex motor activity. When a person is described as *comatose* there is no response to verbal or painful stimuli, and no motor activity is present. If these terms are used without any description of the athlete's status of consciousness, many different individual interpretations may result. Therefore it is better to describe your findings in functional language.

An effective method often used to describe various states of consciousness is the Glasgow Coma Scale (GCS). The advantages of the GCS are that it is a standard guide for rating different athletes' conditions, it saves time because observations are rated numerically, and it allows for easy identification of a change in an athlete's level of consciousness. The GCS evaluates three different

TABLE 13-2
Glasgow Coma Scale

Best eye opening response	Purposeful and spontaneous	4
	To verbal command	3
	To painful stimuli	2
	No response	1
Best motor response	Obeys verbal commands	6
	Localized pain (painful stimuli)	5
	Withdraws from pain	4
	Flexion—abnormal (decorticate rigidity)	3
	Extension—abnormal (decerebrate rigidity)	2
	No response	1
Best verbal response	Oriented and converses	5
	Disoriented and converses	4
	Inappropriate words	3
	Incomplete sounds	2
	No response	1

responses: (1) eye opening, (2) motor responses, and (3) verbal responses. Each is evaluated independently of the others, and each is assigned a numerical value. Higher scores are awarded to athletes who are more responsive. The total score reflects the level of brain functioning. The highest score is 15 and the lowest is 3 (Table 13-2).

The scores for eye opening range from 1 to 4. Spontaneous eye opening indicates that arousal mechanisms in the brain stem are intact and the brain is functioning at a normal level. A score of 4 is recorded for an athlete whose eyes open spontaneously when a person approaches. If an athlete's eyes open in response to verbal stimulus a score of 3 is given. If there is no doubt that an athlete's eyes will not open in response to verbal stimuli, then a painful stimulus is applied. There are several methods of applying a painful stimulus, such as pinching the muscles on the side of the neck, pinching the calf, or applying pressure with the knuckles in a circular motion over the sternum. If an athlete's eyes open in response to a painful stimulus, a score of 2 is given. If all of these methods fail to cause the athlete's eyes to open, the score is 1.

Motor activity is used to assess the functioning state of the central nervous system. A difference between the responsiveness or ability of one limb or another may occur; however, for the purpose of addressing the degree of altered consciousness, the best response is recorded. The scores for motor response range from 1 to 6. An athlete who can follow simple motor commands is given a score of 6. When an athlete cannot follow simple motor commands, a painful stimulus is applied. A 5 is recorded if the athlete localizes the pain by attempts to remove the source of pain or to move away from the pain. If an athlete withdraws because of pain but does not localize it or attempt to remove its source, the score is 4. When decorticate posturing or flexion is the response, 3 is the score. This response is characterized by the arms bent at the elbow and rapidly adducted toward the chest, while the lower extremities are extended and rigid. Decerebration or extension of the extremities in response to stimuli is given a score of 2. In this response the legs are extended with strong plantar flexion and the upper extremities are extended with the wrists hyperpronated and the arms internally rotated. If the athlete does not respond to repeated painful stimuli, a score of 1 is given.

Speech or verbal response indicates a high degree of integration within the central nervous system. Scores in this category range from 1 to 5, with the highest score reflecting the person who is fully oriented. This athlete is aware of personal identity, location, the reason for the location in that particular situation, and the time or the date. A disoriented athlete may memorize responses; therefore it is important to vary the questioning slightly. An athlete whose attention can be held but whose responses are confused is given a score of 4. This person may be able to carry on a conversation, but the responses are often inappropriate or disoriented. A score of 3 is given to an athlete who may be able to articulate but only in a random fashion without complete sentences. This person may converse with only inappropriate words. When an athlete's best verbal response is a moan or cry, a score of 2 is given. This athlete's attempts to articulate are unsuccessful. If no verbal response occurs, even after repeated administration of painful stimuli, the athlete is given a score of 1.

The GCS should not be considered the only factor that can be used in determining an athlete's level of consciousness, but it should be familiar to all athletic trainers. Determine the level of consciousness of the injured athlete and then ascertain any subsequent changes. In most instances the athlete's level of consciousness will improve in a short period of time. If the athlete regains consciousness quickly, the prognosis for a rapid and uneventful recovery is good. If the athlete regains consciousness slowly, the prognosis is more guarded. The athlete who shows minimal or very slow improvement should be referred to a physician or medical facility. A decrease in the level of consciousness is the most sensitive indicator of additional intracranial involvement; anytime the level of consciousness deteriorates, immediate medical attention is indicated.

The American College of Surgeons Committee on Trauma has adopted the "AVPU" method of determining levels of consciousness. This method determines whether the individual is *alert,* responsive to *verbal* stimuli, responsive to *painful* stimuli, or *unresponsive*. Within seconds you can assess the athlete's pupil size and reaction and best motor response. You can note whether the athlete responds appropriately to commands, painful stimuli, or exhibits no movement at all. This method can be used in conjunction with the Glasgow Coma Scale.

Headache. Headache is another frequent symptom of a head injury, and an important consideration that should be discussed while talking with an injured athlete. A headache that becomes progressively more severe is an alarming symptom that may indicate additional intracranial involvement. The persistence of a headache indicates that whatever damage occurred to the brain has not subsided, and the athlete should not return to activity. The cessation of the headache is probably the most reliable indicator that adequate recovery has occurred, and the athlete can return to activity provided there are no other positive neurologic signs. Athletes should resume activity slowly and cautiously to see if they can tolerate the activity without experiencing a headache. As you periodically check the health status of an athlete who has suffered an injury to the head, remember to question the athlete about his or her headache.

In addition to the mechanism of injury, level of consciousness, and headache, you should attempt to gain further information during the history portion of the assessment process. Question the athlete about his or her feelings concerning the head and neck. Is there any pain in the neck? Does the athlete feel any numbness, weakness, or tingling? Does the athlete complain of any ringing in the ears (tinnitus), dizziness, nausea, or blurred or double vision? All this information is important in establishing a neurologic baseline and should be obtained by talking with the injured athlete. In addition, question the athlete about any other painful or tender areas of the body that may require further evaluation.

Observation

An athlete suffering from a head injury requires close observation throughout the assessment process. Watch the athlete carefully as you carry out the history-taking procedures. Notice if the athlete has any difficulty in finding or saying the right words or understanding commands *(aphasia)*. Check for any obvious deformities or abnormal positions of any body parts. Notice if the athlete attempts any movements of the head, neck, or extremities. Does the athlete demonstrate any weakness or paralysis? Watch for neurologic signs that may indicate the existence of expanding intracranial pressure, such as pupillary signs, irregular respirations, seizures, or a decreasing level of consciousness.

Pupils. It is important to check the quality and reaction of the pupils. Both pupils

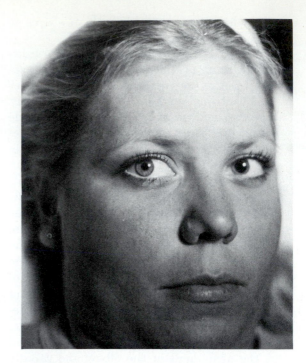

FIGURE 13-9
Athlete exhibiting a dilated pupil following trauma to the head.

should be symmetric in size and react quickly and equally to light. When one pupil becomes larger and shows a decreased response to light, there is strong evidence for increased intracranial pressure (Figure 13-9). The athlete should be referred to a physician. Also observe the eye movements. Normally the eyes gaze straight ahead, unless focused on something. The movement of the eyes should be coordinated; with a head injury, the gaze may be abnormal, or the eyes may turn in different directions. Any abnormal, uncoordinated, or involuntary movement of the eyes may indicate intracranial involvement. If the athlete is conscious, instruct him or her to follow your finger with the eyes and notice whether eye movement is paralyzed or decreased in any direction. For example, an athlete with a fracture of the orbit is usually not able to look upward as far on the fractured side. Involuntary rapid movement of the eyeballs in any direction **(nystagmus)** is another indication of intracranial involvement.

Respirations. Observe the respiratory rate and pattern. A normal respiratory pattern suggests that there is no apparent brain damage, at least at that time. Abnormal breathing patterns may indicate severe brain dysfunction and the need for medical assistance. These abnormal respiratory patterns are discussed in Chapter 12 and outlined in Table 12-1.

Signs of trauma. Look for any signs of trauma; they can give important clues as to the nature and severity of the injury. Examine the head, neck, and face for any deformities, lacerations, contusions, or hemorrhaging. Cuts and bruises are reliable signs that strong forces have been applied to the athlete's head. Watch for discharge from the ears or nose. Look for unusual or abnormal positions of any part of the body, which may indicate additional injuries.

Physical Examination

Much of the information necessary to establish a neurologic baseline will be gained during the history and observation portion of the assessment process. However, once the injured athlete is stable, additional information can be gained through additional physical examination procedures.

Palpation

Pulse. It is important to evaluate the rate and nature of the pulse in an athlete who has suffered an injury to the head. The pulse should be felt periodically during the evaluation. Remember, the development of an unusually slow heart rate after the athlete has calmed down may be another sign of increasing intracranial involvement.

Blood pressure. In addition to heart rate, blood pressure should be measured periodically during the evaluation of a head injury. Increased blood pressure and decreased pulse rate are danger signs and should alert the athletic trainer to the possibility of intracranial bleeding. The rise in blood pressure is compensatory, maintaining blood flow through the cranium as intracranial pressure increases. Low blood pressure or hypotension rarely occurs as the result of bleeding into the cranium alone.

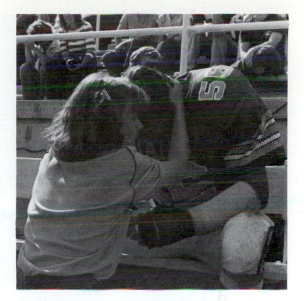

FIGURE 13-10
Palpating the head and neck for signs of trauma.

Bleeding within the skull is usually a relatively small volume because of the confined space. Therefore low blood pressure in a head injury almost always indicates the presence of a spinal cord injury or serious blood loss from another injury in some other area of the body.

Signs of trauma. Along with observing the head and neck for signs of trauma, you can also palpate these areas. Gently feel any painful areas indicated by the athlete for deformities, irregularities, tenderness, or swelling (Figure 13-10). By carefully cupping your hand under the neck, the cervical spinous processes can be palpated with your fingertips to detect any localized deformity or pain. Tenderness or increased pain over these spinous processes is sufficient reason to suspect an associated cervical spine injury. The athlete should be handled appropriately.

Neurological evaluations

Sensory functions. To evaluate sensory ability, gently touch or lightly scratch various parts of the athlete's body while he or she keeps eyes closed. Ask if the athlete can feel the touch and identify its location. If

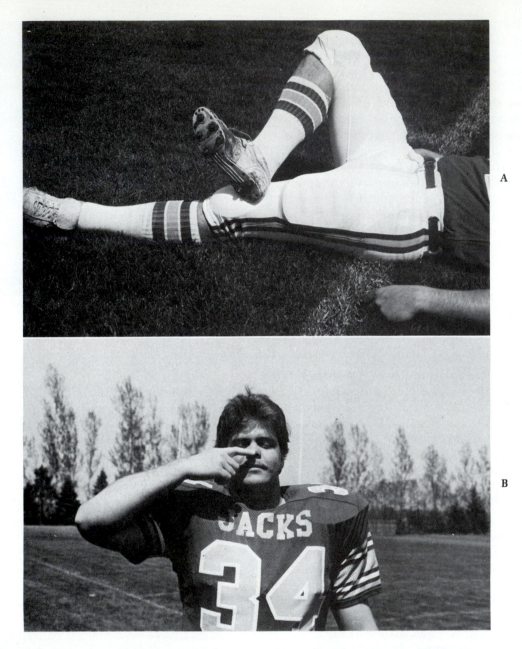

FIGURE 13-11
Athlete performing coordination exercises. **A**, Touching knee with opposite heel and **B**, touching nose with index finger with eyes closed.

sensations are intact, an athlete should correctly identify location of touch with eyes closed.

Coordination and balance. As an athlete recovers from a head injury, there are a few activities you can have the athlete perform to evaluate and monitor progress. Begin by focusing on a basic neurologic as-

sessment of functions controlled by the higher centers of the brain, the cerebrum and cerebellum, for testing the athlete's coordination and balance. For coordination have the athlete touch one knee with the opposite heel with the eyes closed (Figure 13-11, *A*). Have the athlete touch the nose or ear with each index finger while the eyes are closed (Figure 13-11, *B*). These maneuvers should be repeated with increasing speed. Have the athlete touch each finger with the thumb of the same hand as rapidly as possible. Normally an athlete should be able to perform each of these maneuvers easily and quickly. Anything less than this indicates prolonged involvement, and the athletic trainer should continue to monitor the athlete. Another activity that may be used to monitor an athlete's balance and strength is to have him or her stand with arms outstretched and eyes closed. If there is a tendency for one of the arms to drift outward and downward, it may indicate an expanding intracranial lesion on the side of the brain opposite the weak arm. To test the lower extremity, have the athlete sit on the edge of a table or in a chair and hold both legs out in front for 10 to 20 seconds. If there is a lower extremity weakness, the affected leg should begin to drop or drift. An additional test often used on an athlete following a head injury is a check for a positive **Romberg's sign.** This is accomplished by having the athlete stand with his or her feet together, arms at the side, and eyes closed (Figure 13-12). Normally a person can stand still in this position, but a tendency to sway or fall to one side is a positive Romberg's sign, which indicates continued intracranial involvement.

Cranial nerve assessment. Other tests that can be included in a neurological evaluation assess specific motor and sensory functions of the cranial nerves. Testing of cranial nerves would normally not be performed on an athlete suffering a moderate-to-severe head injury and who is going to be referred to medical attention. However, the cranial nerves can be tested in a conscious athlete who has suffered a mild head injury to rule out an isolated injury. Table 13-3 lists various tests that an athletic trainer can perform to evaluate the cranial nerves. Athletic trainers need not be concerned with conducting detailed assessments of each nerve. A positive test for any of the following indicates the need for medical consultation.

The olfactory (I) cranial nerve controls the sense of smell. To check this nerve, test the

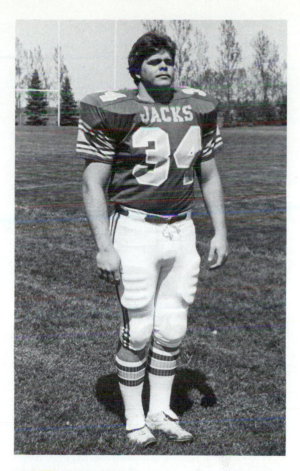

FIGURE 13-12
Athlete performing Romberg's test. The ability to maintain correct posture while standing with feet together, arms at sides, and eyes closed is interpreted as negative.

athlete's sense of smell or ability to detect odor. Test one nostril at a time, and be sure the athlete's eyes are closed so that the object smelled cannot be seen. Any item that has a distinct smell can be used, such as coffee, peppermint, soap, balm, or lemon. Items with strong pungent odors such as alcohol or ammonia capsules may irritate the athlete's nasal mucosa and should not be used during testing.

The optic (II) cranial nerve controls visual acuity and the visual field, and two tests must be conducted. When conducting both tests it is important to assess each eye individually and both eyes together. To test acuity hold up a few fingers and ask the ath-

TABLE 13-3

Cranial Nerve Assessment

Nerve	Name	Function	Test
I	Olfactory	Smell	Have athlete identify familiar odors applied to each nostril
II	Optic	Visual acuity	Have athlete identify number of fingers held up and/or read from magazine
		Visual field	Approach athlete's eye from the side using your hand
III	Oculomotor	Pupillary reaction	Shine light in each eye and note reactions
IV	Trochlear	Eye movements	Have athlete follow your finger without moving head
V	Trigeminal	Facial sensation	Have athlete identify where touch is applied about the face
		Motor	Have athlete hold mouth open as you attempt to close it
VI	Abducens	Motor	Lateral eye movements
VII	Facial	Motor	Have athlete smile, wrinkle forehead, wink, or puff cheeks
		Sensory	Have athlete identify tastes
VIII	Acoustic	Hearing	Have athlete identify sounds in both ears
		Balance	Have athlete put finger to nose, touch knee with heel, perform Romberg's test, or walk
IX	Glossopharyngeal	Swallowing	Have athlete say "ah," swallow, or test for gag reflex
		Voice	
X	Vagus	Gag reflex	Tested along with the glossopharyngeal
XI	Spinal	Neck strength	Apply resistance against shoulder shrugging and turning of the head
XII	Hypoglossal	Tongue movement and strength	Have athlete stick out tongue and move it around rapidly; apply resistance against it with a tongue depressor

lete to identify the number of fingers. Repeat this procedure using the opposite eye. Also position a magazine or newspaper 12 to 18 inches from the athlete and instruct him or her to read aloud items from different sizes of print. Repeat using the opposite eye and then using both eyes. For the visual fields test, the athlete should look straight at you while covering one eye. Extend your hand to the side being tested and out of the field of vision. Slowly bring your hand into the field of vision and have the athlete state when the moving hand is first seen. Examine the opposite eye in the same manner.

The oculomotor (III) cranial nerve controls pupillary reactions. To test this function make sure that both of the athlete's pupils are the same size and are receiving the same amount of light. Then, instruct the athlete to fix eyes on an object while you shine a beam of light directly into each pupil. Note the size, shape, and reaction of the pupils to the light stimulus. When conducting this test the pupil not receiving the light

stimulus should also constrict because of the communication fibers between the two oculomotor nerves. This reaction is called the **consensual light reflex.**

The oculomotor nerve also functions with the trochlear (IV) and abducens (VI) cranial nerves to control extraocular movements. Therefore these three cranial nerves are usually assessed simultaneously. To test these nerves instruct the athlete to follow your finger without any head movement. Move your finger upward, downward, to the left, and to the right. Observe for limited eye movement and the presence of *nystagmus,* involuntary movement of the eyeball. Closely observe for lagging of any eye movements while the eyes are following your finger. Also evaluate for the presence of **diplopia** or double vision. This can be done by holding up fingers and having the athlete identify the number of fingers extended. If there is double vision have the athlete look from side to side and state if the double vision is increased; diplopia should increase when looking toward the damaged side.

The trigeminal (V) cranial nerve has both sensory and motor components and controls facial sensation and jaw movements. To evaluate sensory function instruct the athlete to close the eyes as you gently touch various parts of the face and to identify where the touch is applied each time. Motor function is evaluated by asking the athlete to tightly hold open his or her mouth while you attempt to close the mouth with your hands.

The facial (VII) cranial nerve has both motor and sensory functions. This nerve controls facial muscles and supplies taste fibers to the anterior two thirds of the tongue. To test the motor function of the facial nerve, have the athlete smile showing the teeth, wink, or wrinkle the forehead. Observe for symmetrical movements. To test sensory function, have the athlete close the eyes while you put a little salt or sugar on the tip of his or her tongue. Have the athlete identify the taste.

The auditory (VIII) cranial nerve controls hearing and the sense of balance. Testing for balance has already been described. To assess the sense of hearing, hold a ticking watch or rub your fingers together 1 or 2 inches from the athlete's ear. Note the athlete's ability to hear sounds in both ears.

The glossopharyngeal (IX) and vagus (X) cranial nerves control swallowing, the gag reflex, and articulation. To assess these functions, ask the athlete to say "ah." The palate should rise promptly and symmetrically. Note any hoarseness. Assess the gag reflex by asking the athlete to stick out the tongue while you gently touch the back of the throat with a tongue depressor. The athlete should feel a gagging reflex. Swallowing can be evaluated by watching the athlete slowly drink some water.

The spinal accessory (XI) cranial nerve controls the trapezius and sternocleidomastoid muscles. These muscles can be evaluated by putting resistance against shoulder shrugging and turning of the head.

The hypoglossal (XII) cranial nerve controls tongue movement and strength. Ask the athlete to stick out his or her tongue. It should protrude along the midline. Instruct the athlete to move the tongue rapidly from side to side. To test strength, hold a tongue depressor against one side of the tongue and ask the athlete to push the tongue against the blade. Repeat with the tongue depressor against the opposite side of the tongue.

Movement procedures

Some movements by the injured athlete may be necessary to determine if there is associated spinal cord involvement. This is discussed further in Chapter 15 and should not be attempted until the steps of history, observation, and physical examination described in this chapter have been carried out and you have some indication of the nature and severity of the injury. If the signs and symptoms already observed indicate a possible increasing intracranial lesion or spinal cord involvement, it is not necessary to subject the athlete to any movement or manipulation. Instead the athlete should be immediately protected from further trauma and referred to a physician or medical facility.

Evaluation of Findings

Because of the potential seriousness of trauma to the head, athletic trainers must be able to recognize the signs and symptoms that may indicate severe injury. Failure to do so may result in permanent damage, paralysis, or even death to the athlete. Serious head injuries occur infrequently in athletics, but the mechanism for a catastrophic injury is present in most athletic activities.

The importance of the information gained during the assessment of a head injury cannot be overemphasized. This information indicates what emergency care should be provided for the athlete and provides clues to the nature and severity of the injury. This information also establishes the neurologic baseline for the physician's diagnosis and treatment plan and must be documented and passed along whenever the injured athlete is referred to medical assistance.

When to refer the athlete

The athlete with an injury to the head, whose physical signs continue to improve or appear normal, may be handled by the athletic trainer. Remember that intracranial in-

South Dakota State University Training Room

This is a medical follow-up sheet for your health and safety. Quite often, signs of head injury do not appear immediately after trauma but hours after the injury. The purpose of this fact sheet is to alert you to the symptoms of significant head injuries, symptoms that may occur several hours after you leave the training room.

If you experience one or more of the following symptoms following a head injury, medical help should be sought.

1. Difficulty remembering recent events or meaningful facts
2. Severe headache, particularly at a specific location
3. Stiffening of the neck
4. Bleeding or clear fluid dripping from the ears or nose
5. Mental confusion or strangeness
6. Nausea or vomiting
7. Dizziness, poor balance, or unsteadiness
8. Weakness in either arm or leg
9. Abnormal drowsiness or sleepiness
10. Convulsions
11. Unequal pupils
12. Loss of appetite
13. Persistent ringing of the ears
14. Slurring of speech

The appearance of any of the above symptoms tells you that you have had a significant head injury that *requires medical attention*. If any of the symptoms appear, contact J. Booher, B. Janicki, X. Gaglias or report to the Brookings Hospital Emergency Room.

REMEMBER: Your health depends on how much you care about proper medical attention.

THE SDSU ATHLETIC TRAINING STAFF

Athletic Injury Assessment Checklist: Head Injuries

Primary survey

_____ Responsiveness
_____ Airway
_____ Breathing
_____ Circulation

Secondary survey

_____ History
    _____ Mechanism of injury
    _____ Level of consciousness
    _____ Headache
    _____ Pain
    _____ Sensations (numbness, weakness, paralysis, tinnitus, dizziness, nausea, blurred or double vision)

_____ Observation
    _____ Aphasia
    _____ Obvious deformities
    _____ Position and alignment
    _____ Movement in extremities
    _____ Pupil equality and symmetry
    _____ Eye movements
    _____ Respiratory rate and pattern
    _____ Signs of trauma

_____ Physical Examination

Palpation

    _____ Rate and character of pulse
    _____ Blood pressure
    _____ Signs of trauma (deformities, irregularities, tenderness, or swelling)

Neurologic Evaluations

    _____ Sensory functions
    _____ Coordination and balance
    _____ Active motion in extremities
    _____ Romberg's sign
    _____ Muscle strength
    _____ Cranial nerve assessment

When to Refer the Athlete ...

Rapid loss of consciousness or progressive development of coma

Prolonged mental confusion

Prolonged amnesia

Increasing headache

Unequal size of pupils or their failure to react to light

Ucoordinated or involuntary movement of the eyes

Abnormal breathing patterns

Signs about the head indicating possible skull fracture (clear fluid or blood coming from the ears, Battles's sign, racoon eyes, skull depressions)

Unusual slowing of the heart rate and increasing blood pressuree

A positive test for any of the cranial nerves

Doubt regarding the presence of an intracranial lesion

---

volvement may develop over a period of time. Repeated evaluations must be performed to note the progression of physical signs and symptoms associated with a head injury. If the athlete is not referred to a physician, it is important to inform someone who will be with the athlete for a period of time after the injury, such as the parents or roommates, of the importance of continued observation. Give this person a list of signs to watch for that includes information concerning the nature of the injury, the physical signs that may indicate an expanding intracranial lesion, and what to do or who to notify if these signs develop. A sample watch list is presented on p. 288.

Physical signs indicating that an athlete with a head injury should be referred to a physician for additional assessment and treatment are critically important. The list of conditions in the box, should they appear, require that the athlete be referred to medical assistance.

REFERENCES

American Academy of Orthopaedic Surgeons: *Emergency care and transportation of the sick and injured,* ed 5, Chicago, 1992, The Academy.

Arnheim DD, Prentice WE: *Principles of athletic training,* ed 8, St. Louis, 1993, Mosby.

Casson IR: Brain damage in modern boxers, *JAMA* 251(20):2663, 1984.

Diamond S: Treating athletes who have posttraumatic headaches, *Phys Sportsmed* 20(9):167, 1992.

Grant HD, Murray RH, Berberon JD: *Emergency care,* ed 5, Englewood Cliffs, 1990, Prentice Hall.

Hargarten KM: Rapid injury assessment: how to identify life-threatening emergencies, *Phys Sportsmed* 21(2):33, 1993.

Kelly JP: Concussion in sports: guidelines for the prevention of catastrophic outcome, *JAMA* 266(20):2867, 1991.

Knight RL: The Glasgow Coma Scale: ten years after, *Critical Care Nurse* 6(3):65, 1986.

Maroon JC, and others: Assessing closed head injuries, *Phys Sportsmed* 20(4):37, 1992.

McSherry JA: Cognitive impairment after head injury, *AFP* 40(4):186, 1989.

Montgomery J: Overview of head injuries, *Phys Ther* 63:1945, 1983.

O'Donoghue DH: *Treatment of injuries to athletes,* ed 4, Philadelphia, 1984, Saunders.

Parcel GS: *Basic emergency care,* ed 4, St. Louis, 1989, Mosby.

Pons PT: Head trauma. In Rosen P and others, editors: *Emergency medicine: concepts and clinical practice,* ed 3, St. Louis, 1992, Mosby.

Saunders RL, Harbaugh RE: The second impact in catastrophic contact-sports head trauma, *JAMA* 252(4):538, 1984.

Torg JS: *Athletic injuries to the head, neck and face,* ed 2, St. Louis, 1991, Mosby.

Walleck CA: A neurologic assessment procedure that won't make you nervous, *Nursing* 12(12):50, 1982.

SUGGESTED READINGS

Cantu RC: Guidelines for return to contact sports after a cerebral concussion, *Phys Sportsmed* 14(10):75, 1986.
Discusses a practical grading scheme for identifying cerebral concussions in contact sports. Also discusses management and guidelines for determining when an athlete can return to activity.

Cantu RC: Second impact syndrome: immediate management, *Phys Sportsmed* 20(9):55, 1992.
Discusses the importance of understanding the second impact syndrome and not allowing athletes who are symptomatic from a head injury to return to activity.

Nelson WE, and others: Athletic head injuries, *Ath Training* 19(2):95, 1984.
Reviews anatomy, physiology, mechanism, classification, and management of head injuries.

Price MB, DeVroom HL: A quick and easy guide to neurological assessment, *Neurosurg Nurs* 17:313, 1985.
A basic guide to neurological assessment including pictorial descriptions for evaluating the cranial nerves and motor and sensory functions.

Roberts WO: Who plays? who sits? managing concussions on the sidelines, *Phys Sportsmed* 20(6):66, 1992.
Discusses carefully evaluating and monitoring an athlete who sustains a concussion to determine whether the athlete can safely return to play.

$\mathcal{C}$HAPTER 14

Face injuries

After you have completed this chapter, you should be able to:
- Describe the common facial injuries that can occur in athletic activity.
- Describe specific assessment procedures that should be performed after injuries to the jaw, nose, ear, teeth, or eyes.
- List the signs and symptoms that indicate an athlete suffering a facial injury should be referred to medical assistance.

Although head and facial trauma may occur simultaneously, facial injuries are discussed separately because of the importance of recognizing trauma to the head. The remainder of this chapter discusses the anatomy for each area of the face, the common injuries or conditions that may result from athletic activity, and the associated signs and symptoms an athletic trainer should recognize during the assessment process.

Facial injuries are fairly common in athletic activity. However, their frequency and severity have declined in recent years because more sports are requiring the use of protective devices such as mouth guards, eye guards, ear guards, and face masks. Athletes in many sports, however, have no protection for the face, and various facial injuries can occur. Remember, any facial injury is indicative of trauma to the head, which can also result in injuries to the brain or spinal cord. Because of the great vascularity of the face, profuse bleeding can result in dramatic-appearing injuries (Figure 14-1). Do not concentrate on facial trauma to the exclusion of possible associated injuries to the head or neck, which may be more serious.

ANATOMY OF THE FACE
The face is made up of 14 bones. Refer to Table 14-1 and Figure 14-2 to identify and review these bones. Figure 14-3 illustrates the surface anatomy of the face. The facial bones are largely subcutaneous and readily palpable. Identify and note the position of the following surface structures or bony landmarks on your own face.
1. *Supraorbital margin:* This is the portion of the frontal bone that forms the upper margin, or ridge, over each eye orbit.

2. *Nasion:* This is a depression just above the nose, midway between the two supraorbital margins.

3. *Glabella:* This structure is felt as a prominent ridge of bone just above the nasion.

4. *Lateral orbital margins:* The sharp lateral (outer) margin of each eye orbit formed by the edge of the malar or zygomatic bone.

5. *Zygomatic arch:* This is the prominent portion of the cheek bone. The outline of the arch is easily traced by pressing gently along the undersurface of the orbit. The superficial temporal artery crosses the posterior extremity of this bony landmark. You should be able to feel the pulse at the point where the artery crosses the arch.

6. *Angle of mandible:* Area of mandible where this bone changes direction.

7. *Lower border of mandible:* Bony ridge of the jawbone.

Soft tissue injuries

Common facial injuries are contusions, abrasions, and lacerations of the skin. These injuries are treated much as they would be if located anywhere else on the body; however, the need for optimal cosmetic results demands careful evaluation and care. Athletes who have isolated injuries to the skin of the face can normally return to activity after receiving primary wound care and bleeding has been controlled. If lacerations are carefully cleaned and protected, suturing can be delayed as long as 6 hours after the primary injury. Careful inspections and palpation of the bony structures underlying lacerations, contusions, and abrasions are very important to rule out fractures of the face, nose, or skull. Any suggestion of frac-

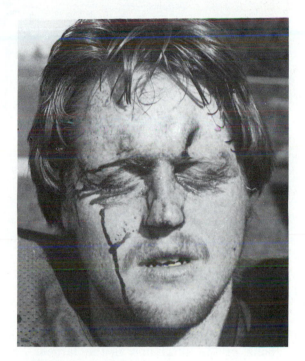

FIGURE 14-1
Facial bleeding following forehead laceration.

TABLE 14-1

Bones of the Face

Name	Number	Description
Nasal	2	Small bones that form upper part of bridge of nose
Maxillary	2	Upper jawbones; also help form roof of mouth, floor, and side walls of nose and floor of orbit; large cavity in maxillary bone is *maxillary sinus*
Zygoma (malar)	2	Cheek bones; also help form orbit
Mandible	1	Lower jawbone
Lacrimal	2	Small bone; helps form medial wall of eye socket and side wall of nasal cavity
Palatine	2	Form back part of roof of mouth and floor and side walls of nose and part of floor of orbit
Inferior turbinate	2	Form curved "ledge" long inside of side wall of nose, below middle turbinate
Vomer	1	Forms lower, back part of nasal septum

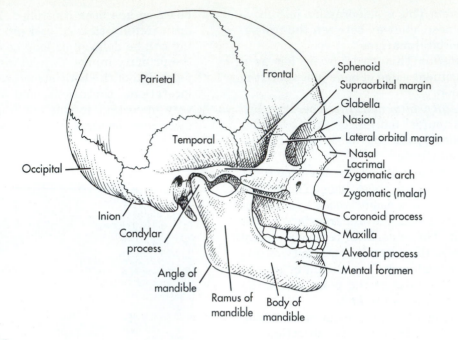

FIGURE 14-2
Bony anatomy of the skull, face, and jaw.

ture should promptly be referred to medical assistance.

Jaw

The jaw is composed of an upper jaw, or maxilla, and a lower jaw, or mandible (Figure 14-2). The mandible is the only movable bone in the skull and is the largest and strongest of the group. This bone has bony contact with the rest of the skull only at the *temporomandibular* (TMJ) joints and the teeth. The mandible consists of a curved, horseshoe-shaped body and two perpendicular rami that project upward at each end. Each flat ramus is joined to the body at the angle of the mandible. The upper border of the body bears the alveolar border, with 16 dental sockets for the teeth. Each ramus has two bony processes: (1) the posterior condyloid process, or head, that articulates with the undersurface of the skull in the temporomandibular joint, and (2) the anterior coronoid process, which serves as an attachment for muscles. The coronoid process is thin and triangular. The mental foramen can be seen on the external surface of the body of the mandible just below the second premolar tooth on each side.

The temporomandibular joint is the only synovial, or diarthrotic, joint of the skull. The joint lies between the condyloid process of the mandible and the articular fossa on the undersurface of the temporal bone. The articular surfaces of both bones in the joint are covered by a unique type of fibrous (not hyaline) cartilage. A fibrocartilaginous articular disc divides the joint cavity into an upper and lower compartment. Each compartment is surrounded by a synovial membrane. You can palpate the joint by placing your finger just in front of the ear as you open and close the mouth.

The temporomandibular joint is enclosed in a thin, loose articular capsule that is weakly reinforced by support ligaments. The mandible can be elevated, depressed, protruded, retracted, and moved from side to side.

Jaw injuries

❖ **Mandible fractures.** Injuries to the jaw normally occur as the result of a direct blow.

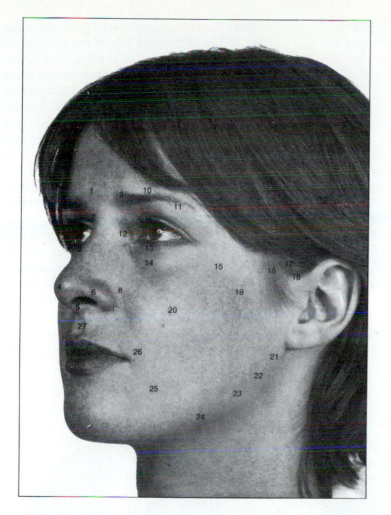

1 Glabella
2 Root
3 Dorsum
4 Apex
5 Septum   } of external nose
6 Ala
7 External aperture
8 Alar groove
9 Frontal notch and supratrochlear nerve and vessels
10 Supraorbital notch (or foramen), nerve, and vessels
11 Lateral part of supraorbital margin
12 Medial palpebral ligament in front of lacrimal sac
13 Infraorbital margin
14 Infraorbital foramen, nerve, and vessels
15 Zygomatic arch
16 Head of mandible
17 Auriculotemporal nerve and superficial temporal vessels
18 Tragus
19 Parotid duct emerging from gland
20 Parotid duct turning medially at anterior border of masseter
21 Angle of mandible
22 Lower border of ramus of mandible
23 Anterior border of masseter and facial artery and vein
24 Lower border of body of mandible
25 Mental foramen, nerve, and vessels
26 Lateral angle of mouth
27 Philtrum

FIGURE 14-3
Surface markings on the front and left side of the face.

Fractures to the mandible are more common than fractures to the maxilla or dislocations of the temporomandibular joint. The most common fracture of the mandible is near the angle of the lower jaw. Any contusion or suspected fracture of the mandible should be carefully palpated along the body to determine areas of point tenderness, swelling, or deformity. If there is no obvious deformity or abnormal movement observed, ask the athlete to open and close his or her mouth and appose the teeth. Does the jaw open and close normally on both sides? Do the teeth line up correctly? Palpate the temporomandibular joint as the athlete moves the jaw. If there is malocclusion of the teeth or increased pain on movement, the athlete should be referred to a physician for further assessment.

❖ **Zygoma fractures.** The most common fracture to the upper jaw involves the zygoma, or cheekbone. The most common fracture site is at its attachments to the temporal, frontal, and maxillary bones and is often called a tripod or trimalar fracture. This fracture normally results from blunt trauma to the cheekbone or side of the face. If the zygomatic arch is fractured, the cheek will be depressed. In assessing potential facial injury, the athletic trainer should always look down over the forehead from behind the athlete (Figure 14-4). Subtle differences in symmetry, indicating fracture, are often more apparent when the face is viewed from above and behind. Palpation of the involved bone can help supplement the over-head inspection because tenderness and crepitus are common with zygomatic fractures.

Maxilla fractures. This is an uncommon athletic-related injury because it requires significant force to fracture the maxilla. However, a high velocity impact to the mid-portion of the face can cause fractures of the maxilla. This results in varying degrees of deformity and mobility of the fractured pieces.

Temporomandibular dislocation. A dislocation of the temporomandibular joint does not occur often in athletic activity. However, when it does occur, it is normally the result of a blow to the side of the jaw with the mouth open. Uncomplicated dislocation of the jaw occurs only in a forward direction. Upward dislocation can only occur in association with extensive fracture of the base of the skull, and backward dislocation occurs with smashing of the bony portion of the auditory canal, which lies immediately behind the joint. The major signs to recognize in a temporomandibular joint dislocation are loss of jaw movement and malocclusion of the teeth (Figure 14-5). Athletes with these signs should be referred to a physician for reduction.

Temporomandibular joint dysfunction. Pain and limitation of jaw movement may occur as a result of trauma to the mouth, chin, or side of the head. Symptoms can result from various of conditions such as traumatic arthritis, bony or fibrous ankylosis of the TMJ, spasm of the muscles of mastication, condylar fracture, or displacement of the articular disk. Chronic TMJ pain and/or dysfunction following trauma to this area should be referred for further evaluation procedures.

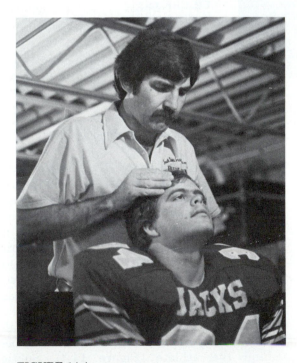

FIGURE 14-4
Looking over the forehead of an athlete to note any subtle differences in symmetry.

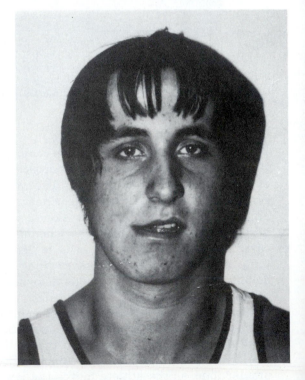

FIGURE 14-5
Temporomandibular joint dislocation. Note malocclusion of the teeth.

Nose

The nose consists of an external and internal portion. The external portion, the part that protrudes from the face, consists of a bony and cartilaginous framework overlaid by skin that contains many sebaceous glands. The two nasal bones meet at the nasion, where they are surrounded by the frontal bone to form the root of the nose. The nasal bones are surrounded by the maxilla laterally and inferiorly at the base of the nose. The flaring cartilaginous expansion forming the outer side of each nostril is called the *ala.*

The fact that the skin of the external nose contains many sebaceous glands has great clinical significance. If these glands become blocked, it is possible for infectious material to pass from facial veins in the area to the intracranial cavernous sinus. For this reason, the triangular zone surrounding the external nose is often known as the "danger area of the face."

The internal nose, or nasal cavity, lies over the roof of the mouth and is divided into right-left cavities by a midline nasal septum. The nasal septum is made up of three structures: the perpendicular plate of the ethmoid bone above, the vomer bone, and the nasal cartilage below. The septum can be deviated (**deviated septum**) to one side or the other, interfering with respiration and with drainage of the nose and sinuses.

Each nasal cavity communicates with the outside through the nostril, or anterior nares, and opens into the nasopharynx behind, through the posterior nares. The nasal cavity also communicates with the middle ear through the eustachian tube and with the paranasal air sinuses—frontal, maxillary, sphenoid, and ethmoid—through their respective orifices. Communication with the conjunctiva of the eye exists through the nasolacrimal duct. These extensive relations of the nasal cavity are important in the spread of infection.

The roof of the nose is separated from the cranial cavity by a portion of the ethmoid bone called the *cribriform plate.* The cribriform plate is perforated by many small openings, which permit branches of the olfactory nerve responsible for the special sense of smell to enter the cranial cavity and reach the brain.

Separation of the nasal and cranial cavities by a thin, perforated plate of bone presents real hazards. If the cribriform plate is damaged as a result of trauma to the nose, it is possible for potentially infectious material to pass directly from the nasal cavity into the cranial fossa. If fragments of a fractured nasal bone are pushed through the cribriform plate and tear the dura, cerebrospinal rhinorrhea can result.

There are five paranasal air sinuses in the skull that communicate directly with the nose. The *frontal sinuses,* which are located inside the frontal bone, are perhaps the most important from the standpoint of potential for complications after a skull fracture. Note the close relationship of the frontal lobe of the brain to the wall of the frontal sinus (Figure 14-6).

A skull fracture involving the sinus may tear the dura and injure the brain. If this occurs, a passageway is formed that will permit exchange of air and cerebrospinal fluid between the brain and nasal cavity. Air that enters and becomes trapped in the brain produces a condition called **pneumocephalus** (Figure 14-6). As discussed previously, discharge of cerebrospinal fluid from the nose is called cerebrospinal rhinorrhea and is cause for immediate referral to a physician or medical facility.

Rhinitis. Rhinitis is an inflammation of the mucosa of the nasal cavity. It is commonly caused by a viral infection, as in the common cold or flu. Rhinitis can also be caused by nasal irritants or an allergic reaction to airborne allergens. Allergic rhinitis, or **hay fever,** occurs in sensitive individuals in a seasonal pattern, depending on the allergens involved (pollen for example). Excessive mucus production that results from the inflammatory response involved in rhinitis can cause fluid to drip down the pharynx and into the esophagus and lower respiratory tract. This dripping can cause sore throat, coughing, and upset stomach.

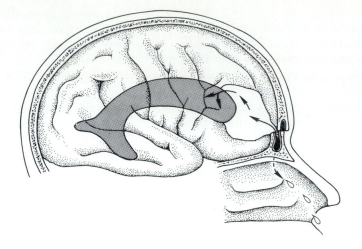

FIGURE 14-6
Skull fracture involving the frontal sinus. Solid arrows indicate path of air, resulting in pneumocephalus; broken arrows indicate path of cerebrospinal fluid, resulting in cerebrospinal rhinorrhea.

Irritation of the nasal mucosa often triggers the sneeze reflex. Elimination of the causative factor, rest, and the use of antihistamines and decongestants usually relieve these symptoms.

❖ **Sinusitis.** Sinusitis is an inflammation of the mucous lining of the sinuses. Because the upper respiratory mucosa is continuous with the mucous lining of the sinuses, eustachian tube, middle ear, and lower respiratory tract, it is not uncommon to see a common cold progress to a sinus infection or middle ear infection.

Nose injuries

❖ **Nosebleeds (epistaxis).** Hemorrhage from the nose is common in athletic facial injuries. Nosebleeds rarely become serious enough to jeopardize the life of the athlete. Because the nasal cavity is a bony space, even serious hemorrhage usually can be controlled by packing the cavity with gauze or cotton and applying pressure to the nostril of the bleeding side (Figure 14-7). Cold compresses also can be applied to the nasal area in an attempt to constrict the blood vessels. Nosebleeds occur most often as a result of septal contusions caused by a direct blow to the nose.

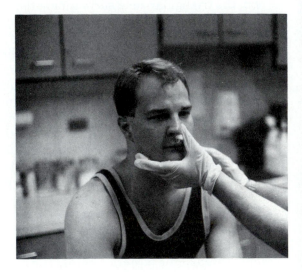

FIGURE 14-7
Applying pressure to control a nosebleed.

Occasionally, the presence of insects or debris in the nose will produce inflammation or irritation and subsequent hemorrhage. If the presence of foreign bodies in the nose is suspected, the nasal interior should be examined and the athlete instructed to gently blow his or her nose while the unaffected nostril is pinched shut. If this does not rid the nostril of the foreign body, the athlete

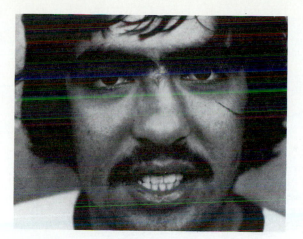

FIGURE 14-8
Nasal fracture.

should be referred to a physician. Violently blowing the nose or probing for the foreign body may cause increased irritation.

❖ **Nasal fractures.** The two nasal bones are the most frequently fractured bones in the face. Nasal fractures result from a blow to the nose; bleeding may be profuse and must be controlled. It is best to evaluate the nose as soon after injury as possible. Swelling is likely to occur, and once the area becomes swollen, important signs indicating a nasal fracture may be masked.

Begin the evaluation by carefully observing the nasal area for any deformity. A nasal fracture should be suspected with any abnormal deviation of the nose (Figure 14-8). Whenever there is a question about the abnormal deviation of an injured nose, it is a good practice to allow the athlete to view his or her nose in a mirror to evaluate the normal alignment and contour. Another method used to observe for any deviation is to view the injured nose by looking down the forehead and across the bridge of the nose when standing behind the athlete, as previously discussed. You can also look at the nasal openings from underneath to assess symmetry.

If obvious abnormal deviation is not present, the injured area should be gently palpated. Carefully feel the two nasal bones be-

tween your thumb and forefingers to locate the areas of pain and tenderness. Palpation may also reveal deformity, increased mobility, or crepitation. All obvious and suspected nasal fractures should be promptly referred to a physician for further evaluation and reduction of the fracture.

After controlling bleeding or evaluating the external structures of the nose, the internal structures should also be examined. All too often this portion of the assessment of nasal injuries is neglected. Nasal trauma can result in injuries to the septum, which, if not recognized and treated properly, can result in complications. Injuries involving the blood vessels adjacent to the nasal septum can cause blood to be trapped in the space between the septum and the mucous membrane, which is called a **septal hematoma.** This can lead to destruction of the septal cartilage and bone or replacement by fibrous tissue. Another complication of an injured septum is a septal abscess. Septal trauma can have devastating effects on the nasal complex by affecting the airway passage and breathing. In extreme situations, it can even be life threatening. Adequate treatment begins with a thorough nasal examination.

Internal examination of the nasal structures involves evaluation of the nasal septum for trauma. This evaluation requires the use of a light and a clear passageway. Look for and attempt to locate sites of bleeding. Inspect the nasal septum for the presence of a septal hematoma, which is characterized by a widening of the septum. You may also see a discolored area filled with fluid, which can be depressed with a cotton-tipped applicator. An abscess may be identified by a fluctuant, purulent (pus-filled) blister. This abscess will be painful to palpation, and the athlete may have an increase in body temperature. Also evaluate the nasal septum for any angulation or deviation. A **deviated septum** may result in a narrowing of one air passage with a compensatory widening of the other. If any of these conditions are recognized, the athlete should be referred to medical assistance.

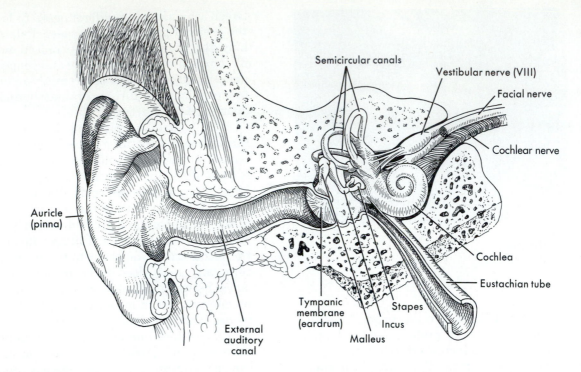

FIGURE 14-9
Components of the ear. Note in particular the external ear, consisting of the auricle (pinna), external auditory canal, and tympanic membrane (eardrum).

Ear

As an organ of special sense the ear is the organ of hearing and of balance, or equilibrium. It is divided into three parts (Figure 14-9).

1. The external ear, consisting of (1) the auricle, or pinna, (2) the external auditory canal, or meatus, and (3) the tympanic membrane, or eardrum.
2. The middle ear cavity, containing (1) the ear ossicles and (2) the opening of the eustachian tube, which permits equalization of pressure on both sides of the eardrum.
3. The inner ear, containing (1) the semicircular canals involved in maintenance of balance (equilibrium) and (2) the cochlea, which is the sensory organ for the perception of sound.

The visible part of the external ear is called the auricle, or pinna (Figure 14-10). Except for the ear lobe, which is composed of connective tissue and fat, the auricle consists of fibroelastic cartilage with a very thin layer of tightly adhered and sensitive skin. It is important to realize that there is little or no subcutaneous tissue between the cartilaginous plates of the external ear and the overlying skin. As a result, there is no room between the skin and underlying cartilage to permit diffuse accumulation of tissue fluid or blood after an injury. Deformity occurs as blood or fluid accumulates in very localized areas.

The auditory canal, or meatus, is a tube-like structure about $1\frac{1}{4}$ inches long. It extends from the auricle into the temporal bone of the skull. The outer (lateral) third of the tube is cartilaginous, and the inner (medial) two thirds is bony. The canal terminates internally at the tympanic membrane, or eardrum. The skin that lines the canal is tightly adherent and very thin over the inner bony part and thicker over the outer

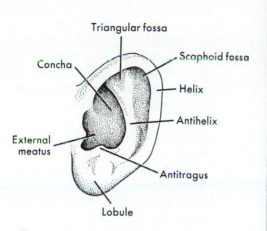

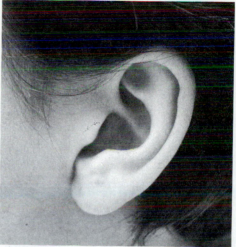

FIGURE 14-10
The external ear, showing the component parts of the auricle (pinna).

cartilaginous portion, where it contains hair and sebaceous and ceruminous (wax) glands. It is in the outer portion of the tube that infections are most likely to occur, involving the sebaceous glands or hair cells.

The auditory canal is not a straight tube; the bony portion is directed downward and forward. This anatomic fact explains why it is necessary to draw the auricle upward and backward to align the cartilaginous portion with the nonmovable bony portion. When the canal is straightened out it is possible to inspect its entire length for lacerations, foreign bodies such as insects, excess cerumen (earwax), **impacted cerumen**, and infections. An otoscope is used to examine the auditory canal and eardrum (Figure 14-11).

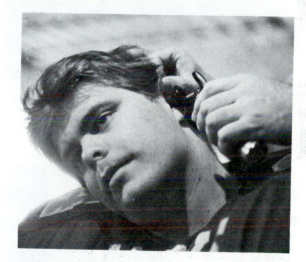

FIGURE 14-11
Using an otoscope to examine an ear.

Ear injuries

Sports-related ear injuries are limited almost invariably to the components of the external ear. However, symptoms involving the middle and inner ear may be described by an athlete after an injury or sickness. These symptoms include defective hearing, tinnitus, **vertigo** (sensations of movement), or sensations of sudden fullness in the ear. Athletes expressing these symptoms should be referred to a physician or medical facility.

Assessment of the ear for potential injury after any type of head trauma should be a standard component of your examination sequence. You will need good illumination, proper positioning, and physical control of the athlete to complete a detailed assessment in this area. Always begin with palpation and examination of the surrounding mastoid and temporal areas of the skull. Look for ecchymosis, swelling, tenderness, and signs of localized trauma such as lacerations or deformity.

As you focus your attention on the ear itself, look first for evidence of hemorrhage and carefully inspect the opening into the auditory canal for the presence of a foreign body (Figure 14-12). If bleeding is noted after an injury, you should always consider the possibility of a basilar or temporal bone skull fracture. Leakage of cerebrospinal fluid (cerebrospinal otorrhea) from the ear after injury necessitates immediate referral. Most bleeding from the external ear is the result of simple canal lacerations. Although sometimes very painful, they are seldom serious.

❖ **Cauliflower ear (hematoma auris).** Repeated contusions and twisting or friction-type injuries to the external ear, especially in the absence of protective ear guards, may result in a hematoma formation between the skin and underlying cartilage. If the hematoma remains untreated and is allowed to "organize," it becomes fibrotic and results in a **keloid.** A keloid is a raised nodular deformity that can only be removed by surgery. A cauliflower ear is the end result of keloid formation between the skin and underlying cartilage of an injured external ear, generally in the scaphoid fossa or concha areas (Figure 14-13).

If assessment reveals continued swelling

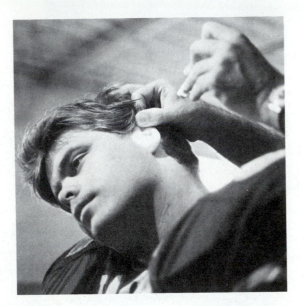

FIGURE 14-12
Inspecting the external ear and auditory canal.

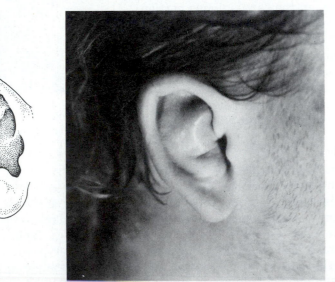

FIGURE 14-13
A, Hematoma auris (cauliflower ear), resulting in keloid formation in the scaphoid fossa. **B,** Onset of hematoma auris after acute trauma.

or hemorrhage of an ear injury after initial treatment with a cold pack and compression, the athlete should be referred to a physician. Ear deformity resulting from keloid formation can be avoided by timely aspiration of the hematoma and prompt initiation of compression therapy.

✤ **Swimmer's ear (otitis externa).** External otitis, or swimmer's ear, is a common infection of the external ear in athletes. It can be bacterial or fungal in origin and is usually associated with prolonged exposure to water or excessive moisture. This condition is particularly prevalent in hot, humid climates, and during the summer. The S-shaped auditory canal is designed to protect the ear against invasion by foreign objects also prevents water from escaping. This retained moisture is the main predisposing factor in most cases of swimmer's ear. The infection generally involves the auditory canal and perhaps the auricle. Ear pain is the most common symptom of swimmer's ear. In early stages the pain is usually mild and may be accompanied by itching. In later stages, pain can be severe and there may be a discharge from the ear. The ear as a whole is tender, and pressure may cause pain. The canal is red and swollen. The athlete may report a feeling of "fullness" in the ear. Swimmer's ear generally responds quickly to treatment. It normally involves cleaning out the auditory canal, the use of antibiotic therapy, and perhaps prescription analgesics to alleviate the pain and itching. Early referral to a physician is recommended. Any treatment routine should include prevention techniques so that athletes who spend long hours in the water learn to care for their ears to avoid recurring infections.

Eardrum perforations. Traumatic rupture of the tympanic membrane can be caused by the penetration of a sharp object or a sudden blow across the ear. You should also suspect eardrum damage if hemorrhage is noted after a diving or altitude-related sports injury. Such injuries may be characterized by sharp pain, slight hearing impairment, tinnitus, and slight bleeding. Ruptured eardrums normally heal sponta-

neously but should be under a physician's care.

✤ **Otitis media.** Otitis media is an infection of the middle ear, most common in children 6 to 36 months of age. It is probably the most common pediatric illness. Its incidence decreases with maturation of the eustachian tube and is much less common in adults. Otitis media is more common in winter and often accompanies a viral upper respiratory infection. Symptoms in children often include earache, hearing loss, vertigo, tinnitus, or behavior changes. Otitis media may also include fever, otorrhea, rhinitis, cough, or conjunctivitis. Treatment normally involves antibiotics. Otitis media can usually be differentiated from swimmer's ear by manipulating the auricle or pressing on the cartilage plate. Either of these maneuvers will normally cause increased pain in swimmer's ear but not in otitis media.

Frostbite. Athletes who participate in cold-weather sports are susceptible to frostbite. Superficial facial frostbite generally involves the ears, nose, and cheeks; the ears are particularly susceptible. Symptoms include burning, numbness, tingling, and blanching of the skin. Frostbite was discussed in more detail in Chapter 8.

Teeth

There are 32 permanent teeth in the adult. Each tooth is composed of three main parts: crown, neck and root (Figure 14-14). The crown is the exposed portion of the tooth and is covered by enamel. The neck is that portion surrounded by the soft gingiva, or gum tissue. It is the root of each tooth that articulates with the jaw bone in the specialized gomphosis joint described in Chapter 4 (see Figure 4-1).

There are four types of teeth, which are easy to identify by direct inspection or by doing a little exploring with your tongue (Figure 14-15):

1. *Incisors:* There are four chiseled, wedge-shaped incisors on top and four below.
2. *Canines:* The four canine, or eye teeth, are the longer, sharp teeth found on

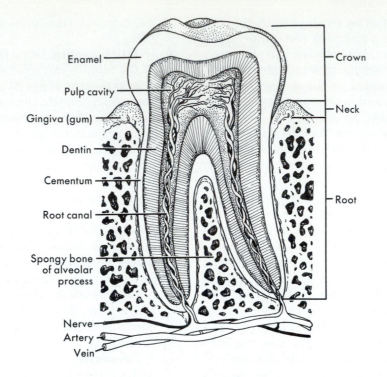

FIGURE 14-14
A molar (tricuspid) tooth sectioned to show its bony socket and details of its three main parts:
crown, neck, and root.

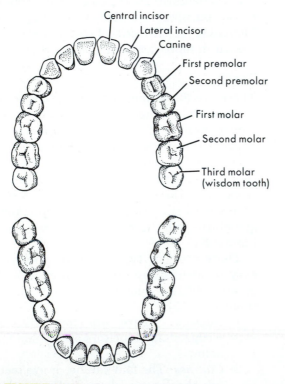

FIGURE 14-15
The 32 permanent teeth.

either side of the incisors; they are particularly prominent above but are found on both upper and lower jaws.

3. *Premolars (bicuspids):* Each premolar, or bicuspid tooth, has two points, or cusps, on the biting surface. There are two premolar teeth on each side, upper and lower, just behind the canines.

4. *Molars (tricuspids):* Each molar, or tricuspid tooth, has three major points (cusps) on the biting surface. There are three molar teeth on each side, top and bottom. The third molars, or wisdom teeth, usually erupt between the ages of 16 and 23 and often come in twisted or misaligned.

Dental injuries

Acquiring accurate and complete dental information should be an important goal of the preseason assessment process. Knowing about an athlete's dental crowns, bridges, and other appliances such as partial dentures before an injury occurs will greatly facilitate rapid assessment and treatment of an obstructed airway if these structures enter the respiratory passages following a facial injury.

Athletic-related dental injuries have decreased over the years as a result of the use of mouth guards and face masks. However, dental injuries still occur, particularly in the sports that do not require mouth protection. It is important that the athletic trainer know the proper techniques of caring for dental injuries to prevent the loss of permanent teeth or later complications. This is especially true when teeth are displaced from their normal position or knocked out of the mouth. The extent of trauma involved in dental injuries can be difficult to assess because the injury may not be readily visible.

The first step in evaluating a dental injury is to locate the source of bleeding. Use a gauze pad to wipe away most of the blood around the teeth, gums, and lips. If there is little or no bleeding from the soft tissues and the seepage of blood seems to be coming from around the tooth, the tooth may be injured. Test the tooth by applying mild finger pressure inward and outward (Figure 14-16). If the movement of the tooth is similar to surrounding teeth and the tooth is not painful, numb, or fractured, the bleeding probably involves only the gum tissues surrounding the tooth. If the tooth is painful, numb, or seems depressed, the athlete should be referred to a dentist. If these symptoms are not expressed by the athlete, he or she can resume activity provided no further care is required for any soft tissue injuries.

❖ **Dental caries.** Dental caries (decay or cavities) is the most frequent cause for pain originating from the teeth. Although this is not an athletic-related injury, athletic trainers must occasionally counsel and advise athletes experiencing the symptoms of dental caries. Athletes may give a variable history of a sudden or gradual onset of a sharp-to-dull throbbing pain. Usually an athlete can indicate the specific tooth involved, but sometimes the pain may be generalized or referred to other areas of the face. Occasionally the dental decay will progress to form a

❖ pocket of pus **(dental abscess).** Suspected

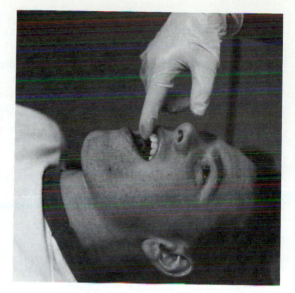

FIGURE 14-16
Applying mild finger pressure to an injured tooth.

dental caries should be referred to a dentist for follow-up care.

❖ **Tooth Fractures.** The anterior teeth are most frequently traumatized from falls or direct blows to the teeth during athletic activity. Forceful blows to the mandible may result in fractures of the premolars and molars. Fractures are managed on the basis of the type of fracture and its relation to the pulp of the tooth. The most common fracture involves only the enamel portion of the tooth. These injuries are usually minor unless a sharp portion of the tooth causes soft tissue trauma. The sharp edge may be smoothed and/or the tooth can be restored to its natural appearance with the use of enamel-bonding materials.

If there is a small corner fracture or chip off a tooth that is not sensitive to air when the athlete inhales vigorously, athletic activity can continue. However, if the fracture is sufficient enough to expose the dentin, it is usually sensitive to air, unless numbed by the trauma. Inspect the broken tooth carefully to see if the fracture cuts across the tip of the pulp or if the pink pulp is visible. A drop of blood on the tooth will also indicate exposure of the pulp. If the pulp is exposed, the athlete should receive immediate dental treatment. If the pulp is not exposed but the tooth is sensitive to air, the athlete may be permitted to continue activity as he or she desires. Tooth injuries that are sensitive to air should be referred to dental treatment within 2 to 3 hours after the trauma. An athlete who exhibits a severe fracture of a tooth should be referred to dental treatment immediately.

✤ **Tooth Subluxations and Avulsions.** Teeth that are loosened in their sockets as a result of trauma are referred to as subluxated. They may or may not be associated with fractures. If a tooth is loosened and shifted in the bone, the blood supply may be compromised. Within months this tooth may turn grey and require a root canal. A tooth that is protruding or extending outward
✤ more than normal is called a **tooth extrusion.** A tooth that is projecting inward or upward more than normal is called a **tooth**
✤ **intrusion.** Teeth that have shifted should be quickly repositioned by firm finger pressure and referred to a dentist. If dental referral and proper treatment is delayed longer than 24 hours, the tooth may eventually turn grey.

Any tooth that is knocked out intact (avulsed) should be saved, cleaned, and either put back into the socket or transported with the athlete to a dentist as soon as possible. Dental research has shown that almost any avulsed tooth can be replanted and retained if the ligamentous components of the tooth are kept viable. When a tooth is avulsed, half of the periodontal ligament remains in the socket and half remains attached to the tooth. The portion that remains in the socket continues to be viable because it is bathed in a pool of blood that fills the socket. The problem area is the portion of the ligament that remains on the tooth root. If this portion remains viable, it will reattach to the periodontal ligament fibers remaining in the socket when replanted. Treatment must therefore center on maintaining the viability of the periodontal ligament still attached to the tooth. The best possible method of creating this environment is by placing the tooth back in the socket immediately. If replanted within 15 to 30 minutes, there is a 90% chance of saving the tooth. After this time, the periodontal ligament cells may have dried out and successful reattachment diminishes rapidly. If the tooth is not replanted at the scene, the success rate of saving the tooth almost totally depends on how the tooth is stored, preserved, and handled. Do not touch the tooth on the root portion because the cells can be crushed and destroyed. The avulsed tooth must not be allowed to dry out and should be kept in a medium compatible with the ligament cells. There are emergency tooth preserving systems on the market and they should be required in every training room. These kits contain a solution to store the avulsed tooth that can keep the cells viable for 4 to 12 hours. These solutions do not require refrigeration and can be kept on the shelf for long periods of time. Saliva can be used as a storage medium for short periods of time (less than 1 hour). Milk is an acceptable storage medium for short periods of time, providing it is available, cold, and whole. Powdered, skim, or sour milk are damaging to the periodontal ligament. Sterile saline is also damaging to the tooth cells if the avulsed tooth is allowed to soak in it for more than 1 hour. Avoid allowing the tooth to dry out or soak in tap water. The athlete should be referred to a dentist as soon as possible. X-rays should be taken within 24 to 48 hours to rule out a fracture, and follow-up films should be taken within 1 to 3 months.

✤ **Gingivitis.** Inflammation of the gingiva is generally the result of an inflammatory response to an irritant such as dental bacterial plaque and organic matter deposited on the surfaces of the teeth. With continuation of the inflammation, there is ultimately loss of alveolar bone, which is termed
✤ **periodontitis.** If this process is allowed to continue, it can result in marked mobility of the teeth and eventual loss of the attachment apparatus. The gingiva can also become inflamed and swollen from the eruption of the third molar, or "wisdom teeth."

✤ This condition is called **pericoronitis** and can be extremely painful as an individual bites down on tender tissues or distends these tissues when opening the mandible.

Eye

The external structures visible in an anterior view of the eye are shown in Figure 14-17. The structures of the eyelids and globe of the eye are illustrated in Figures 14-18 and 14-19. As you view a person's eye from the front you see only a portion of the whole structure. Note in Figure 14-17 that the upper lid normally covers a small portion of the colored *iris* when the eyes are open. The space between the upper and lower lid margins is called the *palpebral fissure*. This distance should be equal in both eyes. The eyelids, or palpebrae, consist of voluntary muscle fibers and fat with a ridge of connective tissue, the *tarsal plate,* at the free edge. The overlying skin is very thin, with the eyelashes distributed evenly along the lid edges. A localized, painful infection of the small glands or hair follicles around the eyelashes

✤ at the lid margins is called a **sty** (Figure 14-20).

A specialized membrane, the *conjunctiva,* lines the eyelids and covers the white (sclera) portion of the eyeball in front. Note in Figure 14-19 that this membrane is divided into two portions: the shiny-pink *palpebral* portion that recesses into the superior and inferior fornix under the lids, and the *bulbar* portion over the eye itself. The bulbar portion is transparent but looks white because of the sclera below it.

Tiny blood vessels in the conjunctiva often become noticeable after periods of sleeplessness or stress. They often rupture in such situations, producing a small **subconjunctival hemorrhage.** Such hemorrhages sometimes occur after minimal stress such as that produced by an episode of repeated sneezing or coughing. Subconjunctival hemorrhages can also result from trauma to the eye, such as that causing a contusion or abrasion. The red blood contrasted with the white sclera (called red eye) make these injuries appear to be more serious than they actually are. It is important to determine if red eye is associated with other, more serious eye injuries.

Eye injuries

Significant numbers of sports-related eye injuries occur as a result of head or facial trauma. Increased popularity and participation in tennis and racquetball, for example, have resulted in a dramatic increase in the number of eye contusion injuries. Most of these injuries could be prevented by wearing protective eye wear and following a few safety rules. Athletic trainers should encourage the use of eye protection whenever possible. When an eye injury occurs, a

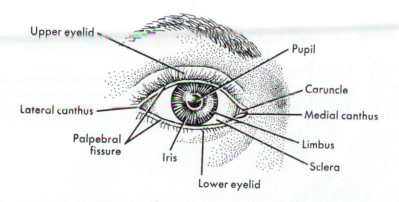

FIGURE 14-17
Anterior view of the eye.

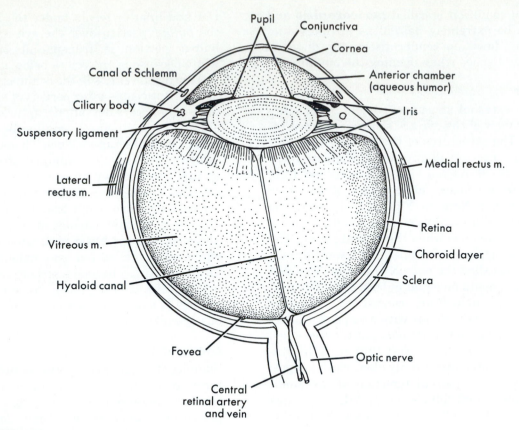

FIGURE 14-18
Horizontal section through left eyeball.

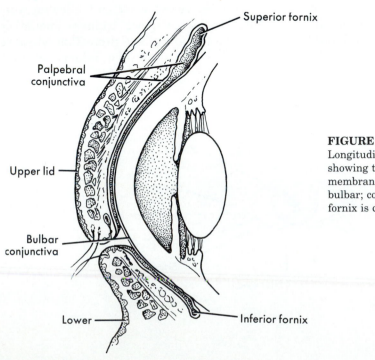

FIGURE 14-19
Longitudinal section through eyeball and eyelids, showing the conjunctiva, a lining of mucous membrane. Conjunctiva covering the cornea is called bulbar; conjunctiva lining the superior and inferior fornix is called the palpebral conjunctiva.

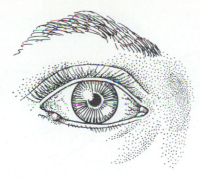

FIGURE 14-20
Lower lid sty.

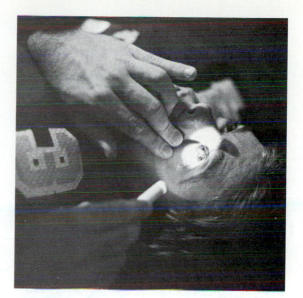

FIGURE 14-21
Examining the inferior fornix of the eye.

knowledge of ocular assessment techniques permits rapid screening of eye injuries or related complaints and facilitates rapid referral of the athlete to medical assistance when required.

Eye assessment is generally initiated as a result of complaints by an athlete of visual loss or ocular pain following head trauma or localized eye injury. The athlete's chief complaint and account of any injury will greatly assist in an accurate evaluation. In addition, the athletic trainer is often called on to assess ocular conditions that are not related to accident or injury. Examples of such noninjury problems include acute red eye and recentering of displaced contact lenses.

The conjunctiva lining the inferior fornix can be examined by moving the lower lid downward. The lid should be pressed and held gently against the lower ridge of the bony orbit without exerting pressure on the eyeball. After the lid is moved downward, ask the athlete to look up and to each side as you examine the inferior fornix (Figure 14-21).

The conjunctiva lining the superior fornix is examined by eversion of the upper eyelid. The steps in everting the upper eyelid are illustrated in Figure 14-22.

1. Ask the athlete to look downward but to keep the eyes open.
2. Grasp the eyelashes and the tarsal plate near the edge of the lid and pull gently downward. DO NOT pull the lid upward or outward.
3. Place a cotton-tipped applicator or lid evertor just above the tarsal plate of the lid and, while still holding the eyelashes, pull the lid over the applicator.
4. Hold the edge of the everted lid against the upper bony ridge of the orbit and examine the area for abrasions or the presence of a foreign body. DO NOT push against the eyeball.
5. The lid will return easily to its normal position when released if the athlete is asked to look upward and blink.

Foreign bodies and abrasions. Foreign bodies and abrasions are among the more common conditions of the eye to be managed during athletic activity. Athletes often express the feeling of having something in the eye. **Corneal abrasions** can occur when an athlete gets "poked" in the eye such as with a finger (Figure 14-23). It is important to know that foreign bodies in the eye and abrasion injuries of the conjunctiva and cornea produce almost identical symptoms, that is, pain, increased tearing, and the sensation of something in the eye. To examine the eye for foreign bodies and abrasions, a penlight for illumination, a magnifying glass, cotton-tipped applicators or lid ever-

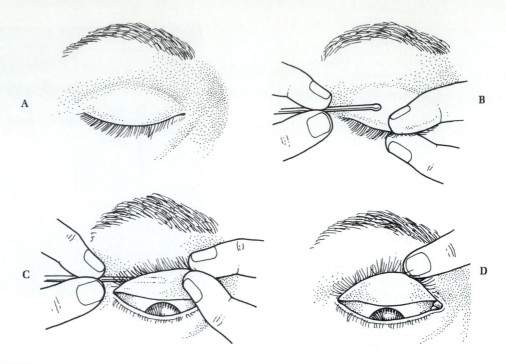

FIGURE 14-22
Steps in everting the upper eyelid. **A**, Athlete looks downward; **B**, grasp the eyelashes and tarsal plate and pull downward; **C**, pull the lid over applicator; and **D**, hold the edge of the everted lid against the upper bony ridge of the orbit.

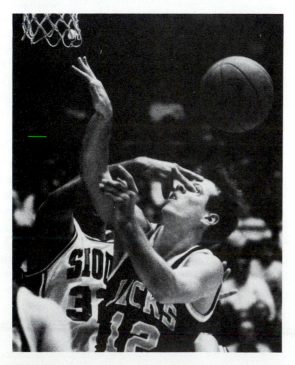

FIGURE 14-23
Athlete getting poked in the eye.

tors, and an appropriate irrigating solution should be available.

Note in Figure 14-18 that the cornea lies just below the bulbar conjunctiva and above the so-called anterior chamber of the eye. It covers the pupil and colored iris. Foreign bodies are often washed free from the cornea by the profuse tearing that occurs as a result of the initial irritation. Although a foreign body may not be present, the athlete who has suffered a corneal abrasion will continue to insist that something is in the eye. In these cases the abrasion and not the foreign body is responsible for the symptoms.

Examine the cornea by directing the penlight at it obliquely from several different positions. The iris should be fully visible, and the corneal surface should be smooth and free of irregularities. Superficial foreign bodies may be removed with a moistened cotton-tipped applicator or ophthalmic irrigating solution. If the foreign body cannot be removed or appears to be imbedded, the

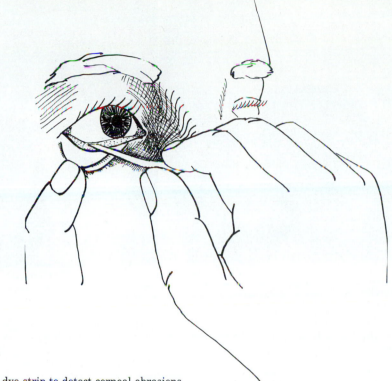

FIGURE 14-24
Use of fluorescein dye strip to detect corneal abrasions.

athlete should be referred to an ophthalmologist or medical facility.

If no foreign bodies can be located on the corneal surface, the conjunctiva lining the inferior and especially the superior fornix should be examined carefully. If no foreign body can be located after the examination is completed, the presence of an abrasion should be suspected and, if symptoms continue, the athlete should be referred to a physician. It is also possible to check for a corneal abrasion by using a fluorescein dye strip (Figure 14-24). The abraded area will be outlined by the dye when the lower fornix is touched by the moistened strip. Superficial abrasions normally heal without scarring or visual impairment.

Lacerations. The seriousness of lacerations involving the eye and surrounding tissues varies greatly. Any laceration of the eyeball itself is a serious injury with potentially grave consequences. The athlete will usually complain of pain in the eye and de-

creased vision. In looking at the eye, you may see the **corneal laceration,** or the pupil may appear tear-shaped. If a laceration of the eyeball is noted, further examination in this area should stop. Reassure the athlete and refer him or her immediately to an ophthalmologist after placing a protective pad or shield over the eye. Often it is helpful to cover both eyes at the same time to reduce eye movement and lower the likelihood of further irritation. Do not exert any pressure on the eye.

Minor horizontal lacerations to the skin of the eyelid that do not involve the lid margin are generally not a serious problem. The cut edges are relatively easy to approximate, and after repair and healing the residual scar is minimal. If the margin of the eyelid is cut, the injury is much more serious. All lacerations that involve the upper or lower lid margin should be referred to an ophthalmologist. Such lacerations may cut through the tarsal plate and lead to a "notched" lid,

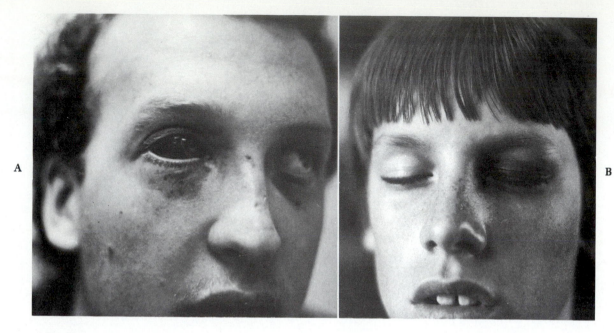

FIGURE 14-25
Blunt-bow injuries to the eye. **A**, Subconjunctival hemorrhage (red eye) and, **B**, periorbital contusion (black eye).

which can be disfiguring. In addition, persistent and troublesome tearing can also result from lacerations that cut the lower lid margin. In these cases the healed but notched tarsal plate interrupts the normal flow and direction of tears over the eye. Instead of flowing naturally toward the medial ducts, which drain fluid into the nose, the tears escape from the eye. If the lower lid margin is cut near the nose (medial aspect) there is the added possibility that the duct, which drains tears into the nose, has also been cut. Such injuries require immediate referral so that the cut ends of the duct can be found and repaired. If the lower lid margin is lacerated near the nose, it should be assumed until proved otherwise that the tear duct has also been cut.

✛ **Conjunctivitis.** Conjunctivitis is an inflammation or infection of the conjunctiva, the membrane covering the anterior eyeball and inner surface of the eyelids. There can be a number of causes including bacteria, viruses, chemicals, and allergies. Symptoms include redness of the eye, a foreign body sensation, and fullness of the eyelids. There

may be some itching and the eyelids may be stuck together on awakening. Physical examination signs include redness of the eye, tearing, some discharge, and swelling of the eyelids.

✛ **Keratitis.** Keratitis is an inflammation or infection of the cornea. It is normally caused by a herpes simplex infection. The individual will have foreign body sensation, tearing, clear discharge, decreased visual acuity, and an intolerance to light. An ophthalmologic consultation is needed.

Blunt-blow injuries. The anatomy of the bony orbit makes the eye quite resistant to serious blunt-blow injuries. Contusion-type blunt-blow injuries can occur quite frequently, however, as a result of racquetball and handball injuries. It is fortunate that in
✛ most cases damage is limited to **subconjunctival hemorrhage (red eye)** and
✛ **periorbital contusion (black eye)** (Figure 14-25).

Hemorrhage into the anterior chamber of
✛ the eye after a blunt blow is called **hyphema.** Assessment of this condition is usually not difficult because the blood can be

seen through the cornea as it collects in a pool in the lower portion of the anterior chamber of the eye (Figure 14-26). The athlete may also complain of pain in the eye and fuzzy vision. Although this condition clears spontaneously in almost all cases, referral to a physician is required because of the possibility of secondary hemorrhage.

A serious injury that can result from blunt-blow trauma to the eye is called an

✤ **orbital blow-out fracture.** If the eye has been subjected to a severe blunt blow (such as from a baseball or hockey puck), the possibility of a fractured orbit should always be considered. In blow-out fractures, the floor of the orbit is pushed into the maxillary sinus. As a result of the fracture, the mobility of the affected eye is restricted. This occurs because the ocular muscles are often trapped or pinched at the fracture site. If

there is restriction of eye movement (especially an inability to look upward), or if the athlete complains of double vision *(diplopia)* following a severe blunt-blow injury to the eye or face, an orbital fracture should be considered (Figure 14-27). In most cases of or-

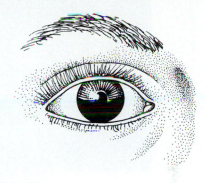

FIGURE 14-26
Blood pooling in the lower portion of the anterior chamber of the eye following injury (hyphema).

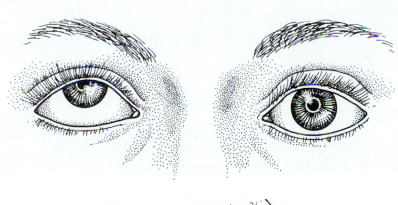

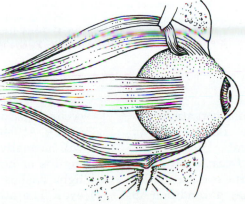

FIGURE 14-27
A blow-out fracture of the left eye orbit. Inability to look upward on the injured side is the result of ocular muscles being trapped or pinched at the fracture site.

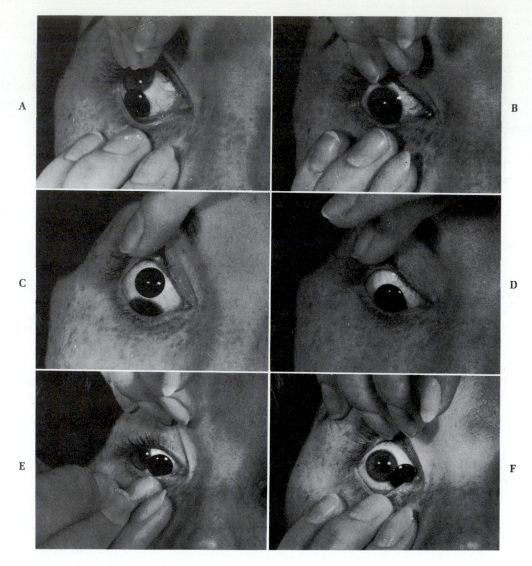

FIGURE 14-28
Recentering of displaced contact lens. For purposes of illustration an opaque lens has been used. **A,** Lens is first located by pulling lids away from globe and looking in various directions. **B,** By pressing lens with lids, lens may be manipulated onto cornea. **C,** Lens displaced above. **D,** Lens recentered from displacement above. **E,** Lens displaced nasally. **F,** Eye is directed toward lens.

bital fracture, multiple and potentially serious eye injuries occur. Referral to an ophthalmologist is essential.

✢   **Retinal detachment.** Occasionally, athletes suffering trauma to the eye may suffer detachment of the retina, a condition in which the inner layers of the retina are separated from the pigment layer. This may occur days, weeks, or even months after an injury. Athletes suffering a detached retina will normally complain of a "curtain" blocking his or her field of vision, together with light flashes or dark spots in front of the eyes. The athlete should be referred to an ophthalmologist immediately.

Displaced contact lenses. The use of

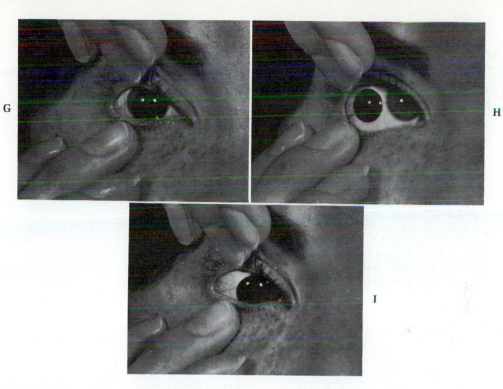

FIGURE 14-28, cont'd
G, Lens is recentered from nasal displacement. **H**, Lens displaced temporally. **I**, Lens recentered from temporal displacement.

contact lenses by athletes has greatly increased and presents some problems for the athletic trainer. Hard contact lenses are more likely than the newer soft lenses to cause eye abrasions, slip around, pop out, and become lost. The athletic trainer is often involved with locating and recentering displaced contact lenses (Figure 14-28). To care for an athlete wearing contact lenses, wetting solution, lens cases, and a mirror should be available.

Evaluation of Findings

The face is the most important cosmetic area of the body and the area involved with the senses of sight, smell, taste, and sound. A variety of athletic trauma can occur to the face. Facial trauma is an obvious area of concern and necessitates a careful, accurate assessment (see p. 314). Athletic trainers must remember that injuries to the face indicate trauma to the head, which can also result in injuries to the brain or spinal cord. Do not concentrate on facial trauma to the extent that associated injuries, which may be more serious, are overlooked.

When to refer the athlete

Because of the great vascularity of the face, injuries can appear very dramatic and sensational, although the underlying injuries may be minimal. Conversely, the appearance of facial trauma may not reflect the magnitude or seriousness of the injury. Therefore athletic trainers must carefully and accurately evaluate each facial injury. Medical assistance should be readily obtained for facial trauma whenever a significant injury is recognized or suspected. Athletic trainers who decide, incorrectly, that a facial injury is not serious enough to warrant medical referral place themselves and the athlete at risk. Conditions that indicate an athlete should be referred to medical assistance are listed in the box on page 315.

Athletic Injury Assessment Checklist: Facial Injuries

Secondary survey

_____ History

    _____ Primary complaint

    _____ Mechanism of injury

    _____ Pain

    _____ Sensations (numbness, crepitation, dizziness, tinnitus, vertigo, loss of hearing, burning, tingling, loose teeth, visual loss, something in the eye)

_____ Observation

Jaw

    _____ Obvious deformity

    _____ Swelling

    _____ Signs of trauma

    _____ Malocclusion of teeth

    _____ Symmetry

    _____ Jaw movement

Nose

    _____ Epistaxis

    _____ Foreign body

    _____ Swelling

    _____ Deformity

    _____ Rhinorrhea

Ear

    _____ Hemorrhage

    _____ Foreign body

    _____ Otorrhea

    _____ Swelling

    _____ Infection or inflammation

    _____ Blanching of the skin

Teeth

    _____ Bleeding around teeth

    _____ Loosened or shifted

    _____ Chipped, cracked, broken, or dislodged

    _____ Malocclusion

Eye

    _____ Foreign body

    _____ Abrasion

    _____ Increased tearing

    _____ Laceration

    _____ Pupil equality and symmetry

    _____ Red eye

    _____ Black eye

    _____ Hyphema

    _____ Diplopia

_____ Physical examination

    _____ Tenderness

    _____ Swelling

    _____ Deformities

    _____ Crepitation

    _____ Abnormal movements

When to Refer the Athlete . . .

Skin
  Lacerations requiring sutures
Facial bones (suspected fractures)
  Teeth do not fit together normally
  Deformity observed
  Pain at the site of injury, which is increased by
    palpation, forcefully biting down, or stress applied
    away from the site of trauma
  Crepitation
Temporomandibular joint (suspected dislocation)
  Loss of jaw movement
  Malocclusion of the teeth
Nose
  Discharge of cerebrospinal fluid
  Foreign body that cannot be easily removed
  Nasal deformity
  Crepitation or increased mobility on palpation
  Septal abnormalities
Ear
  Discharge of crebrospinal fluid
  Foreign body that cannot be easily removed
  Athlete reports sensations of tinnitus, vertigo, or a
    sudden fullness in the ear that does not readily
    go away
  Hematoma formation
  Appearance of infection or inflammation
  Sudden hearing impairment
Teeth
  Chipped, cracked, broken, or dislodged
  Tooth painful, numb, loosened, or depressed
  Athlete reporting continued sensitivity to biting
    down or extremes of temperature
Eye
  Loss of vision
  Ocular pain
  Imbedded foreign body
  Suspected abrasion on eyeball
  Laceration of eyeball or eyelid margin
  Irregularly shaped pupil
  Hemorrhage into anterior chamber
  Restricted eye movements
  Double vision
Doubt regarding facial injuries

REFERENCES

Amsterdam JT: Dental disorders. In Rosen P and others, editors: *Emergency medicine: concepts and clinical practice,* ed 3, St. Louis, 1992, Mosby.

Crow RW: Sports-related lacerations: promoting healing and limiting scarring, *Phys Sportsmed* 21(2):143, 1993.

Erie JC: Eye injuries: prevention, evaluation, and treatment, *Phys Sportsmed* 19(11):108, 1991.

Ghezzi K, Renner GS: Ophthalmologic disorders. In Rosen P and others, editors: *Emergency medicine: concepts and clinical practice,* ed 3, St. Louis, 1992, Mosby.

Lowery DW, Waeckerle JF: Soft tissue trauma of the head and neck, *Phys Sportsmed* 19(10):21, 1991.

MacAfee DA: Immediate care of facial trauma, *Phys Sportsmed* 29(7):79, 1992.

Schelkun PH: Swimmer's ear: getting patients back in the water, *Phys Sportsmed* 19(7):85, 1991.

Sitler M: Nasal septal injuries, *Ath Train* 21(1):10, 1986.

Stair TO: Otolaryngologic disorders. In Rosen P and others, editors: *Emergency medicine: concepts and clinical practice,* ed 3, St. Louis, 1992, Mosby.

Torg JS: *Athletic injuries to the head, neck and face,* ed 2, St. Louis, 1991, Mosby.

Vision, eye care, and the athlete: a round table, *Phys Sportsmed* 13(6):132, 1985.

SUGGESTED READINGS

Cantrill SV: Facial trauma. In Rosen P, and others, editors: *Emergency medicine: concepts and clinical practice,* ed 3, St. Louis, 1992, Mosby.
  This chapter discusses various aspects of evaluating and treating a variety of facial injuries.

Castaldi CR: First aid for sports-related dental injuries, *Phys Sportsmed* 15(9):81, 1987.
  Provides an excellent presentation on evaluation procedures and emergency care of dental injuries, including guidelines to which all athletic trainers should refer when assessing injured teeth.

Krasner P: The athletic trainer's role in saving avulsed teeth, *Ath Train* 24(2):139, 1989.
  An excellent article reviewing all known methods and devices for the storage, preservation, and transportation of avulsed teeth. Specific recommendations are made for athletic trainers to use to save avulsed teeth.

Whyte JD: Eye injuries, *Ath Train* 22(3):207, 1987.
  Reviews the mechanism of injury, signs, symptoms, and the immediate treatment for many types of eye injuries or conditions that can result from athletic activity.

CHAPTER 15

Spine injuries

After you have completed this chapter, you should be able to:

- Identify the basic anatomy of the spine.
- Compare the types of vertebrae found in each area of the spinal column.
- Describe the common types of athletic injuries that may occur to the spine.
- Describe the assessment process for an athlete suffering a spinal injury.
- Explain how to perform a neurologic examination to evaluate muscle function and sensations for each nerve root segment.
- List the signs and symptoms that indicate an athlete suffering a spine injury should be referred to medical assistance.

The human spine is a remarkable structure. During athletic activity the spine is able to withstand tremendous stresses and forces and at the same time remain quite flexible and mobile. The spine, or vertebral column, encases and provides protection for the spinal cord. Trauma to the spine can produce devastating athletic injuries. These injuries can be fatal or can cause irreversible damage to the spinal cord that result in permanent paralysis. To accurately assess and care for injuries to this area of the body, it is imperative that the athletic trainer possess a thorough understanding of the anatomic and mechanical characteristics of the spine.

ANATOMY OF THE SPINE

The spine consists of 33 vertebrae, which are subdivided into seven cervical, twelve thoracic, five lumbar, five sacral (fused), and four coccygeal (fused) vertebrae. The 24 nonfused vertebrae lying superior to the sacrum increase in size from the first cervical through the fifth lumbar. Between each of these vertebrae is an intervertebral disc. Discs act as shock absorbers and allow movement between adjacent vertebrae.

Intervertebral Discs

Each intervertebral disc consists of two structures, the tough outer **annulus fibrosus** and the semisolid central **nucleus pulposus** (Figure 15-1). The annulus fibrosus connects the bodies of adjacent vertebrae through obliquely arranged layers of fibrocartilage. Each layer of fibers is perpendicular to the adjacent layers. This arrangement gives the disc strength and elasticity. The annulus fibrosus is thicker anteriorly and laterally. This fact explains the larger number of posterior disc herniations. The

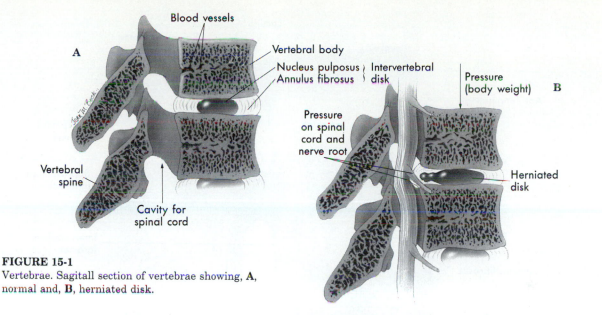

FIGURE 15-1
Vertebrae. Sagitall section of vertebrae showing, **A,** normal and, **B,** herniated disk.

nucleus pulposus is a gelatinous substance located in the center of the disc. It contains a high percentage of water (70% to 80%), which allows the disc to change shape easily during movement of the vertebral column. The intervertebral discs are subject to dehydration as a result of pressure placed on them. Minute quantities of water can be squeezed out of each disc and are absorbed into the bloodstream during a day's activity. This can result in an individual losing up to 2 cm of height during a day. During rest and sleep, when the pressure on the discs is least, water is reabsorbed from the bloodstream and original height is regained. However, as age advances, the water content in the nucleus pulposus becomes somewhat less and the discs become slightly thinner. Although the resultant loss of depth in each disc is small, it may amount to an overall decrease of 2 to 3 cm in length of the vertebral column.

Ligaments of the Vertebral Column

The bodies of adjacent vertebrae are connected by strong ligaments (Figure 15-2). Two important longitudinal ligaments can be identified through the entire length of the spinal column. The *anterior longitudinal lig-*

ament is a strong, bandlike structure composed of several layers of fibers that extends along and is firmly attached to the anterior surface of each vertebral body. It extends from the base of the skull to the sacrum. The *posterior longitudinal ligament* lies on the inside of the vertebral canal on the posterior surface of the bodies of the vertebrae. It is principally a structure that serves to connect the intervertebral discs. It consists of smooth, glistening fibers that commence on the body of the axis and continue downward to the sacrum.

In addition, the *ligamentum flavum* bind the laminae of adjacent vertebrae firmly together. Spinous processes are connected by *interspinous ligaments.* The transverse processes of adjacent vertebrae are connected by *intertransverse ligaments.* The tips of the spinous processes of the cervical vertebrae are connected by the specialized *ligamentum nuchae,* which extends downward from the external occipital protuberance at the base of the skull to join the spinous processes of all seven cervical vertebrae. This strong and important fan-shaped ligament lies in the midline and forms a septum between the neck muscles. The extension of this ligament, the *supraspinous ligament,* connects

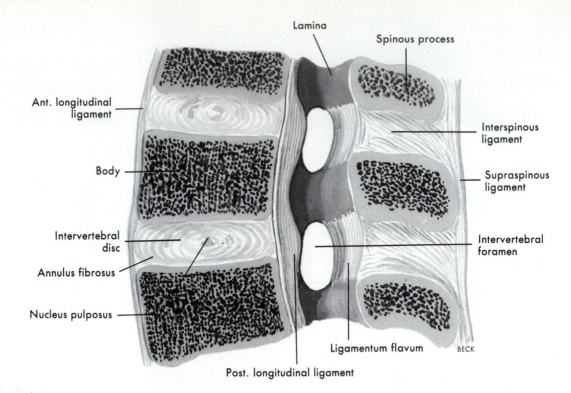

FIGURE 15-2
Sagittal section of vertebral column and ligaments.

the tips of the rest of the vertebrae down to the sacrum.

Spinal Cord

The spinal cord (Figure 15-3) is a continuation of the motor and sensory pathways from the brain to the body and the extremities. It is oval and less than ½ inch in diameter. It tapers slightly from above downward and is extremely sensitive to injury. For example, it is said that if you were to drop a quarter on an exposed spinal cord from a height of 12 inches, neural function distal to the point of impact would be severely impaired. It is encased and protected within the bony spinal canal. The spinal cord is surrounded by the meninges, cerebrospinal fluid, a cushion of adipose tissue, and blood vessels. The cord extends from the foramen magnum to the lower border of the first lumbar vertebra, an average distance of 17 to 18 inches in the adult. Although the spinal cord terminates at the level of the first lumbar vertebrae, lumbar, sacral, and coccygeal nerve roots

continue to descend in the canal. This gives the lower end of the spinal cord, with its attached spinal nerve roots, the appearance of a horse's tail, and prompted early anatomists to describe it as the **cauda equina.**

✜   **Meningitis.** Meningitis is an inflammation of the membranes (meninges) of the spinal cord or brain. It is most often caused by a bacteria, however, viral infections, fungal infections, and tumors may also cause inflammation of the meninges. It most often involves the arachnoid and pia mater. Symptoms are usually fever, severe headache, nausea, vomiting, and neck pain. Depending on the primary cause, meningitis may be mild and self-limiting or may progress to a severe, perhaps fatal, condition. If only the spinal meninges are involved, the condition is called *spinal meningitis.*

Spinal Nerves

The nerves arising from the spinal cord connect the central nervous system to the rest of the body. A nerve root is that portion of

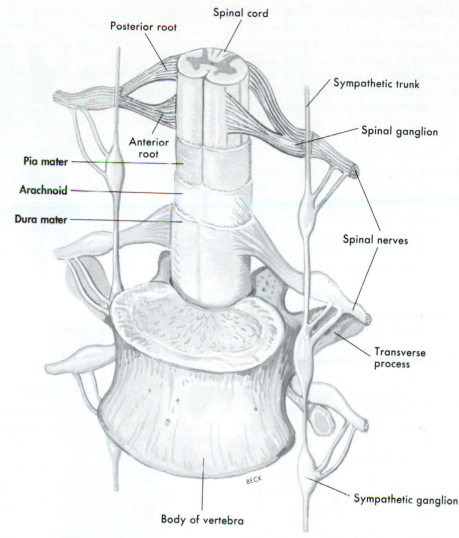

FIGURE 15-3
Spinal cord surrounded by the three meningeal layers: dura mater, arachnoid, and pia mater.
Note also the formation of spinal nerves.

the nerve that connects it to the spinal cord and is the most proximal segment of the peripheral nervous system. A nerve root is made up of a ventral (anterior) part, which is motor, and a dorsal (posterior) part, which is sensory, that unite near or in the intervertebral foramen to form a single nerve root or spinal nerve. There are 31 pairs of spinal nerves connected to the spinal cord. They have no special names but are merely numbered according to the level of the spinal column at which they emerge. Thus, there are eight cervical, twelve thoracic, five lumbar, five sacral, and one coccygeal pair of spinal nerves. These spinal nerves leave the spinal cavity horizontally through the intervertebral foramina of their respective vertebrae and branch out to innervate the various parts of the body. Refer to Table 6-4 for a review of the spinal nerves, their plexuses, and peripheral branches.

As discussed in Chapter 6, each spinal nerve supplies sensory fibers to the areas of skin on the body surface that are arranged in a definite segmented pattern. Each strip of skin supplied by a given spinal nerve is called a **dermatome.** Although there is considerable overlap in the innervation of each dermatome, sensation in each band is associated with a particular spinal nerve; loss of sensation in a dermatome segment suggests injury to the spinal nerve supplying that segment. Refer to Figure 6-15 for a dermatome map of the body.

Myotomes are a group of muscles innervated by a single nerve root. Because most muscles receive innervation from more than one nerve segment, only subtle motor dysfunction is usually noted with a lesion of a single nerve root. However, a lesion of a peripheral nerve may lead to complete motor dysfunction of the muscles supplied by that nerve. Athletic trainers should test for dermatomes and myotomes anytime nerve involvement is suspected.

Muscles Acting on the Vertebral Column

The vertebral column, in part or as a whole, may be moved or acted upon by numerous muscles or muscle groups. Some muscles have both origin and insertion on the spine (intrinsic) and act directly on the column, whereas others act only indirectly on the spine and have their origin or insertion on some other bone or soft tissue component (extrinsic).

The complex deep, or intrinsic muscles of the back, extend from the base of the skull to the pelvis on each side of the body. They control the movements of the vertebral column. These muscles acting on the spine are extremely complex in morphologic detail and specific mechanisms of action. The *short intrinsic muscles* tend to steady adjoining vertebrae during movements of the column as a whole. The *long intrinsic muscles* or muscle groups are more involved in gross movements of the entire spine. From a functional standpoint there is little reason to subdivide the intrinsic back musculature in any detail because these muscles usually work together in most movements of the vertebral column. Refer to Table 5-2 for a review of

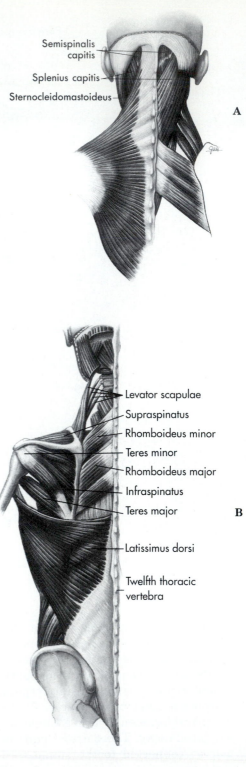

FIGURE 15-4
Muscles of the back that move the, **A**, head and, **B**, upper arm.

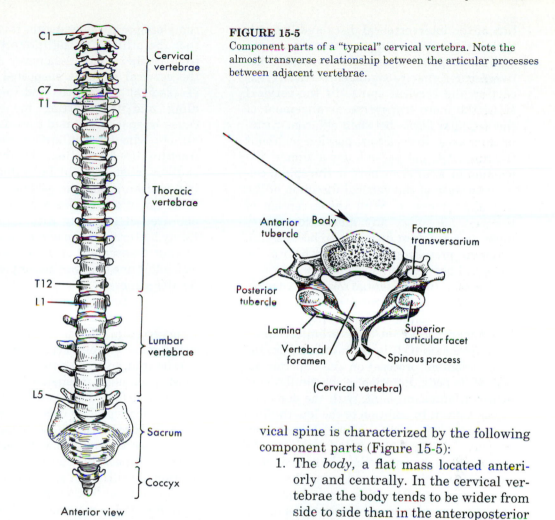

C1

Cervical
vertebrae

C7

T1

Thoracic
vertebrae

T12

L1

Lumbar
vertebrae

L5

Sacrum

Coccyx

Anterior view

FIGURE 15-5

Component parts of a "typical" cervical vertebra. Note the almost transverse relationship between the articular processes between adjacent vertebrae.

Anterior
tubercle   Body

Foramen
transversarium

Posterior
tubercle

Lamina

Vertebral
foramen

Superior
articular facet

Spinous process

(Cervical vertebra)

the muscles that move the vertebral column.

The superficial muscles of the back are, as a group, muscles that move the head or upper limbs (Figure 15-4). These muscles will be discussed in more detail in later chapters.

Cervical Spine

The cervical spine is of paramount importance to the athletic trainer. This area of the spine has greater flexibility than any other vertebral segment. There are seven cervical (neck) vertebrae, which can be distinguished from other vertebrae by the presence of a foramen through their transverse processes. With the exception of the first cervical vertebra, or atlas, each component of the cer-

vical spine is characterized by the following component parts (Figure 15-5):

1. The *body,* a flat mass located anteriorly and centrally. In the cervical vertebrae the body tends to be wider from side to side than in the anteroposterior diameter.
2. Two *transverse processes,* which project laterally from each vertebra.
3. The *spinous process,* a sharp palpable process that projects posteriorly and inferiorly from each vertebra.
4. Two *lamina,* join the spinous process on each side with the body.
5. A central opening called the *vertebral foramen,* formed by the junction of the lamina with the body. This is the opening through which the spinal cord passes.
6. *Superior articular facets,* which are directed superiorly and posteriorly.
7. *Inferior articular facets,* which are directed anteriorly and inferiorly.

The bodies of adjacent vertebrae articulate with each other through the intervention of the intervertebral discs and through their articular facets or processes. The upper and lower pairs of articular processes between vertebrae are arranged vertically, except in the cervical spine. In the cervical spine the more transverse arrangement of the articular facets between adjacent vertebrae makes dislocation possible without fracture. It is not possible for a simple dislocation to occur elsewhere in the spinal column because of the vertical direction of the articular processes. With the exception of the cervical spine, any dislocation injury must be a fracture dislocation, because the articular processes must break before the vertebral bodies can be separated.

The atlas (C1) has large oval and concave facets that articulate with the occipital condyles of the skull. Flexion and extension movements occur at the atlantooccipital joint. The axis (C2) is characterized by the dens (odontoid process) on the superior aspect of its body. Rotation of the skull occurs at the atlantoaxial joint, with the dens acting as a pivot. In addition to the longitudinal ligaments and articular capsules, a number of specialized ligaments help to stabilize the articulations between the skull and atlas and between the atlas and axis. The *transverse ligament of the atlas,* for example, protects the spinal cord in certain types of cervical fractures by limiting backward displacement of the dens into the vertebral canal. Rotation of the skull is limited by the lateral odontoid or "check" ligaments. These very strong fibrous bands extend from each occipital condyle at the base of the skull to the dens, or odontoid process, of the axis.

The seventh cervical vertebra (C7) is called the *vertebra prominens* because of its relatively long and easily palpated spinous process. It is the first clearly palpable spine as you run your fingers downward along the vertebral crests, although the spine of the first thoracic vertebra (T1) immediately below it is in fact more prominent.

Cervical spine injuries

Injuries to the cervical spine can be the most serious of athletic injuries. These injuries range in severity from minor neck pain to complete paralysis or death. It is imperative that the athletic trainer protect the athlete from further injury whenever an injury to the cervical spine is suspected. Ill-advised assessment procedures and improper handling and transporting maneuvers may cause irreparable spinal cord damage to an athlete who has suffered a cervical spine fracture or dislocation. Therefore utmost caution must be used in evaluating, treating, and handling the athlete who has suffered an injury to the neck region. This is one area of the body with which it is certainly better to be conservative and cautious in your assessment of injury rather than to risk a lifetime of paralysis, or possibly death, for the athlete.

Mechanisms of injury to the cervical spine can involve the vertebrae, facet joints, intervertebral discs, ligaments, muscles, nerve roots, or spinal cord. These structures can be injured by various mechanisms. The most common mechanism of injury to the neck is forced movements of the head on the cervical spine or excessive motion of the neck (Figure 15-6). This can occur when the athlete receives a blow to the head that forces the neck beyond its normal limits of motion, resulting in forced hyperextension, flexion, lateral flexion, rotation, or a combination of these movements. The contractile tissue surrounding the cervical spine may be stretched or strained while attempting to resist this forced movement. If forced movement is severe or violent enough, serious injuries to the neck, such as fractures or dislocations, may occur. The most serious injuries to the cervical spine occur most often as the result of axial loading or cervical compression. This may happen when an athlete receives a head-on blow to the top or crown of the head, especially when the neck is slightly flexed. In this position, the cervical lordosis is straightened and the force is transmitted directly through the cervical spine. This mechanism may cause a fracture of the vertebra or the articular facets to slide away from each other, resulting in a vertebral dislocation. The neck can also be injured by a direct blow. This mechanism usually results in contusions or bruising about

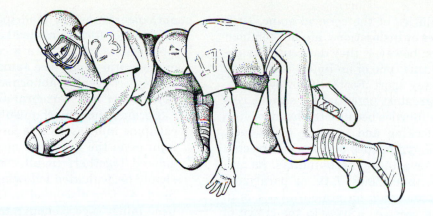

FIGURE 15-6
Possible mechanism of neck injury. The cervical spine is forced beyond its normal limits of motion.

the neck, but can result in a serious spinal injury, depending on the force of the blow, the object involved, and the position of the cervical spine.

❖ **Cervical sprains and strains.** Some of the more common injuries to the neck are cervical sprains and strains that often occur simultaneously. These injuries vary in severity. Slight trauma may result in mild injuries of little consequence. In these cases, the athlete will express no feelings of weakness or instability. Although there may be tenderness and pain at the site of the injury, the athlete can easily demonstrate a normal range of motion (ROM) in the neck. In moderate sprains and strains, the athlete may have limited motion of the cervical spine, but without radiation of pain or paresthesia. Neurologic examination is negative and radiographic studies normal. In more severe injuries, the athlete will usually resist moving the neck through a full ROM. With the more severe injuries there will be localized pain and muscle spasm, and the athlete may complain of an insecure feeling about the neck. Any athlete with less than a full, pain-free range of cervical motion, persistent paresthesia, or weakness should be protected and excluded from further athletic activity. These injuries should be referred to a physician for further radiographic and neurologic evaluations.

❖ **Cervical nerve syndrome.** Another common athletic injury to the neck is a cervical nerve syndrome. This is an injury resulting from forced lateral flexion, causing the nerve roots to be either stretched or impinged. This is commonly known as a "pinched nerve," "burner," "stinger," or "hot shot" and is characterized by sharp, burning, radiating pain. When the cervical plexus is involved, the athlete may complain of pain shooting into the posterior scalp, behind the ear, around the neck, or down the top of the shoulder. If the brachial plexus is involved, the athlete may complain of radiating pain, numbness, and loss of function of the arm and possibly the hand. Brachial plexus injuries are discussed in more detail in Chapter 20. Symptoms of a cervical nerve syndrome usually subside in minutes, but such injuries may leave residual soreness and paresthetic areas. Pain radiating into a specific dermatome is more likely the result of an isolated nerve root injury, whereas pain that persists in the entire upper extremity is most likely associated with a brachial plexus injury. Athletes whose paresthesia completely subsides, who demonstrate full muscle strength in the muscles of the upper extremity, and exhibit full, pain-free range of cervical motion, may return to athletic activity. Severe or repeated cervical nerve syndrome episodes should be evaluated by a physician. These athletes may have congenital or posttraumatic cervical spine abnormalities.

❖ **Cervical fractures and subluxations.**

Serious injuries of the cervical spine, such as fractures or dislocations, are not common in athletics; however, they do occur. The potential for this type of an injury is inherent in almost any sport. Football, however, provides the greatest potential for serious cervical spine injuries because the head is often used in blocking and tackling techniques. Diving and gymnastics also provide mechanisms for devastating neck injuries. As previously discussed, most fatal or paralyzing injuries occur when an athlete's neck is in flexion and receives a blow to the crown of the head, such as putting the head down and using the top of the head to make contact with an opponent. This type of mechanism can cause either a fracture or subluxations of the vertebrae, which may produce lesions to the spinal cord. The spinal cord may be completely or partially **transected, contused, or concussed.** A spinal cord contusion can cause edematous swelling within the cord, resulting in various degrees of temporary or permanent damage. A spinal cord concussion may cause transitory paralysis and symptoms, but complete recovery is usual. The major signs and symptoms that may indicate serious neck injuries include unremitting neck pain, muscle spasms, and evidence of spinal cord involvement such as numbness, loss of sensations, weakness, *paresthesia* (abnormal sensations such as burning or prickling), and partial or complete paralysis of the limbs. The athletic trainer must be aware of the significance of these important clues. They may indicate a serious spinal injury and require proper care and transportation of the injured athlete. It is especially important to provide proper care and transportation when a spinal injury is suspected.

Athletes may experience transient **quadriparesis** or quadriplegia from a cervical spine injury. This is also called **neurapraxia,** which means the cessation of function of a nerve without degenerative changes occurring. Symptoms may include burning pain, numbness, tingling, loss of sensation, weakness, or complete paralysis. Recovery of complete motor and sensory function usually occurs within a few minutes but may take 36 to 48 hours. Athletes exhibiting neur-apraxia or transient quadriparesis should be referred for further medical evaluation. Possible causes, other than a cervical fracture or dislocation, may be a spinal stenosis (narrowing), congenital abnormality, cervical instability, or intervertebral disk herniation.

Because most mechanisms causing cervical spine injuries involve forces to the head, injuries to the head and neck must be considered together. In all cases, both areas should be evaluated following trauma to the head. As was discussed in Chapter 12, any head injury severe enough to render an athlete unconscious must be handled as if there is also associated cervical spine involvement. Whenever there is any question concerning a neck injury, treat the athlete as if he or she has a serious cervical spine injury until proved otherwise.

Thoracic Spine

The basic anatomic characteristics typical of vertebrae in general are easily identified in the 12 components of the thoracic spine. The thoracic vertebra shows the least modification of the basic pattern. Figure 15-7 illustrates the anatomic components of a typical thoracic vertebra (T8). Transitional changes in appearance occur in individual vertebra toward the cervical and lumbar ends of the thoracic region. The first and twelfth thoracic vertebrae are distinctly transitional. Whereas T1 has a long and almost horizontal spinous process, the spine on T12 is short and broadened. The remaining spinous processes of thoracic vertebrae are long and tend to slope sharply downward.

The heart-shaped body of a typical thoracic vertebra is intermediate in size between those of the cervical and lumbar segments. Unique *costal facets* are found on each side of thoracic vertebrae at the junction of the body and lamina. Adjacent facets of contiguous (touching) vertebrae form an articular socket for the head of a rib. These facets are found only on thoracic vertebrae.

The thoracic spine is the most stable section of the vertebral column. Although a considerable ROM is possible, including flexion, extension, rotation, and lateral bending movements, the actual displacement between vertebrae is limited. Stability of the

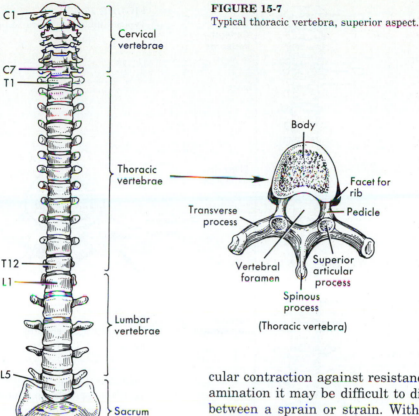

FIGURE 15-7
Typical thoracic vertebra, superior aspect.

Body

Facet for rib

Transverse process

Pedicle

Vertebral foramen

Superior articular process

Spinous process

(Thoracic vertebra)

thoracic spine results from the obliquely set articular facets, the thin intervertebral discs, the overlapping of the long spinous processes, and the attachment of the ribs. In addition, the well-developed anterior longitudinal and posterior longitudinal ligaments effectively limit motion. The functional price paid for stability in this region is restricted motion between individual vertebrae.

Thoracic spine injuries

Common athletic injuries to the thoracic spine are contusions, sprains, and strains. Contusions caused by a blow to the thoracic area commonly involve the paraspinal muscles, the muscles lateral to the spinous processes. Sprains and strains may be caused by overstretching the soft tissue surrounding the thoracic vertebrae or by violent mus-

cular contraction against resistance. On examination it may be difficult to distinguish between a sprain or strain. With either of these injuries there may be tenderness, spasm, and increased pain on active contraction or stretching. An athlete with a moderate to severe injury may exhibit a very stiff back and may resist any motion or movement of the thoracic spine.

Serious injuries to the thoracic spine are extremely rare in athletic activity. Fractures or dislocations are unusual because of the stable anatomy previously described. The most common serious injury is a compression fracture to the body of one of the thoracic vertebrae. The mechanism of injury is usually forced forward flexion of the thoracic spine, which compresses the anterior portion of adjacent vertebral bodies. Typically, the athlete will give a history of sharp forward flexion, resulting in a jackknifing effect. This can occur as an athlete falls violently on the buttocks or is forced into extreme flexion of the thoracic spine. An athlete with a compression fracture will usually have no neurologic complaints and will be able to move around and even walk. However, the athlete will complain of constant localized pain, which may be increased with

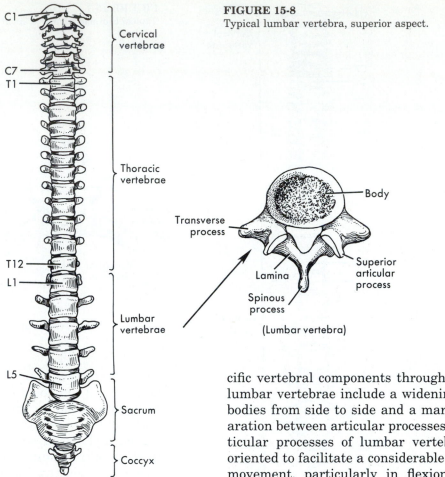

C1

Cervical vertebrae

C7

T1

Thoracic vertebrae

T12

L1

Lumbar vertebrae

L5

Sacrum

Coccyx

Anterior view

FIGURE 15-8
Typical lumbar vertebra, superior aspect.

Body

Transverse process

Superior articular process

Lamina

Spinous process

(Lumbar vertebra)

any movement of this area of the spine and should be referred for further evaluation and radiographs.

Lumbar Spine

The five lumbar vertebrae differ from the thoracic vertebrae in their larger size and absence of costal facets. A typical lumbar vertebra (L3) is shown in Figure 15-8. The massive bodies of these vertebrae are designed to stabilize and accommodate the increasing body weight that must be supported toward the lower end of the spinal column. The prominent lumbar curve, an anterior convexity somewhat deeper in women than men, helps project the weight of the torso onto the lower limbs.

Progressive changes in appearance of spe-

cific vertebral components through the five lumbar vertebrae include a widening of the bodies from side to side and a marked separation between articular processes. The articular processes of lumbar vertebrae are oriented to facilitate a considerable range of movement, particularly in flexion, extension, and side-to-side bending. Rotation in the lumbar region is very limited because of the positions of these articular facets.

The hatchet-shaped spinous processes of lumbar vertebrae are horizontal and extend posteriorly from a triangular vertebral foramen. The horizontal orientation of the spinous processes makes it possible to insert a needle between two adjacent vertebrae and enter the vertebral canal to sample cerebrospinal fluid. This process, usually accomplished between L3 and L4, is known as a **lumbar puncture.**

Lumbosacral joint

The body weight is supported by the opposing surfaces of the first sacral and fifth lumbar vertebra and by the two articulations between the superior sacral and inferior lumbar articular processes. Articulations between the last, or fifth, lumbar vertebra and the sacrum are similar to the joints that exist between the movable vertebrae in the spine above. However, the intervertebral disc located between L5 and the sacrum is very thick, especially along its anterior border. This articulation is the meeting place of the movable lumbar spine above with the fixed and rigid sacrum below. It is notorious as a frequent site of pain. The lumbosacral angle has a rather extensive normal range of variation but averages about 120° in most adults.

The anterior surface of the lumbosacral joint lies in a straight line directly below the occipital condyles when the body is erect and the posture normal. The joint also marks the termination of the lumbar convexity (which begins at T12) and the commencement of the sacral concavity. The fifth lumbar vertebra may be joined in whole or in part to the sacrum. This is known as **sacralization** of the fifth lumbar vertebra. The condition is often devoid of symptoms but may be the cause of back pain in some athletes.

The two bones entering into the lumbosacral articulation are held together by a host of very strong ligaments. Sprains are common, however, if this body area is subjected to direct blows or sudden twisting movements. Lordosis increases the possibility of ligament sprains in this area. The major ligaments associated with the lumbosacral junction can be evaluated by asking the athlete to lie supine on a table and hyperflex both thighs on the abdomen. This position stresses the ligaments and elicits point tenderness and pain if ligament injuries are present.

The lumbosacral trunk (fourth and fifth lumbar nerves) is in close approximation to each side of the lumbosacral joint. Both the fourth and fifth lumbar nerves emerge from the spine through long bony canals, or tunnels, and are subject to compression injuries that may be caused by muscle spasms or direct trauma in the joint area. Because the fourth and fifth lumbar nerves are the principal constituents of the sciatic nerve (L4, L5; S1, S2, S3), irritation to L4 or L5 can cause or contribute to the pain syndrome commonly called **sciatica**.

Lumbar spine injuries

The lumbar spine, or lower back, is an area that is subjected to many types of stresses and forces during athletic, as well as nonathletic, activity. The lower back is very susceptible to injury, and athletes frequently complain of pain in this area. The majority of low back pain in athletes is caused by either acute trauma or chronic stresses. Occasionally, low back pain is caused by structural defects in the vertebrae or intervertebral discs. All conditions affecting the lumbar spine can be aggravated by various contributing factors such as inadequate or inappropriate conditioning, inflexibility, congenital anomalies, or poor postural habits. Each of these factors should be kept in mind when evaluating injuries to the lumbar spine area.

Common athletic injuries to the lower back are contusions, sprains, and strains. Contusions are more common in the paraspinal muscles but may also occur over the subcutaneous spinous processes. The athlete will often have a history of a direct blow to the lumbar area, with localized tenderness and pain on movement. Sprains and strains are common in the multiplicity of muscles and ligaments in the lower back; these injuries can be caused by the same types of mechanisms and may occur simultaneously. Violent muscle contractions against resistance, overuse, and overstretching are common mechanisms resulting in sprains or strains in the soft tissues along the spine. The complex anatomy of the lower back makes it very difficult to stress and evaluate specific muscles and ligaments. As a result, it is difficult to differentiate between a sprain and a strain in this area. Fortunately, it is also usually unnecessary because both of these injuries are treated symptomatically.

Severe injuries to the lumbar spine such as fractures or dislocations are extremely rare in athletic activity. Neurologic damage as a result of such an injury is also not as likely as in the cervical spine because the spinal cord ends at about the first lumbar vertebrae and the peripheral nerves in the cauda equina are more mobile and resistant

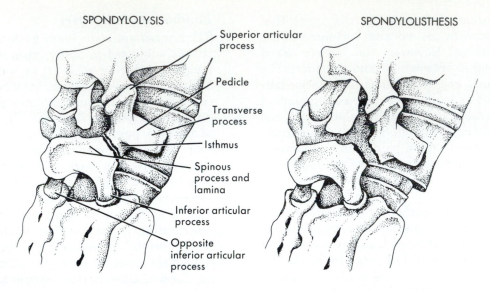

FIGURE 15-9
Spondylolysis and spondylolisthesis. Refer to text for description.

to trauma. Compression fractures, as previously described in the thoracic spine, can also occur to the bodies of the lumbar vertebrae. However, the most common fractures in the lower back involve the spinous or transverse processes. These can occur as a result of a direct blow or violent muscle contraction. Fractures of this type are at times indistinguishable from severe strains or contusions without radiographs.

❖   **Spondylolysis.** The most common structural defect of the lumbar spine in athletes is a condition called spondylolysis, which is a defect in the pars interarticularis of the vertebrae (Figure 15-9). If this defect is bilateral, it may allow that vertebra to slip forward on the vertebra or sacrum below, a con-
❖ dition called **spondylolisthesis.** It may develop in athletes involved in strenuous exercise or competition. Many authorities consider this condition to be a stress fracture and the result of repeated trauma and stress rather than an acute fracture. It is also believed that spondylolysis and spondylolisthesis can be congenital. The athlete with spondylolisthesis will usually complain of low back pain associated with increased activity. With rest or inactivity the pain di-

minishes, only to return again when activity is resumed. In addition to the pain in the lower back, the athlete may complain of pain radiating into the buttocks and upper thighs. The appearance of radiating pain, as well as recurrent episodes of low back pain with activity, should alert the athletic trainer to refer this athlete for further diagnosis and radiographs. Occasionally the pain level remains tolerable and the athlete continues activity without ever knowing about the spondylolisthesis.

❖   **Intervertebral disc herniation.** Another structural defect that may occur in the lumbar spine of an athlete is intervertebral disc herniation. In this condition the nucleus pulposus herniates through the annulus fibrosus and presses against the spinal cord
❖ or the spinal nerve roots (**nerve root compression**). Although this condition is more common in people in their 30s and 40s, it can also occur in younger athletes. The athlete with a ruptured or herniated disc will normally have extreme pain and stiffness in the lower back, pain in the buttocks, and a unique type of radiating leg pain if the compression is severe. This leg pain is usually unilateral and follows the route of the sciatic

nerve, which is formed by the fourth and fifth lumbar nerves and the first, second, and third sacral nerves. Pain may radiate down into the thigh, calf, and foot, depending on the nerve roots involved. Sitting for prolonged periods of time, standing with both legs straight, or bending over will be especially uncomfortable for these athletes. Additional signs that may indicate a herniated disc include unilateral muscle weakness, sensory loss, or reflex loss in the leg. Athletes with signs and symptoms of this type must be referred for further evaluation.

✤ Additional terms with which an athletic trainer should be familiar are **spondylitis,** which is an inflammation of the vertebrae,
✤ and **spondylosis,** which refers to degenerative changes of the vertebrae and can include bony (osteophyte) formation at the disc spaces. This can lead to nerve root entrapment at the spinal foramina.

Spina bifida occulta. Congenital anomalies are more common in the lumbar area than in any other segment of the spine. The most common of these is spina bifida occulta, which is a defect in the bony spinal canal without involvement of the spinal cord or meninges. This condition is usually noted only on a radiograph and, unless it is quite severe, causes only intermittent and moderate discomfort in the lower back. Athletes with spina bifida occulta have a higher incidence of low back pain and should be instructed in proper techniques to help protect this vulnerable area. Proper techniques include appropriate exercise and strength training, correct lifting procedures, and avoidance of sudden stressful loads on the lumbar spine.

Sacrum and Coccyx

The sacral and coccygeal portions of the spine are often referred to as the false, or fixed, vertebrae (Chapter 3). Together, the sacrum and coccyx form the terminal portion of the spinal column. In addition, they form the strong wedge-shaped posterior portion of the bony pelvis. Numerous ligaments of the sacrum and coccyx attach to portions of the lumbar vertebrae above and to points on the bony pelvis laterally and below.

The sacrum (Figure 15-10) is a large wedge-shaped structure formed by the fusion of five vertebrae. The inner (pelvic) surface of the sacrum is smooth and concave, whereas the outer (posterior) surface is convex and rough. The upper portion (base) articulates with the body of the fifth lumbar vertebra, and the lower portion (apex) articulates with the coccyx below. The concave inner surface is grooved by four *transverse ridges* that show the points of separation between the original bodies of the five sacral vertebrae before fusion. At each end of the transverse ridges are large openings (sacral foramina), which accommodate the sacral nerves and arteries. The prominent *sacral promontory* is a bony prominence projecting from the anterior border of the base.

The coccyx forms the bony tip of the spine. It is generally a single, triangular bone fused from four rudimentary vertebrae. These vertebrae are very small and consist of only the fused body and poorly developed transverse processes. No laminae or spinous processes are present. Occasionally, the first element, or vertebra, in the coccyx may be separate from the rest. The upper (superior) portion of the coccyx, called the base, articulates with the sacrum. The coccyx diminishes in size until it reaches the tip (apex). Athletic injuries to the coccyx are not common but may occur from a direct blow to the area, such as a kick or a fall to a sitting position. Although these injuries may be painful, they generally are not disabling and require only routine treatment procedures.

Sacroiliac joints

The sacroiliac joint is formed by the articulation between the sacrum and the iliac portion of the hip bones (innominate bones) on each side of the pelvis. It is a true synovial joint, but movement is limited by the presence of interlocking facets of bone and by extremely strong and dense ligaments. There is no direct muscle control at this joint. However, the sacroiliac joints are influenced by the action of the muscles moving the lumbar spine and hip because many of these muscles attach to the sacrum and pelvis. Any appreciable movement in either or

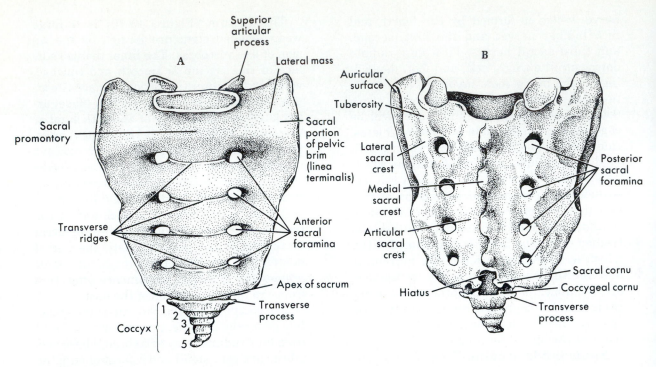

FIGURE 15-10
Sacrum and coccyx. **A**, Anterior view; **B**, posterior view.

both of the sacroiliac joints leads to gross instability in the erect posture. In the sitting or standing position, the full weight of the body above the pelvis passes through these joints. Therefore freedom of motion must be sacrificed for stability. The slight movement that does occur at the sacroiliac joints decreases with age and an individual becomes stiffer.

The sacrum hangs from the sacroiliac joints and is kept from being pushed forward into the pelvis by the interlocking facets of bone and by the *posterior sacroiliac ligaments*, which are among the strongest in the body. The dimple on each side immediately above the buttock is a useful external surface landmark that defines the center of the sacroiliac joint in most young adults. True sacroiliac sprains rarely occur as a result of athletic activity, especially in a young athlete.

Sacroiliac sprains may occur as a result of acute or chronic trauma. They may result from a single maneuver, twist, or awkward movement, or from overuse associated with poor posture, lifting techniques, or strenuous maneuvers repeated many times. Symptoms of a sacroiliac sprain include stiffness or a consistent soreness of the sacroiliac joint area that is better in the morning but gets worse as the day goes on. There are no neurologic signs, but there may be referred pain into the back of the thigh, groin, or hamstrings. Heat and activity may diminish the discomfort during activity, but the pain returns as soon as the athlete cools down.

ATHLETIC INJURY ASSESSMENT PROCESS

The potential for spinal injuries resulting in neurologic damage such as permanent paralysis or death is present in most athletic activities, especially contact sports. With any injury involving the spine, it is extremely important for the athletic trainer to recognize the possibilities for neurologic involvement as quickly as possible. Selection of appropriate assessment procedures, handling maneuvers, and transportation techniques depends on the possibility of involvement of the spinal cord. Added neurologic damage can occur during improper positioning or movement of an injured athlete. At no time in the assessment of athletic injuries is the principle "do no harm" more important than when evaluating and caring for injuries involving the spine.

Athletic trainers should have an emergency action plan developed with local emergency personnel for proper handling of a spine injury. This plan should be prepared in advance of any emergency and practiced periodically to ensure it will work effectively and smoothly if needed.

Athletes suffering an injury to the spine generally present themselves in one of two modes. The athlete may suffer a traumatic injury and remain lying on the court or field. In these instances the injured athlete should be treated as though he or she has sustained a serious spinal cord injury until proved otherwise. This includes protecting the injured athlete from any unnecessary movement during the assessment process until you can be sure there is no spinal cord involvement. It is common, however, for athletes with an injury to the back or neck to be moving about. They often walk into the training room complaining of pain. In dealing with injuries of this type, it is relatively safe to assume there is no serious neurologic involvement. This large group of injuries includes those caused by acute trauma and chronic stresses.

Primary survey

The primary survey is of utmost importance when an injured athlete remains down and appears to be unresponsive or unconscious. Maintenance of airway, breathing, and circulation must then be primary considerations. Remember, whenever a neck injury is suspected, movement of the cervical spine must not occur. If the athlete is unconscious and a neck injury is suspected, the jaw-thrust method of opening the airway is the safest technique to use. If the injured athlete is lying face down and must be moved to a

face-up position, it is extremely important that he or she be rolled or moved as a unit to avoid any unnecessary movements of the spine. The safest and easiest procedure to accomplish this is to logroll the athlete into a face-up position. This procedure requires several individuals to be accomplished effectively. A leader must immobilize the head and neck and command the other individuals who are positioned along the side of the injured athlete. They must maintain the body in line with the head and spine during the roll. All athletic trainers should be familiar with and practice the logroll procedure. After assurance that the respiratory and circulatory states of the injured athlete are adequate, proceed to the secondary survey and a more detailed neurologic evaluation.

Secondary survey

The evaluation procedures used during the secondary survey depend on the responsiveness and position of the injured athlete. A quick glance at the overall picture will generally determine the direction in which the athletic trainer will proceed with the secondary survey. It is important to maintain a high index of suspicion whenever assessing spine injuries because there may be associated damage to the spinal cord or peripheral nerve roots. It can be very difficult for the athletic trainer to determine which spine injuries threaten nerve function and which do not. Therefore it is best to consider all spine injuries as potentially dangerous and handle them accordingly.

Caring for an athlete with a potentially serious spinal injury can manifest many distracting factors, such as those from family, teammates, coaches, and officials. Athletic trainers must remain calm and take control of emergency situations in which others may panic, offer well-meaning advice, or attempt to hurry the process for any reason.

The unconscious athlete must be managed as if a spinal injury has occurred, as discussed in Chapter 12. The athlete who is responsive but remains lying on the floor or ground following a traumatic injury must also be evaluated and handled with utmost caution in the position he or she is found. If a spinal injury is unstable, the vertebral column is no longer able to protect the spinal cord and may actually cause added neurologic damage during any type of positioning or movement. If necessary, the entire secondary survey can be accomplished with the athlete remaining in the original position. Remember, whenever neurologic involvement is recognized or suspected, it is not necessary to continue the assessment process; it is time to seek medical assistance or activate the emergency medical system. It is of paramount importance to protect the injured athlete from further aggravation of any neurologic involvement. Do not move the injured athlete unless it is absolutely necessary. Examination of the neck and immobilization of the spine should precede all other maneuvers of the secondary survey in circumstances in which there is reason to believe that a spinal injury may have occurred. The initial assessment of possible neurologic involvement consists of motor and sensory testing.

Paralysis. Is there any paralysis? Paralysis is the most reliable sign of spinal cord injury. Spinal cord injuries in the neck may cause paralysis of all four extremities **(quadriplegia)** and breathing impairment. Spinal cord injuries below the neck may cause paralysis of the lower extremities **(paraplegia),** with no impairment of breathing functions. However, a spinal cord injury may not manifest itself with symptoms of complete paralysis. An athlete may demonstrate a partial, or incomplete, paralysis **(paresis).**

Muscle function. Test muscle function by requesting very gentle active movements, such as asking the athlete to carefully move his or her fingers or toes. Then proceed to the larger joints such as the wrists, elbows, shoulders, ankles, knees, and hips. Table 15-1 lists nerve root distributions and key movements to test each spinal nerve. Muscles are often supplied by more than one nerve segment; however, only the primary nerve root source is listed. If the athlete has

TABLE 15-1

Segmental Nerve Root Distributions

Segment	Key movements to test	Key sensory areas to test
C1-C4	Neck flexion	Head and face
C3	Neck lateral flexion	Lateral neck
C4	Shoulder elevation	Top of shoulder
C5	Shoulder abduction	Lateral arm and forearm
C6	Elbow flexion, wrist extension	Thumb and index finger
C7	Elbow extension, wrist flexion	Middle finger
C8	Ulnar deviation, thumb extension	Ring and small finger
T1	Approximation of fingers	Medial forearm
L1-L2	Hip flexion	Front of thigh
L3	Knee extension	Front of knee
L4	Ankle dorsiflexion	Medial leg
L5	Toe extension	Lateral leg
S1	Ankle plantar flexion	Sole of foot
S2	Knee flexion	Back of thigh

normal motion in the extremities, proceed to check the speed and strength of movements. The speed of movement can be evaluated by having the athlete open and close the fingers or move the toes quickly. Strength can be evaluated by putting resistance against the active motion. Any demonstrable weakness or loss of function should be considered and managed as a spinal cord injury. Remember to always compare extremities on both sides of the body to note any difference in motion, speed, or strength. It is possible the spinal injury involved nerves on only one side of the body.

Sensations. The loss of voluntary movement in the extremities is usually accompanied by loss of sensations. Sensory function can be evaluated by stimulating the skin of the arms, trunk, and legs with a light touch or sharp object such as a safety pin. Does the athlete perceive the touch and/or pain stimulus appropriately and symmetrically? Are sensations absent *(anesthesia),* decreased, exaggerated, or delayed? Recalling the distribution of dermatomes allows you to locate the dermatomes where sensations are altered (Table 15-1). Try to test as many dermatomes as possible by distributing the stimuli over the body. An athlete may also complain of abnormal sensations *(paresthesia)* such as burning, tingling, or prickling in the extremities. These paresthesias may follow a specific dermatome pattern. It is important that these be recognized as symptoms of possible spinal cord injury and appropriate emergency care measures initiated. It may take a detailed neurologic evaluation to detect minor neural problems, but if the injured athlete has normal sensations, motion, speed, and strength in the extremities, it can be assumed that no serious spinal cord injury has occurred.

Fortunately, the majority of the athletic injuries involving the spine are not serious and consist of contusions, sprains, and strains. In these instances, the secondary survey can provide information necessary to recognize the structures involved and the extent of injury. In addition, the secondary survey can assist the athletic trainer to determine if referral and further evaluation is necessary, which treatment procedures to follow, and when the athlete can safely return to activity.

Always remember that a cervical spine injury can occur with a head injury. Both areas should be evaluated simultaneously. As discussed in the previous chapter, it is important to establish and monitor an athlete's level of consciousness to recognize possible intracranial involvement associated with a head injury.

History

The history of an injury involving the spine is very important. If the athlete remains down after an injury, the initial questioning must be directed at determining the nature and the site of the injury. If the head, neck, or back is involved in the injury, questioning must be directed at recognizing any possible neurologic involvement, as previously discussed. For the athlete who does not appear to have any spinal cord involvement, attempt to gain as much information sur-

rounding the circumstances of the injury as possible. Begin by asking the athlete to express his or her feelings and sensations.

Pain. Question the athlete about pain associated with the injury. Is there any pain in the neck or back? Where is the pain located? How severe is the pain? The athlete with unremitting neck or back pain should be handled as if there is spinal cord involvement. Occasionally, the injured athlete, lying very still, will not complain of much pain until movement of the injured area of the spine is attempted. If pain is increased significantly when an athlete attempts to move, he or she should be managed as if the spinal cord is involved. The athletic trainer should encourage an athlete with possible neck or back injuries to remain motionless.

At this time it may be necessary to palpate and localize the painful or tender areas. Avoid moving the injured athlete during this process. The spinous processes can be palpated by carefully placing your hand under the neck or back. Localized deformity, tenderness, or increased pain detected immediately over the spinous processes is sufficient reason to suspect an injury to the spinal column, and the athlete should be handled as if there is spinal cord involvement.

Continue to investigate the tender and painful areas. Are there muscle spasms or tightness associated with the pain? If possible, ask the athlete to point to the painful areas. Notice if the athlete can localize the pain or if it appears to cover a large area. Also notice if the athlete is complaining of pain in the soft tissues along either side of the spine or over the bony spinous processes. Does the athlete have a difficult time specifying where the pain is? Ask for a description and the location of the pain. For example, is the pain sharp, burning, or a dull ache? Is the pain constant or intermittent? Is there any radiating pain into the arms, shoulders, thighs, or legs? Are there certain types of movements or exercises that aggravate or increase the pain? Is the pain relieved by rest or certain positions?

Mechanism of injury. Attempt to determine the mechanism of injury, including the type of forces or stresses that occurred. Does the injury appear to be the result of an acute traumatic episode or the accumulation of chronic stresses that have developed over a period of time? Was the injury caused by a direct blow or was the spine stretched, strained, or twisted?

Previous history. Many injuries to the spine are chronic conditions that do not arise from a single acute injury. These chronic conditions represent an aggravation of previously existing circumstances, such as congenital abnormalities, structural deviations, postural habits, or previous injuries. Therefore a complete history of any previous neck or back complaints should be sought. The history should include information that might link previous injuries to the current problem. Ask how the symptoms began and what has occurred from the time of onset until the present. How did the pain first start? Was the athlete injured? Are the symptoms affected by posture, rest, or activity? What treatment procedures have been carried out on the injured athlete, and have they helped? Knowing the past history and behavior of symptoms gives the athletic trainer important information to assist in recognizing possible causes and determining treatment procedures.

Observation

Initial observations are extremely important in determining which assessment procedures to use and in what sequence. Watch very carefully as you approach an injured athlete. Is the athlete lying motionless? If so, you should expect and treat the athlete as if he or she has suffered a serious spinal injury until proved otherwise. Is the athlete attempting any movement of the neck or extremities? Remember, an athlete who has suffered a serious cervical spine injury will be very cautious and defensive of any movements of the neck.

Deformities. Watch closely as you complete the history process and talk with the injured athlete. Look for obvious deformities or abnormal positions. Observations may be difficult because of the position of the ath-

lete. For example, if the athlete is lying on his or her back, it is extremely difficult to view the spine without some movement. Uniforms and equipment may also conceal the injured area. If the area can be viewed, look for any deformity of the spine. The spinous processes may appear crooked or out of place, which is an extremely reliable sign. However, the spine rarely appears deformed, even with very severe injuries, and the absence of deformity does not rule out the possibility of a fracture or dislocation.

Signs of trauma. Look for any signs of trauma that may give additional clues to the nature and severity of the injury. If the areas can be viewed, look for cuts and bruises about the head, face, shoulders, back, and abdomen. These physical signs can indicate what types of forces have been applied to the athlete's body and help establish the mechanism of injury. Also watch for any signs that may indicate neurologic involvement such as paralysis or weakness.

Movements and positions. If the athlete is moving about and spinal cord involvement is not suspected, observe his or her movements and the positions preferred. Voluntary movements can be revealing when the athlete is unaware you are examining his or her actions. During an obvious and intentional examination of gait or posture, an athlete may intentionally move or assume a position considered proper or one that depicts an extremely painful state. Either of these may not accurately reflect the symptoms associated with the injured neck or back. Every athletic trainer should develop a protocol for observing the main postures and positions of the body during all types of activity.

Watch the athlete's gait pattern and willingness to move about. Does the athlete appear to (1) stand, walk, and move about normally and without pain, (2) move very cautiously as if in pain, or (3) avoid bending, twisting, or other motions that could be painful? Can the athlete relax, or does he or she seem to have a difficult time finding a comfortable position? Which standing, sitting, or lying positions does the injured athlete prefer or consciously avoid?

Alignment of the neck and back. Evaluating an athlete's postural alignment may reveal underlying causes of neck or back conditions. This is especially true of chronic or overuse conditions affecting the lower back. Athletic injuries and painful conditions can result from malalignments and poor postural habits, which are intensified by heavy or intense athletic activities. Therefore an athletic trainer should understand the fundamental concepts of body alignment and posture.

Posture. Posture is an individual matter. There is no single best or most appropriate posture for all persons. For each athlete, the best posture is that in which the body segments are balanced in the position of least strain and most support. Posture and body mechanics must be considered from the standpoint of the athlete's body build and the activities in which the athlete is involved. Minor postural differences in healthy active athletes are usually of little consequence because the body has a remarkable ability to compensate for deviations from the norm. Athletic activity can lead to postural adaptations, but these do not necessarily cause injuries. Each individual instance requires careful professional judgment. An athletic trainer should be able to recognize moderate to severe deviations in alignment or posture that may be associated with an injury or painful condition. The ability to recognize these factors allows the athletic trainer to refer the athlete for more definitive diagnosis or develop effective exercise programs designed to increase strength or flexibility and to aid in preparing strategies to change body mechanics or improve poor postural habits.

This evaluation of alignment or posture is also important when an injury alters an athlete's posture. Pain and muscle spasms associated with an athletic injury can change the positioning and posture of an athlete. As long as symptoms persist, normal posture may not be possible. Occasionally a faulty postural habit is established that may continue after the injury has healed. Therefore

continuing evaluation of body alignment or posture can serve as a basis for measuring future progress and improving faulty postural habits resulting from injury.

Evaluate the alignment or posture with the athlete standing in shorts or other brief clothing so that the back is bare. For women, this is best performed with the athlete in a two-piece swim suit or halter top. Observe the general body build and development of the athlete. Notice if the athlete can stand evenly with both feet flat on the floor. Occasionally, because of pain, an athlete will be unable to bear weight equally on both feet and the bodyweight will be shifted toward one side.

The athlete should be viewed from the back, front, and side. When evaluating injuries to the spine, it is probably most revealing to view the athlete from the back first. Standing behind the athlete, survey the entire spine, as well as the relationship of the head, shoulders, and pelvis. Normal alignment of the body when viewed from the rear is illustrated in Figure 15-11. An imaginary vertical line should bisect the body into symmetric halves. Any irregularities in symmetry should be noted because they may indicate circumstances that contributed to the injury or painful condition, such as a short leg, muscle weakness, or spinal curvature. Remember, irregularities in symmetry can also result directly from an injury and may be caused by muscle spasms or pain.

When viewing the athlete's spine from the back, you should first consider the level of the pelvis. The pelvis is the "keystone," or foundation, of the spine. When the pelvis is not level, the spine and upper body must compensate in an attempt to keep the body alignment balanced. Determining the level of the pelvis can be accomplished by several methods. The easiest method is to place your fingertips on each iliac crest and check the horizontal level of your fingers or the relative heights of each anterior superior iliac spine (Figure 15-12). Another method to determine relative heights of each side of the pelvis is to palpate both posterior superior

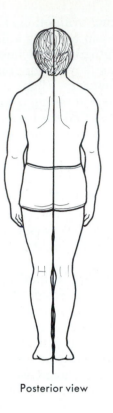

Posterior view

FIGURE 15-11
Normal alignment of the body when viewed from the back.

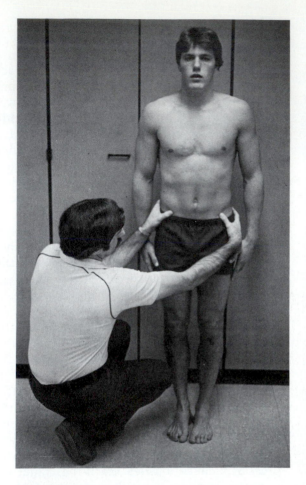

FIGURE 15-12
Palpating anterior superior iliac spines to determine level of pelvis.

iliac spines simultaneously to determine if they are in the same horizontal plane.

Whenever a pelvic obliquity is observed, a discrepancy in leg length should be suspected and evaluated further. A discrepancy in leg length, either actual or functional, can cause an imbalance and contribute to an injury or produce overuse symptoms in the back, pelvis, or lower extremities. To determine if a leg length discrepancy exists, have the athlete lie supine, place both legs in a neutral position, and observe the medial malleoli (Figure 15-13). If the malleoli do not appear to match, a difference in leg length should be suspected. To determine if there is an actual discrepancy in leg length, measure and compare the distance from the anterior superior iliac spine to the medial malleolus of each ankle (Figure 15-14). Unequal distances between these bony landmarks indicate an actual difference in leg length. If

the length of the legs is the same, but the level of the pelvis is uneven, the pelvis is tilted laterally, resulting in one leg being functionally shorter. This pelvic obliquity can be caused by an injury or problem in the back, hips, knees, or feet.

It is doubtful that minor leg length discrepancies cause significant injury symptoms. However, when a leg length discrepancy is encountered, the relevance of the discrepancy to the athlete's symptoms should be investigated further. For example, is pain associated with the condition increased by standing and walking? If not, the difference in leg length is likely to be irrelevant. If pain is produced by standing and

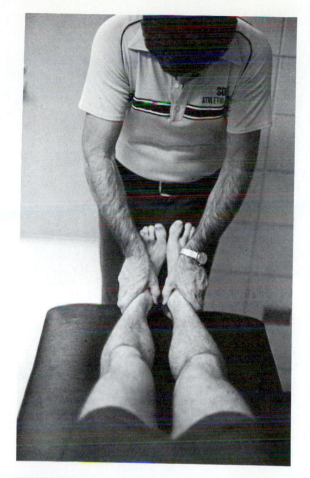

FIGURE 15-13
Observing alignment of medial malleoli to determine
if a leg length discrepancy exists.

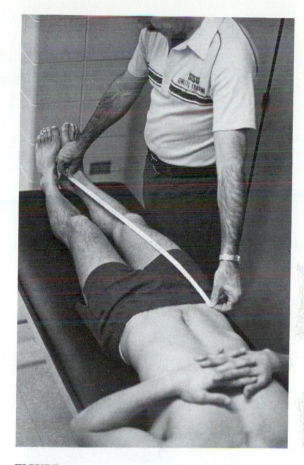

FIGURE 15-14
Measuring distance between the anterior superior
iliac spine to the medial malleolus. Compare both
sides to determine if an actual leg length discrepancy
exists.

walking, perhaps the leg length discrepancy
has an effect on the athlete's symptoms and
the athlete should be referred for medical
evaluation.

The back view can also indicate whether
the spine appears straight. The spinous processes of each vertebra should appear in a
straight line from top to bottom. Any lateral
deviation of the spinal column is called **scoliosis** (Figure 15-15). It is among the most
serious of postural deviations. Later stages
of scoliosis can cause asymmetry of the
upper extremities, shoulders, thorax, pelvis,
and lower extremities. Minor lateral deviations of the vertebral column can result from
athletic activity that uses one side of the
body more than the other, or from symptoms
of an acute injury. Unilateral spasm of vertebral muscles caused by the pull of a ski
tow rope, for example, would result in such
lateral deviation. Lateral deviations that remain after the cessation of injury symptoms,
and especially those found in young athletes,
should be referred to a physician for further
diagnosis and treatment. The early stages of
scoliosis can be corrected by proper treatment.

Additional postural alignments that
should be viewed from the back of an athlete
include positioning of the shoulders and
scapulae. Both shoulders should be at an
equal height or in the same horizontal plane.

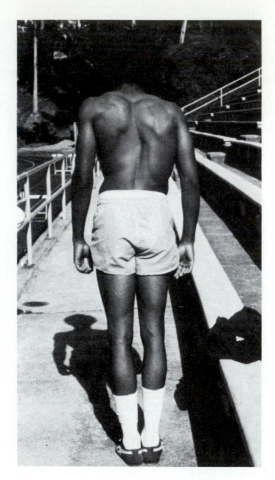

FIGURE 15-15
Athlete with a scoliosis.

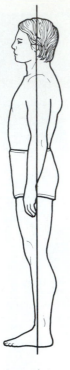

Lateral view

FIGURE 15-16
Normal alignment of the body when viewed from the side.

Unequal height of the shoulders may result from such conditions as lateral curvature of the spine, unequal development of the shoulder girdle musculature, or injury symptoms. It is important to determine whether the unequal shoulder height is caused by local injury or by such remote conditions as leg length discrepancy or lateral curvature of the spine. Both scapulae should also be level and positioned an equal distance from the vertebral column. Occasionally, both scapulae will be a greater distance from the vertebral column than is considered normal. This condition results in the scapula pulling away from the rib cage and is called **winged scapula.** It is usually caused by muscular

weakness and can generally be improved with an exercise program.

When viewing the back of an athlete, head position is an important consideration in assessing spinal alignment. The head should be held in a level, well-balanced position. Occasionally, because of pain and muscle spasms in the cervical musculature, an athlete's neck may be slightly twisted, resulting in the head being held in an unnatural position. This is called **torticollis,** or wryneck.

When evaluating the alignment or posture of the body, the athlete should also be viewed from the side. Normal alignment of the body when viewed from the side is illustrated in Figure 15-16. An imaginary vertical line should pass through the ear lobe, tip of the shoulder, and greater trochanter of the femur, posterior to the patella, and anterior to the lateral malleolus. This side view of

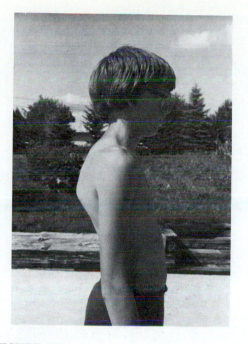

FIGURE 15-17
Young athlete exhibiting rounded shoulders (kyphosis).

body alignment allows the athletic trainer to analyze the anteroposterior curvatures of the spine. Normal spinal curvatures include a concave curve at the cervical and lumbar spine areas and a convex curve of the thoracic spine.

A common postural deviation in athletes is an accentuation of the forward curve of the lumbar spine. This is called **lumbar lordosis** and usually results in forward tilting of the pelvis. Lumbar lordosis is usually associated with weakened and elongated abdominal muscles and contracted and tight muscles of the lower back. This muscular imbalance results in tilting the pelvis anteriorly, creating the common swayback or hollow back appearance. Lumbar lordosis can be improved or overcome by an exercise program involving stretching the lower back muscles, strengthening the abdominals, and making a concerted effort to reestablish proper pelvic alignment.

An exaggerated curve in the thoracic spine is called **kyphosis,** which is an abnormal rounding of the upper back (Figure 15-

17). This condition is often associated with **forward shoulders,** in which the shoulders are carried abnormally forward of the imaginary vertical line described previously. These conditions are usually associated with muscular tightness in the chest and stretched, weakened muscles of the upper back region.

The head should be held in a well-balanced position directly above the shoulders. A common deviation from what is considered normal alignment is **forward head.** This condition occurs when an athlete carries his or her head in an abnormal anterior position, which can result in weakened cervical extensor muscles and tightened flexor muscles. The forward head may become realigned by development of **cervical lordosis,** an accentuation of the normal curvature of the cervical spine.

An alternative method of evaluating the alignment of the body is to have the athlete stand with his or her back against a wall (Figure 15-18). Instruct the athlete to stand straight with the heels within 2 inches of the wall. The back of the head, scapular area, and the buttocks should touch the wall. In this position it is easier to recognize anteroposterior problems such as lumbar lordosis, forward shoulders, or forward head. You can also have the athlete actually participate in the evaluation process. Ask the athlete to place a hand in the small of the back to evaluate spinal curvature in this area. Normally a person should be able to slip a hand in between the wall and the lumbar spine. If there is more room than that and one is able to wiggle the hand around freely, there is probably some degree of lordosis. Using the wall in analyzing posture is an excellent method of allowing athletes to evaluate and monitor their own postural habits.

Physical Examination

Some physical examination procedures were already discussed just before the history portion of this assessment process. These procedures were used to evaluate the neurologic status (motor and sensory functions) of the injured athlete. It is important to use these

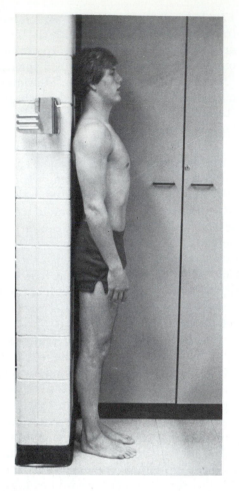

FIGURE 15-18
Wall test to observe anterior posterior alignment of the spine.

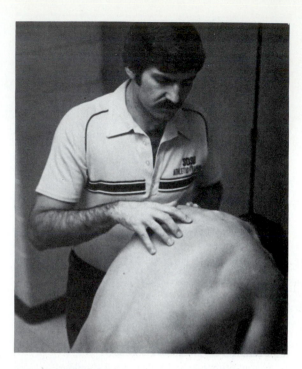

FIGURE 15-19
Palpating spinous processes with the spine in flexion.

procedures early in the assessment of spinal injuries to recognize possible spinal cord involvement. There are many additional assessment techniques used on spinal injuries not suspected of involving the spinal cord. The order in which these techniques are used will depend on the signs and symptoms exhibited by the injured athlete.

Palpation

Palpation procedures are used for the purpose of localizing the injured area. Carefully palpate along the spinous processes, as well as the paraspinal muscles, in an attempt to localize tenderness or muscle spasms associated with the injury. It may be helpful to

have the athlete hunch the shoulders forward or slightly flex the spine so that the spinous processes are more pronounced (Figure 15-19). If the athlete can assist in the examination in this way it will highlight anatomic landmarks in the area and help the examiner localize the injury. Even with this type of help, however, it may be difficult to identify the exact structures involved in an injury because many of the structures about the spine are deep and not subcutaneous. In addition, there may be a great deal of generalized muscle spasm or referred pain associated with the injury, making it difficult to define exactly which structures are injured. Every effort should be made, however, to localize the painful areas as precisely as possible and correlate this information with active and resistive movements described in the next section.

Movement Procedures

Appropriate movement procedures can be very helpful in the assessment of the more

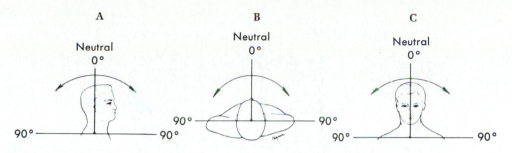

FIGURE 15-20
Active ROM of the cervical spine. **A**, Flexion and extension. These motions can be estimated in degrees or indicated by the distance the chin lacks from touching the chest. **B**, Rotation can be estimated in degrees or in percentages of motion compared in each direction. **C**, Lateral bending can be estimated in degrees or indicated by the number of inches the ear lacks from reaching the shoulders.

common injuries to the spine. It is important to remember that if pain is increased considerably on any attempt to move the spine, or if the athlete aggressively resists moving the spine, he or she should be handled as if there may be serious spinal injury. In these cases the athlete must not be subjected to continued movement or manipulation, but, instead, should be protected from further trauma and referred to a physician.

Active movements. Active movements were already discussed briefly to evaluate muscle function and test spinal nerves. It is important to use active movements early in the assessment of spinal injuries to recognize possible spinal cord or nerve root involvement.

Active movements are certainly the first type of stress maneuvers that should be attempted by any athlete suffering a back injury. Careful movements made by the athlete suffering an acute injury to the spine are not likely to cause spinal cord damage because the athlete will usually cease even the slightest movement on experiencing a significant increase in pain. Do not encourage movement of the spine if pain is increased. The importance of caution when evaluating an acute injury to the spine cannot be overemphasized.

Active movements are also performed to evaluate the flexibility and ROM in various segments of the spine and to localize any pain associated with movement. As the athlete performs each of the movements, observe if the motion is performed smoothly and through a normal ROM. To evaluate the active ROM in the cervical spine, ask the athlete to perform each of the basic movements of the neck (Figure 15-20). To test flexion and extension, ask the athlete to nod the head forward and backward. Normally an athlete should be able to touch the chest with the chin and to look directly upward. To evaluate rotation in the cervical area, ask the athlete to turn his or her head to both sides as far as possible. An athlete should be able to move the head to each side so that the chin is almost in line with the shoulder. Remember to compare motions on each side. To evaluate lateral bending, ask the athlete to move the head from side to side as if to touch the ear to the shoulder. Normally an athlete should be able to tilt the head about 45° toward each shoulder. Again compare motions in each direction and make sure the athlete does not compensate by lifting a shoulder toward the ear.

The active ROM in the thoracic and lumbar areas of the spine is evaluated simultaneously (Figure 15-21). More movement is possible in the lumbar than in the thoracic area, but only a small amount of that movement actually takes place in the spine. As the athlete performs each of the active movements, observe the degree of motion,

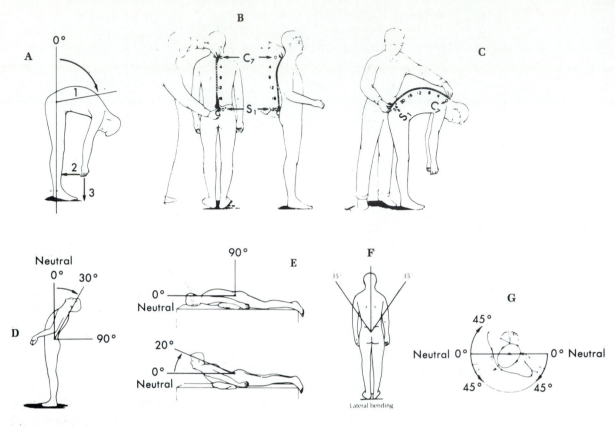

FIGURE 15-21
Active ROM of the thoracic and lumbar spine. **A**, Forward flexion. Motion can be estimated in degrees or measurement of fingertips to leg or from floor. **B** and **C**, Flexible tape measuring method. **D**, Hyperextension with the athlete standing. **E**, Hyperextension with the athlete lying prone. **F**, Lateral bending. **G**, Rotation of the spine.

smoothness of the spinal curve, and symmetry of body areas. To evaluate flexion, ask the athlete to bend forward with the knees straight as if to touch the toes. Although most of this motion occurs at the hip joint, it allows the athletic trainer to observe the movements of the spine. Observe extension as the athlete returns to an upright position.

A more accurate method of measuring true motion of the spine is to use a flexible tape. With the athlete standing, hold the tape over the spinous processes C7 and S1 (Figure 15-21, *B*). As the athlete bends forward, measure the lengthening distance from C7 to S1 (Figure 15-21, *C*). Normally there is an average increase of approxi-

mately 4 inches in forward flexion. The motion in the thoracic and lumbar spines can be further evaluated individually by following the same procedure and measuring the distance from C7 to T12 and T12 to S1. Usually 1 inch of lengthening occurs in the thoracic spine and 3 inches occurs in the lumbar spine.

To test hyperextension, ask the athlete to bend backward as far as possible (Figure 15-21, *D*). Normally an athlete can hyperextend approximately 30°. An alternative method of evaluating hyperextension of the spine is to have the athlete lie prone and raise the head and shoulders (Figure 15-21, *E*). To test lateral bending, ask the athlete to bend to the

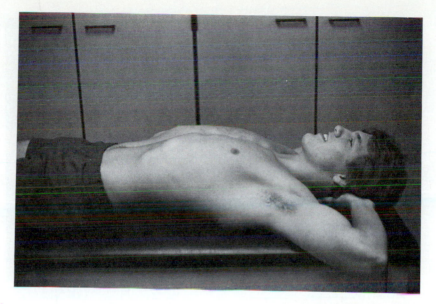

FIGURE 15-22
Evaluating tightness in the shoulder adductor and internal rotator muscles by having the athlete lie supine with hands behind the neck. An athlete should be able to place both elbows on the table.

left and right as far as possible (Figure 15-21, *F*). It may be necessary to stabilize the pelvis because an athlete may compensate by moving the pelvis. Normal range is approximately 35° of lateral bending in each direction. To evaluate trunk rotation, ask the athlete to turn the head and shoulders to both sides (Figure 15-21, *G*). Again, it is important to stabilize the pelvis so that turning of the hips will not compensate for lack of rotation in the spinal area. One method of stabilizing the pelvis is to have the athlete perform trunk rotation while sitting on a table.

In addition to evaluating the flexibility of the spine, active maneuvers can be used to evaluate any limitation of motion in body areas that may affect spinal alignment. Certain muscles and muscle groups are frequently found to be shortened in athletes with apparent abnormal spinal alignment. This may be caused by atypical muscle usage during athletic activity or inappropriate posture. If the athletic trainer suspects that shortening of muscles may be a causative factor in loss of flexibility or decrease in

ROM, muscle groups should be evaluated.

Forward shoulders is usually associated with tight shoulder adductor and internal rotator muscles. To evaluate any limitation of these shoulder motions, instruct the athlete to lie supine with hands behind the neck and elbows on the table (Figure 15-22). Normally an athlete should be able to rest his or her elbows on the table without any strain. If rounded shoulders or kyphosis prevents the elbows from resting on the table, the athlete would probably benefit from an exercise program designed to stretch these muscle groups.

The pelvis is another body area that has a major effect on spinal alignment. Muscular tightness can tilt the pelvis, resulting in compensating curves in the lumbar spine. Hip flexor and hamstring muscle groups are the common sites of muscle tightness about the pelvis. To evaluate the hip flexors, instruct the athlete to lie supine and pull one thigh up against the chest (Figure 15-23). If the hip flexors of the opposite leg are not tight, the extended leg will remain on the table. If the hip flexors are tight, the oppo-

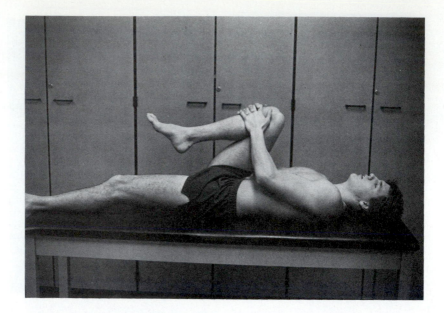

FIGURE 15-23
Thomas test. Evaluating tightness in the hip flexor muscles by having the athlete pull one thigh up against the chest. The opposite leg should remain on the table. Compare both legs.

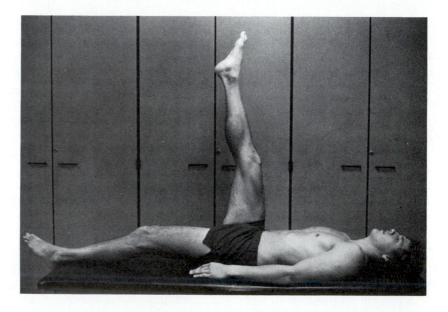

FIGURE 15-24
Evaluating tightness in the hamstring musculature by having the athlete raise one leg as high as possible without flexing the knee. An athlete should be able to obtain approximately 70° of flexion with each leg. Compare both legs.

site thigh will be lifted from the table. Repeat the same procedure using the other leg. This procedure is called a **Thomas test.**

The same supine position can be used to evaluate hamstring tightness. Instruct the athlete to raise one leg as high as possible without flexing the knee (Figure 15-24). The opposite extremity should remain in contact with the table. Repeat the same procedure with the other leg. An athlete should be able to obtain approximately 70° of flexion with each leg. An alternate method of evaluating the hamstrings is to instruct the athlete, in a long sitting position, to reach out as far as possible and try to touch the toes without flexing the knees. Tight hamstrings or lack of spinal flexibility can prevent an athlete from touching the toes.

Another procedure you can ask an athlete to perform, if you suspect a space-occupying lesion of the spinal canal, is the **valsalva maneuver.** The athlete is asked to hold his or her breath and bear down as in moving the bowels. This maneuver increases the pressure within the spinal canal (intrathecal pressure) and may cause pain if there is a space-occupying lesion such as a herniated disc or a tumor. The pain may also be radiated or referred. Use this procedure with caution because an athlete may become dizzy and pass out while performing this maneuver. Similar increased pain may be temporarily reproduced by sneezing or coughing.

Resistive movements. Applying resistance against spinal motions can serve two main purposes: (1) to assist in determining which structures are involved in spinal injury, and (2) to assess the strength of muscles surrounding and supporting the spine. Both of these functions are important in evaluating acute and chronic spinal injuries affecting the spine. Remember, active motion of an injured muscle against resistance will cause pain or increase the severity of existing pain. In addition, applying resistance against active movement allows you to evaluate the relative strength of specific muscles. The strength of muscles surrounding the flexible segments of the vertebral col-

umn is extremely important in supporting the spine and keeping the various segments in proper alignment. Muscle weaknesses and imbalances can cause injury symptoms. This is especially true in the lower back.

The muscles about the cervical spine are evaluated by applying resistance against the neck movements described previously. For each movement, manual resistance is applied. This is accomplished by using one hand to stabilize the shoulder or thorax to prevent any substitute motions and exerting the resistance with the other hand. To evaluate cervical flexion, place the stabilizing hand on the athlete's shoulder and the palm of the resistance hand on the forehead. Instruct the athlete to flex the neck slowly while resistance is increased until the pain is localized or the relative strength of the muscles producing flexion is determined (Figure 15-25, *A*). To test extension, cup the palm of one hand over the back of the athlete's head, stabilize the thorax with the other, and instruct the athlete to slowly extend against resistance (Figure 15-25, *B*). To evaluate lateral flexion of the neck, place the resistance hand against the side of the athlete's head and the stabilizing hand on the shoulder on the same side to prevent elevation (Figure 15-25, *C*). To evaluate rotation of the head to the right, the examiner should stabilize the left shoulder and apply resistance along the right side of the athlete's jaw (Figure 15-25, *D*). To test rotation to the left, reverse hand positions.

Applying resistance against trunk movements can be accomplished by resisting motions in the standing position, as described earlier. However, it is much easier to apply resistance to trunk movements when the athlete is lying down. In these positions, gravity can assist in applying resistance against a particular movement. Remember that movements involving the trunk can be made more or less difficult by varying the weight distribution; for example, placement of the athlete's hands and arms can make the movements easier or harder. Movements can be performed with the athlete's hands at the side, at the abdomen, behind the neck,

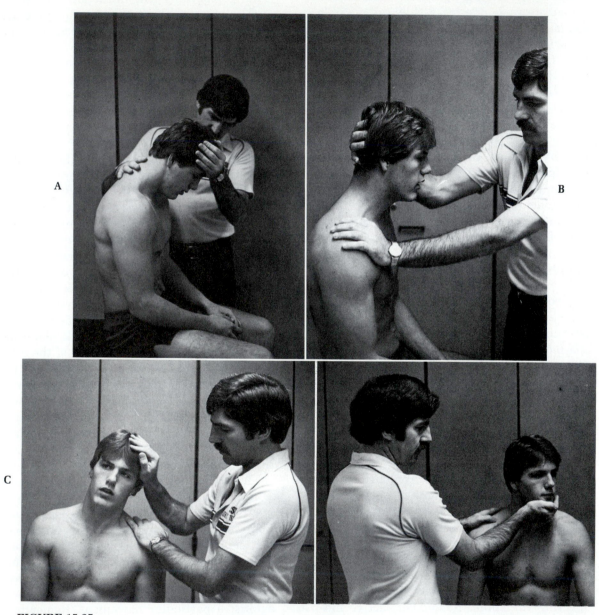

FIGURE 15-25
Applying manual resistance against cervical motion: **A**, flexion; **B**, extension; **C**, lateral bending; and, **D**, rotation.

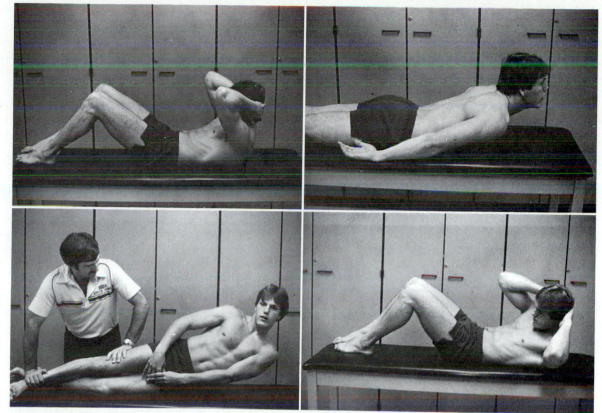

FIGURE 15-26
Active movements resulting in resistance to specific trunk movements: **A**, flexion; **B**, hyperextension; **C**, lateral bending; and, **D**, rotation.

on top of the head, or extended overhead; each of these changes in arm position shifts the center of gravity upward and thereby progressively increases resistance. As techniques are refined and "hands on" experience in the assessment process grows, the student athletic trainer will learn a great deal about the practical aspects of functional anatomy and applied kinesiology. Overall body position and the selective positioning of the extremities during the assessment, for example, will not only shift the center of gravity but may also change the angle of attack of secondary and tertiary movers at a joint, thus significantly altering the athlete's response to a particular test. Therefore functional anatomy and principles involving mechanics of motion must be understood and applied by the athletic trainer during the evaluation process.

The abdominals are an extremely important group of muscles that must be considered when evaluating any lower back condition. These muscles are a key factor in lumbar spine support because they provide anterior stability and active forward flexion of the trunk. Weakness of the abdominals can result in forward tilting of the pelvis, cause an increase in lumbar lordosis, increase the possibility of lumbosacral ligament sprains, and ultimately contribute to lower back pain. The abdominals are one of the most common areas of muscular weaknesses in athletes. To evaluate the strength of the abdominals, have the athlete perform a partial sit-up from the supine position, with knees flexed and feet unsupported (Figure 15-26, A). The hands can be at the side, on the chest, or behind the head, depending on abdominal strength. An athlete with normal abdominal strength should be able to perform this activity with hands behind the head. Instruct the athlete to raise the head and continue to curl the spine upward until the thoracic spine is lifted from the table, approximately 30° to 40°. Motion up to this point is caused predominately by the abdominals, especially the rectus abdominis muscle, and provides a good test of abdominal strength. Athletes who are recognized as having weakened abdominals should be instructed in an abdominal strengthening program. To evaluate trunk rotation, have the athlete perform the same partial sit-up in a rotated position (Figure 15-26, *D*). Instruct the athlete to rotate in the other direction. These tests are designed predominantly to evaluate the oblique abdominal muscles. When the trunk is rotated to the right, this sit-up uses the right external oblique and left internal oblique muscles. When the athlete rotates the trunk to the left, the action is brought about by the opposite muscles.

To apply resistance against extension or hyperextension of the spine, have the athlete lie prone and raise the head and shoulders off the table (Figure 15-26, *B*). The mus-

cles causing lateral flexion of the trunk are evaluated with the athlete lying on one side and the feet stabilized (Figure 15-26, *C*). Additional resistance can be applied against these movements as the athlete raises the hands above the head. The athletic trainer can also apply additional resistance against the athlete's upper back or shoulders. Watch the mechanics of these movements to recognize any increase in pain or muscular weaknesses.

Passive movements. Fewer passive movements are used during the assessment of injuries to the spine, especially injuries to the cervical spine. An athletic trainer normally does not attempt to passively evaluate the ROM in an athlete's spine after an injury. The vertebral column may be unstable, and damage to the spinal cord could result. Remember, passive movements are generally more dangerous, and caution must be used in evaluating injuries to the spine.

A passive maneuver that can be used on the cervical spine is compression and distraction (Figure 15-27). These procedures are used to evaluate the possibility of nerve root involvement. To perform cervical com-

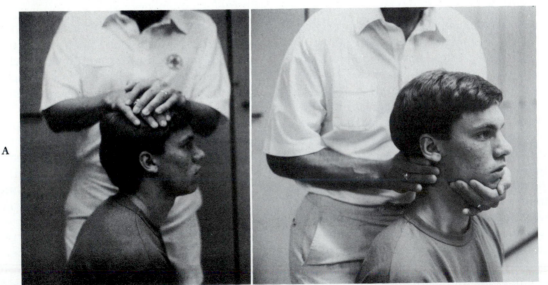

A   B

FIGURE 15-27
Applying passive stress to the cervical spine to evaluate for possible nerve root involvement: **A**, cervical compression and, **B**, cervical distraction.

pression, carefully press straight down on the athlete's head while he or she is sitting. If pain is increased in the cervical spine or radiates into the arm with this maneuver, it may indicate pressure on a nerve root. Note the distribution of the pain or altered sensations. The cervical compression test can also be done with the head rotated to either side and/or laterally flexed before compression. Cervical distraction is performed by placing one hand under the athlete's chin and the other around the occiput and slowly lifting the head. If pain is relieved or decreased when the head is lifted, it is indicative of relieving pressure on a nerve root or facet joint.

Another passive procedure that may assist in evaluating injuries to, or conditions of, the spine is the straight-leg raising test. This test is designed to reproduce back and leg pain to determine its cause. With the athlete lying supine, grasp the athlete's heel with one hand, place your other hand on his or her knee to prevent it from bending, and lift the leg upward until there is discomfort or tightness (Figure 15-28). You should be able to raise the leg approximately 70° to 80°. Straight-leg raising may be limited and painful because of tight hamstrings, lumbosacral or sacroiliac joint injury, or a problem with the sciatic nerve. Determine the location of the pain. Tight hamstrings will produce pain in the posterior thigh. An injury to the lumbosacral or sacroiliac joints should produce pain in those areas of the spine. Sciatic pain can radiate all the way down the leg. To determine if there is a sciatic nerve problem, drop the leg down slightly until there is no pain or discomfort. With the leg held stationary, dorsiflex the foot (Figure 15-29). This maneuver, the **Lasègue's test,** puts no additional stress on the lumbosacral or sacroiliac joints or the hamstrings. It does, however, place additional pull on the sciatic nerve trunk, and increased pain indicates possible sciatic nerve involvement. If sciatic nerve involvement is suspected, the athlete should be referred to a physician for further assessment.

The sacroiliac joints and ligaments can also be evaluated by passive movements. As previously discussed, great care must be taken to localize the pain to the sacroiliac joint. Many of the tests already explained

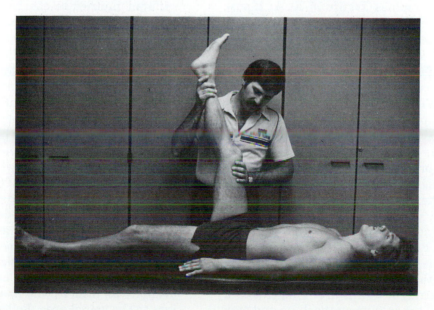

FIGURE 15-28
Straight-leg raising to evaluate hamstring tightness, and lumbosacral, sacroiliac, or sciatic nerve involvement.

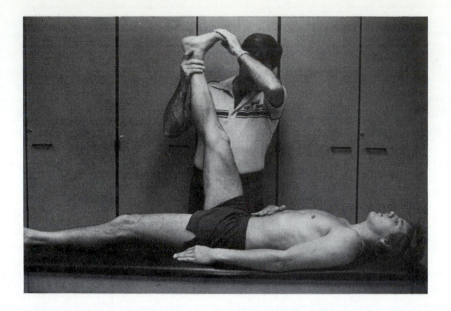

FIGURE 15-29
Lasègue's test. Straight-leg raising with ankle dorsiflexion to determine possible sciatic nerve involvement.

may elicit pain in the sacroiliac joint. The most significant tests for this area of the body are designed to compress or separate the iliac crest. With the athlete lying supine, apply outward pressure against the anterior superior iliac spines (Figure 15-30, *A*). If posterior pain is produced, this may indicate a sprain of the anterior sacroiliac ligaments. The posterior sacroiliac ligaments can be tested by forcibly compressing the anterior superior iliac spines toward the midline of the body (Figure 15-30, *B*). The posterior sacroiliac ligament can also be evaluated with the athlete lying on his or her side. Place your hands over the upper part of the iliac crest and press toward the floor (Figure 15-30, *C*). This maneuver exerts forward pressure on the sacrum and may cause an increase in pain. Another test that may indicate sacroiliac involvement is demonstrated in Figure 15-30, *D*. With the athlete lying prone, place the heel of one of your hands on the apex of the sacrum and apply pressure straight downward. This causes a shearing of the sacrum on the ilium and may produce additional pain if there is involvement at the sacroiliac joint.

Functional movements. Functional movements are used to evaluate the functional abilities of the athlete who has suffered a spinal injury. These are especially important in evaluating athletes who have suffered injuries to the back or neck. The initial functional movements are the same as those described in the stress portion of the assessment process: alignment, flexibility, and strength. The athletic trainer must carefully monitor the treatment and rehabilitation of the injured athlete to ensure that no abnormal alignments, faulty postural habits, or inequality in flexibility and strength occur as an athlete returns to activity, because the athlete who returns to active competition with any of these conditions is subject to reinjury and continued problems. Once the athlete can demonstrate normal alignment, flexibility, and strength, he or she should be observed performing movements or activities specific to his or her sport. The athletic trainer must continue to evaluate an athlete who has suffered an injury to the spinal area. Follow-up care is extremely important to ensure a rapid and safe return to activity.

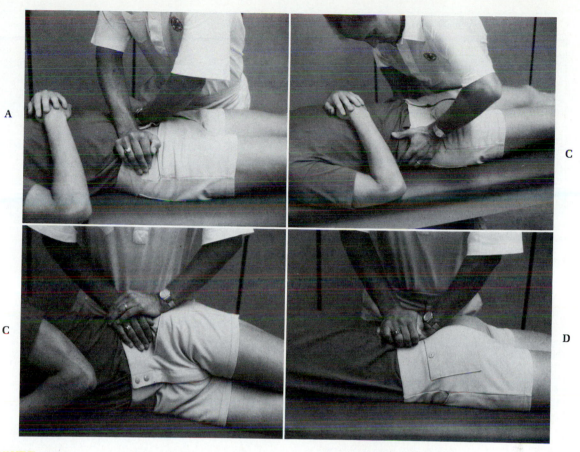

FIGURE 15-30
Applying passive stress to the sacroiliac joints. **A**, Applying outward pressure against the anterior superior iliac spines. **B**, Forcibly compressing the anterior superior iliac spines toward the midline of the body. **C**, Applying downward pressure on the iliac crest. **D**, Applying downward pressure on the apex of the sacrum.

Neurological evaluations

Many of the techniques for testing sensory and motor functions were discussed previously because these procedures should be used initially to help determine if there is any spinal cord or nerve root involvement. Refer to Table 15-1 to review the key myotomes and dermatomes.

Reflexes. Deep tendon reflexes can also be tested to evaluate the state of the nerve or nerve roots supplying that reflex. Reflexes were discussed in more detail in Chapter 6. Commonly assessed reflexes are the biceps (C5), brachioradialis (C6), triceps (C7), patellar (L4), and Achilles (S1). Choose the reflexes that you think are the most pertinent to your assessment. Test each reflex bilaterally before moving to another area of the body. Compare each reflex response symmetrically as you proceed. Remember, reflexes should always be symmetrically equal. Note any differences between the two sides and refer the athlete with unequal reflexes to medical assistance for further evaluation.

Evaluation of Findings

Disastrous and serious athletic injuries that can occur to the spine are fractures or dislocations of the vertebrae with actual or potential damage to the spinal cord. Whenever a severe injury to the spine is recognized or

---

Athletic Injury Assessment Checklist: Spine Injuries

Primary survey

_____ Responsiveness
_____ Airway
_____ Breathing
_____ Circulation

Secondary survey

_____ Paralysis
_____ Muscle function
_____ Sensations

_____ History
_____ Pain
_____ Mechanism of injury
_____ Previous history

_____ Observation
_____ Motionlessness
_____ Deformities
_____ Signs of trauma
_____ Movements and positions
_____ Alignment of neck and back

_____ Physical Examination

Palpation
_____ Tenderness
_____ Muscle spasm
_____ Sensations

Movement Procedures
_____ Active movements
_____ Resistive movements
_____ Passive movements
_____ Functional movements

Neurologic Evaluations
_____ Sensory functions
_____ Motor functions
_____ Reflexes

---

suspected, it is imperative that you make certain the athlete is protected from further trauma to the neural elements. An injury without neurologic involvement must not be converted into one with irreversible spinal cord or peripheral nerve damage by ill-advised evaluation, manipulation, or transportation procedures. The mechanism for a catastrophic injury to the spine is present in most athletic activities. Therefore the assessment of injuries involving the spine are among the most important that you will perform.

The majority of athletic injuries to the spine, however, are not this serious or disastrous and will consist of contusions, sprains, and strains. For most injuries involving the spine, the assessment process will be centered on evaluating the severity of the injury and identifying the structures involved. This usually cannot be accomplished quickly. A complete and accurate evaluation of spinal injuries or related conditions takes considerable time. The information gained during the assessment process is essential in establishing a treatment regimen aimed at relieving acute pain and restoring normal flexibility, strength, and proper body mechanics.

When to refer the athlete

When a serious injury to the spine occurs, the athlete must be referred to medical assistance immediately. You must be able to

---

When to Refer the Athlete . . .

Paralysis—inability to move arms or legs
Loss of normal sensations
Pain, tenderness, or deformity along the
  vertebral column
Unremitting neck or back pain
Weakness noted in the extremities
Loss of coordination of the extremities
Unusual sensations in the extremities or body
  surface
Doubt regarding the presence of spinal cord
  involvement

---

recognize signs and symptoms of severe spinal injuries. Conditions or findings that indicate the athlete has a potentially serious spinal injury and should be protected from further trauma and referred to medical assistance are listed in the box.

REFERENCES

Anderson C: Neck injuries: backboard, bench, or return to play, *Phys Sportsmed* 21(8):23, 1993.

Arnheim DD, Prentice WE: *Principles of athletic training,* ed 8, St. Louis, 1993, Mosby.

Edgelow PI: Physical examination of the lumbosacral complex, *Phys Ther* 59(8):974, 1979.

Fourre M: On-site management of cervical spine injuries, *Phys Sportsmed* 19(4):53, 1991.

Halpren BC, Smith AD: Catching the cause of low-back pain, *Phys Sportsmed* 19(6):71, 1991.

Hartley A: *Practical joint assessment: a sports medicine manual,* St. Louis, 1990, Mosby.

Harvey J, Tanner S: Low back pain in young athletes: a practical approach, *Sports Med* 12(6):394, 1991.

Hockberger RS, Kirshenbaum K, Doris PE: *Spinal trauma.* In Rosen P and others, editors: *Emergency medicine: concept and clinical practice,* ed 3, St. Louis, 1992, Mosby.

Hoppenfeld S: *Physical examination of the spine and extremities,* New York, 1976, Appleton-Century-Crofts.

Jackson DW, Wiltse LL: Low back pain in young athletes, *Phys Sportsmed* 2(11):53, 1974.

Jordan BD, and others: How to evaluate transient quadriparesis, *Phys Sportsmed* 20(2):83, 1992.

Keim HA, Kirkaldy-Willis WH: Low back pain, *CIBA Clin Sym* 32(6), 1980.

Magee DJ: *Orthopedic physical assessment,* ed 2, Philadelphia, 1992, Saunders.

Mueller FO, Blyth CS: Catastrophic head and neck injuries, *Phys Sportsmed* 7(10):71, 1979.

O'Donoghue DH: *Treatment of injuries to athletes,* ed 4, Philadelphia, 1984, Saunders.

Post M: *Physical examination of the musculoskeletal system,* Chicago, 1987, Year Book Medical.

Roy S, Irvin R: *Sports medicine: prevention, evaluation, management, and rehabilitation,* Englewood Cliffs, 1983, Prentice-Hall.

Sward L: The thoracolumbar spine in young elite athletes: current concepts on the effects of physical training, *Sports Med* 13(5):357, 1992.

Tator CH, Edmonds VE: Sports and recreation are a rising cause of spinal cord injury, *Phys Sportsmed* 14(5):157, 1986.

Torg JS: *Athletic injuries to the head, neck and face,* ed 2, St. Louis, 1991, Mosby.

SUGGESTED READINGS

Kalfas IH, and others: Spondylotic C3 radiculopathy in a professional football player, *Phys Sportsmed* 15(7):79, 1987.
  Reviews a case study of a spondylotic C3 radiculopathy resulting from a football injury, and discusses more common football-related injuries to the cervical nerve roots and brachial plexus.

Lehman LB: Nervous system sports-related injuries, *Am J Sports Med* 15(5):494, 1987.
  Reviews the wide range of nervous system injuries resulting from sports activities, and discusses the mechanisms of such injuries and their prevention and management.

Spencer CW: Injuries to the spine, *Clin Sports Med* 5(2), 1986, Saunders.
  Devoted entirely to spine injuries and includes a potpourri of topics concerning areas of spinal pathology.

Torg JS, editor: Head and neck injuries, *Clin Sports Med* 6(1), 1987, Saunders.
  Devoted entirely to head and cervical spine injuries. Articles by various contributors include prevention, evaluation, emergency management, definitive treatment, and rehabilitation.

*C*HAPTER 16

Throat, chest, abdomen, and pelvis injuries

After you have completed this chapter, you should be able to:

- Identify the basic anatomy of the throat, chest, abdomen, and pelvis.
- Describe the common athletic injuries and conditions that may occur to the throat.
- Describe the common athletic injuries that may occur to the chest and list the signs and symptoms that may indicate intrathoracic involvement.
- Describe the various conditions that may affect the respiratory tract.
- Describe the common athletic injuries that may occur to the abdomen and list the signs and symptoms that may indicate intraabdominal involvement.
- Describe the assessment process for an athlete suffering an injury to the throat, chest, abdomen, and pelvis.
- List all conditions or findings that indicate an athlete with a chest or abdominal injury should be referred for medical attention.

The torso of the body is composed of two major areas: (1) the chest, or **thorax,** and (2) the abdomen. The boundary between these two areas is the diaphragm, and each area forms a major body cavity that contains vital life-sustaining organs. Athletic injuries can occur to either the walls of these cavities or their visceral contents. Superficial injuries involving the cavity walls are common during athletic activity and generally are not serious. Fortunately, athletic injuries to the internal contents **(viscera)** or either of these cavities are not common; however, serious and potentially life-threatening injuries can occur to these vital organs. Athletic trainers must be alert to the possibilities of serious internal injuries resulting from athletic activity.

The chest and abdomen contain organs essential for respiration, circulation, and digestion. Structures vital to each of these systems pass through the neck. As a result, athletic injuries or related conditions involving the neck can compromise these body processes. This chapter discusses injuries involving the anterior neck or throat (excluding the cervical spine), chest, abdomen, and pelvis.

THROAT (ANTERIOR NECK)

For purposes of description, the upper limit of the neck is considered to be the lower border of the jaw extending on either side of the mastoid process just behind the ear. The lower limit is defined by the suprasternal notch anteriorly, the clavicles, and a line extending from the acromioclavicular joint on either side to the spinous process of the seventh cervical vertebra posteriorly. The sur-

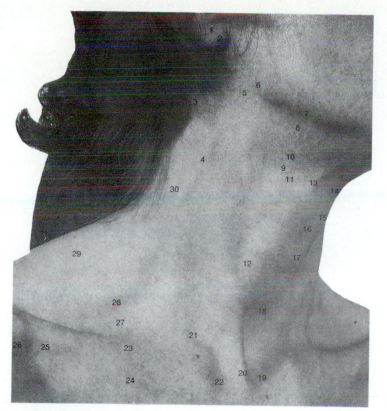

1	Mastoid process
2	Tip of transverse process of atlas
3	Sternocleidomastoid
4	External jugular vein
5	Lowest part of parotid gland
6	Angle of mandible
7	Anterior border of masseter and facial artery
8	Submandibular gland
9	Tip of greater horn of hyoid bone
10	Hypoglossal nerve
11	Internal laryngeal nerve
12	Site for palpation of common carotid artery
13	Anterior jugular vein
14	Body of hyoid bone
15	Laryngeal prominence (Adam's apple)
16	Vocal fold
17	Arch of cricoid cartilage
18	Isthmus of thyroid gland
19	Jugular notch and trachea
20	Sternal head } of sterno-
21	Clavicular head } cleidomastoid
22	Sternoclavicular joint and union of internal jugular and subclavian veins to form brachiocephalic vein
23	Clavicle
24	Pectoralis major
25	Infraclavicular fossa and cephalic vein
26	Deltoid
27	Inferior belly of omohyoid
28	Upper trunk of brachial plexus
29	Acessory nerve passing under anterior border of trapezius
30	Accessory nerve emerging from sternocleidomastoid

FIGURE 16-1
Surface markings on the front and right side of the neck.

face characteristic and contour of the neck vary with age, sex, body type, and level of conditioning. The neck is rounded in women, more angular in men. Landmarks such as the thyroid cartilage (Adam's apple) are more conspicuous and defined in the male. Refer to Figure 16-1 to review the surface markings of the neck.

The numerous visceral structures, blood vessels, and nerves in the neck are relatively exposed and thus vulnerable to traumatic injury. Because of the functional significance of these anatomic structures, proficiency in assessment of injuries in this area is critically important to the athletic trainer.

Neck Muscles

The two major muscles of the neck are the sternocleidomastoid and trapezius muscles. The sternocleidomastoid muscles divide each side of the neck into an anterior and posterior triangle. The athletic trainer should review the points of attachment and the function of the sternocleidomastoid and trapezius muscles in movements of the head and neck. Note in Figure 16-2 that the sternocleidomastoid muscle arises by two heads: a narrow sternal head from the manubrium of the sternum, and a broader clavicular head from the medial third of the clavicle. The small triangular interval between the two heads is quite noticeable in thin athletes and generally appears as a slight depression. The carotid arteries, internal jugular vein, vagus nerve, and portions of the cervical plexus lie beneath the sternocleidomastoid muscle.

Anatomic Structures of the Neck

Major anatomic structures in the midline of the neck include the hyoid bone, the larynx, the trachea, the thyroid gland, and the more

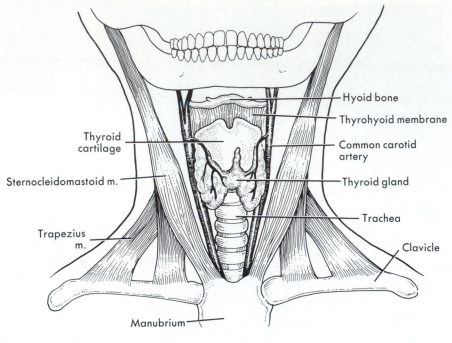

FIGURE 16-2
Anatomic structures of the neck.

deeply placed pharynx and esophagus. The major blood vessels, important nerves, and many lymph nodes are located on the sides of the neck under or around the sternocleidomastoid muscles. The posterior portion of the neck contains the cervical segment of the spinal cord, the cervical vertebrae, and surrounding musculature, which was discussed in Chapter 15.

Locate the hyoid bone in Figure 16-2. This unusually shaped little bone is unique in that it does not articulate with any other bone in the skeleton. It lies at the level of the third cervical vertebra just below the mandible. Located in the musculature and soft tissues at the root of the tongue, the hyoid bone is in close proximity to many major structures in the upper neck. It possesses great mobility but is vulnerable to injury in certain kinds of athletic activity.

The *larynx* (voice box) lies between the root of the tongue and the upper end of the trachea and can be described as the opening into the trachea from the pharynx. It normally extends between the fourth, fifth, and sixth cervical vertebrae but is often somewhat higher in women and in children. The larynx consists of cartilage and muscles. The largest cartilage—the thyroid, or Adam's apple—is normally quite smooth and is an easily palpable landmark in front. The cricoid cartilage forms a complete ring around the larynx and is also easily palpable inferior to the thyroid cartilage. The cricoid lies on a level with the sixth cervical vertebra.

The trachea (windpipe) is a tube about $4\frac{1}{2}$ inches (11 cm) long that extends from the larynx to the bronchi in the thoracic cavity. Its diameter measures about 1 inch (2.5 cm), and its walls are composed of smooth muscles in which C-shaped rings of cartilage are embedded. The cartilaginous rings give firmness to the wall of the trachea, preventing collapse and occlusion of the airway, and are incomplete on the posterior surface. The trachea is easiest to palpate just above the manubrium (suprasternal notch) between the sternal attachment of the two sternocleidomastoid muscles.

In most persons the H-shaped thyroid

gland is not visible during inspection of the neck. However, occasionally the gland can be palpated when the upper trachea or cricoid cartilage is being examined. The right lobe of the thyroid is larger than the left and is sometimes noticed if the athlete swallows during the examination. If felt, the lobes of the thyroid gland are smooth, nontender, and tend to move freely under the skin.

The *pharynx* is a tubelike structure approximately 5 inches (12.5 cm) in length that extends from the base of the skull to the esophagus and lies just anterior to the cervical vertebrae. It is made of muscle and lined with mucous membrane. The pharynx serves as a passageway for the respiratory and digestive tracts; air and food must pass through this structure before reaching their respective tubes.

Lymph nodes in and around the neck are found in serial groups called "chains." There are many chains of lymph nodes in the neck that normally cannot be felt or seen. However, lymph nodes in the neck are often enlarged as a result of head and neck infections. The athlete may complain of "swollen glands" or "lumps."

THROAT INJURIES AND CONDITIONS

Most athletic injuries to the throat are caused by some type of direct blow to the anterior or lateral portions of the neck. This normally results in a contusion with varying degrees of pain, soreness on swallowing, hoarseness, and tenderness to touch. Occasionally the blow results in shortness of breath and the inability to speak, which can cause the athlete to become extremely anxious and apprehensive. A calm and reassuring approach to these athletes is indicated. Symptoms of this type usually subside quickly, but soreness and hoarseness may persist. The athlete should be able to resume activity if normal speech and breathing return. Athletes whose symptoms persist longer than a day should be referred to a physician for a laryngeal examination.

An athletic injury that results in a fracture of the cartilage of the larynx or trachea is quite rare. However, this is a serious and potentially life-threatening injury; therefore the athletic trainer must be prepared to recognize and handle such an emergency. Difficulty in breathing, loss of voice, inability to swallow, bleeding from the throat, and crepitation on palpation are signs and symptoms indicating immediate medical attention is required. After suffering an anterior neck trauma, an athlete may develop a compromised airway as a result of the development of edema or an expanding hematoma. Therefore, trauma to the anterior neck should be carefully monitored for a period of time after the injury to detect the formation of edema or a hematoma.

❖ **Pharyngitis.** A common complaint that the athletic trainer will have to evaluate is the sore throat. Inflammation or infection of the pharynx is called pharyngitis. This condition is indicated by pain on swallowing, dryness, hoarseness, and burning of the throat. If symptoms are severe, persist, and occur along with a fever, chills, and swollen lymph nodes in the neck, strep throat should be suspected, and the athlete should be referred to a physician.

❖ **Laryngitis.** Laryngitis, an inflammation or irritation of the larynx, is another common complaint. This condition may be indicated by hoarseness, loss of voice, dryness and soreness of the throat, cough, and difficulty in swallowing. A period of yelling may cause vocal strain, resulting in swelling and irritation of the vocal cords. If symptoms persist, a physician should be consulted.

❖ **Tonsillitis.** Tonsillitis is an inflammation of the tonsils, which are small almond-shaped masses located in the back of the throat and composed mainly of lymphoid tissue. As a result of an acute inflammation, the tonsils become markedly swollen, narrowing the opening of the throat and causing pain and difficulty in swallowing (**dysphagia**). Tonsillitis usually responds to antibiotic therapy.

❖ **Mumps.** Mumps is an inflammation of the parotid glands that lie just beneath each ear. This is a contagious disease caused by a virus. After an incubation period, symp-

FIGURE 16-3
Anterior view of the thorax (rib cage).

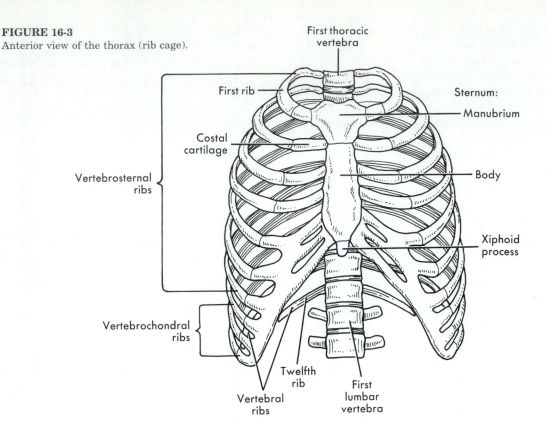

toms appear, including fever, headache, and pain and swelling in the parotid region that often interferes with chewing and swallowing. Symptoms gradually disappear after a few days. This is essentially a disease of childhood, however, when the infection occurs in an adult, it is more likely to involve other organs such as the testis, pancreas, or the meninges.

CHEST

The chest, or **thoracic cavity,** is surrounded by a conical bony cage (Figure 16-3) formed by the sternum and costal cartilages anteriorly, the ribs laterally, and the thoracic vertebrae posteriorly. The anatomy of the thoracic skeleton described in Chapter 3 should be reviewed.

Topographic Anatomy of the Thorax

The athletic trainer must have a sound working knowledge of the topographic, or surface, landmarks of the thorax to properly assess an injury to this area. Anatomic assessment guidelines assist in identifying the location of internal structures and in describing the exact location of injury. Review the surface landmarks in Figure 16-4. Note the lines of reference and placement of internal anatomic structures in Figures 16-5 and 16-6. Anatomic descriptions of many of the muscles that attach to or are an integral part of the thorax are given in the discussion of shoulder injuries in Chapter 20. Muscles of particular interest and importance at this time are the pectoralis major, serratus anterior, latissimus dorsi, trapezius, rectus abdominis, external oblique, intercostals, and superficial back muscles. Review the points of attachment of these muscles described in Chapter 5.

The anterior chest wall is characterized by a shallow midline depression just over the subcutaneous sternum. This shallow median furrow lies between the two pectoralis major muscles and is more prominent in athletes

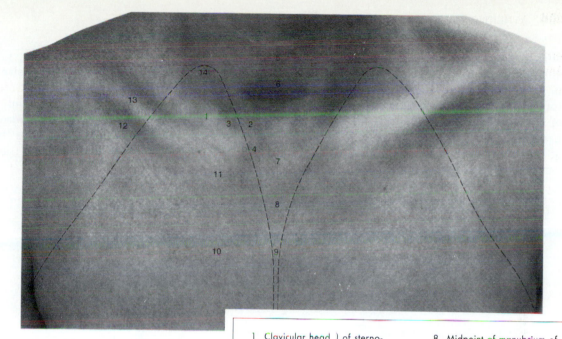

FIGURE 16-4

Surface markings on the lower neck and
upper thorax.

1 Clavicular head ⎱ of sterno-	8 Midpoint of manubrium of
2 Sternal head ⎰ cleidomastoid	sternum
3 Internal jugular vein	9 Manubriosternal joint
4 Sternoclavicular joint	10 Second costal cartilage
5 Cricoid cartilage	11 First costal cartilage
6 Trachea and isthmus of thyroid	12 Infraclavicular fossa
gland	13 Clavicle
7 Jugular notch	14 Apex of pleura and lung

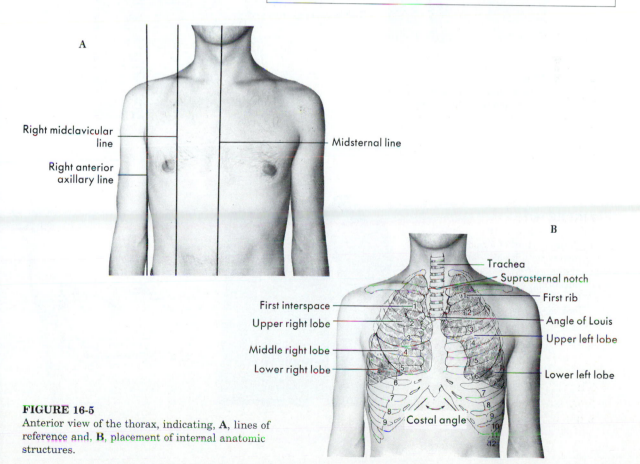

FIGURE 16-5

Anterior view of the thorax, indicating, **A**, lines of
reference and, **B**, placement of internal anatomic
structures.

with good muscular definition and limited subcutaneous fat. The anterior axillary line is formed by the lateral border of the pectoralis major. The toothlike points of origin of the serratus anterior muscle are prominent along the lateral chest wall. The point of origin of the serratus from the fifth rib can be seen just below the pectoralis major.

The *sternal angle,* or *Louis's angle,* is the manubriosternal junction just opposite the sternal end of the second rib. It is an extremely useful aid in rib identification and the most reliable thoracic surface landmark. The lines of reference and surface landmarks should be employed during the assessment process.

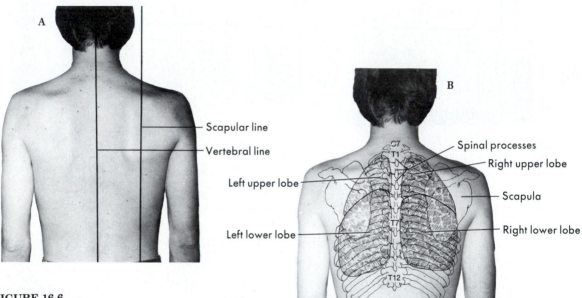

FIGURE 16-6
Posterior view of thorax, indicating **A**, lines of reference and, **B**, placement of internal anatomic structures.

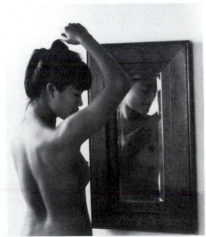
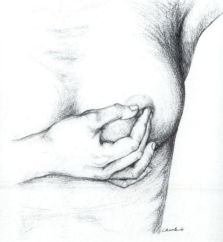

FIGURE 16-7
Breast self-examination.
1. Stand in front of a mirror and inspect both breasts for any discharge from the nipples and puckering or scaling of the skin. Gently squeeze the nipples and look for a discharge.

FIGURE 16-7, cont'd.

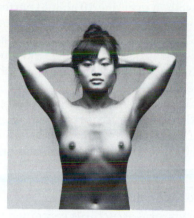

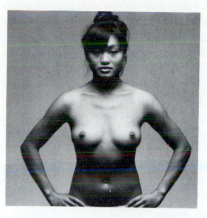

2. Stand in front of a mirror, clasp your hands behind your head, and press hands against head. Note any change in breast shape or contour.

3. Next put hands on hips and press firmly. At the same time, lean your shoulders and elbows forward. Note any change in the shape or contour of the breasts.

4. Raise one arm and use the fingers of the opposite hand to check the breast on that side. Beginning at the outer edge, press the flat part of the fingers together and move them in circles around the breast. Start at the outer margins of the breast and continue to make smaller and smaller circles until you get to the nipples. Feel for any unusual lumps or masses beneath the skin. Repeat the procedure on the other breast.

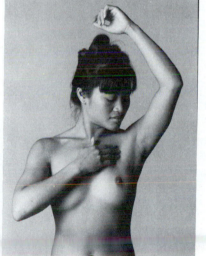

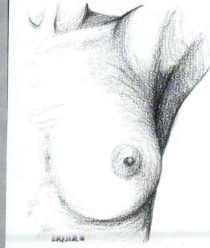

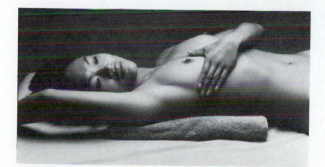

5. Repeat step 4 while lying down with a pillow under the shoulder that is raised. In this position the breast is flattened and easier to examine. Use the same technique with your fingers as described above to examine each breast.

The nipple in the male, and young female who has not borne children (nulliparous female), lies opposite the fourth intercostal space. In the female the breasts lie over the **pectoral** muscles and extend from the second to the sixth or seventh rib and from the lateral border of the sternum to beyond the anterior axillary line. The nipples are bordered by a circular pigmented area, the *areola*. Female breast size is determined more by the amount of adipose (fat) tissue around the glandular tissue than by the amount of glandular tissue itself. Although symmetric, they are usually not absolutely equal in size and shape.

Female breast self-examination

A very important component of self-health for women is a routine breast examination.

The American Cancer Society recommends all women over age 20 should perform breast self-examination monthly. This examination can help a woman know what is normal for her breasts so she can quickly notice any changes. If there are changes, she should consult a physician.

Figure 16-7 illustrates and describes a method of monthly breast self-examination. The best time for this exam is 2 or 3 days after menstruation when the breasts are less likely to be tender or swollen.

Thoracic Viscera

The visceral structures contained in the thoracic (chest) cavity (Figure 16-8) are found in subdivisions called the right and left *pleural cavities* and a region situated between these called the *mediastinum*. Fibrous tis-

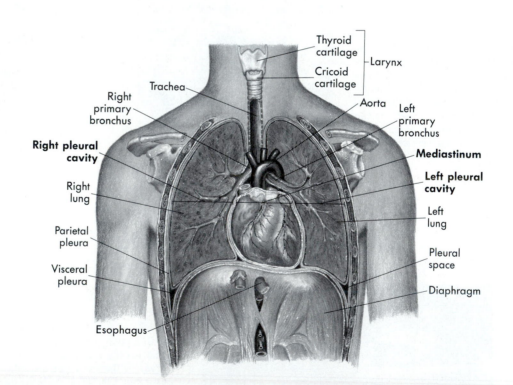

FIGURE 16-8
Thoracic cavity. The thoracic cavity, or "chest cavity," is divided into three subdivisions (left and right pleural cavities and mediastinum) by a partition formed by a serous membrane called the pleura.

sue forms a wall around the mediastinum, completely separating it from the right pleural sac, in which the right lung lies, and from the left pleural sac, which contains the left lung. Contained within the mediastinum are the heart and great vessels, the thymus gland, the trachea and right and left bronchi, the esophagus, the thoracic duct, and other lymphatic vessels and many nerves, arteries, and veins. Thus the only organs in the thoracic cavity that are not located in the mediastinum are the lungs.

The mediastinum is commonly subdivided into four parts. The superior portion lies above a horizontal plane that passes through the great vessels above the heart; the anterior portion lies between the sternum and the heart; the middle portion consists of the heart and its pericardium; and the posterior portion is located between the heart and the bodies of the thoracic vertebrae.

Lungs and Pleura

Paired conical lungs are the essential organs of respiration. Although intricate organs, lungs are essentially a network of branching tubes and air sacs. The lower end of the trachea divides into two *primary bronchi,* which enter each lung. Each primary bronchus divides into smaller branches called *secondary bronchi,* which continue to branch, forming small *bronchioles.* The trachea and the two primary bronchi and their many branches resemble an inverted tree trunk with its branches and are therefore referred to as the *bronchial tree.* The bronchioles subdivide into smaller and smaller tubes, eventually terminating in alveolar sacs, the walls of which consist of numerous *alveoli.* Alveoli are very small air sacs deep in the lungs where oxygen and carbon dioxide are exchanged. This structure can be likened to a bunch of grapes. Some 300 million alveoli are estimated to be present in our two lungs.

Each lung invaginates and fills its pleural cavity. They extend from the diaphragm to a point about ½ to 1 inch (1.5 to 2.5 cm) above the clavicles and lie against the ribs both anteriorly and posteriorly. The medial surface of each lung is roughly concave to allow room for the mediastinal structures and for the heart, but concavity is greater on the left than on the right because of the position of the heart. The primary bronchi and pulmonary blood vessels, bound together by connective tissue to form what is known as the root of the lung, enter each lung through a slit on its medial surface called the *hilum.* Lung tissue is light, spongy in texture, and highly elastic. The right lung contains three lobes, whereas the left lung contains two. The broad inferior surface of each lung, which rests on the diaphragm, is called the base. The pointed upper margin, or apex, projects above the clavicle.

The term **pleura** is used to describe the thin, serous membrane that invests the lungs *(visceral pleura)* and lines the pleural cavity *(parietal pleura)* in which each lung is situated. The visceral pleura adheres so firmly to the lung surface that it is difficult to differentiate from lung tissue.

The parietal layer of the pleura lines the entire thoracic cavity. It adheres to the internal surface of the ribs and the superior surface of the diaphragm, and it partitions the pleural cavities from the mediastinum. A separate pleural sac thus encases each lung. Because the outer surface of each lung is covered by the visceral layer of the pleura, the visceral pleura lies against the parietal pleura, separated only by a potential space (pleural space) that contains just enough pleural fluid for lubrication. Thus when the lungs inflate with air, the smooth, moist visceral pleura adheres to the smooth, moist, parietal pleura, friction is thereby avoided, and respirations are painless. In pleurisy, on the other hand, the pleura is inflamed and respirations become painful.

Mechanism of Pulmonary Ventilation

The thorax plays a major role in ventilation. Because of the elliptic shape of the ribs and the angle of their attachment to the spine, the thorax becomes larger when the chest is raised and elongated and smaller when it is lowered and shortened. It is these changes in thorax size that bring about inspiration and expiration. Lifting up the chest raises the ribs so that they no longer slant downward from the spine, and because of their elliptic shape this enlarges both the depth (front to back) and the width (side to side) of the thorax.

Inspiration

Contraction of the diaphragm alone, or of the diaphragm and the external intercostal muscles, produces quiet inspiration. The diaphragm descends as it contracts, making the thoracic cavity longer. Contraction of the external intercostal muscles pulls the anterior end of each rib up and out. This also elevates the attached sternum and increases the depth and width of the thorax. In addition, contraction of the sternocleidomastoid and serratus anterior muscles can aid in elevation of the sternum and rib cage during forceful inspiration. As the thorax enlarges, it forces the lungs to expand with it because of cohesion between the moist visceral pleura covering the lungs and the moist parietal pleura lining the thorax. As the size of the thorax is enlarged, the pressure inside the chest decreases. This leads to a relative decreased pressure inside the bronchial tubes and alveoli, and this air moves into the lungs.

Expiration

Quiet expiration is ordinarily a passive process that begins when the pressure changes in the thorax that resulted in inspiration are reversed. It is important to remember that lung tissue is highly elastic and tends to return to its original size during expiration. As the thorax decreases in size, the pressure in the bronchial tubes and alveoli increases, and a positive pressure gradient is established from alveoli to atmosphere. This results in expiration as air flows outward through the respiratory passageways. In forced expiration, contraction of the abdominal and internal intercostal muscles can increase the pressure in the thorax far above that produced by the elastic recoil of lung tissue and assist in the outward flow of air.

CHEST INJURIES AND CONDITIONS

Most athletic injuries to the chest are the result of a direct blow. The majority of these injuries are superficial, involving the chest wall or rib cage. Occasionally, athletic injuries may involve the contents of the chest cavity, such as the lungs, heart, or great vessels. These injuries can be life threatening and should be of primary concern to athletic trainers when they occur.

Chest Wall

✤ **Contusions of the chest wall.** Contusions, or bruises, are the most frequent injuries to the chest wall. They may involve the skin, subcutaneous tissues, muscles, or periosteum of the ribs or sternum. On examination, contusions to the chest wall reveal an area of localized tenderness and possibly swelling. In most instances this type of injury does not cause pain during breathing or restrict motion of the rib cage unless very deep respirations are taken.

Breast contusions. Occasionally, a breast tissue contusion, especially to the female breast, will result in fatty necrosis and the formation of a firm nodule of fibrous tissue. These are generally of little consequence but should be examined by a physician for further evaluation. Women participating in collision activities may wear a protective type of brassiere. Another possible cause of breast contusions in women is the significant movement of the breasts during athletic activity, especially in large-breasted women. Constant uncontrolled movement of the breasts over a period of time, can also stretch the Cooper's ligament and cause premature sagging. Today there are various types of support bras designed to prevent excessive breast motion during athletic activity.

Runner's nipple. Runner's nipple is a term given to a irritating and sometimes painful condition caused by the nipple rubbing against a shirt or uniform top. This can normally be prevented by placing a Band-Aid over each nipple before activity.

Strains. A muscle strain is much more likely to involve muscles attached to the rib cage rather than the intercostal muscles within the chest wall. A number of muscles attach to the chest wall and may be strained by overstretching or sudden violent contractions. Injuries to these muscles are discussed in Chapter 18 because disability associated with them is primarily in the use of the arm. Intercostal muscle strains do not occur frequently because these muscles are well protected and usually do not act forcibly enough to stretch their fibers. The signs and symptoms of an intercostal muscle strain resemble those of a chest wall contusion and require similar treatment.

❖ **Rib fracture.** Another fairly common injury to the chest wall resulting from athletic activity is a rib fracture. These are normally caused by a direct blow to the ribs. Less frequently a rib fracture may be caused by forceful compression of the rib cage. An example of this mechanism is an athlete who is involved in a "pile-up" or gives a history of the rib cage being crushed or compressed. The bony integrity may be interrupted anywhere along a rib or ribs because of this general compression of the rib cage; however, ribs tend to break just in front of the angle, which is the weakest point. Ribs 4 through 9 are more liable to fracture because the first three ribs are protected by the shoulder girdle. The lower ribs (10 through 12) also have a greater freedom of movement. Undisplaced fractures, or cracked ribs, are more common in athletic activity than displaced fractures because the ribs are well stabilized by the attachment of the intercostal muscles and the fixation of each rib to its corresponding thoracic vertebra. Signs and symptoms associated with fractured ribs include severe localized pain, which is usually increased on movement of the ribs, breathing deeply, coughing, and sneezing. An athlete with fractured ribs will generally refrain from breathing deeply by taking rapid shallow breaths and may also hold the injured side in an attempt to restrict any painful movement of the chest. During gentle palpation and compression of the ribs, the athlete will indicate pain at the fracture site. If the fracture is displaced, there may also be a pal-pable defect in the rib and crepitation on movement or coughing. Serious complications such as a puncture of thoracic or abdominal visceral structures can occur as a result of rib fractures.

❖ **Costochondral separation.** The mechanisms of injury described for rib fractures are also responsible for costochondral separations. Instead of a rib fracture, there may be a separation or actual dislocation at the articulation between the rib and its articulating cartilage. Signs and symptoms of costochondral separations are similar to rib fractures. In this type of injury, the pain and tenderness are localized over the costochondral junction. If the dislocation is complete, there may be a palpable defect because the tip of the rib rests anteriorly to the costicartilage. In many cases the dislocation will spontaneously reduce, and the athlete may feel a click or snap as the rib dislocates and then almost immediately relocates after the injury. Occasionally this audible and palpable click can be detected on examination (palpation) or will occur during certain voluntary movements of the rib cage. Occasion-

❖ ally an athlete may suffer a **chondrosternal separation** due to a similar mechanism of injury. Tenderness would exist along the chondrosternal junctions. Athletes may also

❖ suffer a sprain of the **costovertebral joints** in the posterior thorax. These may be difficult to distinguish from musculotendinous strains of the thoracic spine. There may be dysfunction of the costovertebral joints, and the athlete may complain of a catch or sharp pain on movement or breathing.

❖ **Fractured sternum.** Injuries involving the sternum do not occur often during athletic activity. Occasionally an athlete may suffer a fractured sternum by a significant direct blow to the sternal area. The signs and symptoms are similar to a rib fracture except that tenderness exists along the sternum. The sternum is thin at the junction of the manubrium with the body, and if fractures do occur, this will be the area most likely involved. If the upper manubrium passes behind the body at the point of fracture, the possibility of an airway obstruction exists. This mechanism of injury may be of sufficient force to potentially involve the heart, lungs, or major blood vessels. It is important that an athlete who receives this type of injury be monitored very carefully for signs of respiratory or circulatory distress.

Intrathoracic Injuries

Intrathoracic (visceral) injuries or conditions occur rarely during athletic activity because of the protection provided by the rib cage and the protective equipment required for various sports. However, these types of injuries can occur as the result of severe trauma to the chest or from complications accompanying rib or sternal fractures. An athlete may also suffer an intrathoracic injury as a result of the penetration of a sharp object. Fortunately, this type of injury rarely occurs during athletic activity. Intrathoracic injuries or conditions can develop rather quickly or insidiously over several hours. Therefore the athletic trainer must be alert to recognize immediate and delayed signs and symptoms associated with chest injuries indicating possible intrathoracic involvement.

✤ **Pneumothorax.** A common intrathoracic complication after a significant chest injury is a pneumothorax; that is, an accumulation of air in the pleural space, that can collapse the lung. This condition may be caused by trauma or the spontaneous rupture of lung tissue. A traumatic pneumothorax can occur when the lung is punctured by a bone fragment resulting from a rib fracture. When lung tissue is lacerated, air from the lung enters the pleural cavity with each inspiration. As this air is trapped in the pleural cavity, the lung separates from the chest wall. With the air continuing to fill the pleural cavity, the volume of the lung is reduced, and the lung can no longer expand normally. This condition is referred to as a collapsed lung and can result in chest pain and shortness of breath. As the uninjured lung fills with air, the trachea may shift or deviate toward the side of the collapsed lung. If the tear in the lung does not seal

itself, the amount of trapped air that cannot escape from the pleural space will continue to increase, and the pressure will continue to build up in the affected pleural cavity. With the increasing pressure, the collapsed lung may be pressed against the uninjured lung and heart, thereby reducing their efficiency. This can develop into a life-threatening situation called a **tension pneumothorax.** A true medical emergency, the tension pneumothorax will usually manifest signs and symptoms of rapidly progressing respiratory distress or breathing difficulty (dyspnea). The trachea shifts or deviates away from the affected or injured side because of the increase in pressure. The importance of following (and completing) a predetermined checklist in the assessment of thoracic injuries is critical. Unless a formal and sequential approach is followed, a serious problem—such as pneumothorax—may be overlooked by athletic trainer and athlete if attention is focused on a painful but non-life-threatening injury such as a broken rib.

Spontaneous pneumothorax. A spontaneous pneumothorax occurs in the absence of trauma or injury. This condition is common in young people between the ages of 15 and 30 and occurs more often in women than men. A spontaneous pneumothorax usually occurs during or immediately after activity when an area of lung tissue ruptures spontaneously, resulting in release of air into a pleural cavity. Spontaneous pneumothorax is characterized by the sudden onset of severe sharp pain in the chest and shortness of breath. It can occur during simple exertions such as coughing.

Hemothorax. A hemothorax is an intrathoracic condition similar to a pneumothorax except that blood, rather than air, collects in the pleural cavity. Hemorrhage may result from injured blood vessels in the chest wall or within the chest cavity. A hemothorax may also be caused by fractured ribs and may occur spontaneously or in conjunction with a pneumothorax (**hemopneumothorax**). A small amount of bleeding will cause few, if any, symptoms. If bleeding is significant, the signs and symptoms are similar to a pneumothorax in that normal lung expansion cannot occur and lung volume is decreased. If bleeding is very severe, the athlete may also show signs of shock from the loss of blood.

Another important sign indicating intrathoracic involvement is coughing of blood or spitting of blood-stained sputum **(hemoptysis).** This may be one of the first signs of injury to the pulmonary structures and must be distinguished from bleeding of the mouth or nose. On occasion an athlete will complain of spitting up blood hours after a traumatic injury to the chest or abdomen. In these cases it is important to differentiate blood-stained sputum from the vomiting of blood **(hematemesis),** which may occur as a result of hemorrhage into the digestive tract. Ask the athlete to bare the teeth; a symptom of true hematemesis is often coagulated blood at the gum line. Any episodes of hemoptysis following injury to the chest should not be ignored. The athlete should seek medical attention for further diagnosis.

Myocardial contusion or concussion. A violent blow or compression of the chest may cause intrathoracic involvement of the cardiovascular system. A heart contusion or concussion can occur following a blow to the anterior chest, such as being hit by a pitched ball. A myocardial concussion is the most acute form of blunt cardiac trauma. This injury is a transitory event that can cause a brief dysrhythmia or loss of consciousness. If the individual survives the initial dysrhythmia, there are no lasting pathological changes. A myocardial contusion results in some degree of cellular injury, may lead to disturbances of the heart's electrical system, and possibly create life-threatening complications. Athletes with severe closed chest trauma need to be closely monitored and perhaps receive medical attention as soon as possible to avoid a fatal outcome.

Conditions Affecting the Respiratory Tract

Common Cold. The common cold is the most frequent viral infection of the respiratory tract. Most individuals will have two or three colds a year, with the peak incidence occurring in the winter months. Symptoms include nasal mucous discharge **coryza**, slight fever and mild chills, generalized malaise, and sometimes a sore throat. Evaluation is based on the above clinical manifestations. The condition is self-limiting, with resolution of symptoms in 7 to 10 days. There is no specific therapy, but bed rest, increased fluid intake, and symptomatic treatment may ease the athlete's discomfort. Antibiotic therapy is indicated only for secondary bacterial infections such as an ear or sinus infection.

Influenza. Influenza (flu) is caused by the influenza virus. Three types have been identified: A, B, and C. Epidemics are associated with Type A and Type B. Type C usually results in a mild sore throat or common cold symptoms. Fever (often as high as 103°F.), runny nose, myalgia (muscular pain), and malaise (uneasiness) occur. Cough and stomach distress usually develop after a few days. Symptoms can be severe. Bed rest, increased fluid intake, and analgesics are important aspects of treatment. Pneumonia is a common complication.

Asthma. Asthma is a common respiratory disease. It is characterized by intermittent episodes of narrowing of the air passages due to muscular constriction of the airway (bronchial tubes). This airway narrowing (often called bronchial spasm) is accompanied by edema of the bronchial wall and excessive bronchial secretions. This restricts air flow to the alveoli. When bronchospasm occurs, an athlete usually experiences wheezing, coughing, and shortness of breath. The wheezes have a characteristic musical quality and are best heard in expiration. The characteristic cough of asthma is usually dry, but may result in the athlete raising large amounts of mucous that is very thick. The shortness of breath varies greatly, depending on the severity of airflow obstruction.

Stimuli that trigger asthma attacks vary from person to person. Some examples are allergens, strong odors or fumes, ingested substances (such as aspirin or certain foods), emotional upset, and stress. Other stimuli are more universal triggers of an asthma attack such as strenuous exercise, cold air, infections, and inhaled irritants such as smoke. Historically, asthma sufferers avoid or have been excluded from athletics or exercise. However, avoiding exercise is unwarranted today and may even be detrimental to an individual with asthma. Medications that allow everyone to be physically active are available to prevent and treat asthmatic attacks.

❖ **Exercise-induced asthma (EIA).** Exercise-induced asthma can occur in an athlete who has asthma but may be present in some athletes only when they are exercising strenuously. An athlete may exercise for several minutes without experiencing any symptoms and then suddenly develop an airway obstruction with the associated symptoms of wheezing, shortness of breath, and chest tightness. An attack usually lasts 5 to 15 minutes, but may last as long as 60 minutes before the obstruction spontaneously resolves. Athletes typically report EIA more often in cold weather. The important factors in inducing an episode of EIA are the level of ventilation during exercise and the temperature and relative humidity of the air. The more intensive the exercise and the colder and drier the inspired air, the greater the airflow obstruction that can develop after exercise. EIA can be controlled in many athletes by observing and adjusting the physical variables that have been linked to this condition. Other approaches include wearing a scarf or mask over the mouth and nose when exercising. Breathing slowly through the nose to warm the air may help. Exercising in repeated spurts of less than 6 minutes each may reduce the development of EIA. Some athletes can "run through" their asthma and continue exercising. Each athlete suffering from EIA must learn how exercise affects his or her body and adjust workouts to avoid attacks. If modifying exercise does not help, medications are available for prevention and treatment of EIA episodes.

Athletes may think an EIA episode is brought on by weakness, exhaustion, or lack of conditioning and may remove themselves from activity. Athletic trainers should be aware of the signs and symptoms of EIA so that more athletes suffering from this condition can be identified and treated. If the athlete, athletic trainer, and physician work together, an athlete can cope with EIA and actively participate in any athletic activity.

❖ **Bronchitis.** Bronchitis (airway inflammation) is an inflammation of the bronchial tubes and can be acute or chronic. Chronic bronchitis is not seen very often in athletic groups. Acute bronchitis is an inflammation of the air passages of the lungs (bronchi and bronchioles) and is caused by an infection. Probably 90% of all cases are caused by viruses and 10% caused by bacteria. The protective functions of the cells lining the bronchial tubes are disturbed by air pollutants such as cigarette smoke, predisposing persons to bronchitis. Symptoms begin with a hacking cough and after 1 to 2 days the person often begins to bring up phlegm, especially if it is a bacterial infection. Other symptoms include malaise, fever, and muscular-type chest wall discomfort. Persons may have clear lungs or they may have wheezing caused by secretions within the large airways. Rest is indicated until the fever subsides; cough suppressants may be helpful. If symptoms do not improve in a few days, a physician should evaluate the athlete to rule out pneumonia or determine the need for antibiotic therapy.

❖ **Infectious Mononucleosis.** Infectious mononucleosis is an infection caused by the Epstein-Barr virus (EBV). EBV infections involve lymphatic cells in the throat. The infection can spread to involve lymphatic tissue in lymph nodes, and often the liver and spleen. Infectious mononucleosis can occur at any age and is very common from age 10 to 25. It is spread by close contact, usually oral to oral contact. This may occur when individuals are asymptomatic. Symptoms may include fever, sore throat, and enlarged and tender cervical lymph nodes. Sometimes the axillary and inguinal nodes and the liver and spleen are tender and/or enlarged. Most cases resolve within 7 to 21 days, although fatigue and weakness may last much longer in some individuals. Athletes suspected of having infectious mononucleosis should be seen by a physician. A blood test is generally required to confirm the diagnosis. Treatment is supportive. Physicians may give cortisone products when complications are suspected. Athletes should refrain from activity until asymptomatic. Splenic rupture is a rare risk factor, especially during the second and third week of the illness.

✤   **Pneumonia.** Pneumonia is generally caused by the same viral or bacterial organisms that cause bronchitis. Pneumonia is an infection of lung tissue, especially the alveoli where oxygen is transported from the air to the red cells in the blood stream. Exposure to the virus or bacteria can occur through the bronchial tubes, by aspiration of foreign material, or direct spread to the alveoli through the blood stream. Before an athlete can develop pneumonia, the body's defense mechanisms are compromised by another infection such as influenza, other medical conditions, or by smoke or noxious fumes. Pneumonia is characterized by coughing, pleurisy, shortness of breath, high fever, chills, malaise, and a toxic appearance. Athletes suspected of pneumonia should be under the care of a physician. Chest x-rays are often used to confirm the diagnosis.

✤   **Coccidioidomycosis.** Coccidioidomycosis is a disease caused by infection of the lungs by a fungus (*Coccidioides immitis*). This fungus is common in dry desert regions and is sometimes called "valley fever" or "desert fever."

ABDOMEN AND PELVIS

The *abdomen* is that portion of the body torso bounded above by the diaphragm and below by the upper pelvis. The abdominal cavity is continuous with the pelvic cavity, and its wall merges with the wall of the pelvis below and the thorax above.

Anatomic Mapping

The method of dividing the abdomen into quadrants (Figure 16-9) or sections for study purposes is discussed in Chapter 2 and should be reviewed. Table 16-1 lists abdominal and pelvic visceral structures located in each of these subdivisions.

Surface Anatomy

In the upper abdomen the costal angle (see Figure 16-5) is formed below the xiphoid process by the diverging cartilages of the sixth to eighth ribs. This area is also known as the epigastrium. The costal margin on the upper and lateral abdominal wall is usually found at the inferior limit of the tenth costal cartilage. Inferiorly, the abdominal wall is bounded by the iliac crest of the hip. The crest ends in front in the anterior superior iliac spine and behind in the posterior superior iliac spine. The *inguinal ligament* (Figure 16-9) in the groin marks the separation between the abdominal wall and the lower extremity.

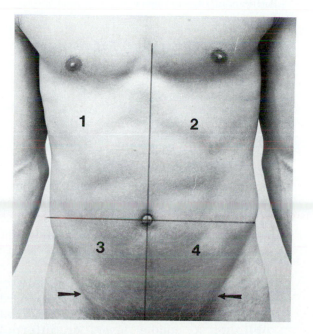

FIGURE 16-9
Division of the abdomen into four quadrants. *1*, Right upper or superior; *2*, left upper or superior; *3*, right lower or inferior; and, *4*, left lower or inferior. Inguinal ligaments are indicated by arrows.

TABLE 16-1

Visceral Structures Located in the Four Abdominal Quadrants

Right upper (superior) quadrant

Right lobe of liver
Gallbladder
Right kidney and adrenal gland
Pylorus of stomach
Duodenum (bulb)
Hepatic flexure of large intestine
Small intestine
Distal (upper) half of ascending colon
Right half of transverse colon
Head of pancreas
Proximal portion of right ureter
Blood vessels, nerves, and lymphatics associated with the
above visceral structures

Left upper (superior) quadrant

Small intestine
Body and fundus of stomach
Spleen
Splenic flexure of large intestine
Tail of pancreas
Left half of transverse colon
Left kidney and adrenal gland
Terminal esophagus
Proximal portion of left ureter
Upper half of descending colon
Blood vessels, nerves, and lymphatics associated with the
above visceral structures

Right lower (inferior) quadrant

Small intestine
Cecum
Appendix
Proximal half of ascending colon
Portion of urinary bladder
Portion of rectum
Distal portion of right ureter
Reproductive structures:
 Female
  Portion of uterus and vagina
  Right ovary
  Right fallopian tube
 Male
  Portion of right vas deferens
  Right seminal vesicle
  Right ejaculatory duct
  Portion of prostate gland
Blood vessels, nerves, and lymphatics associated with the
above visceral structures

Left lower (inferior) quadrant

Small intestine
Distal portion of descending colon
Sigmoid colon
Portion of urinary bladder
Portion of rectum
Distal portion of left ureter
Reproductive structures:
 Female
  Portion of uterus and vagina
  Left ovary
  Left fallopian tube
 Male
  Portion of left vas deferens
  Left seminal vesicle
  Left ejaculatory duct
  Portion of prostate gland
Blood vessels, nerves, and lymphatics associated with the
above visceral structures

The umbilicus is a prominent but somewhat unreliable midline landmark normally located at the level of the intervertebral disc between the third and fourth lumbar vertebrae. In well-developed athletes the anterior abdominal wall is marked by three vertical lines: the *linea alba,* which marks the midline junction between the rectus abdominis muscles, and the two *linea semilunares,* which define the lateral margins of these muscles.

Muscles of the Abdominal Wall

The muscles of the anterior and lateral abdominal wall (Figure 16-10) are arranged in three layers, with the fibers in each layer running in different directions much like the layers of wood in a sheet of plywood. The result is a very strong "girdle" of muscle that covers and supports the abdominal cavity and its internal organs.

The three layers of muscle in the anterolateral (side) abdominal walls are arranged as follows: the outermost layer, or **external oblique;** a middle layer, or **internal oblique;** and the innermost layer, or **transversus abdominis.** In addition to the sheetlike muscles, the band-shaped (or strap-shaped) **rectus abdominis** muscle runs down the midline of the abdomen from

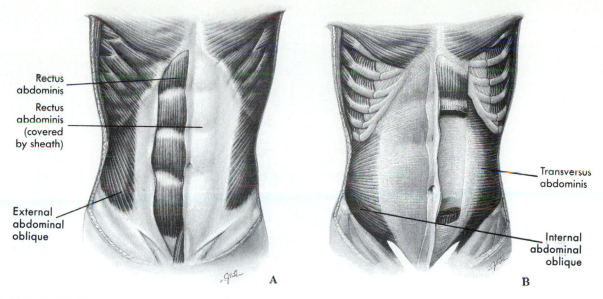

Rectus
abdominis

Rectus
abdominis
(covered
by sheath)

External
abdominal
oblique

Transversus
abdominis

Internal
abdominal
oblique

A

B

FIGURE 16-10
Muscles of the trunk and abdominal wall. **A,** Anterior view showing superficial muscles and, **B,** anterior view showing deeper muscles.

the thorax to the pubis. In addition to protecting the abdominal viscera, the rectus abdominis flexes the spinal column.

Abdominal and Pelvic Anatomy

Division of the abdomen into regions or quadrants makes it easier to locate organs in the abdominopelvic cavity. It is important for the athletic trainer to be able to visualize the placement of these deep visceral structures using external landmarks on the abdominal wall. Review the major internal abdominal organs and their relationships to bony landmarks in Figure 16-11. The abdominal cavity contains the liver, gallbladder, stomach, pancreas, intestines, spleen, kidneys, and ureters. The bladder, certain reproductive organs (uterus, uterine tubes, and ovaries in the female; prostate gland, seminal vesicles, and part of the vas deferens in the male), and part of the large intestine (namely, the sigmoid colon and rectum) lie in the pelvic cavity.

These cavities are lined with a large continuous sheet of serous membrane called the **peritoneum.** The peritoneum lines the walls of the entire abdominal cavity *(pari-etal layer)* and also forms the outer coat for most of the organs *(visceral layer)*. In several places the peritoneum forms reflections, or extensions, that bind abdominal organs together and hold them loosely in place.

ABDOMINAL INJURIES AND CONDITIONS

The abdominal area is vulnerable to injury during most athletic activities, especially contact sports. The muscular abdominal wall is the most commonly involved area. Occasionally, the visceral contents of the abdominal cavity may be involved. Intra-abdominal injuries can be very serious, possibly life threatening. Therefore the athletic trainer must be constantly alert to detect signs and symptoms that may indicate intra-abdominal involvement.

Abdominal Wall

Abdominal strains. Because the abdominal wall is predominately muscular, strains are a common injury. Muscle strains of the abdominal wall are usually the result of a sudden violent contraction, overstretching, or continued overuse. Signs and symptoms

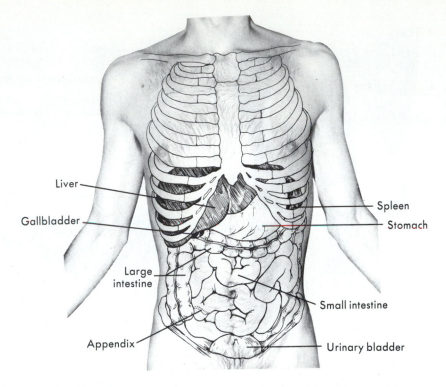

Liver

Gallbladder

Large intestine

Appendix

Spleen

Stomach

Small intestine

Urinary bladder

FIGURE 16-11
Major structures of the abdominal cavity.

associated with strains of the abdominal muscles include localized tenderness, muscle spasm, and rigidity. In strain injuries, the pain will be increased or aggravated by active muscle contraction or passive stretching. For this reason, strains of the abdominal muscles tend to be disabling because these muscles are important when performing most athletic activities. Abdominal strains do not usually involve rupture of the muscle fibers, and recovery is generally rapid. However, when the injury does involve some tearing of muscle fibers or musculotendinous units, the symptoms can be prolonged and disabling. This is especially true if the injury occurs where the abdominal muscles attach to the ribs, iliac crests, or pubis. In these instances, the athlete may continue to aggravate the injured area, and the injury can be self-limiting.

Contusions. Contusions are common injuries to the abdominal muscles, because this area can be subjected to direct blows during many types of athletic activity. Because of the resiliency of the abdominal wall, muscle contusions in this area are generally not severe. No rigid background exists on which an external blow can impact to cause this type of injury. The greatest danger of impact-type trauma to the abdominal wall is injury to the visceral contents within the cavity.

❖ **Iliac crest contusion.** Direct blows to the bony attachments of the abdominal muscles can be severe. For example, a blow to the crest of the ilium can cause both a crushing type of injury, resulting in a localized muscle contusion, and the tearing of some fibers at the point of muscle attachment to bone. This injury, commonly called a **hip pointer**, can be disabling. Athletes will complain of severe and agonizing pain that is aggravated by any type of movement, such as turning, twisting, laughing, coughing, or going to the bathroom. In such cases the athlete should be treated symptomatically, that is, the athlete should be kept inactive until the symptoms subside.

Side ache. Another common condition involving the abdominal wall is a "side ache", or "stitch in the side." The sharp pain and muscle spasms associated with this condition usually occur along the lower rib cage or in the upper abdominal muscles and are often associated with running activities. In many cases the pain will be increased on inspiration, making deep breathing very uncomfortable. Most side ache attacks are short lived, and pain is relieved after cessation of the activity. A side ache also appears to respond well to stretching of the involved side. Several theories have been advanced to explain why an athlete may experience a side ache. Current theories point to local anoxia (lack of oxygen) of the involved muscles or spasm of the diaphragm as causative factors. Athletes who experience repeated side aches may need additional evaluation to determine possible causes contributing to the condition. Level of conditioning, current training program, eating habits, or elimination routines may also be causative factors.

❖ **Hernia.** Protrusion of abdominal viscera through a portion of the abdominal wall is called a hernia. This condition, although generally not caused by an athletic injury, can be aggravated by athletic activity. Intra-abdominal pressure, which increases during weight training or strenuous athletic activity, can produce the signs and symptoms associated with a hernia. Areas of the abdominal wall most susceptible to hernias are the inguinal and femoral canals. The inguinal canal is the point at which the spermatic cord containing blood vessels, nerves, and the vas deferens of the male reproductive system leaves the abdominal cavity and enters the scrotum. In the female, the round ligament of the uterus passes through the canal and terminates in the labia majora. The femoral canal is the point at which the femoral blood vessels and nerves pass from the abdominal cavity into the lower extremity. These two openings are protected by muscular control, much like the shutter of a camera, and may be congenitally weak or weakened by continued intra-abdominal pressure, resulting in abdominal viscera being forced through these canals and out of the abdominal cavity. The resulting hernia can range from a minor problem to a severe abdominal wall defect. Symptoms associated with a hernia are pain and prolonged discomfort and a feeling of weakness or pulling in the groin. A protrusion may also be felt in the groin, which will increase on coughing. In almost every case an athlete with a hernia experiences only minor pain and discomfort, which is tolerated well during athletic activity. However, in a severe hernia, there is always the danger of incarceration of the protruding viscera with the possibility of occluding the blood supply to the tissue. This is called a **strangulated hernia** and needs immediate medical attention. Any time the signs and symptoms of a hernia are increased by athletic activity, the athlete should be referred to a physician.

Intra-abdominal Injuries

Athletic injuries involving the contents of the abdominal cavity occur infrequently. The musculature of the abdominal wall provides adequate protection for the intra-abdominal viscera from most injuries. However, serious athletic injuries to the intra-abdominal contents do occur and can become life threatening. These injuries are usually associated with contact or collision sports and occur as the result of some type of direct trauma to the abdomen or lower back. The structures most often associated with serious intra-abdominal injuries are the solid organs such as the kidneys, spleen, and liver— all organs rich in blood supply. Occasionally the hollow organs, mesentery, peritoneum, or female reproductive organs are involved in an athletic injury. Intra-abdominal injuries or conditions can develop quickly or insidiously over a period of time; therefore the athletic trainer must be alert to signs and symptoms, such as shock, that may indicate possible intra-abdominal involvement.

❖ **Celiac plexus syndrome.** The most common intra-abdominal injury is a blow to the celiac plexus (solar plexus), commonly known as having the "wind knocked out." This network of nerves lies deep in the upper middle region of the abdomen. A blow to this area can cause a transitory paralysis of the diaphragm. Although an athlete may become very anxious, this injury is usually of short duration, and no treatment is necessary because the condition responds to a few moments of rest and reassurance. If complete recovery does not occur within minutes, and pain, tenderness, and signs of shock appear, intra-abdominal injury should be suspected. The athlete should be referred to a physician for further evaluation or treatment. It is important to remember that the signs and symptoms associated with significant intra-abdominal injuries will persist.

Signs and symptoms associated with an injury to the abdominal viscera depend on the organ involved, severity of the injury, and the resulting amount of hemorrhage. For the most part, the abdominal organs are insensitive to pain because they contain few pain fibers. Therefore an injury to the organ itself may cause little if any pain or tenderness unless the covering capsule is involved. An exception to this is the liver, which has a good network of nerves; an injury to the liver will cause acute pain. More often it is hemorrhaging into the capsule of an organ or into the peritoneal cavity that causes pain. For example, bleeding into the capsule surrounding one of the kidneys will cause pain or point tenderness.

Injuries to the hollow organs are extremely uncommon because an athlete's stomach, intestines, and bladder are generally empty during athletic activity. A hollow organ injury may not produce symptoms unless some of the contents within come into contact with the peritoneum and cause irritation or the organ becomes *distended*. A common example of this is the appendix. Many times the symptoms associated with

✤ **appendicitis** are not present until the organ distends or ruptures.

✤   **Peritonitis.** Hollow organs are more susceptible to an athletic injury when they are

TABLE 16-2

Referred Visceral Pain

Organ	Area of body to which pain may be referred
Appendix	Right lower quadrant, umbilicus
Bladder	Lower abdomen and upper thighs
Diaphragm	Anterior shoulders
Esophagus	Along sternum, left upper thorax
Heart	Base of neck, left jaw, and left shoulder and arm
Intestines	Back (backache or sharp pain in the back), umbilicus
Kidney	High in the posterior costovertebral angle and radiating forward around the flank
Liver	Right shoulder
Pancreas	Directly behind pancreas
Spleen	Left shoulder and upper third of arm
Ureter	Costovertebral angle, radiating to lower abdomen, testicles (male), and inner thigh

full of food or waste products. When these hollow structures are injured, they may discharge their contents into the abdominal cavity or adjacent tissues. This may cause an intense, painful inflammatory reaction to the peritoneum called peritonitis. The resulting signs and symptoms may include abdominal pain and tenderness similar to those associated with injuries to solid organs. Additional signs that may indicate an injury to one of the hollow organs are black **tarry stools,** bright red blood in the fecal discharge, or bloody vomitus (hematemesis).

Another important symptom that must be remembered when evaluating abdominal injuries is referred pain. Many injuries affecting abdominal viscera will cause pain in a part of the body removed from an injured area. For example, an injured spleen may cause pain in the left shoulder and upper arm **(Kehr's sign).** An injury to the liver may refer pain to the right shoulder, and an injury to one of the kidneys may be felt high in the posterior costovertebral angle, as well as radiating forward. Table 16-2 lists the common referral sites for pain corresponding to injured viscera. It is not necessary for the athletic trainer to remember all the referral sites of pain. However, it is important to understand the phenomenon of referred visceral pain, which often accompanies an intra-abdominal injury, and to be able to recognize this symptom.

The "visceral pain" that arises in an injured abdominal organ is generally poorly localized at the actual site of injury. Instead, referred pain is felt at a distant site that is innervated by the same spinal segment as the injured visceral structure. Although the exact mechanism of referred pain is still unknown, the most accepted theory suggests that visceral pain fibers synapse with neurons in the spinal cord that receive pain fibers from the skin in the referred area. When a visceral structure is injured and pain fibers are stimulated, the pain sensations spread to neurons that normally conduct pain sensations from the skin, and the athlete has the feeling that the pain sensations actually originate in the skin of the referred pain area. The location of the referred pain on the body surface is in the same dermatome of the segment from which the injured visceral organ was originally derived during embryonic development. Some types of referred pain also result from reflex muscular spasm. A bruised ureter, for example, will cause reflex spasm of the lumbar muscles on the side of injury.

❖ **Kidney, spleen, and liver injuries.** Of the solid organs, the kidneys are most frequently injured, followed by the spleen and liver. When these organs are injured during athletic activity, the mechanism is usually some type of direct blow to the abdomen or back. These organs may be contused or lacerated. A ruptured spleen is the most frequent cause of death among athletes who sustain blunt abdominal injuries. The universal symptom of a spleen injury is constant left upper quadrant or left flank pain that is aggravated with movement or deep inspiration. Athletes may also feel shoulder pain (Kehr's sign). They are often cold or clammy or show signs of shock, as well as being nauseated and vomiting.

The primary danger of any solid organ injury is the possibility of severe hemorrhaging into the abdominal cavity. Bleeding can occur rapidly or very slowly and insidiously. Occasionally the bleeding will stop a short time after the injury, only to start again hours, days, or possibly weeks later. Therefore the athletic trainer must be alert for delayed symptoms occurring with abdominal injuries. The injured athlete must also be made aware of possible delayed symptoms that, if they occur, should be reported immediately.

The signs and symptoms associated with an injury to a solid organ usually include pain, localized tenderness, rebound tenderness, abdominal rigidity, nausea, and vomiting. If hemorrhaging is severe, the athlete will also exhibit signs of blood loss or shock. These signs include pallor, rapid pulse, low blood pressure, dizziness, and fainting. An injury to the kidneys usually produces blood in the urine (**hematuria**). The amount of blood in the urine may be such that it is easily recognized on inspection or so minor that the urine looks normal *(microscopic hematuria)*. Therefore, after a suspected injury to the kidneys, all urine passed should be checked visually and microscopically for blood.

Gastrointestinal Conditions

Athletic trainers should also be alert for signs and symptoms that may indicate the presence of an infection or inflammatory process in the gastrointestinal system. If present, these are not necessarily associated with an athletic injury but may indicate the athlete should be referred to a physician for further diagnosis. Some of the common gastrointestinal conditions are as follows.

Vomiting. Vomiting, or *throwing up,* is a common response of the stomach to a stimulus such as irritation, obstruction, or infection. As previously discussed, an injury or blow to the abdomen may also cause an athlete to vomit. Vomiting is always serious and an important sign. It is normally not an emergency in itself unless it goes on for several days and the athlete has not eaten or drunk enough fluids to replace that lost in the vomitus.

❖ **Diarrhea.** Diarrhea is a condition of abnormally frequent and liquid bowel movements. Many conditions such as anxiety, gastroenteritis, bacterial infections, parasitic infestations, and inflammatory processes in the bowel can cause an athlete to have diarrhea. Like vomiting, diarrhea is not normally an emergency unless it continues for several days and the athlete has not eaten or drunk sufficient fluids to replace those lost.

❖ **Constipation.** Constipation is an infrequent or difficult evacuation of the feces. It can be caused by some disease or condition of the gastrointestinal tract, lack of sufficient roughage and bulk in the diet, overuse of laxatives, and nervousness and anxiety. Constipation may also be due to bad habits. If the desire to defecate is neglected or suppressed, the urge passes and water is absorbed from the fecal mass, which becomes hard and dry. Constipation is not normally a problem in the athletic age group. However, it should become a concern if there is a change from an athlete's normal pattern in such things as a sudden decrease in frequency of defecation, sudden and persistent change in the character or amount of stools, or problems expelling the stool.

❖ **Indigestion.** Indigestion (*dyspepsia*) is a lack or failure of normal digestion. There can be many causes. In athletes, indigestion is often associated with emotional stress associated with competition, idiosyncrasies in eating habits, or inflammation of the mucous membranes of the esophagus and stomach. Constant indigestion can lead to chronic disorders such as gastritis, gastroenteritis, or ulcers. Anxious, high-strung athletes who exhibit chronic indigestion should be seen by a physician.

❖ **Gastroenteritis.** Gastroenteritis is an inflammation of the stomach and intestines. It is usually of viral or bacterial origin and a very common cause of vomiting.

❖ **Gastritis.** Gastritis is an inflammation of the lining of the stomach. Some of the possible causes of this condition are the use of aspirin, alcohol, some medications, and stress. The result is gastric bleeding that may vary from slight to massive. An athlete with gastritis normally has vague, indefinite pain in the upper left quadrant or epigastrium.

❖ **Ulcer.** An ulcer of the gastrointestinal tract is the disintegration and necrosis of the mucous membrane caused by the acid gastric juices. An ulcer of the stomach is called a *peptic ulcer,* and an ulcer in the duodenum next to the stomach is called a *duodenal ulcer*. When for any reason a small area of gastric or duodenal mucous membrane is injured and becomes necrotic, the acid gastric juice digests the dead tissue just as it would a piece of meat. In this way a depression or hole is made that extends into the wall of the stomach or duodenum. Often an athlete with an ulcer is high-strung, nervous, irritable, prone to worry, and stressful. The primary symptom of an ulcer is pain. The pain is often relieved by taking food but usually returns within an hour. An alkali such as sodium bicarbonate may also relieve the pain by neutralizing the acid. Athletes with ulcers must often be treated symptomatically during various athletic activities.

❖ **Colitis.** Colitis is an inflammation of the colon. A common cause of bowel disease, ulcerative colitis affects all age groups and often starts in young adult life. The condition generally begins with an acute attack of abdominal pain accompanied by diarrhea and the passage of blood, mucus, and pus in the feces. Fever and malaise are also present. This is often a chronic condition characterized by alternating periods of exacerbations and remissions.

❖ **Hemorrhoids.** Hemorrhoids, or piles, is a condition in which the veins at the lower end of the rectum become varicose (swollen) and enlarged. *Internal hemorrhoids* are those covered by the mucous membrane of the lower end of the rectum. They may "come down" through the anal opening and appear on the surface, although they can be replaced by pressure. *External hemorrhoids* are covered by the skin in the neighborhood of the anus. Chronic constipation, heredity, and increased pressure due to straining during a bowel movement can cause these varicose veins. The result may be a protrusion and/or bleeding of the veins of the anus. Most hemorrhoids are self-limiting but occasionally an athlete must be referred to a physician for care and perhaps surgery.

Additional Abdominal Conditions

❖ **Pancreatitis.** Pancreatitis is an inflammation of the pancreas that can be mild and lead to vague abdominal symptoms or severe with intense pain, often referred to as an "acute abdomen." It can be caused by an infectious agent. Often it appears to be due to the sudden release of active pancreatic enzymes within the organ itself. Attacks often occur after a large meal or an alcoholic spree. Intense pain is the outstanding symptom. More painful than ulcers, often the individual remains motionless, appears to be in shock, turns blue in the face. Immediate medical referral is indicated.

❖ **Hepatitis.** Hepatitis is an inflammation of the liver. Commonly it is a result of viral infection, but it can be secondary to bacterial, fungal, or parasitic infection, a result of toxic exposure, a side effect of a prescribed medication, or a consequence of an immunologic disorder. Symptoms of hepatitis are variable. Common symptoms are malaise, fever, loss of appetite, and jaundice, followed by nausea, vomiting, abdominal discomfort, and diarrhea. **Jaundice** is a yellow coloring to the skin or the sclera. Infectious hepatitis is extremely contagious and precautions should be taken to avoid infection.

❖ **Sickle cell anemia.** Although sickle cell anemia is a condition of the blood, it is discussed at this time because of its abdominal symptoms and possible involvement with the spleen. Sickle cell anemia is a hereditary, genetically determined, sometimes fatal disease that is characterized by an abnormal type of hemoglobin. It is largely confined to the black population. An individual who inherits only one defective gene develops a form of the disease called *sickle cell trait*. In sickle cell trait, red blood cells contain a small proportion of a type of hemoglobin that is less soluble than normal. If two defective genes are inherited (one from each

parent), then more of the defective hemoglobin is produced and the distortion of red blood cells becomes severe. An athlete may never experience any complications from having sickle cell trait. However, an acute crisis may occur and can be a recurrent, painful, and frustrating problem. Precipitating factors may be high altitudes, fever, infections, cold exposure, and stress. Symptoms include fatigue, muscle weakness, pallor, and severe pain, often in the abdomen, chest, back, and extremities. The disease may mimic an acute abdomen. In the most severe cases, death may occur.

❖ **Diabetes mellitus.** Diabetes mellitus can be defined as a disorder of carbohydrate and fat metabolism that is due to an absolute or relative lack of insulin. Insulin is a hormone secreted by the pancreas and is essential in the metabolism of glucose. Insulin deficiency prevents synthesis of glucose and causes a rise in the blood glucose level (**hyperglycemia**). When blood sugar levels rise above normal, glucose escapes into the urine (**glycosuria**), which leads to an increased secretion of urine (**polyuria**). Additional signs and symptoms of untreated diabetes are excessive thirst and hunger, marked weakness, and loss of weight.

Diabetes mellitus is classified into two types. Insulin-dependent diabetes (IDD) is also known as type I or juvenile-onset diabetes. This form of diabetes can occur at any age, but primarily affects children and young adults and is due to a failure of the pancreas to secrete insulin. These individuals must have insulin injected daily. Non-insulin-dependent diabetes (NIDD) is also known as type II or adult-onset diabetes. This form of diabetes occurs in the middle-aged and elderly. These individuals have impaired insulin function and can usually control the condition by a combination of diet, exercise, and medications.

Athletic trainers must be familiar with the two acute emergency situations that may develop from diabetes. **Diabetic coma** is caused by an increase of acid waste products in the blood (**ketoacidosis**) and the loss of body fluids. This condition develops slowly, usually over a period of several days. Precipitating factors may be infections or illness, dietary mistakes, and failure to take insulin or prescribed medications. As blood sugar levels rise the individual may become listless, dehydrated, with rapid and deep breathing, a rapid and weak pulse, and a sweet or fruity odor on their breath. Without treatment the individual will eventually become unresponsiveness and comatose. This individual needs medical attention and insulin. This condition will be rarely seen in an actively exercising diabetic athlete.

Insulin shock is seen in an individual who has taken too much insulin, not enough food, or has exercised too much and used up all available glucose. In this situation, not enough sugar remains in the blood to provide the continuous supply needed for the brain. Insulin shock develops much more quickly than diabetic coma, perhaps in a matter of minutes. The signs and symptoms associated with insufficient sugar in the blood (**hypoglycemia**), include irritability, hunger, dizziness, sweating, apprehension, confusion, headache, and possibly convulsions and coma. Athletes in insulin shock need sugar immediately. This can be in the form of sugar cubes, candy, juice, fruit, or sweetened soft drinks. The symptoms will be reversed within several minutes. An athlete who cannot swallow should be transported immediately to medical assistance where intravenous glucose can be given.

Most diabetic athletes are well versed in controlling their blood glucose levels and can participate in athletic activity. However, athletic trainers should always know which athletes are diabetic so they can be monitored for signs and symptoms of diabetic conditions. This is especially true early in any season when an athlete is adjusting his or her activity level with diet and insulin or medication requirements.

Eating Disorders

Eating disorders have become prominent in society, as well as in athletics, especially in sports in which low bodyweight is viewed as enhancing optimal performance. The two nutritional disorders with which all athletic trainers should be familiar are anorexia nervosa and bulimia.

❖ **Anorexia nervosa.** Anorexia nervosa is an eating disorder with symptoms of self-starvation, a refusal to maintain normal bodyweight, and an intense fear of gaining weight or becoming fat. The result is bodyweight at least 15% below that expected for age and height. Anorexia is primarily found in young women and is frequently associated with menstrual disorders. Often an intense exercise program is strictly adhered to as an additional means of burning calories and as a way to distract oneself from feelings of hunger. Anorexia is a serious disorder because an individual can die from self-starvation.

❖ **Bulimia.** Bulimia is a disorder including episodes of binge eating followed by self-induced vomiting, use of laxatives or diuretics, strict dieting and fasting, or vigorous exercise to undo the effects of the binge episode to prevent weight gain. These individuals usually have a more normal weight. Vomiting can become addictive and uncontrollable.

Athletes with anorexia or bulimia portray a poor body image and are overly concerned about body shape and weight. These individuals may need intervention and counseling. Table 16-3 lists warning signs an athletic trainer can look for to assist in recognizing an athlete with an eating disorder.

THE GENITALIA

Male

The external genitalia in the male consist of the scrotum and penis (Figure 16-12). The scrotum is a skin-covered pouch suspended from the perineal region. Internally it is divided into two sacs by a septum; each sac contains a testis, epididymis, and lower part of a spermatic cord. The testes are small ovoid glands somewhat flattened from side to side. The left testis is generally located about 1 cm lower in the scrotal sac than the right. Both testes are suspended in the pouch by attachment to scrotal tissue and by the spermatic cords, which ascend from

TABLE 16-3
Warning Signs for Eating Disorders

Anorexia nervosa

Dramatic loss in weight

A preoccupation with food, calories, body image, and weight

Wearing baggy or layered clothing

Relentless, excessive exercise

Disruption or change in usual eating patterns, such as skipping meals, eating alone, unusual food choices, etc.

Denial or defensive behavior when confronted with changes in eating patterns, weight, appearance, etc.

Mood swings

Changes in school or work performance

Changes in menstrual cycle

Avoiding food-related social activities

Bulimia

A noticeable weight loss or gain

Persistent overconcern with body shape and weight

Bathroom visits after meals

Depressive moods

Strict dieting followed by eating binges

Increasing criticism of one's body

Continual episodes of overeating not accompanied by weight gain

Regular use of self-induced vomiting, laxatives, and diuretics

Sores at the corners of the mouth that do not heal

Sudden increase in frequency or number of dental cavities

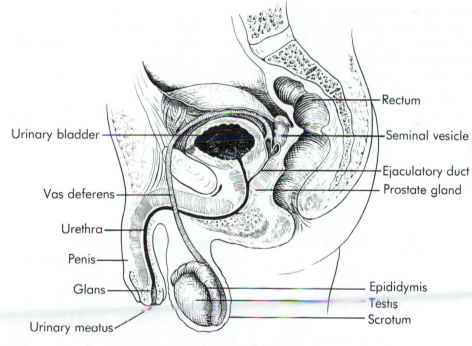

FIGURE 16-12
Sagittal section through the male pelvis.

the scrotum and enter the abdomen by passing through the inguinal canals. The muscular vas deferens, a component of the spermatic cord, can be palpated through the scrotal wall as a firm and rounded cord.

The penis is composed of three cylindrical masses of erectile, or cavernous, tissue, enclosed in separate fibrous coverings and held together by a covering of skin. The two larger and uppermost of these cylinders are named the corpora cavernosa penis, whereas the smaller, lower one, which contains the urethra, is called the corpus cavernosum urethrae (corpus spongiosum).

The distal part of the corpus cavernosum urethrae overlaps the terminal end of the two corpora cavernosa penis to form a slightly bulging structure, the glans penis, over which, in the uncircumcised male, the skin is folded doubly to form a more or less loose-fitting, retractable casing known as the prepuce or foreskin. The opening of the urethra at the tip of the glans is called the external urinary meatus.

Female

The term *vulva* is used to describe structures that constitute the female external genitalia (Figure 16-13). The vulva consists of the mons pubis, labia majora, labia minora, clitoris, urinary meatus (external orifice), and vaginal orifice. Ducts from the greater vestibular (Bartholin's) and lesser vestibular (Skene's) glands also open into the vulva.

The mons pubis is a skin-covered pad of fat over the symphysis pubis. Pubic hair appears on this structure at puberty. The labia majora (large lips) are covered with pigmented skin and hair on the outer surface and are smooth and free from hair on the inner surface.

The labia minora (small lips) are located within the labia majora and are covered with modified skin. These two lips come together anteriorly in the midline. The area between the labia minora is the vestibule.

The clitoris is a small organ composed of erectile tissue, located just behind the junction of the labia minora; it is homologous to the corpora cavernosa and glans penis. The prepuce, or foreskin, covers the clitoris, as it does the glans penis in the male. The urinary meatus (urethral orifice) is the small opening of the urethra, situated between the clitoris and the vaginal orifice. The vaginal orifice is located posterior to the external urinary meatus.

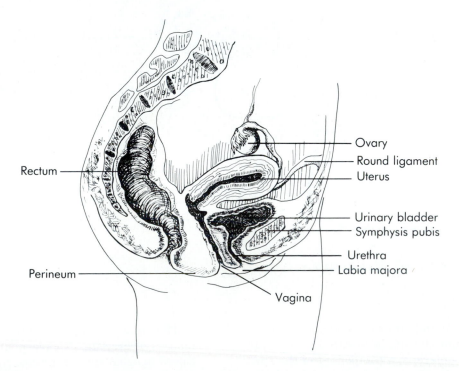

FIGURE 16-13
Sagittal section through the female pelvis.

GENITALIA INJURIES AND CONDITIONS

Athletic injuries to the genitalia, and especially to the internal reproductive organs, are extremely uncommon. The female reproductive structures, almost entirely internal and well protected by the bony pelvis and abdominal musculature, are seldom injured. Occasionally the vulva is injured as the result of a fall astride some object such as a balance beam or uneven parallel bar. The resulting injury is normally a contusion and should be treated as any other injury of this nature. Contusions should be treated with a cold pack to minimize hemorrhaging, and lacerations should be referred for suturing to minimize scarring. Even relatively small lacerations involving the skin-covered muscular region (perineum) between the vaginal orifice and the anus are potentially dangerous and should always be referred to a physician for treatment. In women the perineum and perineal body form an important support structure in the pelvic floor and, if weakened, may result in partial uterine or vaginal prolapse.

✤ **Vaginitis.** Vaginitis is common in women and is usually caused by a yeast or parasitic infection. It normally has a gradual onset with painful urination **(dysuria),** vaginal discharge, vaginal odor, and itching. Women with these symptoms should be referred for an examination and proper treatment.

✤ **Testicle contusion.** The external genitalia is a common injury site for the male athlete. The testes are fairly vulnerable to injury during many types of athletic activity. These injuries usually occur as the result of a direct blow to the scrotum. The resulting contusion can range from very mild to an extremely painful, nauseating, and disabling injury for the athlete. In most cases, pain from these injuries is short lived. Occasionally there will be a significant amount of bleeding associated with a testicular contusion, which requires the application of an ice pack to the scrotal area. An athlete may also complain of a drawing sensation as the muscles attached to the testes go into spasm.

Following a blow to the scrotum, the athlete must be put at ease and testicular spasm reduced. One method of reducing testicular spasm is to instruct or assist the athlete in bringing both knees up toward his chest (Figure 16-14). This assists in relaxing the muscle spasms and reducing discomfort. Another procedure that helps reduce testicular spasm is the **Valsalva maneuver.** This is accomplished when the athlete forcibly exhales against a closed glottis, thereby building up intra-abdominal pressure. Examine for or have the athlete check for normal positioning and appearance of the testes following a blow to the scrotum. It is possible that torsion of the spermatic cord can occur by a testicle revolving in the scrotum as a result of trauma. If this condition occurs, the scrotum may appear to be a cluster of swollen veins, and the athlete may experience a dull pain combined with a heavy, dragging sensation in the scrotal region. An athlete with these signs and symptoms should receive immediate medical attention. Usually the signs and symptoms associated with most scrotal injuries subside in a few minutes and require no further evaluation. If the trauma results in residual pain and swelling, the athlete should use an athletic supporter for scrotal support during the recovery phase. Continue to monitor this athlete, and if symptoms persist or become worse, the athlete should be referred to medical assistance for further evaluation and treatment.

✤ **Hydrocele.** A hydrocele is fluid in the tunica vaginalis which is the membrane covering the front and sides of the testis and epididymis. The cause is an inflammatory condition of the testis or epididymis, a tumor, or trauma. When trauma is involved there may be blood present as well; this is called a **hematocele.**

✤ **Varicocele.** A varicocele is a varicose condition of the veins from the testicle and epididymis forming a swelling that feels like a "bag of worms." This may appear bluish through the skin of the scrotum and is accompanied by a constant pulling, dragging, or dull pain in the scrotum.

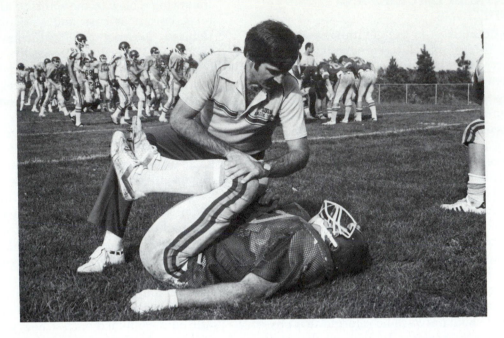

FIGURE 16-14
Method of reducing testicular spasm by bringing both knees up to the chest.

Testicular cancer. All athletic trainers should possess knowledge about testicular cancer and the signs and symptoms that may indicate a testicular tumor. Cancer of the testes is the most common type of tumor cancer in men 15 to 35 years of age. It accounts for 12% of all cancer deaths in this age group. However, it is difficult to get an accurate estimate of total cases because often testicular cancer has metastasized before being discovered and will then be reported under the later site. Early detection is the basis of effective treatment, but it is often delayed as a result of an individual's fear and lack of knowledge of this condition. If discovered and treated promptly in its early stages, testicular cancer can be treated effectively.

A painless scrotal mass is the most common symptom of a testicular tumor. Other symptoms include: (1) a slight enlargement of one of the testes or a change in its consistency, (2) a dull ache in the lower abdomen, and (3) a sensation of dragging or heaviness in the scrotum. The incidence of testicular cancer is higher among males with an undescended testicle. Although it is unlikely

that testicular cancer is caused by an athletic injury, trauma is another of the possible risk factors for individuals having testicular tumors. Testicular tumors can be confused with other conditions of the testes, such as epididymitis, hydrocele, hematoma, spermatocele, or varicocele. An athlete with any testicular or scrotal mass should be referred to a physician immediately. Athletic trainers should monitor an athlete under treatment for any of these conditions and, if there is no improvement, refer the athlete again for further medical consultation.

The best method for early detection of testicular cancer is testicular self-examination (TSE) and education. All young males should be taught how to perform monthly TSE and be made aware of signs and symptoms that indicate further evaluation is necessary. Figure 16-15 illustrates testicular self-examination. The best time to check for abnormal lumps in the testicles is after a hot bath or shower. The hot water causes the scrotal muscles to relax, and the testicles and related structures within the scrotum are easily felt. Each testicle should be checked separately using the tips of the fin-

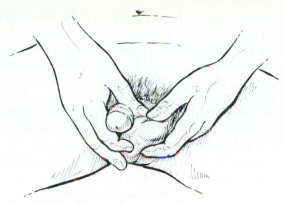

FIGURE 16-15
Testicular self-examination. Note that each testicle is checked using fingertips and thumb.

gers and thumb. Males should learn what feels normal and know what the epididymis feels like. If any lumps are felt, a physician should check the suspected growth. The American Cancer Society has material available to the public on testicular cancer and TSE. In addition, a careful examination of the testes by a physician should be part of any physical examination of young male athletes.

Menstrual Dysfunctions

Menstrual irregularities seem to be more prevalent in physically active women. Although the exact mechanism has not been established, there are a variety of proposed mechanisms related to menstrual disturbances. These include body composition, training regimen, reproductive maturity, diet, psychologic stress, and pathologic conditions.

❖ **Amenorrhea.** Amenorrhea is the absence or abnormal stoppage of the menses.
❖ **Oligomenorrhea** is abnormally infrequent or scanty menstruation. Primary amenorrhea is the delay in menarche beyond age 16; secondary amenorrhea is the absence of menstruation in women who previously were periodically menstrual.
❖ **Dysmenorrhea.** Dysmenorrhea is painful menstruation. It is a less frequent menstrual disturbance and inconclusive whether athletic activity can lessen or produce dys-

menorrhea. All women who demonstrate any of these menstrual irregularities should be referred for medical examination and specific treatment.

Sexually Transmitted Diseases

Sexually transmitted diseases are common, and any athlete with urethral discharge should be referred to medical assistance. These diseases can become chronic and have devastating, long-term effects for the individual.

❖ **Chlamydia.** Chlamydia is a genus of microorganisms that are intracellular parasites that cause a wide variety of diseases. Chlamydia trachomatis causes genital infections in males and females and is the most common sexually transmitted pathogen. In males the inflammation occurs with pus (purulent) discharge 1 to 4 weeks after intercourse. Occasionally, painful urination and traces of blood in the urine result. This is the most common cause of **urethritis** (inflammation of the urethra) in the male. In females the infection is often asymptomatic but may cause a vaginal discharge, painful urination, and a painful pelvis. These individuals should be referred to medical assistance for evaluation and treatment.

❖ **Gonorrhea.** Gonorrhea, commonly called the *clap,* is caused by the gonococcal bacteria and is normally spread through sexual intercourse. In the male, an acute urethritis appears 2 to 8 days after infection. A purulent discharge is the main symptom and is combined with difficulty and pain on passing urine. If treated promptly the disease usually clears up rapidly. If untreated, the infection can spread to involve the seminal vesicles and epididymis. In the female, gonorrhea causes acute urethritis and cervicitis, but symptoms are frequently ignored or absent, and the infection goes unnoticed. The infection can spread to the fallopian tubes and lead to an associated peritonitis. These individuals should be under a physician's care.

❖ **Syphilis.** Syphilis is caused by the spirochete *Treponema pallidum,* a slender, spiral, parasitic microorganism. A small papule develops at the site of inoculation 10 to 90 days after exposure. This papule then becomes a painless ulcer, the classic *chancre*. The chancre heals without treatment in 4 to 5 days and leaves little scarring. Its occurrence can easily be missed, particularly in women in whom the lesion can be on the cervix or vaginal vault. Within 2 to 3 months of exposure, the disease becomes clinically generalized and a rash of secondary syphilis appears. This is seen as a non-itching rash and can affect the whole body, including the palms and soles. A slight fever, headaches, and joint pain may be noted at this stage. These individuals should be under a physician's care.

ATHLETIC INJURY ASSESSMENT PROCESS

Potentially serious and life-threatening injuries involving the chest or abdomen can occur during athletic activity. The chest contains the heart and lungs, the most vital life-sustaining organs. Any trauma to the chest that seriously compromises the function of these organs can pose an immediate threat to survival. The abdomen contains several organs richly supplied with blood, to which trauma can cause severe and possibly fatal hemorrhaging. Although most athletic injuries involving the chest and abdomen are not serious or life threatening, the possibility always exists. Therefore the athletic trainer must be aware of the possible types of chest and abdominal injuries that can occur and be alert for signs and symptoms indicative of life-threatening situations to ensure appropriate assessment and emergency treatment.

Primary survey

During the primary survey, evaluation of the respiratory and circulatory status of the athlete is of utmost importance. As stated previously, you must be sure the athlete has a patent (unobstructed) airway, is breathing, and has a pulse. An athlete suffering from a significant injury to the chest may have difficult or labored breathing (dyspnea). This can be a serious condition and terrifying for the athlete. The athletic

trainer must have a calm and reassuring approach to these athletes to help them relax and breathe more easily. Assisting these athletes may include (1) making certain the airway remains clear of blood and vomitus, (2) helping the athlete find the most comfortable position for breathing, (3) being ready to help the athlete control vomiting, (4) being prepared to provide artificial ventilation and circulation if necessary, and (5) providing prompt transportation to emergency medical services. When these conditions or problems are under control, you can proceed to the secondary survey.

Secondary survey

The evaluation of athletic injuries to the chest and abdomen is of major importance because of the possibility of internal bleeding or involvement of internal organs. As previously mentioned, most athletic injuries affect the chest or abdominal wall. It is important, however, for the athletic trainer to determine as quickly as possible if there are any associated intrathoracic or intra-abdominal injuries. An athlete exhibiting signs and symptoms that may indicate internal involvement should be referred to medical attention immediately. A "wait and see" approach should not be practiced because an internal injury can quickly develop into a serious and complicated condition. Follow-up examinations are also important to detection of slowly developing intrathoracic or intra-abdominal problems. For example, an injured spleen may splint itself only to go into a delayed hemorrhage hours or days after the injury. For this reason, it is important that the athlete who has suffered direct trauma to the chest or abdomen and does not initially exhibit signs and symptoms indicating internal injuries be instructed to immediately report further complications that may develop. This is also true for the athlete whose signs and symptoms subside only to recur. Signs and symptoms that may indicate internal involvement are discussed throughout this chapter and listed in the box on p. 393.

Another important point to remember is that athletes who have suffered acute

Athletic Injury Assessment Checklist: Throat, Chest, and Abdomen Injuries

Primary survey

_____ Airway
_____ Breathing
_____ Circulation

Secondary survey

_____ History
        _____ Mechanism of injury
        _____ Location of injury
        _____ Pain
        _____ Sensations
        _____ Progression of signs and symptoms

_____ Observation
        _____ Position and movements
        _____ Respiratory rate and rhythm
        _____ Symmetry
        _____ Signs of trauma

_____ Physical examination

Palpation

        _____ Tenderness
        _____ Deformities
        _____ Swelling
        _____ Crepitation
        _____ Symmetry
        _____ Muscle rigidity
        _____ Rebound tenderness

Movement procedures

        _____ Active ROM
        _____ Resistive movements
        _____ Passive stress on rib cage

trauma to the abdomen, or in whom intra-abdominal involvement is suspected, should not be allowed to eat or drink anything after the injury. The ingestion of food or fluids may aggravate the symptoms, and if surgery is required, the presence of food in the digestive tract will make the operation more dangerous. In addition, the athlete should not be given any medication for the pain because some of the symptoms may be masked. A physician examining the athlete must know both the location and the intensity of the pain.

History

The history of an injury to the chest or abdomen is extremely important as an indication of the nature of the injury and what has happened since the injury occurred. Begin by determining the mechanism of injury. Most injuries to the chest and abdomen occur during contact sports and are caused by some type of direct trauma, such as a direct blow or forcible contact with an object or another athlete. Question the athlete to get a detailed description of how the injury occurred. Was there a direct blow, and if so, by what? How large was the area of contact? Attempt to determine the severity of the blow or force. In addition to the mechanism, determine the location of the injury. Was the trauma to the back, chest, or abdominal area? Attempt to localize the site of the trauma as precisely as possible.

Next, question the athlete about any pain associated with the injury. Ask the athlete to localize the painful or tender areas. How severe is the pain? Is it constant or intermittent? Is the pain increased during respiration or movement? Does the athlete feel the pain is located in the chest or abdominal wall, or does he or she believe it is deeper, or inside the cavity? Does there appear to be any radiating or referred pain? Remember, an injury involving a visceral organ may cause no other symptom other than referred pain. Correlating the mechanism of injury to the exact location of all painful areas and realizing that visceral pain may be referred are very important in assessing injuries of the chest and abdomen.

Inquire about any additional symptoms the athlete may have experienced. Does the athlete express any crepitation that may accompany a fractured rib or costochondral separation? Does he or she feel any tightness, cramping, or rigidity of the abdominal muscles, which may indicate peritoneal irritation? Is there a pulling sensation in the groin or abdominal musculature? Does the athlete feel nauseated or complain of trouble with breathing? Allow the athlete to describe his or her impression of the injury. Does the athlete think the injury is of a serious nature?

If the athlete was not evaluated immediately after the injury, inquire about what has happened to any signs or symptoms since the injury first occurred. Have they improved, deteriorated, or stayed about the same? Has the athlete urinated or defecated since the injury? If so, was there any indication of blood in the urine or stool? If the athlete failed to check or has not yet eliminated, he or she should be instructed to look for blood after the next elimination. Remember, blood in the urine or stool should be reported immediately. Inability to urinate after abdominal trauma should also be reported.

Additional information that may be important to you or the physician assessing abdominal trauma concerns the status of the hollow organs before and after the injury. Was the athlete participating on a full stomach? Was the bladder full or empty? If a period of time has elapsed since the injury, has the athlete eaten recently? Did the symptoms appear worse or better after eating?

Observation

Observations made during assessment of chest and abdomen injuries are beneficial in determining the site, nature, and severity of the injury. These observations begin as soon as you see the athlete and continue throughout the assessment process. If the athlete is seen immediately after the trauma or remains lying on the court or field, assess first the respiratory and circulatory systems as described during the primary survey. Once the adequacy of these systems is assured, evaluate all signs and symptoms associated with the injury. It is extremely important to watch for the development of signs that may indicate intrathoracic or intra-abdominal involvement.

Begin by noting the position of the injured athlete. If the athlete remains lying on the court or field, notice if the athlete is moving about. Remember, if there is pain, he or she will usually not want to perform any movement that will increase that pain. Is the athlete holding an area of the chest or abdomen? Are his or her knees drawn up toward the chest? This position takes stress off the abdominal muscles and is generally more comfortable for a person who has suffered an injury to the abdomen. The athlete may also be taking rapid shallow breaths in an attempt to avoid pain caused by thoracic or abdominal movement. If the athlete is up and moving around, notice his or her gait and willingness to move. Is the athlete leaning toward or favoring one side of the body or appear to be in much pain during movement? Is the athlete avoiding any position or movements that may increase the pain? These initial observations can be very helpful in determining what further assessment procedures will be used.

When evaluating trauma to the torso, especially the chest, monitor the athlete's respiratory rate and rhythm. Does either appear to be abnormal or irregular? Is the athlete having a difficult time breathing or catching his or her breath? If the athlete has had the "wind knocked out," normal breathing will return rapidly, and most signs and symptoms will subside quickly. However, if signs and symptoms persist, additional intrathoracic or intra-abdominal involvement must be suspected and the injury must be evaluated further. Note if the breathing appears to be painful or if the athlete is holding an area of the chest wall. Does the athlete avoid taking any deep breaths, which may increase the pain? While observing the rate and rhythm of the respirations, inspect the chest for symmetry of movements. Both sides of the chest should move equally with each breath. Also look at the trachea to note any change in position. Normally the trachea lies in the midline of the neck and does not move during respirations. Note also the symmetry of the abdomen. Is there abnormal distention or protrusion? Are there overlying contusions? Does the abdomen appear to be rigid? Any signs that may indicate intrathoracic or intra-abdominal involvement must be carefully and continually monitored.

Bilateral symmetry of the neck should be judged with the head centered and muscles relaxed. Look for head tilting, muscle shortening, and masses. Inspect the anterior and posterior chest, noting the general shape of the thorax and its symmetry (Figure 16-16). Observe skin color and integrity; look for cy-

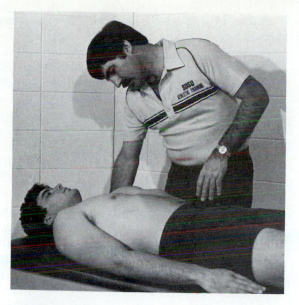

FIGURE 16-16
Inspecting the anterior chest and the abdomen.

anosis, pallor, or for obvious signs of traumatic injury. To do this, clothing or equipment should be removed. Look for deformities, contusions, abrasions, bleeding, or swelling. These observations can indicate the site of the trauma and provide important clues as to which structures may be involved. These signs may also indicate the severity of the direct trauma. Are there any areas of ecchymoses about the abdomen, which may suggest internal hemorrhaging? Periumbilical ecchymosis (Cullen's sign) is indicative of intraperitoneal bleeding; flank ecchymosis (Grey-Turner's sign) indicates retroperitoneal hemorrhage. Do the painful areas correlate with the site of trauma? That is, are the injured structures lying immediately below the site of trauma, or is pain expressed at an area away from the direct trauma? Examples of the latter could be forceful compression of the rib cage, resulting in a fracture or separation away from the site of direct trauma, as well as referred visceral pain.

In addition to these observations, an athlete with an injury to the chest or abdomen should be watched particularly for signs of impending shock or internal involvement. Signs of shock include pallor; cool, clammy skin; and a weak, rapid pulse. These signs and symptoms, along with others that suggest hemorrhaging or additional internal complications, are important to recognize. The rapidity with which the signs and symptoms develop after a torso injury is extremely important. Signs and symptoms developing quickly indicate a medical emergency requiring immediate attention by a physician. Remember, an athlete may appear to be doing well but may actually have a serious internal condition that becomes symptomatic hours or even days after the injury. You must continue to observe and reassess the health status of athletes who suffer trauma to the chest or abdomen.

Physical Examination

Palpation

Careful palpation techniques can be beneficial in evaluating injuries to the chest or abdomen. They can be used to confirm or investigate findings or suspicions gained during the history and observation portions of the assessment process. Remember to begin all palpation techniques very gently to elicit the athlete's cooperation and to avoid inflicting any unnecessary pain.

When palpating the chest, gently feel the site of the trauma and all painful areas expressed by the athlete (Figure 16-17). Locate as precisely as possible the tender areas. Note the anatomic structures you are palpating, such as along a rib, between two ribs, at the costochondral junction, or along the sternum or trachea. Do you feel any obvious deformities, crepitation, or swelling? Remember, if an obvious deformity or injury is recognized, it is not necessary to continue the assessment process; the appropriate treatment or transfer procedures should be initiated. Rib or costochondral injuries that are not obvious but are suspected because of the site of the pain can be evaluated by stress procedures described later.

You can also evaluate the symmetry of respirations by placing your hands on the athlete's rib cage. Anteriorly, place the tips of your thumbs on the xiphoid process and spread your hands over the lower rib cage (Figure 16-18). Posteriorly, place your thumbs along a lower thoracic spinous process and spread your hands over the posterior lateral rib cage. Both hands should move equally with each breath. If one side does not move as much, and the athlete exhibits signs of breathing difficulty, there may be intrathoracic involvement. In addition, you should palpate the trachea during respirations to note any shifting that may accompany an intrathoracic condition such as pneumothorax.

Palpation of the abdomen should be performed with the athlete lying supine and as relaxed as possible. It is best to have the athlete's arms along either side of the torso, rather than behind the head. The hips should be flexed. The place where the examination is conducted should be sufficiently warm so the athlete does not shiver. Instruct the athlete to relax and breathe quietly and slowly. Everything should be done to avoid tensing the abdominal muscles. If these muscles are contracted or tense, it is difficult to accurately palpate the abdomen. Avoid using cold hands or quick pokes into the abdomen because both can cause the athlete to tighten, or guard, the abdominal muscles. Palpation techniques should be performed with the flats of the fingers with the palm of the hand lying lightly on the abdomen (Figure 16-19).

Palpate the abdomen gently to prevent unnecessary pain or further injury. It is a good practice to palpate the uninjured areas of the abdomen first, to gain the athlete's cooperation and assist in relaxing the abdominal muscles. Feel for any tightness or muscle rigidity. Remember, peritoneal irritation is indicated by a rigid abdomen. However, an athlete with tenderness in the abdomen may guard the painful area by tightening or contracting the abdominal muscles. This rigidity can be distinguished from peritoneal rigidity by careful palpation; voluntary guarding of the muscles by the athlete can be relaxed, whereas peritoneal rigidity cannot. Continue to palpate the tensed area while instructing the athlete to relax and breathe slowly. If you feel a relaxation of the muscle rigidity, it is voluntary guarding. Occasionally, distracting the athlete may also help overcome the voluntary guarding. A truly rigid abdomen resulting

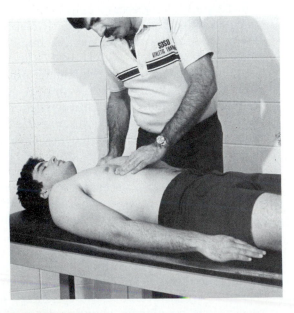

FIGURE 16-17
Palpating the site of trauma on the chest.

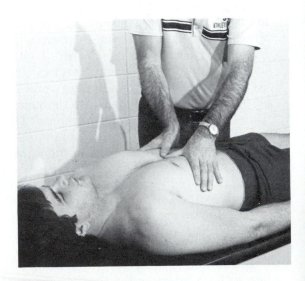

FIGURE 16-18
Feeling for symmetry of respirations.

from peritoneal irritation will not be affected and may feel boardlike.

Rebound tenderness is also present with peritoneal irritation. This is elicited by putting firm pressure on the abdomen and then quickly releasing the pressure. The release of pressure will cause a sharp, severe pain. For example, rebound tenderness in the lower right quadrant of the abdomen is a classic sign of acute appendicitis. It is normally unnecessary to perform this procedure and cause the athlete additional pain. However, it is important to understand that this phenomenon does occur with peritoneal irritation and that an athlete may experience this sudden stabbing pain with any unexpected movement, such as coughing or being jolted.

If the abdomen is not rigid and tense, you can continue palpating for tenderness in each of the four quadrants. Feel about the spleen, liver, and kidneys. Locate any areas of tenderness. Remember to palpate gently to begin with; then, if there is no pain, you can proceed with deeper palpation. While palpating, feel for masses, swelling, protrusions, or other deficits in the continuity of the abdominal wall. If the athlete suffered a blow to the crest of the ilium, palpate along this bony ridge (Figure 16-20).

Movement procedures

The majority of the assessment process to evaluate injuries to the chest and abdomen is completed by using history, observation, and palpation procedures as described. Very few movement or stress maneuvers are performed. When these techniques are utilized they are used to assist the assessment of in-

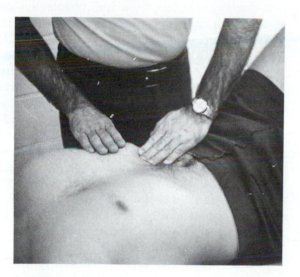

FIGURE 16-19
Palpating an athlete's abdomen.

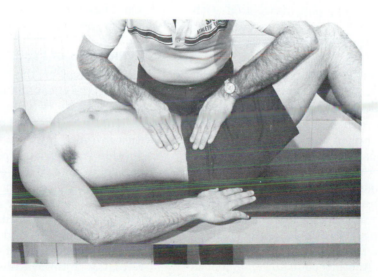

FIGURE 16-20
Palpating the crest of the ilium.

juries to the chest or abdominal walls.

Active movements. Assessment of injuries to the neck includes an evaluation of active motion (see Chapter 15). Evaluate the normal range of motion (ROM) of the neck for flexion, hyperextension, lateral bending, and rotation. In checking for adequacy of lateral bending movements, make certain that the athlete moves the side of the head toward the shoulder, not the shoulder up to the ear. Look for ratchety or tremulous movements. Is there pain associated with any movement or at any particular point during movement? Is muscle spasm apparent? Is there a limited ROM? Always remember, *never* initiate passive ROM assessment techniques in the presence of a traumatic neck injury.

The integrity of the abdominal wall, which is composed primarily of muscles, can be further evaluated by having the athlete actively contract the abdominals. Remember, pain associated with a muscle strain is usually aggravated by active contraction or stretching of the muscle. When an abdominal muscle strain is suspected, instruct the athlete to perform a series of ROM exercises for the trunk. The normal ROM of the trunk in flexion, hyperextension, lateral bending, and rotation is discussed and illustrated in Chapter 15. Can the athlete perform these movements? Is there pain associated with any active movement or at any particular point during motion? Is there a limited ROM?

Resistive movements. Resistance can be applied against these active movements to further evaluate the integrity of the contractile unit. With cervical motion, resistance is easily applied manually, as described in the previous chapter. For trunk movements, instruct the athlete to perform a partial sit-up (Figure 16-21, *A*). If pain is increased significantly, note the exact location. The oblique muscles may be better evaluated by having the athlete perform some twisting of the trunk during the sit-up (Figure 16-21, *B*). Another point to remember is that performing a sit-up will increase the

intra-abdominal pressure, which may also increase the symptoms associated with a hernia or other internal injury.

Passive movements. The integrity of the chest wall, composed primarily of the ribs, sternum, and rib cartilages, can be further evaluated by applying passive stress to these structures. When a bone or costochondral injury is not obvious but is indicated or suspected, you can apply stress to the structures by gently compressing the rib cage. If a fracture is suspected along the lateral side of the rib cage, apply gentle compression in an anteroposterior direction (Figure 16-22, *A*). Each rib can be stressed in this manner. If pain is increased at the suspected site, the continuity of the rib is probably interrupted and referral is indicated. Remember, a bruise or other injury to the intercostal muscles does not result in a significant increase of pain during this maneuver. If pain is expressed along the costochondral margin, apply gentle compression on the rib cage in a transverse direction (Figure 16-22, *B*). Again, stress can be applied to each rib. If pain is increased at the costochondral junction, the athlete has probably suffered a separation at this area. It cannot be overemphasized that these passive stress maneuvers must be performed gently to begin with so as not to cause any additional damage. They are only performed after thorough history, observation, and palpation.

Evaluation of Findings

As stated earlier, the majority of athletic injuries to the chest and abdomen involves the walls of these two major body cavities. Occasionally the visceral contents of these cavities are also injured. Visceral injuries can develop into serious, possibly life-threatening, conditions. When evaluating injuries to the chest or abdomen, the athletic trainer must also be alert for signs and symptoms that may indicate an intrathoracic or intra-abdominal injury, and be prepared to provide emergency care if necessary, as well as refer the injured athlete to a physician or medical facility.

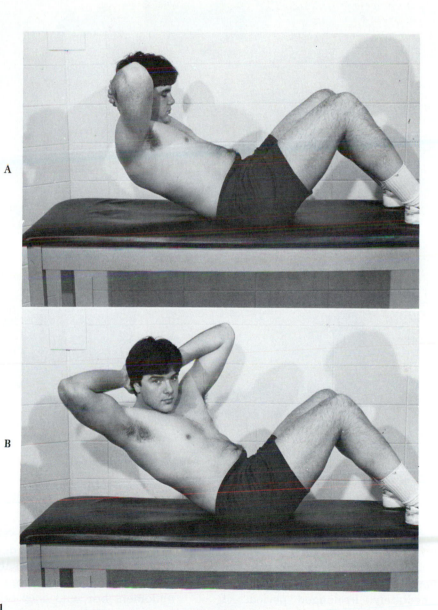

FIGURE 16-21
Athlete performing, **A**, partial sit-up to stress the abdominal muscles and, **B**, partial sit-up with trunk rotation to apply more resistance to the oblique muscles.

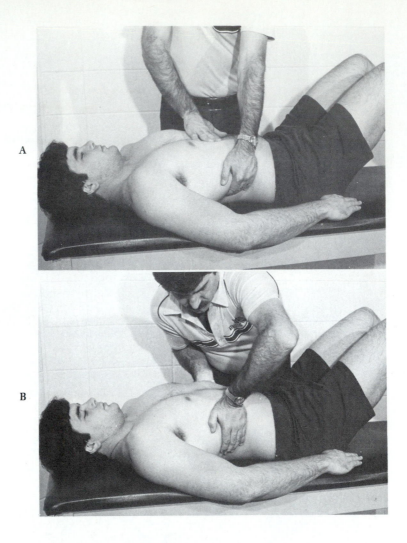

FIGURE 16-22
Applying compression to the rib cage. **A**, Anteroposterior compression to evaluate bony
integrity. **B**, Transverse compression to evaluate costochondral junctions.

When to refer the athlete

Whenever intrathoracic or intra-abdominal
involvement is indicated or suspected, the
athlete should be referred to medical assistance immediately. Prolonged periods of
watching and waiting can allow internal
conditions to become more serious. Therefore the athletic trainer must be constantly
alert for signs and symptoms that may indicate internal injuries. Remember also that
internal complications may develop hours,
days, or possibly weeks after significant
trauma to the chest or abdomen. An athlete
may appear to be doing very well, only to
have delayed symptoms develop later. For
this reason, any athlete suffering what appears to be severe trauma to the chest or
abdomen, but who does not show signs of
internal complications, should be instructed
to immediately report any unusual signs
and symptoms that may develop later. Give
the athlete a list of signs and symptoms to
watch for, which includes information concerning the nature of the injury, the physical
signs that may indicate intrathoracic or
intra-abdominal involvement, and what to

South Dakota State University Training Room

This is a medical follow-up sheet for your health and safety. Signs of a chest or abdominal injury may not appear immediately following trauma but can develop hours after the injury. The purpose of this fact sheet is to alert you to the symptoms of significant chest or abdominal injuries which may develop several hours after you leave the training room.

If you experience one or more of the following symptoms, medical help should be sought:

Chest injuries
 1. Difficulty in breathing
 2. Shortness of breath—inability to catch breath
 3. Pain increasing in chest
 4. Vomiting or coughing up blood

Abdominal injuries
 1. Pain or discomfort increasing in abdomen
 2. Rigidity and spasm of abdominal muscles
 3. Blood in the urine or stool
 4. Vomiting
 5. Increasing nausea
 6. Painful urination

The appearance of any of the above symptoms tells you that you may have sustained a significant chest or abdominal injury that *requires medical attention*.

If any of these symptoms appear, contact Jim Booher, Bernadette Janicki, or Xristos Gaglias, or report to the Brookings Hospital Emergency Room

REMEMBER: Your health depends on how much you care about proper medical attention.

THE SDSU ATHLETIC TRAINING STAFF

When to Refer the Athlete. . .

Throat injuries or conditions
 Persistent soreness, hoarseness, or loss of voice
 Difficulty in breathing
 Inability to swallow
 Bleeding from the throat
 Crepitation on palpation
 Suspected inflammation or infection of throat structures
 Doubt regarding the nature and severity of the throat injury or condition

Chest injuries
 Difficult or labored breathing
 Shortness of breath—inability to catch breath
 Severe pain in chest
 Diminished chest movement on affected side
 Shifting or moving of trachea with each breath
 Vomiting or coughing up blood
 Suspected rib fracture or costochondral separation
 Signs of shock
 Doubt regarding the nature and severity of the chest injury

Abdominal and pelvic injuries
 Severe pain in abdomen
 Presence of what appears to be radiating or referred pain
 Tenderness, rigidity, and spasm of the abdominal muscles
 Blood in the urine or stool
 Signs of shock
 Rebound tenderness
 Prolonged discomfort, sensation of weakness or pulling in groin
 Superficial protrusion or palpable mass
 Increasing nausea
 Vomiting
 Persistent symptoms following a blow to the scrotum
 Menstrual irregularities
 Any perineal laceration (women)
 Doubt regarding the nature and severity of the abdominal injury

do or who to notify should these signs develop. A sample medical follow-up sheet with instructions to follow immediately should any of the signs and symptoms develop is at the top of p. 393. Conditions or findings that indicate a chest or abdominal injury should be attended by a physician are listed in the box at bottom of p. 393.

REFERENCES

Affleck TP: Severe sports-related spleen injury: not all patients require surgery, *Phys Sportsmed* 20(9):109, 1992.

American Academy of Orthopaedic Surgeons: *Emergency care and transportation of the sick and injured,* ed 5, Chicago, 1992, The Academy.

Arnheim DD, Prentice WE: *Principles of athletic training,* ed 8, St. Louis, 1993, Mosby.

Barsan WG, Wolf LR:Disorders of the upper gastrointestinal tract. In Rosen P, and others, editors: *Emergency medicine: concept and clinical practice,* ed 3, St. Louis, 1992, Mosby.

Berman BM and others: Spleen injury in sports: part I: what diagnostic imaging can reveal, *Phys Sportsmed* 20(3):168, 1992.

Boyd CE: Referred visceral pain in athletics, *Ath Train* 15(1):20, 1980.

Brown LM and others: Testicular cancer in the United States: trends in incidence and mortality, *Int J Epidemiol* 15(2):164, 1986.

Budassi SA, Barber JM: *Mosby's manual of emergency care: practices and procedures,* St. Louis, 1984, Mosby.

Colucciello SA, Plotka M: Abdominal trauma: occult injury may be life threatening, *Phys Sportsmed* 21(6):33, 1993.

Eichelberger MR: Torso injuries in athletes, *Phys Sportsmed* 9(3):87, 1981.

Floyd RT, Tew M: Injury on impact—thoracic injuries due to sport-related contact, *Sports Med Update* 10, 1991.

Harwood-Nuss AL, Hollard RW: Genitourinary disease. In Rosen P, and others, editors: *Emergency medicine: concept and clinical practice,* ed 3, St. Louis, 1992, Mosby.

Henderson JM: Ruling out danger: differential diagnosis of thoracic pain, *Phys Sportsmed* 20(9):124, 1992.

Johnson C, Tobin DL: The diagnosis and treatment of anorexia nervosa and bulimia among athletes, *JNATA* 26(2):119, 1991.

Leon GR: Eating disorders in female athletes, *Sports Med* 12(4):219, 1991.

Loucks AB, Horvath SM: Athletic amenorrhea: a review, *Med Sci Sports Exerc* 17(1):56, 1985.

Malasanos L, Barkauskas V, Stoltenberg-Allen K: *Health assessment,* ed 4, St. Louis, 1986, Mosby.

Miles JW, Barrett GR: Rib fractures in athletes, *Sports Med* 12(1):66, 1991.

Morden RS and others: Spleen injury in sports: part II: avoiding splenectomy, *Phys Sportsmed* 20(4):126, 1992.

Morton AR and others: Physical activity and the asthmatic, *Phys Sportsmed* 9(3):51, 1981.

Myburgh KH, Watkin VA, Noakes TD: Are risk factors for menstrual dysfunction cumulative, *Phys Sportsmed* 20(4):115, 1992.

O'Donoghue DH: *Treatment of injuries to athletes,* ed 4, Philadelphia, 1984, Saunders.

Stamford B: Exercise-induced asthma: taking the wheeze out of your workout, *Phys Sportsmed* 19(8):139, 1991.

SUGGESTED READINGS

Belis JA: Testicular tumors, *Hospital Med* 18:37, 1982.
Discusses testicular cancer and the importance of early detection.

Haycock CE: How I manage abdominal injuries, *Phys Sportsmed* 14(6):86, 1986.
Reviews the common injuries that may occur to the abdomen and discusses the proper recognition and treatment of these injuries to minimize complications and ensure the athlete's speedy return to activity.

Katz RM: Coping with exercise-induced asthma in sports, *Phys Sportsmed* 15(7):101, 1987.
Reviews the history and pathophysiology of exercise-induced asthma and discusses various treatment procedures and drugs that are effective against this condition.

McCutcheon ML, Anderson JL: How I manage sports injuries to the larynx, *Phys Sportsmed* 13(4):100, 1985.
Discusses laryngeal trauma, which can compromise the airway and create a true emergency for the physician and athletic trainer.

Shangold MM: How I manage exercise-related menstrual disturbances, *Phys Sportsmed* 14(3):113, 1986.
Discuss the prevalence of amenorrhea and oligomenorrhea in heavy exercise, as well as the evaluation and treatment of these conditions.

Wichmann S, Martin DR: Eating disorders in athletes: weighing the risks, *Phys Sportsmed* 21(5):216, 1993.
Discusses the warning signs of eating disorders and the need to convince athletes to get medical treatment to overcome them.

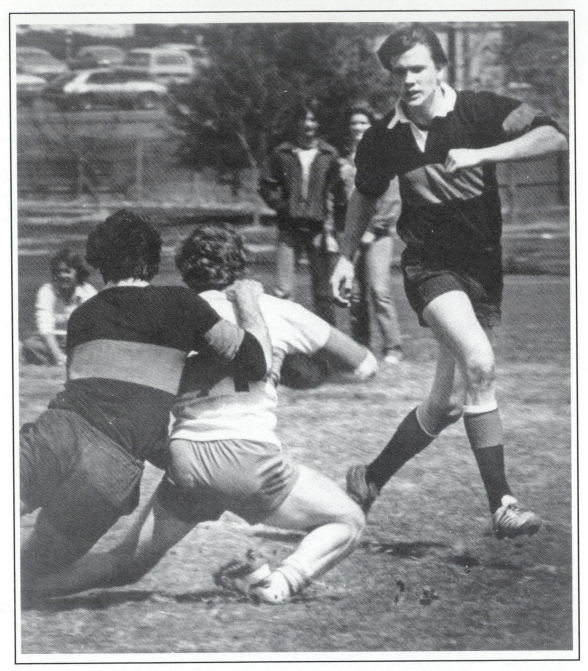

Athletic Injuries of the Lower Extremities

The lower extremities are complex functioning units which are extremely important to almost every type of athletic endeavor. There are few athletic activities that do not require the use of the lower extremities in one manner or another. Because of its high and diversified utilization, this area of the body is continually subjected to many traumatic stresses. Athletes involved in running and jumping are especially at risk. All sports participants however, are susceptible to sustaining some type of injury to this area of the body. Considered as a functioning unit, the lower extremity is impaired more frequently and is subject to more injury-related conditions or problems than any other area of the body. Athletic trainers are constantly expected to handle injuries and disorders involving the lower extremities. The professional athletic trainer must continue to improve and broaden assessment skills related to evaluation and treatment of injuries to this important area of the body.

17 Foot, ankle, and leg injuries
18 Knee injuries
19 Thigh and hip injuries

$\mathcal{C}$HAPTER 17

Foot, ankle, and leg injuries

After you have completed this chapter, you should be able to:

- Identify the basic anatomy of the foot, ankle, and leg.
- List the criteria of a normal foot.
- Describe the three foot types commonly associated with overuse injuries.
- Describe the common athletic injuries and conditions that may occur to the foot, ankle, and leg.
- Describe the assessment process for an athlete suffering an injury to the foot, ankle, or leg.
- List the signs and symptoms that indicate an athlete with a foot, ankle, or leg injury should be referred for medical assistance.

The feet, ankles, and legs form the foundation for the body. Just as buildings and structures are only as strong as their foundations, athletes are only as sturdy and effective as their base of support.

The body's foundation originates with the feet, which support the body weight in a myriad of positions and function over a multitude of surfaces and contours. Most athletic activity begins with and is dependent on the feet. As such, the feet continually bear the brunt of physical stresses and rapidly changing forces thrust on them from all directions. The ankle joint is the fulcrum between the foot and leg, and as such is subjected to tremendous amounts of physical stress and many types of potentially damaging forces. The leg is the functional unit that transmits muscular power to the foot and ankle. Combined, the leg, ankle, and foot constitute the area of the body most frequently involved with athletic injuries. Therefore athletic trainers must possess the knowledge and skills necessary to accurately assess and effectively manage athletic injuries of the foot, ankle, and leg. This effective management begins with a fundamental understanding of the anatomy, functional mechanics, and possible mechanisms of athletic injury involving this region of the body.

ANATOMY OF THE FOOT AND ANKLE

The structure of the foot is similar to that of the hand, with certain differences that adapt it for locomotion and supporting weight. Refer to the surface anatomy illustrated in Figure 17-1 as you review the anatomy of the foot and ankle.

The skeleton of the foot is composed of tarsal, metatarsal, and phalangeal bones

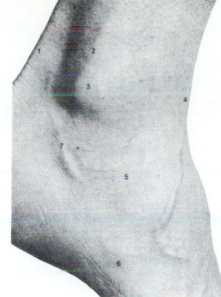

FIGURE 17-1
Surface anatomy of the right ankle and foot from the
A, lateral side and **B**, medial side.

1	Extensor hallucis longus
2	Tibialis anterior
3	Great saphenous vein
4	Medial malleolus
5	Posterior tibial artery
6	Tendo calcaneus (Achilles tendon)
7	Tibialis posterior
8	Calcaneus
9	Tuberosity of navicular
10	Head of first metatarsal
11	Dorsal venous arch
12	Extensor digitorum longus
13	Extensor digitorum brevis
14	Dorsalis pedis artery

(Figure 17-2). The word **tarsus** is a collective term used to describe the seven bones that constitute the midfoot and hindfoot: talus, calcaneus, navicular, cuboid, and the three cuneiform bones. Although the calcaneus, or heel bone, is the largest and strongest tarsal, it supports only about half of the total weight transmitted from the talus during walking or running. The remaining weight is transmitted evenly to the other tarsals.

The calcaneus projects backward behind the ankle, and provides leverage for the **triceps surae,** (gastrocnemius and soleus muscles), which inserts on its posterior sur-

face. The lateral surface of the calcaneus is almost entirely subcutaneous. It can be palpated easily just distal to the lateral malleolus and can be followed forward from the back of the heel for approximately 2 inches. The upper surface of the calcaneus has articular facets for the talus, the largest being the medially projecting ledge called the **sustentaculum tali.** Between the talus and the calcaneus is the important subtalar joint, and at the anterior ends of these bones is the transverse tarsal joint. These two joints allow inversion and eversion to occur. The upper end of the talus is called the **trochlea.**

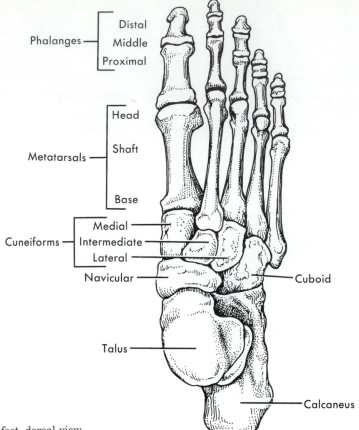

FIGURE 17-2
Bones of the ankle and foot, dorsal view.

It is this bony process that articulates with the tibia and fibula. The anterior end of the talus articulates with the navicular bone. The navicular has a rather large process (tuberosity) on its medial side. The tuberosity of the navicular can be palpated easily as a prominence about an inch diagonally below and in front of the medial malleolus. It lies about midway between the back of the heel and the base of the great toe and serves as a useful landmark during the assessment process. Practice locating these bony landmarks in the healthy, noninjured foot. The more practical experience you have in mentally visualizing underlying anatomic structures, the more accurate you will become in identification of specific types of injury in this complex area.

The **metatarsus** consists of five bones named and numbered 1 to 5 from the medial to the lateral position. The metatarsals re-

semble the metacarpales of the hand; each has a proximal base, a body or shaft, and a distal head. Identify the proximal and distal points or articulation of the metatarsals in Figure 17-2. The bases of the first three metatarsals articulate with the cuneiforms, whereas the fourth and fifth articulate with the cuboid. The head of each metatarsal articulates with the base of its corresponding proximal phalanx. Note also in Figure 17-2 that the body (shaft) of the first metatarsal is thicker than the other four—a structural adaptation that permits it to bear more weight.

Like the fingers, there are 14 phalanges in the toes—three for each digit except the big toe, which as two. The phalanges are designated as proximal, middle, and distal. Normally the tarsals and metatarsals play the major role in the functioning of the foot as a supporting structure, with the phalan-

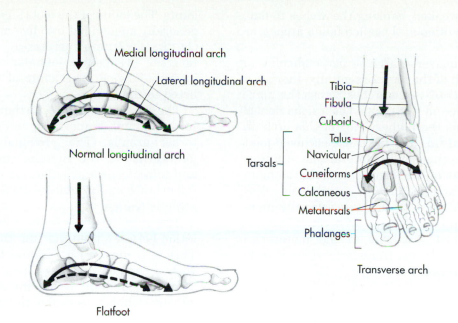

Normal longitudinal arch

Flatfoot

Transverse arch

FIGURE 17-3
Arches of the foot.

Accessory Bones

Accessory bones occur in both the hands and feet but are of much greater practical importance in the feet. Over 20 types of accessory bones can be found in the feet, and they occur in about 25% of the population. They are easily mistaken on X-ray film for bone fragments, which would indicate a fracture. For this reason physicians will sometimes conduct radiographic examinations of both feet when only one foot is injured. As a group, accessory bones are divided into two classes: (1) sesamoids and (2) true accessory bones, which are almost always bilateral in their appearance (hence the need for examining both feet by radiography).

Arches

The bones of the feet are held together in such a way as to form springy lengthwise and crosswise arches. The longitudinal and transverse arches (Figure 17-3) of the feet

ges being relatively unimportant. In the hand, where manipulation rather than support is the main function, the reverse is true.

provide a highly stable and resilient base to bear the body's weight and also yield as weight is applied to aid in absorbing the shocks associates with walking and running. The longitudinal arch has an inner (medial) portion and an outer (lateral) portion, both of which are formed by the tarsals and metatarsals. The medial longitudinal arch is sometimes referred to as the "arch of movement." It is high, easily seen in most people, and is made up of the calcaneus, talus, navicular, and three cuneiforms, and the first, second, and third metatarsals. In the medial longitudinal arch the principal weight-bearing points are the heel and the metatarsal heads. The apex of this arch is the talus.

The calcaneus and cuboid, plus the fourth and fifth metatarsals, shape the lateral longitudinal arch. The cuboid is the apex of this arch. It is low, however, and permits the outer border of the foot to touch the ground along its entire length. The longitudinal arch is formed by the placement of the metatarsals and tarsals. The result is a convexity formed on the top (dorsum) and a concavity on the sole (*plantar aspect*) of the foot. Strong ligaments and tendons from muscles originating in the leg normally hold the bones of the foot firmly in their arched positions, but it is not uncommon for these bones to weaken, causing the arches to flatten, a condition aptly called fallen arches, or flatfeet.

The transverse arch is perpendicular to the length of the foot. Essentially, there is a series of transverse arches across the plantar surface of the foot. The talonavicular joint forms the highest part of this arch on the medial side and the calcaneocuboid joint the highest part on the lateral side. Anterior to the peak of the transverse arch, the plantar surface becomes successively less arched. Athletic trainers occasionally manage painful transverse arch conditions occurring just proximal to the metatarsal heads. This area is frequently referred to as the metatarsal arch.

Joints

The many interlocking bones of the ankle and foot result in the formation of numerous joints. The joints of the foot (Figure 17-4) are generally subdivided into five major groups: (1) tarsal, (2) tarsometatarsal, (3) intermetatarsal, (4) metatarsophalangeal, and (5) interphalangeal. The joints of the foot are listed in the box.

The tarsal joints are further subdivided into proximal, transverse, and distal intertarsal groups. The proximal intertarsal joints, that is, the subtalar (talocalcaneal) and talocalcaneonavicular, are of particular importance and practical significance to the athletic trainer.

The subtalar joint is the point of articulation between the talus and the calcaneus. This is a diarthrotic, gliding type of joint with a capsule and a synovial membrane. The subtalar joint is not the only point of articulation between the talus and calcaneus; inversion and eversion movements of the foot on the talus occur simultaneously at

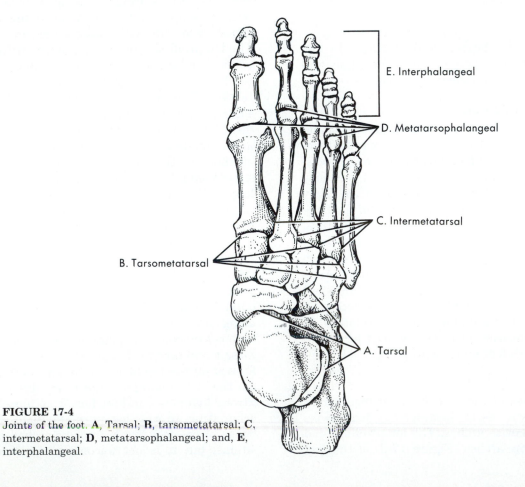

FIGURE 17-4
Joints of the foot. **A,** Tarsal; **B,** tarsometatarsal; **C,** intermetatarsal; **D,** metatarsophalangeal; and, **E,** interphalangeal.

Joints of the Foot

Tarsal
  Proximal intertarsal joints
    Subtalar (talocalcaneal)
    Talocalcaneonavicular
  Transverse intertarsal joints
    Calcaneocuboid
    Talonavicular
  Distal intertarsal joints
    Cuneonavicular
    Intercuneiform
    Cuneocuboid
  Tarsometatarsal
  Intermetatarsal
  Metatarsophalangeal
  Interphalangeal

---

both the subtalar and talocalcaneonavicular joints. A limited range of inversion and eversion are extremely important to the athlete. It enables the body to move sideways over the foot while the foot itself remains fixed. The muscles producing inversion are the tibialis anterior and tibialis posterior. Eversion movements are produced by the peroneus longus, brevis, and tertius muscles.

As the name implies, the talocalcaneonavicular joint is really a complex of synovial joints between the talus, navicular, and calcaneus bones. In addition, the calcaneonavicular, or *spring ligament,* also enters into the formation of this important and frequently injured joint. The spring ligament attaches the calcaneus to the navicular bone and limits the flattening of the medial longitudinal arch of the foot.

The distal intertarsal, tarsometatarsal, and intermetatarsal joints are all plane-type, synovial joints. Although several of them form single joint cavities, they are, individually, of only limited importance to the athletic trainer. As a group these joints permit only limited gliding movements. The joint between the medial cuneiform and the metatarsal of the great toe is somewhat unique in that it allows a greater range of plantar flexion and dorsiflexion to occur. Some rotary movements are also available at this joint.

The arrangement of the metatarsophalangeal and interphalangeal joints is on the same basic plan as in the hand. Metatarsophalangeal joints are of the ellipsoid type. They permit plantar flexion, dorsiflexion, and some abduction and adduction. The interphalangeal joints are classified as hinge joints and permit only flexion and extension.

Foot Types

The structure and alignment of the foot is an extremely important consideration when assessing injuries to the lower extremities, and especially when evaluating injuries caused by overuse. The shape of the foot is subject to as many individual variations as any other area of the body. These variations are the culmination of the development of the foot and result from a variety of causes, such as functional demands, structural deformities, injuries, heredity, body type, and postural faults. Significant foot variations are considered the most common form of physical impairment among athletes. Before an athletic trainer can recognize variations of the foot that may predispose an athlete to injuries, he or she must have a conception of what is considered to be a "normal" foot. An accurate definition of the ideal or normal foot is elusive. However, there are criteria established for a normal foot (see box), and the athletic trainer should be familiar with these characteristics and alert to any significant variations.

Most people have varying degrees and types of deviation from the ideal foot type. These deviations seldom cause problems in normal everyday activities. However, because of the nature of sporting activities, these variations are magnified and become much more significant in athletes. The greater the degree of variation, the more susceptible an athlete is to problems. Also, the greater the continued repetitive nature of the athletic activity, the more susceptible an athlete is to developing overuse problems. For example, runners who train many miles a week are more susceptible to overuse injuries caused by variations on their feet than are athletes who participate in sports

---

Criteria for a Normal Foot

1. The anatomic contours should appear in neutral positions.
2. The calcaneus should be centrally located below the leg and perpendicular to the floor.
3. The medial border of the foot should lie in a reasonably straight line from the heel to the great toe.
4. Each toe should be flexible and in straight alignment.
5. The medial longitudinal arch should form a gentle, smooth curve.
6. A normal range of active motion at the ankle joint should be available.
7. There should appear to be good tone and balanced strength of the leg muscles.
8. The contact of the foot should be distributed between the heel and the ball of the foot, during weight bearing. All metatarsal heads should rest firmly on the floor.
9. The feet should be asymptomatic under most conditions. That is, an athlete with normal alignment and structure of the feet should have a very low incidence of injury symptoms when following a sensible training program. Of course, this precludes traumatic injuries such as those caused by twisting or collision.

---

that require less constant running. The athletic trainer should be able to recognize a foot that is more susceptible to overuse injuries. The athletic trainer should also be alert to signs about the feet and shoes that may indicate malalignment or imbalance conditions. These signs include such things as excess callus formation on the foot, blisters, clawed toes, bunions, and shoes that wear unevenly.

There are three foot types commonly associated with overuse injuries: (1) the pronated foot, (2) the cavus foot, and (3) Morton's foot. The athletic trainer should be able to recognize each of these foot types and understand something about the mechanics associated with each. Again, the athletic trainer is not expected to be an expert on evaluating foot types; however, he or he should be able to recognize gross abnormalities of the foot. Recognizing these foot types can provide the athletic trainer with sufficient information to refer the athlete to a foot specialist, or plan treatment strategies designed to alleviate the symptoms.

Pronated foot

Pronation of the foot is a combination of abduction, dorsiflexion, and eversion. These motions take place in the tarsal joints and especially the subtalar joint. Some pronation is normal, but excessive pronation, or hyperpronation during weight bearing, is a common condition found in athletes who exhibit overuse problems of the feet and legs. In fact, this defect is considered to be the most common cause of chronic overuse injuries in runners. **Pes planus** is commonly associated with foot pronation; however, the two are separate deviations. Pes planus, or flatfoot, is a static structural abnormality in which the position of the bones relative to each other has been altered, resulting in a lowering of the longitudinal arch.

The hyperpronated foot is considered to be a very flexible foot with excessive motion at the subtalar joint. When the foot pronates, the weight line falls to the medial side of the foot, the medial longitudinal arch depresses, and the toes tend to be directed outward (Figure 17-5). Other common signs of a pronated foot include an inward tilting of the heel, causing a medial curving of the Achilles tendon and a more pronounced medial malleolus. These deviations result in an abnormal relationship between the talus, calcaneus, and tarsal articulations with each foot strike, and a variety of chronic overuse syndromes in the foot, leg, and knee can result.

The amount of pronation of the foot can range from quite mild to very severe. The mildly pronated foot may present fatigue and pain in the arch as well as a generalized postural fatigue, especially with running activities. The moderately pronated foot has increased mobility and poorer shock-absorbing qualities at heel strike. The toes are more unstable, and the intrinsic muscles fatigue more quickly. There is a higher incidence of overuse injuries such as plantar fascial strains, heel bruises, calcaneal spurs,

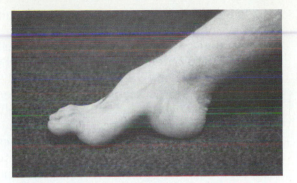

FIGURE 17-6
Cavus foot with a rigid high arch.

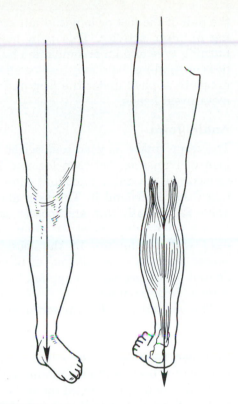

FIGURE 17-5
Pronated foot.

bursitis, tendinitis, and stress fractures. The severely pronated foot is a hypermobile flatfoot with very little longitudinal arch visible during weight bearing. All the symptoms are accentuated and occur frequently during athletic activity. The athlete with severely pronated feet may even exhibit pain and symptoms without athletic activity.

Cavus foot

 The cavus foot or **pes cavus** has a high longitudinal arch with limited tarsal motion (Figure 17-6). This is considered to be an inflexible foot that does not adequately absorb shock or adapt easily to various surfaces. The cavus foot is usually associated with heavy callus formation on the ball of the foot or heel caused by additional stresses placed on these areas. Clawing of the toes and pain along the bottom of the foot or under the metatarsal heads is typical. Lateral tilting of the calcaneus, or rearfoot varus, is often associated with this type of foot. In addition,

the cavus foot transmits increased shock to the ankle, leg, knee, thigh, hip, or back, and creates an increased incidence of overuse injuries.

The cavus foot can range from a flexible foot to one that is very rigid. The flexible cavus foot has a high arch when it is not bearing weight. The toes also appear to be mildly clawed when there is no weight on the foot, but straighten out during weight bearing. The flexible cavus foot has somewhat limited shock-absorbing qualities, which predisposes it to overuse injuries such as plantar fasciitis, heel bruises, Achilles tendinitis, shin splints, and stress fractures. The flexible cavus foot may progress to a rigid cavus foot deformity despite treatment strategies.

As the cavus foot becomes more rigid, the high arch and claw toes become less flexible. The arch will flatten only mildly and the claw toes do not straighten completely with weight bearing. This foot has more callus build-up and frequent pain under the metatarsal heads because increased abnormal stresses transmitted to this area are common. Dorsiflexion of the ankle is limited to a greater degree, and the intrinsic muscles of the foot are tighter. This type of foot, called a *semiflexible* or *moderate cavus* foot, has more limited shock-absorbing properties, which result in more stress being transmitted to the lower extremity and lower back. There is also a related increase in overuse injuries.

The rigid cavus foot is the most difficult foot to manage. This foot has a very high longitudinal arch and clawed toes at rest and when bearing weight. It has a tight plantar fascia, and painful calluses usually develop under the metatarsal heads. The rigid cavus foot does not absorb shock well, adapts to surfaces very poorly, and is inadequately suited for athletic activity. Athletes with this type of foot are more susceptible to sprained ankles, Achilles tendon problems, arch conditions, stress fractures, and a variety of overuse injuries.

Morton's foot

Morton's foot is characterized by a congenitally short, hypermobile first metatarsal. This results in an imbalance in the transverse metatarsal arch because more stress is placed on the longer second metatarsal. There is often thickening of the second metatarsal shaft as a result of more weight being transferred to the second toe. Normally the second metatarsal is just slightly longer than the first. When the first metatarsal is significantly shorter, the foot must adapt to this abnormal condition. The great toe does not bear weight until later in the gait cycle, and the second metatarsal must absorb more stress during weight bearing. This can increase the incidence of overuse injuries. The foot may attempt to compensate for this by pronating or rolling inward so that the first metatarsal can more quickly contact the surface. The magnitude of overuse problems associated with excessive pronation was previously discussed.

An accurate diagnosis of Morton's foot normally involves a radiographic study. However, the athletic trainer should be familiar with the common signs that may indicate Morton's foot. A rough estimate of the length of the metatarsals can be observed while the athlete flexes the toes. The head of the first metatarsal will sit back farther than the second. When the second metatarsal is longer, there often will be a callus buildup under the head of the second metatarsal as the result of increased stress to this area. The athlete may complain of pain in the ball of the foot or longitudinal arch during or after activity. This pain may be a burning type of pain accompanied by numbness or tingling. Pain may also be elicited by pressure applied under the first and second metatarsal heads.

Ankle Joint

The term "ankle" is used to describe the region of transition between leg and foot. It consists of the ankle joint and those structures that surround it. The skin about the ankle is normally thin and loosely attached to the underlying parts. If edema occurs, fluid will accumulate in the loose tissue spaces, and the skin will "pit" or become indented, when pressure is applied by the fingertips during palpation.

The medial and lateral *malleoli,* which are the distal ends of the tibia and fibula, respectively, can be palpated at the ankle. However, the lateral one is less prominent, lies farther back, and extends more distally than the medial. The distal tip of the lateral malleolus projects a half inch below and behind its palpable bony prominence. The ankle joint is located about one-half inch above the tip of the medial malleolus, which serves as the most prominent of the medial bony landmarks in this region. The Achilles tendon is the prominent landmark at the back of the ankle. It is important to realize that blood vessels, nerves, and tendons, which all have a vertical orientation in the leg, must turn forward and assume a horizontal orientation in order to enter the foot. Although specialized connective tissue bands (retinacula) hold these structures against the bones of the ankle and foot to prevent "bowstringing," they are still vulnerable to injury in this area.

The ankle joint is a uniaxial, diarthrotic hinge joint. It is often described as a three-sided box-like or mortise joint made up of the tibia, fibula, and talus. The ankle joint is designed for weight bearing and has great strength and stability. The top and sides of the box-shaped socket are formed by the medial and lateral malleoli and the distal articular surface of the tibia. This socket articulates with the trochlea of the talus below.

The active movements permitted at the ankle joint include dorsiflexion and plantar flexion. In dorsiflexion the forepart of the foot is raised and the angle between the front of the leg and the top of the foot is decreased; in plantar flexion the foot is lowered and the angle is increased as the toes are pointed downward. If the foot is forcibly plantar flexed, the talus will be pushed forward and become prominent just in front of the lateral malleolus. In the normal range of movement, the two malleoli project downward and tightly grasp the sides of the talus. As a result, only very slight lateral or medial movement is possible.

Ankle Ligaments

The bones that compose the ankle are held together by a strong fibrous capsule that is attached to the articular margins of the tibia and fibula above and to the talus below. In addition to the capsule, the distal ends of the tibia and fibula are tightly bound to each other by ligaments at the distal tibiofibular articulation just above the ankle. This distal tibiofibular articulation is a fibrous type of joint, called a *syndesmosis*. Stability of the distal tibiofibular syndesmosis is maintained by the anterior and posterior tibiofibular ligaments and the interosseous membrane. Occasionally athletes will suffer syndesmosis sprains of the ankle.

The capsule of the ankle joint proper is subdivided into four ligaments: (1) anterior, (2) posterior, (3) medial (deltoid), and (4) lateral (Figure 17-7). The requirement of free movement in flexion and extension results in the anterior and posterior ligaments of the capsule being loose and weak. The medial (deltoid) and lateral (collateral) ligaments of the capsule are tight and strong. The individual components of the articular capsule are listed in the box.

The deltoid, or medial collateral, ligament is triangular, thick, and very strong. Its apex is attached to the medial malleolus and its base to bones and ligaments in the foot. It supports the talus and braces the spring lig-

---

Capsule of the Ankle

Anterior Ligament
Posterior Ligament
Collateral ligaments
   Medial (deltoid) ligament
   Lateral ligament
      Anterior talofibular ligament
      Posterior talofibular ligament
      Calcaneofibular ligament

---

ament between the calcaneus and navicular bones, thus helping to preserve the medial longitudinal arch of the foot. In extreme and forced eversion of the foot, the deltoid ligament may tear away from or fracture the medial malleolus rather than tear or rupture itself.

The lateral collateral ligament comprises three separate ligaments. These three components of the lateral ligament are not as strong as the single deltoid ligament on the medial side of the ankle; as a result, sprains occur more frequently when the ankle is turned inward (inverted).

FOOT AND ANKLE INJURIES/CONDITIONS

Athletic injuries involving the foot and ankle are very common and vary widely in terms of structural damage or functional loss. Because of the high utilization of the foot in most types of athletic activity, acute traumatic injuries are as prevalent as overuse injuries. Injuries involving an athlete's feet are often magnified in severity because the feet are weight bearing structures. A relatively minor injury of the foot can impair an athlete's performance as dramatically as a major injury to another body area. Unfortunately, athletes often abuse or neglect their feet until conditions or symptoms interfere with their performance. Proper and adequate care should be given all injuries and athletic related conditions of the feet, no matter how minor they may appear. This discussion of the more common foot injuries and conditions includes injuries to the ankle joint.

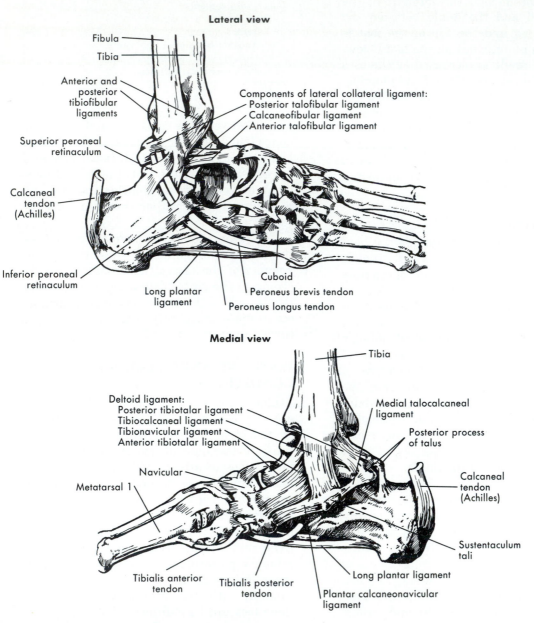

FIGURE 17-7
Ligaments of the ankle and tarsal joints.

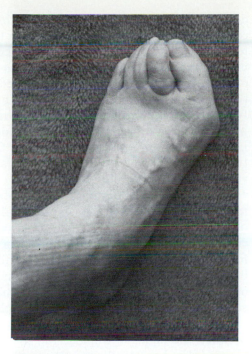

FIGURE 17-8
Bunion (hallucis valgus).

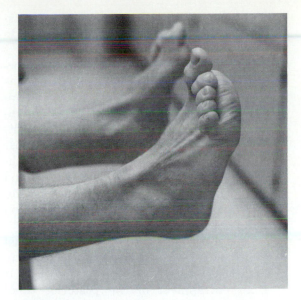

FIGURE 17-9
Hammertoes.

Foot Conditions

✤ **Bunion (hallux valgus).** A bunion is an inflammation and thickening of the bursa of the metatarsophalangeal joint of the great toe, usually associated with abnormal enlargement of the joint and lateral displacement of the toe (Figure 17-8). The normal cause is chronic irritation and pressure from poorly fitted shoes or structural anomalies. A bunionlike enlargement of the metatarsophalangeal joint of the fifth toe is called a **bunionette** or *tailor's bunion.*

✤ **Hammertoe.** A hammertoe is an extension deformity of the metatarsophalangeal joint and flexion deformity of the proximal interphalangeal joint of the lesser toes (Figure 17-9). Occasionally this condition involves flexion of the distal interphalangeal joints as well. Some authorities call this last circumstance, *claw toes,* while others define the terms hammertoes and claw toes as synonymous.

✤ **Morton's neuroma (plantar neuroma).** Involves one of the digital nerves which lie between the metatarsal heads. The nerve becomes entrapped, pinched, or squeezed and swelling occurs. The result is a tumor or mass of nerve fibers called a **neuroma.** This condition occurs more commonly with repetitive trauma, especially in a hypermobile foot. The nerve between the third and fourth metatarsal is affected most often. A sharp, burning pain is present in the region of the third web space and is accentuated by activity. The pain may radiate into the third and fourth toes. Tight shoes aggravate the condition, and the pain is often relieved by removing the shoe. The condition is recognized by squeezing the ball of the foot together, which drives the metatarsals against the swollen nerve, or by palpating directly between the metatarsal heads.

✤ **Corn.** A hard corn is a localized hardening and thickening of the skin produced by friction and pressure. The most common location is over the dorsum of the toes, especially the dorsal aspect of the proximal interphalangeal joint of the fifth toe. A corn has a conical shaped core that extends into the dermis, and causes pain and irritation. A **soft corn** is a thickening of the epidermis between the toes caused by pressure between two prominent phalangeal condyles.

This type of corn is kept softened by moisture and maceration, and often leads to painful inflammation beneath the corn.

❖ **Ingrown toenail.** An ingrown toenail occurs when the skin of the nail fold receives pressure from the nail edge, causing inflammation and pain. It can be caused by improperly trimming of the toenail or poor fitting shoes. Ingrown toenails occur most often in the great toe. In a competitive athlete this condition can be aggravating and even disabling. In a chronic stage, an ingrown toenail may require a wedge resection of the involved nail.

❖ **Tarsal tunnel syndrome.** Tarsal tunnel syndrome of the foot and ankle is similar to the carpal tunnel syndrome of the wrist. It is an entrapment of the posterior tibial nerve within the tarsal tunnel, which is located behind the medial malleolus and covered by the flexor retinaculum. The structures passing through the tarsal tunnel are the posterior tibial, flexor digitorum longus, and flexor hallucis longus tendons with their separate synovial sheaths and the tibial nerve, artery, and vein. Any condition that compromises the contents of the tarsal tunnel may lead to a tarsal tunnel syndrome. Causes may be chronic tendinitis or residuals from a fracture or sprain. Symptoms may be a burning, numbness, tingling, prickling, or cutting pain in the plantar aspect of the foot. There may be some radiating pain. Medial heel and arch pain, often aggravated by athletic activity, are typical of tarsal tunnel syndrome. On the other hand, pain from plantar fasciitis is more likely to occur at the origin of the plantar fascia and to diminish with stretching and running. Weakness and atrophy may occur if tarsal tunnel syndrome continues to progress.

Contusions

Contusions about the foot resulting from various types of direct impacts are common occurrences in athletics. The skin over the dorsum of the foot is thin and only loosely attached to the underlying structures. Further, the subcutaneous placement and exposed nature of most structures near the dorsum of the foot make them susceptible to contusion injuries. Injuries in this area tend to be painful even if actual tissue damage is minor. However, all direct trauma to the dorsum of the foot should be evaluated for the presence of significant damage to underlying structures such as bones, tendons, or nerves. In most instances, although painful initially, such injuries are not serious. Contusions that do not heal promptly must be reevaluated periodically.

Contusions to the plantar, or weight-bearing, surface of the foot can be particularly bothersome and handicapping. These injuries, common to the plantar aspect of the heel and ball of the foot, are normally caused by direct trauma such as repeated pounding on a hard surface, a faulty spike or cleat, stepping on an object, or even a wrinkle in the athlete's sock. The subcutaneous tissue between the bones of the foot and the thick plantar skin becomes bruised and inflamed. This injury, often called a **stone bruise,** or heel bruise, may become quite painful and disabling during weight bearing and athletic competition. Localized tenderness at the site of trauma may persist until weight bearing is relieved. Contusions of this type may develop into a chronic inflammatory process and recur throughout the athletic season.

Strains

Strains involving the foot are common occurrences in athletics. These injuries may involve the intrinsic muscles, the tendons, and tendinous attachments of the extrinsic muscles, and the **plantar aponeurosis** (plantar fascia). Strains may occur to any of the intrinsic muscles of the foot as a result of excessive overuse or violent stresses applied to muscles during athletic activity. Symptomatically, these injuries usually cause cramping or fatigue of the involved muscles and are painful during resistive movements. Symptoms normally subside when activity is reduced or discontinued.

Athletic trainers are more often expected to manage strains involving the extrinsic muscles of the foot or those muscles that originate about the leg. These injuries are discussed in more detail along with injuries of the leg. Because the tendons and tendinous attachments of these extrinsic muscles are in and about the foot and ankle, injuries involving these structures produce symptoms similar to foot and ankle sprains. Therefore each must be accurately evaluated. Strains of these extrinsic tendons cause tenderness at the site of injury and increased pain on active and resistive contractions of the muscle or muscles involved.

❖ **Plantar fasciitis.** Another common strain of the foot occurs to the plantar aponeurosis or fascia. These strong bands of fibrous connective tissue originate on the calcaneal tuberosities and insert into the sides of the metatarsal heads and into the flexor digital tendon sheaths. This tough fascia surrounds the soft tissue structures of the sole of the foot and acts as one of the primary supports for the longitudinal arch. It is often described as a "tie rod" for the longitudinal arch because it serves to connect its ends and prevent their spread. The plantar fascia is subjected to many stresses and forces during athletic activity, which may result in a strain injury that often becomes chronic. The pain associated with this type of an injury can be acute and handicapping. In many cases the pain is most severe when the athlete first puts weight on the foot, for example, when getting out of bed in the morning or at the beginning of activity. The pain generally diminishes during activity, only to increase when activity stops or when the athlete is "cooling down." Point tenderness is usually located toward the calcaneal end of the aponeurosis and very often over the anterior medial tuberosity of the calcaneus. Occasionally the pain can be reproduced by having the athlete stand on the toes. Plantar fasciitis is often aggravated by excessive pronation of the foot, obesity, or an abnormally high arch.

❖ **Heel spur.** A bony growth (exostosis) that arises at the plantar aspect of the calcaneal tuberosity. This may accompany or result from severe cases of plantar fasciitis and be present on a radiograph. However, heel spurs may be present with or without any painful symptoms.

❖ **Talotibial spurs.** Exostoses or bone spurs are common about the foot and ankle. These bony prominences represent localized overgrowth of bone that develops secondary to direct trauma, avulsion of ligaments, chronic synovitis, and fractures. Bone spurs are common on the anterior lip of the tibia and the adjacent talus due to repetitive compression in this area. Athletes may complain of pain in the anterior aspect of the ankle in dorsiflexion because of mechanical impingement. The athlete may have difficulty in "driving off" because the anterior end of the talus cannot enter the mortise normally.

Sprains

Injuries involving the ligaments or ligamentous capsules surrounding the various joints of the foot are common in athletic activity. This is especially true of the ankle joint. Sprains frequently result from forced motion at a joint, especially torsion movements, which can stress any of the supporting ligaments and cause various degrees of damage. Although it must be remembered that the human body is a chain-linkage system, sprains will be discussed in three segments that correspond to divisions of the foot: (1) forefoot, (2) midfoot, and (3) hindfoot, which includes the ankle joint. An injury in any one of these segments can cause problems or affect the others.

Forefoot

The forefoot is composed of the metatarsals and phalanges. This part of the foot is used in the pushing-off phase of the gait cycle and as such is subjected to stresses that may result in various types of sprains. The interphalangeal and metatarsophalangeal joints are most often injured by extreme dorsiflexion or plantar flexion forces.

❖ **Great toe sprain.** The metatarsophalangeal joint of the great toe is a common site for a sprain type of an injury, which is often referred to as a **turf toe.** A sprain of this joint can be debilitating in that the great toe is very important in weight bearing and must bear the brunt of every step. Symptomatically, sprains about the toes will be tender at the site of injury with an increase in pain on reproduction of the stress that caused the injury. In addition, there are normally varying amounts of swelling, stiffness, and soreness surrounding the articulations. Depending on the amount of ligamentous damage, there may be varying amounts of instability associated with the injury. If instability is recognized, the athlete should be referred to medical assistance. Various instability tests are discussed in the assessment portion of this chapter.

❖ **Transverse arch sprain.** The metatarsal bones are joined by a complex mechanism of ligaments. Occasionally the ligaments and supporting tissues of the metatarsal heads will be injured. The mechanism of injury is varied but usually is associated with prolonged activity on hard surfaces or with overuse. Physical findings normally include tenderness and swelling under the heads of the metatarsals and pain upon weight bearing. Sprains involving the tarsometatarsal joints sometimes occur as a result of a twisting mechanism or direct stress, such as the athlete stepping on someone or something. This type of forefoot sprain can be very disabling because of the increased tenderness and pain upon weight bearing. Return to full activity may take up to 4 weeks or longer with this type of injury.

Midfoot

The midfoot is composed of the navicular, cuboid, and three cuneiform bones. The midtarsal and tarsometatarsal joints are supported by a strong ligamentous system that is not injured often. Figure 17-7 illustrates the many small ligaments in the midfoot area. However, **midfoot sprains** can result from severe twisting mechanisms or forceful direct trauma that causes a subluxation of the involved tarsals or metatarsals. These sprains produce tenderness at the site of injury, and often weight bearing is extremely painful. Tenderness may be elicited at the involved joint by gentle passive pronation and abduction of the forefoot. Midfoot sprains can prevent an athlete from normal activity for a considerable length of time. If

recovery is slow, it is often beneficial to place the foot in a firm-soled shoe or firm orthotic to decrease the stress across the midfoot and promote healing.

❖ **Longitudinal arch sprains.** The ligaments that support the longitudinal arch are also subjected to many stresses during athletic activity and can become inflamed, stretched, or torn. The mechanisms of injury and symptoms are very similar to plantar fasciitis that was previously discussed.

Hindfoot

The hindfoot is composed of the calcaneus and talus. These bones serve as attachments for the medial and lateral ligaments that support the ankle joint; therefore injuries to the hindfoot include sprains of the ankle.

❖ **Ankle sprains.** Ankle sprains are among the most commonly treated injuries that occur to athletes. The frequency of ankle injuries results from the anatomic structure, the weight-bearing function, and the violent forces applied to this joint during high-speed athletic activity. As previously discussed, the talus fits into a mortise formed by the distal ends of the tibia and fibula. The medial and lateral malleoli project downward to articulate with the sides of the talus. The talus is narrower posteriorly than anteriorly. This anatomic fact explains the slight looseness or increased amount of motion of the ankle joint in plantar flexion. The talus fits more snugly into the mortise during dorsiflexion. The ankle joint is designed to function as a hinge joint permitting only dorsal and plantar flexion. Ankle injuries occur when this joint is forced to the extremes of motion or in an abnormal direction.

One of the most common mechanisms of ankle sprains is forced inversion with some degree of plantar flexion. Plantar flexion brings the narrower portion of the talus between the malleoli and increases laxity of the ankle joint. This makes the ankle more susceptible to injury. Because of the shorter medial malleolus, inversion occurs more readily than eversion. In fact, during forced inversion, the short medial malleolus may become a fulcrum, causing further inversion.

Most athletic activity predisposes a participant to inversion injuries. This occurs because most cutting and turning maneuvers are initiated from the foot opposite the direction of the turn. For example, if an athlete wants to cut right, the maneuver begins with a lateral push-off from the left foot, which forces the ankle into inversion, external rotation, and plantar flexion. This stresses the lateral ligament complex, especially the anterior talofibular ligament, which is the most frequently injured ligament in the ankle. Additional factors that accentuate the ankle's normal tendency to go into inversion occur if the foot strikes an irregular or uneven surface, such as coming down on another athlete's foot (Figure 17-10).

The opposite mechanism of injury, forced eversion, occurs less frequently during athletic activity. This can occur when the leg is hit laterally with the foot fixed. Because the lateral malleolus is as long as the talus is high, it is very difficult for the lower end of the fibula to act as a fulcrum during this type of an injury. This fact, along with the strength of the medial ligaments, explains why athletic trainers seldom see isolated injuries to the deltoid ligament. Sprains to the medial side of the ankle are often severe and involve additional structures such as a fractured fibula.

Syndesmosis ankle sprain. Syndesmosis sprains of the ankle are uncommon injuries. This injury occurs as the tibia and fibula are forced apart injuring the ligaments that bind these bones together. Often the mechanism causing a syndesmosis ankle sprain is forced dorsiflexion. As the foot is forced into dorsiflexion, the broad part of the talus is located firmly between the malleoli and may force the bones apart, thus injuring the ligaments of the distal tibiofibular joint. A similar injury can result from forced rotation of the leg with the foot firmly fixed. In these cases the shape of the talus acts as

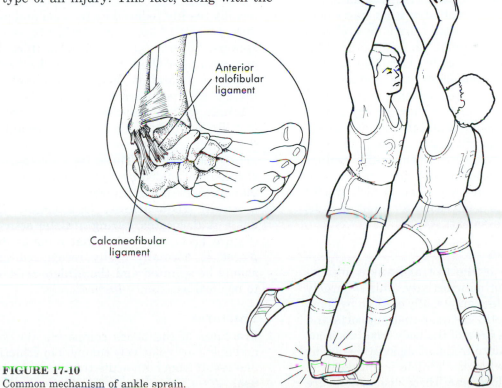

Anterior
talofibular
ligament

Calcaneofibular
ligament

FIGURE 17-10
Common mechanism of ankle sprain.

a fulcrum forcing the tibia and fibula apart. It is important to differentiate the syndesmosis sprain from the more common lateral ligament sprain because this sprain often causes more disabling symptoms and has a prolonged recovery time. Symptoms include point tenderness and swelling localized over the anterior and posterior tibiofibular ligaments. There may be some pain over the medial malleolus and/or the interosseous area. Bimalleolar compression usually produces pain to the syndesmosis. The athlete will often prefer to walk on his or her toes and complain of an inability to "push off." Initial complaints may appear out of proportion to your objective findings.

In light of the many and varied mechanisms that can cause ankle sprains, it is easy to understand the importance of an accurate history in evaluation of these injuries. The information gained in a thorough history assists the athetic trainer in focusing on those anatomic structures that might be involved. A good history always includes a review of the forces and stresses associated with the injury and a careful evaluation of the athlete's description of what happened. Significant ankle sprains are almost always accompanied by immediate pain and difficulty in bearing weight. Localized tenderness will be exhibited over the ligaments involved, and there may or may not be initial swelling. Ankle motion may or may not be restricted. It is important to evaluate the severity of the sprain before swelling develops and motion is restricted. On initial evaluation, the athletic trainer must attempt to recognize an unstable ankle, which should be referred to a physician for additional diagnostic assessment.

Dislocations

Dislocations of the foot and ankle are uncommon in athletic activity. This is largely because the feet are usually covered by some type of athletic footwear that supports and protects this area of the body from dislocating forces. More frequent dislocations occur to the toes when the athlete is not wearing any type of footwear. These dislocations are

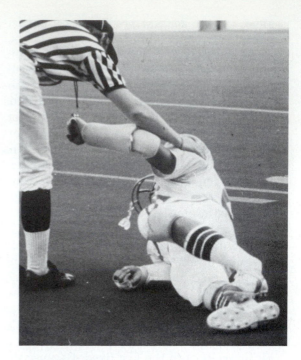

FIGURE 17-11
Athlete with ankle dislocation.

usually readily reduced by traction and produce periods of disability similar to severe sprains. Severe injuries, such as third-degree sprains of the forefoot or midfoot, may result in separation of the metatarsals or tarsals with significant ligament damage. The only symptom may be a painful, swollen foot. Radiographic studies are important in evaluating a swollen foot to assess bone and joint relationships. These types of injuries should be attended by a physician skilled in management of foot injuries.

✛   **Ankle dislocations.** Occasionally the ankle is dislocated during athletic activity (Figure 17-11). An ankle that remains displaced is normally easily recognized and should be splinted and the athlete referred to medical assistance *immediately.*

Fractures

Fractures of the bones composing the foot and ankle are relatively common in athletics and result from both acute trauma and over-use.

✤ **Forefoot fractures.** The forefoot, composed of the long bones of the metatarsals and phalanges, is by far the most common area for fractures in the foot. These fractures can result from a direct blow to the area or by indirect trauma produced when harmful forces are transmitted along the shaft of these bones. Symptomatically these fractures demonstrate point tenderness over the injured site and increased pain during longitudinal stress. Swelling, discoloration, crepitation, and deformity may also be present. Figure 17-12 illustrates a fracture of the middle phalanx of the second toe.

Jones' fracture. A Jones' fracture is a fracture of the base of the fifth metatarsal distal to the tuberosity. This fracture is a possible management problem in that it often requires prolonged immobilization, has a high propensity for nonunion, and commonly refractures after union is obtained by conservative treatment. In competitive athletics, Jones' fractures with delayed union or nonunion should be treated operatively. Athletic trainers should be alert to recognize the difference between a Jones fracture and a styloid fracture. A Jones' fracture is often caused by a forceful load being applied to the ball of the foot laterally, such as during pivoting or landing on the lateral part of the forefoot. The styloid fractures most often during forced inversion causing avulsion of the insertion of the peroneus brevis tendon. These two fractures should not be treated the same.

✤ **Stress fractures.** The current emphasis on cardiovascular fitness and long-distance running has increased the incidence of overuse injuries, including stress or fatigue fractures. Athletes who have stress fractures almost always have a history of high-intensity training, and they frequently have increased their training regimen abruptly in the recent past. Stress fractures may involve any bone in the foot, but more commonly involve the second, third, or fourth metatarsal. These fractures, occasionally called **march fractures,** occur with repetitive trauma. Excessive foot pronation or a high and rigid arched foot may contribute to the incidence

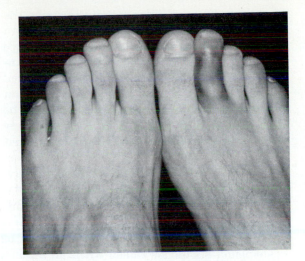

FIGURE 17-12
Fracture of the middle phalanx of the second toe.

of stress fractures. Symptomatically, stress fractures often exhibit a gradual increase in forefoot pain that is aggravated by activity and relieved by rest. X-ray films may be negative initially. If symptoms persist, the foot should be reexamined by radiography in a few weeks. At that time callus formation may indicate the presence of a stress fracture.

Fractures involving the midfoot and hindfoot during athletic activity are not nearly as common as those in the forefoot. When fractures do occur in these areas of the foot, they are usually associated with severe torsion or compression forces and result in major foot injuries. Fractures about the ankle are usually to the medial or lateral malleoli. These are caused by the same forces that cause ankle sprains and have tenderness and swelling in the area of the malleolus. Malleolar fractures are often recognized by the associated instability exhibited during lateral or medial stress.

✤ **Chondral/osteochondral fracture.** An acute or chronic subluxation of the talus in the ankle mortise can allow the edges of the talus to impinge against the fibula or tibia. In dorsiflexion, an inversion force can cause the lateral talar margin to strike the fibula. In plantar flexion, an inversion force can cause the medial talar margin to strike the bottom of the tibia. These mechanisms can result in compression fractures that cause the articular cartilage and possibly the underlying bone to crack and even be chipped away, creating fragments that can float freely in the ankle joint. Symptoms can be quite varied and nonspecific. Athletes may not complain of pain if the ligaments are not involved or injured. Athletes may report pain with activity, weakness, popping, giving out, locking, swelling, and/or stiffness. These lesions to the talar dome may be difficult to detect upon initial evaluation and even following radiographs. Your index of suspicion should be raised when an athlete has prolonged pain and the sprained ankle does not seem to be responding in a routine fashion to standard treatments and protocols. Additional imaging studies are indicated. A nondisplaced fragment can heal with ankle immobilization and rest. A displaced fragment may cause locking and should be removed surgically. It is also possible for a segment of the subchondral bone of the talus to undergo avascular necrosis

❖ **(osteochondritis dissecans).**

❖ **Epiphyseal fracture.** Fractures of the ankle and foot are rare in the growing athlete. An open epiphyseal plate **(physis)** does not mean the young athlete will have more fractures of the ankle than sprains. However, fractures that do occur to the foot and ankle in the growing athlete usually involve the epiphyseal plate and are treated the same as any epiphyseal separation. For example, in a skeletally immature athlete, the mechanism that causes a syndesmosis ankle sprain may result in an avulsion fracture of the distal tibial physis as the ligaments remain intact.

ANATOMY OF THE LEG

The leg is that part of the anatomy from the knee to the ankle. It is composed of the tibia and fibula, which furnish points of attachment for both thigh and leg muscles and transmit the body weight to the ankle and foot.

Tibia and Fibula

The tibia is the larger and stronger and the more medially and superficially located of the two lower leg bones. It can be divided into a shaft separated by proximal and distal ends. The larger proximal end is prismatic in shape and overhangs the shaft. It consists of a tuberosity and medial and lateral condyles (Figure 17-13). The expanded proximal end provides a good weight-bearing surface for the distal end of the femur. The subcutaneous tibial tuberosity can be palpated on the anterior aspect of the bone just distal to the condyle, about an inch from the top of the bone in most adults. In addition to the tibial tuberosity, both condyles of the tibia can be readily palpated at the sides of the bone. The condyles form most of the proximal end of the bone. The anterior border of the tibial shaft (shin) can be easily palpated because it is located very near the surface of the skin. Usually the shaft can be palpated from the tibial tuberosity to the medial malleolus. In some athletes, however, the shin may be somewhat indistinct in its lower third. The distal (lower) end of the tibia projects medially and downward as the medial malleolus of the ankle.

The fibula, the lateral of the two leg bones, is long and slender and lies parallel to the tibia. It is attached proximally and distally to the lateral aspect of the tibia but does not bear any weight. With the tibia it aids in forming the ankle joint and also serves as the site of attachment for muscles. Like the tibia it can be divided into proximal and distal ends and a shaft. It is the pointed distal end of the fibula that forms the lateral malleolus. The lateral malleolus descends about 1.5 cm beyond the medial malleolus of the tibia. Distally the fibula articulates with the tibia and the talus. The latter fits into a box-like socket (ankle joint) formed by the medial and lateral malleoli.

Tibiofibular Joints

The two leg bones articulate with each other at their proximal and distal ends. Additionally a very strong interosseous membrane

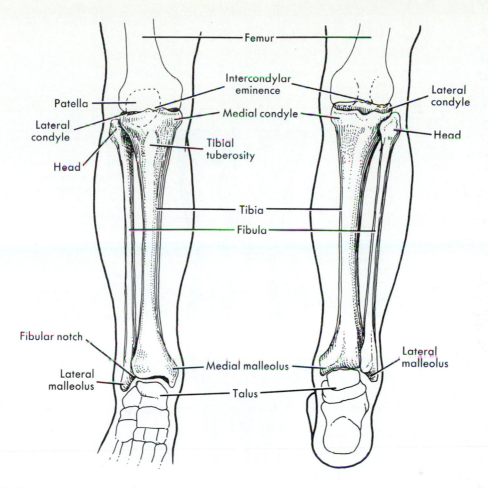

FIGURE 17-13
Right tibia and fibula.

joins the bones throughout their length. The proximal (superior tibiofibular) joint is a diarthrotic (synovial) joint that permits some gliding movements. It is formed by the articulation between the lateral condyle of the tibia and the head of the fibula. The joint is surrounded by a tough fibrous capsule reinforced by both anterior and posterior ligaments. The actual capsule surrounding the joint is much stronger in front than behind, and in about 10% of the population the synovial membrane of the joint is continuous with that of the knee joint.

The inferior tibiofibular joint is a fibrous articulation between the lateral malleolus and the inferior end of the tibia. It is a strong joint reinforced by numerous ligaments, in-

cluding the anterior and posterior tibiofibular ligaments. Occasionally a part of the synovial cavity of the ankle joint extends upward between the lower end of the tibia and fibula, converting this joint into a diarthrotic joint.

Muscles of the Leg
Refer to Figures 17-14 and 17-15 to review the muscles of the leg. The leg muscles and their primary actions and nerve innervations are listed in Table 17-1. The muscles of the leg are divided by thick fascial sheaths into four distinct compartments. (Figure 17-16). The *anterior compartment* contains the tibialis anterior, extensor hallucis longus, and extensor digitorum muscles, as well as

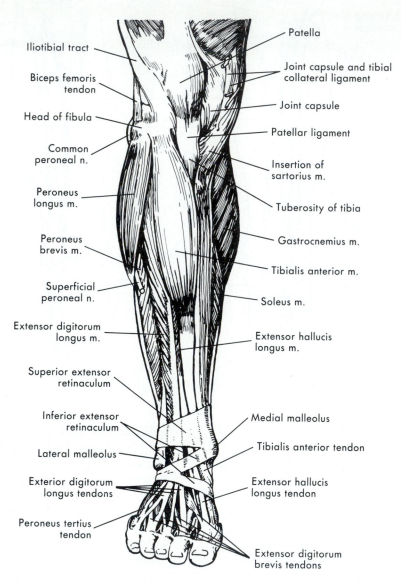

FIGURE 17-14
Anatomy of anterior right leg.

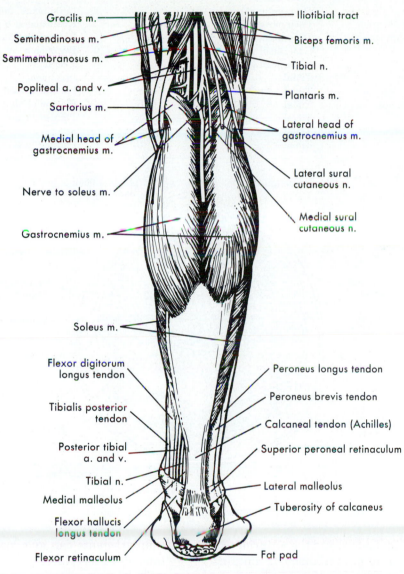

Gracilis m.

Semitendinosus m.

Semimembranosus m.

Popliteal a. and v.

Sartorius m.

Medial head of
gastrocnemius m.

Nerve to soleus m.

Gastrocnemius m.

Soleus m.

Flexor digitorum
longus tendon

Tibialis posterior
tendon

Posterior tibial
a. and v.

Tibial n.

Medial malleolus

Flexor hallucis
longus tendon

Flexor retinaculum

Iliotibial tract

Biceps femoris m.

Tibial n.

Plantaris m.

Lateral head of
gastrocnemius m.

Lateral sural
cutaneous n.

Medial sural
cutaneous n.

Peroneus longus tendon

Peroneus brevis tendon

Calcaneal tendon (Achilles)

Superior peroneal retinaculum

Lateral malleolus

Tuberosity of calcaneus

Fat pad

FIGURE 17-15
Anatomy of posterior right leg.

TABLE 17-1

Muscles of the Leg

Muscle	Nerve	Segmental innervation	Primary action(s)
Tibialis anterior	Deep peroneal	L_4-S_1	Dorsiflexion and inversion
Extensor hallucis longus	Deep peroneal	L_4-S_1	Extension of big toe and dorsiflexion
Extensor digitorum longus	Deep peroneal	L_4-S_1	Extension of toes and dorsiflexion
Peroneus longus	Superficial peroneal	L_4-S_1	Eversion
Peroneus brevis	Superficial peroneal	L_4-S_1	Eversion
Tibialis posterior	Tibial	L_5-S_1	Inversion
Flexor digitorum longus	Tibial	L_5-S_1	Flexion of toes
Flexor hallucis longus	Tibial	L_5-S_2	Flexion of big toe
Gastrocnemius	Tibial	S_1-S_2	Plantar flexion
Soleus	Tibial	S_1-S_2	Plantar flexion
Plantaris	Tibial	L_4-S_1	Plantar flexion

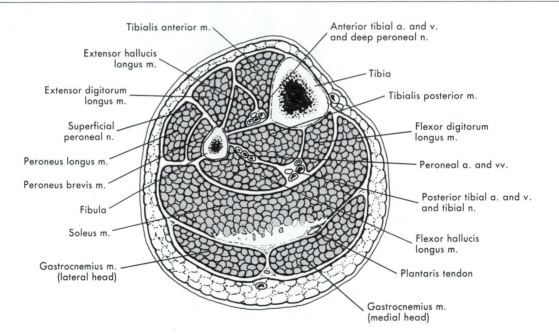

FIGURE 17-16
Cross section of leg showing the four compartments.

the deep peroneal nerve and the anterior tibial artery. The *lateral compartment* contains the peroneal muscles and the superficial peroneal nerve. The *deep posterior compartment* contains the tibialis posterior, flexor digitorum longus, and flexor hallucis longus muscles, as well as the tibial nerve and the posterior tibial artery. The *superficial posterior compartment* contains the gastrocnemius, soleus, and plantaris muscles. Excessive pressure developing within these compartments can give rise to injury symptoms described later.

The largest tendon in the body, the Achilles, is the common attachment for the gastrocnemius and soleus muscles. This tendon runs from approximately two thirds of the way down the lower leg, where it attaches the calf muscles to the calcaneus. Two bursae surround the Achilles attachment, the superficial subcutaneous between the skin and the Achilles tendon and the deep retrocalcaneal between the calcaneus and the tendon. Either of these bursae can be irritated during athletic activity.

Alignment of the lower extremity

With any injury involving the lower extremity, and especially those of a chronic or overuse nature, it is important to appraise the alignment and structure of the lower extremity as a whole. The lower extremity functions optimally when each segment is in proper alignment and there are no structural abnormalities. This area of the body is especially susceptible to injuries resulting from malalignment and structural abnormalities. These conditions can produce abnormal stresses in the musculoskeletal structures of the lower extremity and affect other areas of the body, such as the hips and back. The alignment and structure of the lower extremities is therefore an important indicator of the soundness of the skeletal framework and muscular system in this area.

Evaluating the alignment of the lower extremities can be accomplished while the athlete is sitting or lying down with both legs in an extended and neutral position. However, it is usually easier to observe alignment when the athlete stands with his or her feet together. An important advantage of having the athlete stand is that most abnormal conditions are magnified with weight bearing and therefore more easily recognized. The athlete should be viewed from the front, side, and back. During the initial evaluation it is important to observe the pelvic area and the spine in addition to the lower extremities because abnormalities may be manifested in these body areas. While viewing the athlete, look for any obvious malalignments or structural faults. The common malalignment problems of the lower extremity are listed in the box. Conditions involving the knee are discussed in more detail in Chapter 18.

When observing an athlete, an important consideration is the length of the legs. A discrepancy in leg length, either actual or functional, can cause an imbalance and produce

---

Common Malalignments of the Lower Extremity
Thigh
Leg length
Knee
Genu varum
Genu valgum
Q angle
Patella alta
Squinting patella
Genu recurvatum
Leg
Internal tibial torsion
External tibial torsion
Ankle
Ankle varus
Ankle valgus
Foot types
Pronated foot
Pes cavus
Morton's foot
Toe deformities
Bunions
Hammertoes

---

symptoms of overuse syndromes in the lower extremities, pelvis, or back. Whenever a difference in the level of the hips is observed, a discrepancy in leg length should be suspected. Determining leg length discrepancies was previously discussed and illustrated in Chapter 15 along with spinal alignment, but is reviewed in this chapter. To determine if the hips are level, have the athlete stand. Look to see if both anterior superior iliac spines are in the same horizontal plane. If the iliac spines appear to be uneven, there may be a difference in the length of the athlete's legs. With the athlete lying down, place both legs in a neutral position and observe the medial malleoli. If the malleoli do not appear to match, a difference in leg length should be suspected. To determine if there is an actual discrepancy in leg length, have the athlete lie supine with both legs in a neutral position. Measure the distance from the anterior superior iliac spines to the medial malleoli of both ankles. Unequal distances between these bony landmarks indicate an actual difference in leg length. If the legs are the same length but the iliac spines

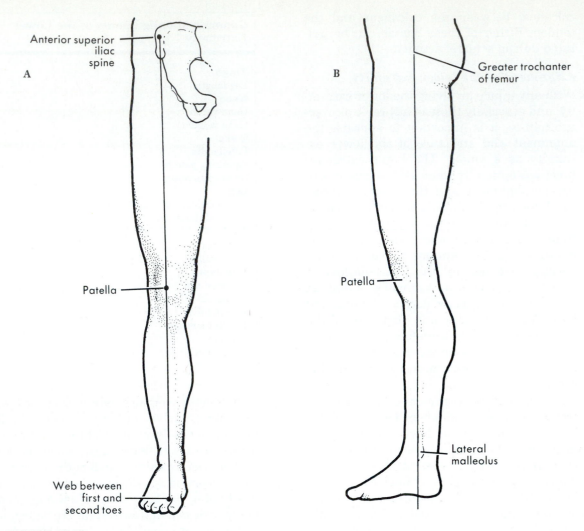

FIGURE 17-17
Normal alignment of the lower extremity when viewed **A**, anteriorly and **B**, laterally.

appear to be uneven, the pelvis is tilted laterally, resulting in one leg being functionally shorter. This may be caused by a problem in the back, hips, knees, or feet. Leg length discrepancies may or may not cause problems for an athlete or produce symptoms. In many cases, minor differences in leg length remain asymptomatic.

The normal alignment of the lower extremity when viewed anteriorly with the athlete standing is illustrated in Figure 17-17, *A*. When observing the lower extremity from the front, three landmarks are impor-

tant: (1) the anterior superior iliac spine, (2) the patella, and (3) the web space between the first and second toes. The lower extremity of the athlete is considered to be in normal alignment when these three landmarks appear to be in a straight line. This straight vertical alignment results in a mechanically straightforward position of the feet during walking and running. This position allows the most efficient and powerful action of the leg muscles in propulsion of the body. When these three landmarks do not lie in a straight line, a malalignment is indicated.

The greater the deviation from a straight line, the greater the degree of malalignment. Any deviation from a straight line imposes abnormal stresses on the joints, ligaments, tendons, and muscles of the lower extremities and feet.

The normal alignment of the lower extremity when viewed laterally is illustrated in Figure 17-17, *B*. When observing the lower extremity from the side, again three landmarks are important: (1) the greater trochanter of the femur, (2) the patella, and (3) the lateral malleolus. The lower extremity is considered in normal alignment when an imaginary vertical line extends from the greater trochanter, posterior to the patella and anterior to the lateral malleolus. The most common fault in lateral alignment of the lower extremity is hyperextension of the knee (Figure 17-18). This is also known as **genu recurvatum** or back knee. Some degree of genu recurvatum should be considered normal in certain persons. However, a severe form of alignment discrepancy of this type can contribute to stability problems in the vulnerable knee joint. Hyperextension of the knee can result from structural defects, muscular imbalance, and compensation for functional faults.

Viewing an athlete from the back is extremely useful in determining the alignment of the spine and pelvic area, as was discussed in Chapter 15, and can also be used to evaluate the alignment of the knees. In assessment of the lower extremity, this view is most useful in observing alignment between the leg and foot. The midline of the Achilles tendon should extend downward to the calcaneus without curving medially or laterally (Figure 17-19). The midline of the calcaneus should also be perpendicular to the surface on which the athlete is standing. Any deviation from this line is usually associated with a malalignment of the foot and was discussed with the various types of feet.

Mechanics of the foot, ankle, and leg

The mechanics of a body area involve the function of that part during motion and the forces acting upon it. To further understand

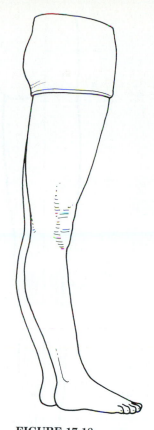

FIGURE 17-18
Hyperextension of the knee.

the function of the lower extremity and conditions that may contribute to overuse injuries, the athletic trainer should possess basic knowledge of the mechanics involved. Understanding these mechanics allows the athletic trainer to more accurately evaluate injuries affecting the lower extremities. The mechanical function of the foot and ankle reflects the mechanics of the entire lower extremity.

The alignment and structure of the lower extremity is certainly an indication of the functional relationship and mechanical efficiency of each segment. Variations and abnormalities observed while the athlete is sitting or standing will also be present during activity. In fact, these conditions may be further magnified and more easily recognized during motion because of additional stress applied to the area. Observing an athlete

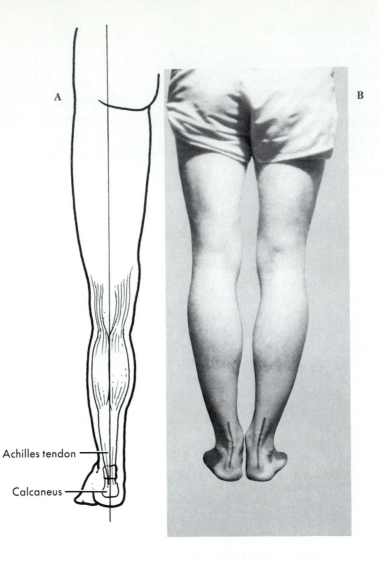

FIGURE 17-19
Alignment of the lower extremity when viewed posteriorly. **A**, Diagram showing normal
alignment; **B**, photograph showing bilateral curvature of the Achilles tendons medially.

who is walking or running can help the athletic trainer determine if there are functional reasons for the athlete's particular injury. A complete examination of the lower extremity, designed to recognize all possible conditions that may contribute to overuse injuries, will often include an observation of the athlete walking or running.

Walking and running gaits are divided into two major phases: (1) the stance phase and (2) the swing phase. The stance phase begins with the foot in contact with the ground and is subdivided into three basic portions: (1) foot strike, beginning at the time the foot touches the ground; (2) mid-stance, when the weight is directly over the foot; and (3) push off, when the body is being propelled forward. The swing phase begins when the foot is off the ground and the leg is moving to another point of contact. One cycle of gait is from foot strike until that same foot strikes the ground again. During walking one foot is always in contact with the ground, and there is a period of time when both feet are simultaneously in contact with the ground. Running differs in that there is a period of time when neither foot is in contact with the ground.

To understand and correlate the function of the foot and ankle during walking and running, the athletic trainer should first have an understanding of what is considered by experts to be normal mechanical function. Remember that any variations observed while the athlete is walking will also occur when the athlete is running and performing other types of athletic activity. When watching an athlete walk, the athletic trainer should first look for the previously described characteristics of normal standing alignment of the lower extremity. The same criteria for neutral positions and straight alignments are used to determine if the athlete's feet, ankles, and legs appear to be mechanically sound. The characteristics of normal standing alignment should be present at midstance during walking and running.

In addition to observing the athlete at midstance, the athletic trainer should be aware of some normal functions of the foot and be alert for any deviations that may occur during the cycle. The foot needs to be flexible on contact and rigid on push off. This is accomplished by pronation and supination during weight bearing. Immediately after heel strike, the foot begins to pronate. This pronation unlocks the midtarsal joints, dampens the shock of heel strike, and allows the forefoot to become more flexible to adapt to various surfaces. This is very important in dissipating the constant stress of foot contact and serves to absorb shock. As the body moves over the fixed foot into midstance, the foot begins to supinate. This supination locks the midtarsal joints, stabilizes the forefoot, and provides a rigid lever for push off. The foot usually remains in supination during the swing phase until the next heel strike. These motions are necessary for the foot to change from a mobile adapter at foot strike to a rigid lever at push off.

Difficulties can arise when pronation continues past midstance and into the propulsive phase. This limits the effectiveness of the propulsive action. Excessive and prolonged pronation also flattens the medial longitudinal arch and transfers abnormal stresses and torques to the lower extremities. This can lead to overuse syndromes, fatigue, and a less efficient athletic performance.

To discuss all the components involved with the complicated mechanics of the foot, ankle, and leg is beyond the realm of this text. We recommend that athletic trainers seek additional information concerning the mechanics of the foot, ankle, and leg and continue to develop their assessment skills by observing and analyzing the various foot mechanics of their athletes.

Circulation and Nerve Supply

The femoral artery in each lower extremity enters the leg at the back of the knee as the popliteal artery. The popliteal artery becomes the posterior tibial artery as it courses between the knee and ankle. The peroneal and anterior tibial arteries branch off the posterior tibial artery in the lower leg near the ankle. It is the anterior tibial artery that is continued beyond the line of the ankle joint, as the dorsalis pedis. The posterior tibial divides into the lateral and medial plantar arteries, which anastomose with the **dorsalis pedis** in supplying blood to the foot.

Blood from the foot is returned by both superficial and deep veins. The great saphenous vein enters the lower leg from the foot just in front of the medial malleolus and then ascends from this constant anterior position along the medial surface of the leg. The small saphenous vein enters the lower leg by passing behind the lateral malleolus and then upward under the skin of the back of the calf to empty into the popliteal vein behind the knee.

The sciatic nerve enters the lower extremity and divides into two terminal divisions called the tibial and common peroneal nerves. The tibial is the larger of the two divisions. After passing between the heads of the gastrocnemius it descends to the ankle, providing branches to the leg musculature, knee, and ankle joints. Branches of the tibial nerve are distributed to the skin of the heel and sole of the foot. In addition, digital branches of the tibial nerve supply the deep muscles of the foot and adjacent sides of the toes. Branches terminate in the base of the toes and structures around the nails.

The common peroneal nerve, the smaller of the two sciatic divisions, divides into superficial and deep branches. Both branches have muscular and cutaneous components. The muscles on the anterior surface of the leg are supplied by the deep peroneal, those on the lateral surface by the superficial peroneal. The superficial branch of the peroneal nerve also provides sensory innervation to the dorsum of the foot and digits, except for the area between the great and second toes. An interosseous branch of the deep peroneal nerve supplies the metatarsophalangeal joint of the great toe and the skin between the great and second toes.

LEG INJURIES

Injuries involving the leg are common in all athletic activities. Many of the injuries which occur to the distal portion of the leg were discussed along with ankle injuries. Those athletic injuries occurring to the proximal portion of the leg are discussed in the following chapter on knee injuries. In addition to the high incidence of athletic injuries occurring about the ankle and knee joints, the leg proper is also subject to a significant amount of athletic related trauma.

Contusions

The lower leg is exposed to various types of direct trauma during athletic activity and is therefore subjected to frequent contusions. Contusions occur most often over the shin, where the anteromedial tibia lies subcutaneously (Figure 17-20). Bone periosteum is extremely sensitive, and a blow to this area of the leg can be very painful and disabling. There is hardly ever a doubt as to the mechanism of injury, that is, a history of direct impact. Contusions to the shin are often associated with abrasions or lacerations resulting from the direct trauma. Once the possibility of direct bone injury has been

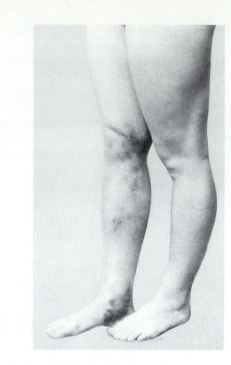

FIGURE 17-20
Contusion to the shin of a gymnast who hit the right leg on the uneven parallel bars. Note swelling and ecchymosis of the right leg. Note also hyperextension of the opposite knee.

eliminated by the evaluation process, the area should be treated using standard treatment procedures and protected from further trauma.

Contusions can also involve the muscular areas of the leg. A possible complication of a severe contusion to any of the leg muscles is significant swelling within the various compartments. In these closed spaces, swelling is not only uncomfortable but may also lead to a compartment syndrome, which is discussed in greater detail later in this section. Another possible complication of a direct blow to the leg is damage to the peroneal nerve. This nerve is particularly vulnerable because it passes around the head of the fibula. A severe blow to this area may cause peroneal nerve injury, with pain radiating throughout the distribution of the nerve. Transient tingling and numbness to the lateral surface of the leg or dorsal surface of the foot may remain for a period of time.

Occasionally peroneal nerve damage will result in loss of function to the dorsiflexors and evertors of the foot, resulting in **footdrop.** These symptoms are often temporary and recovery is usually complete.

Strains

The lower leg is the site of origin for the primary muscles responsible for transmitting power to the foot and ankle. The explosive and repetitive nature of various athletic activities subjects these muscles to extremely dynamic forces. Frequent and powerful use of the leg muscles commonly results in injuries. Strains can occur anywhere along these contractile units and normally result from a violent contraction, overstretching, or continued overuse. Symptoms may be present in the leg, about the ankle, or in the foot.

The most common leg strains occur to the calf muscles because of the forcible contractions of these muscles during most athletic activities. Strains usually occur in the area of the musculotendinous junction or at the insertion of the Achilles tendon into the calcaneus. These injuries may result from repetitive overuse or a single violent contraction. Acute strains to the Achilles tendon have a tendency to become chronic and frequently are complicated by tendinitis.

❖ **Achilles tendinitis.** Achilles tendinitis is a common disorder, especially in distance runners. The Achilles tendon is surrounded by a sheath of loose areolar and adipose peritenon tissue, which contains lubricating fluids. Inflammation between the tendon and its sheathlike covering is sometimes referred to as *Achilles tenosynovitis.* Achilles tendinitis can result in a thickening of the surrounding tissue and loss of the smooth gliding movements (Figure 17-21). This inflammation can cause tenderness on palpation along the tendon and an increase of pain with activity. Often there is also swelling along the tendon, crepitation with movement, and a stiffness or lack of normal motion, especially dorsiflexion.

❖ **Retrocalcaneal bursitis.** Inflammation of the retrocalcaneal bursa, which is located

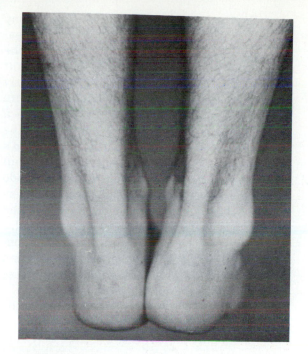

FIGURE 17-21
Chronic Achilles tendinitis. Note swelling of left Achilles tendon.

between the Achilles tendon insertion and the calcaneus. With repeated trauma, the bursa may become inflamed and hypertrophied. An athlete with a prominent superior tuberosity of the calcaneous is more susceptible to retrocalcaneal bursitis. Symptoms consist of pain and tenderness in the retrocalcaneal region. Retrocalcaneal bursitis may be difficult to differentiate from Achilles tendinitis. Careful examination demonstrates that the area of tenderness is anterior to the Achilles tendon.

❖ **Calcaneal apophysitis. Apophysitis** is an inflammation of an **apophysis** which is a bony projection or outgrowth. Calcaneal apophysitis is at the attachment of the Achilles tendon to the calcaneus in young, adolescent athletes. Symptoms include pain and tenderness on the posterior heel below the attachment of the Achilles tendon. Pain is made worse with activity. Calcaneal apophysitis, also known as *Sever's disease,* normally goes away as the calcaneal apophysis ossifies in the young athlete.

Pump bump. A pump bump is a bony growth in the area of the posterior calcaneal tuberosity, which is the attachment of the Achilles tendon. These bumps usually result from local irritation caused by rigid, poorly fitting heel counters. These bumps are more likely to occur in individuals who have a prominent posterosuperior surface of the calcaneus, a condition known as *Haglund's deformity*. The athlete will demonstrate pain and swelling of the heel, which is made worse by exercise. Palpation reveals tenderness, thickening of the overlying skin, and signs of local inflammation. The Achilles tendon may be tender and thickened. Continued irritation of this bony prominence can cause bursitis or Achilles tendinitis. These exostoses are often bilateral.

✣ **Achilles tendon rupture.** Contractile and connective tissue components in the calf muscles may be partially or completely rup-tured during athletic activity. This can result from a single violent contraction or repeated strains. Serious tears occur most frequently in the musculotendinous junction, through the tendon itself, or at the tendinous attachment to the calcaneus (Figure 17-22). Any calf strain should be evaluated for the possibility of Achilles tendon rupture. Symptomatically, calf strains will produce tenderness at the site of injury and an increase in pain on active contraction, resistive movements, and passive stretching. A complete rupture of the Achilles tendon is rare in young athletes and occurs more often in middle-aged recreational athletes. When it does occur, it should be readily recognized, because there is often a palpable gap in the tendon and loss of function of the calf muscle. The athlete will also exhibit a positive Thompson test, which is described and illustrated in Figure 17-33, *D*.

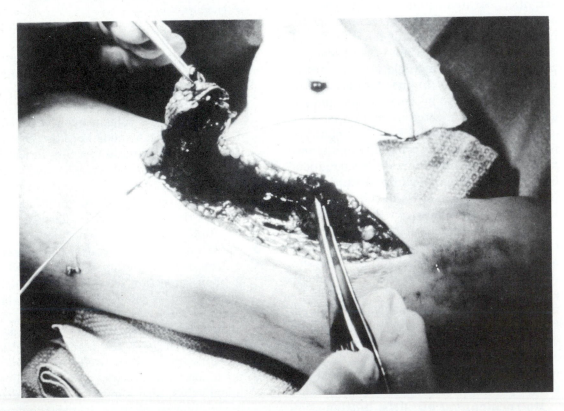

FIGURE 17-22
Complete rupture of the Achilles tendon.

❖ **Plantaris muscle rupture.** The plantaris muscle arises from the posterior lateral femoral condyle, runs between the gastrocnemius and soleus muscles, and inserts just medial to the Achilles tendon on the calcaneus. The belly of this muscle is only 3 to 4 inches in length and is attached by a very small, ribbonlike tendon, which begins high in the leg. The plantaris is comparable to the palmaris longus of the forearm and is absent in a small percent of the population. A plantaris muscle strain or rupture may be indicated when an athlete feels a sudden sharp or tearing pain in the upper midcalf during strenuous activities. These symptoms also accompany a strain of one of the gastrocnemius muscle heads. The athlete with a gastrocnemius strain will have tenderness over the head of the muscle with varying degrees of swelling and ecchymosis. The plantaris muscle strain or rupture will probably not cause significant swelling or ecchymosis. Strains to the plantaris or gastrocnemius muscles are more common in middle-aged athletes.

❖ **Subluxation of the peroneal tendons.** Occasionally athletes will dislocate or sublux their peroneal tendons as they pass behind the fibula. The peroneus brevis and longus muscle tendons pass downward in close conjunction and enter a common synovial tendon sheath above the ankle before passing behind the lateral malleolus. These tendons are held in a groove posterior to the fibula by the superior peroneal retinaculum. Some individuals have anatomic variations in this groove resulting in the sulcus being narrow or flat, which may lead to instability of the peroneal tendons. Peroneal tendon dislocation may occur due to a rupture of the superior retinaculum or because the retinaculum pulls away from the periosteum of the lateral malleolus allowing the tendons to cross over the distal end of the fibula. The mechanism causing this injury may be a sudden, forceful contraction of the peroneal muscles or inversion of a plantar flexed foot. This later mechanism can also cause an ankle sprain and the symptoms may be similar. The symptoms for a subluxation of the peroneal tendons will be swelling and perhaps ecchymosis in the posterior malleolar area with tenderness over the peroneal tendons. Instructing the athlete to actively evert the foot, you may observe the tendons actually sublux. This may not be feasible immediately following an injury, but is often possible after the acute symptoms have subsided in a few days.

❖ **Shin splints.** A term unique to the leg is shin splints, which is a catchall term for chronic painful conditions. Shin splints most often occur early in a training program or after training has been discontinued for a period of time and then resumed. It appears to be associated with repetitive activity on hard surfaces or forcible excessive use of the leg muscles, especially in running and jumping activities. There is disagreement as to the exact nature and cause of this extremely common condition; however, shin splints are considered to be an overuse syndrome generally limited to the musculotendinous components. Pain associated with shin splints may occur anywhere in the leg and occasionally will become totally disabling. Tenderness is most often found along the medial border of the tibia, which is the origin for the tibialis posterior muscle. There are many causes of shin splints, such as muscle inflexibility, a fallen longitudinal arch, a pronated foot, ill-fitting footwear, training techniques, and playing surfaces. All evaluations of shin splints must take into consideration all possible causes of the pain and discomfort in the athlete's leg and rule out stress fractures and ischemic disorders. Treatment procedures must emphasize the correction or modification of possible causes. There is no one best treatment for shin splints, and athletic trainers cannot simply treat the symptoms. This overuse syndrome certainly emphasizes the importance of a thorough and accurate injury assessment.

Tibial stress syndrome. Tibial stress syndrome is recurrent discomfort along the medial border of the middle and distal tibia. It is a common cause of shin splints. The pain is intensified by exercise and not completely relieved by rest. The syndrome is caused by a stress reaction of the fascia, periosteum, or bone along the posteromedial aspect of the tibia. It can also be a combination of any of these. It is often located at the posterior tibialis or soleus muscle attachments to the posterior medial tibia. Physical examination reveals tenderness along the posteromedial border of the tibia, often extending several inches. There should be no vascular or neurologic involvement. Radiographs are frequently normal and a bone scan may be needed to confirm the diagnosis.

✤   **Compartment syndromes.** Other important conditions that must be recognized by athletic trainers and properly managed are **compartment syndromes.** These are disorders of the extremities in which increased tissue pressure compromises the muscles, nerves, or blood vessels within the space and distal to the compartment. Compartment syndromes are more common in the lower leg, where four natural compartments exist. Refer to Figure 17-16 to review the anatomy of each compartment. The superficial posterior compartment is a more loosely contained space not subjected to the constriction forces placed on the anterior, deep posterior, and lateral compartments. The anterior compartment is more frequently involved, followed by the deep posterior. The tight binding of fascia that forms these compartments does not allow for significant swelling within their confines.

Compartment syndromes can develop whenever there is swelling within these tightly closed spaces. Swelling may be caused by excessive exercise, overuse, contusion, localized infection, or overstretching of a particular muscle group. Anything that causes an inflammatory response or uncontrolled swelling may result in increased pressure within one of these compartments. Another possible cause of compartment syndrome is muscle hypertrophy. As muscles in these tightly confined compartments become bigger as a result of repetitive use or exercise, the relative space decreases, which may give rise to constriction forces. Depending on the cause of the condition there may be sudden or gradual onset of symptoms in the involved leg. There will be swelling accompanied by point tenderness and pain in the affected muscle group. In the later stages, numbness, weakness, and the inability to use the affected muscle may develop. Regardless of how or why the symptoms develop, it is important to recognize them early and seek medical attention quickly. Any delay in treatment may result in permanent neurologic disability. Acute compartment syndromes with severe pain as the result of muscle and nerve **ischemia** should be readily recognized. However, many compartment syndromes develop slowly, with symptoms similar to shin splints, stress fractures, muscle strains, or cramps.

The assessment of chronic compartment syndrome is based on a thorough history and physical examination. An athlete with a chronic compartment syndrome typically complains of lower leg pain and tightness that occurs only with physical activity. The pain is usually brought on by approximately the same amount of exercise each time; however, some athletes relate that the amount of exercise that can be performed without pain is less on successive days. The symptoms usually resolve with a day of rest but return with resumption of exercise. Physical examination may reveal weakness and mild tenderness in the muscles of the respective compartments. For example, weakness may be detected on dorsiflexion and toe extension (anterior compartment), eversion (lateral compartment), inversion and toe flexion (deep posterior compartment), or plantar flexion (superficial posterior compartment). Abnormal sensations or paresthesia may be present along the course of the involved nerve. Chronic compartment syndrome can be confirmed by measuring compartment pressures during exercise (Figure 17-23). Conservative care has been shown to be ineffective and severe or persistent cases often require surgery to return an athlete to activity.

Fractures

The tibia and fibula are susceptible to fractures associated with athletic activity (Figure 17-24). The tibia, which is not fractured

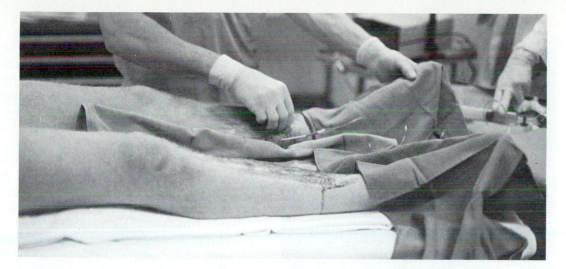

FIGURE 17-23
Compression test performed on the deep posterior compartment of the leg. A catheter is inserted into the compartment to record internal pressure.

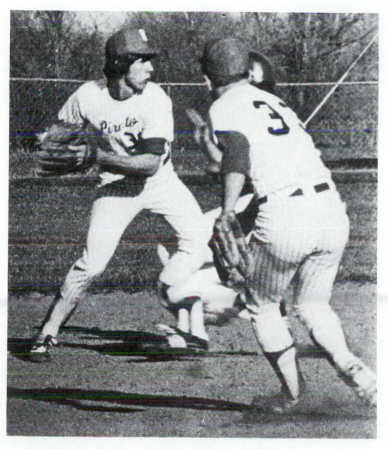

FIGURE 17-24
Fracture of the left tibia and fibula. Picture was taken at the moment of fracture.

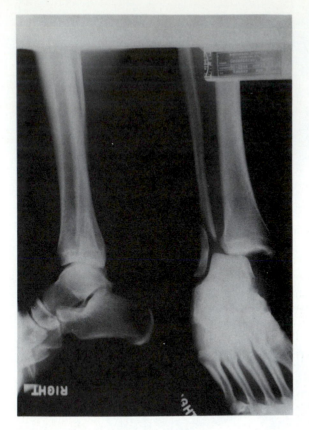

FIGURE 17-25
Fractured fibula with an intact tibiofibular
syndesmosis. Note widening of ankle mortise
medially, indicating deltoid ligament injury.

nearly as often as the fibula, can be fractured as the result of a direct blow, a twisting force, or occasionally from repetitive
overuse, which produces a stress fracture.
Acute tibial fractures are usually readily
recognized because this is the weight-bearing bone in the leg, and symptoms are normally severe enough to mandate radiographic studies. Stress fractures may be
indicated by local tenderness over the bone
and persistent aching pain. The initial pain
may be diffused but eventually becomes localized. Symptoms will be intensified by impact activities such as jumping. Normally,
an athlete who sustains a stress fracture
will report a recent change in routine, running surface, or shoes.

The fibula is normally fractured by a direct blow to the outside of the leg but is also
prone to stress fractures. Because this is not
a weight-bearing bone, the athlete may not
exhibit severe disability and may be able to
walk or even finish a practice or contest.
Symptomatically, fractures of the fibula reveal tenderness at the site of injury, local
swelling, and increased pain on any manipulation of the bone. The tenderness and
swelling might be mistaken for a contusion
because the athlete is able to walk. A fracture of the lower fibula that also involves the
tibial articulation is called a **Pott's fracture.** This type of fracture usually results in
a chipping off of a portion of the medial malleolus or a rupture of the deltoid ligament.
A fracture of the distal fibula with an intact
tibiofibular syndesmosis may have an accompanying injury to the deltoid ligament
(Figure 17-25). A severe eversion and external rotation injury of the ankle resulting in
a deltoid ligament injury, with an intact tibiofibular syndesmosis, may cause an associated fracture of the proximal shaft of the fibula **(Maisonneuve fracture)** (Figure 17-
26). Remember to always palpate the entire
length of the fibula on significant ankle injuries.

ATHLETIC INJURY ASSESSMENT PROCESS

As segments of the lower extremity, the foot,
ankle, and leg form a complex unit that must
function efficiently and be in proper alignment for optimum athletic performance. The
lower extremities are the functional basis for
many of the important motor skills required
for most athletic activity. They allow athletes to run, jump, cut, push, throw, strike,
deliver a blow, and perform in numerous
other ways. Athletic activities place tremendous demands and physical stresses on the
lower extremities, which can result in various types and degrees of severity of injuries
to the foot, ankle, and leg. In addition, with
the intensity of modern training techniques
and the growing interest in physical fitness,
there is a continuing increase in overuse injuries affecting the lower extremities of athletes in all sports.

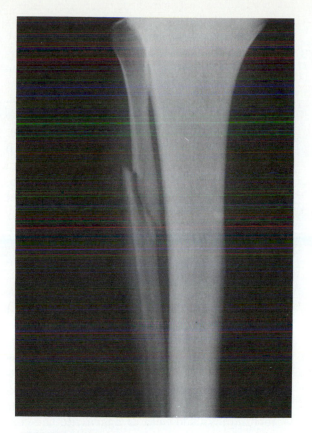

FIGURE 17-26
Maisonneuve fracture. This ankle sprain resulted in a
fracture of the proximal fibula.

Secondary survey

In assessing athletic injuries involving the
foot, ankle, and leg, the athletic trainer must
consider the functional interrelationships of
the lower extremity as a whole. The many
factors that can predispose or increase the
frequency of athletic injuries to the lower extremities must be considered individually
and as a group. Among the more common
factors that can influence injuries to the
lower extremities are malalignments, structural abnormalities, faulty foot and leg mechanics, improper training techniques, and
footwear problems. All of these factors can
be interrelated and affect one another; for
example, faulty foot mechanics can cause an
injury to the knee or hip. A comprehensive
assessment of any injury occurring to one
segment of the lower extremity should include an evaluation of the entire lower extremity in an attempt to recognize all the
associated and potentially interrelated factors.

Remember that deviation from proper
alignment and normal function in one area
of the body may cause a compensation in another area. The greater the deviation, the
greater the susceptibility to problems and
symptoms of injury. However, not all malalignments, abnormalities, or functional
faults result in injuries or produce symptoms. The body has the remarkable ability
to adapt or to compensate for the various
stresses and demands imposed on it. Many
athletes with varying degrees of malalignments, structural abnormalities, or functional faults perform quite well athletically
without overt problems or complications.

The athletic trainer is not expected to be
able to evaluate all the various alignmental,
structural, and functional problems that
may be present in the lower extremity. Some
of these conditions will be minor and only
detected by someone highly specialized in
their recognition. However, the more information the athletic trainer possesses concerning these factors, the more proficient he
or she will become in assessing injuries to
the lower extremity. The ability to recognize
these factors allows the athletic trainer to
develop more effective exercise programs designed to increase strength and flexibility
and also aids in preparing strategies to
change mechanics, training techniques, or
shoes. It is important for the athletic trainer
to continually develop assessment skills in
order to accurately recognize conditions and
problems in the lower extremities and recognize factors that predispose an athlete to
various types of injuries.

History

The history component of the assessment of
foot, ankle, or leg injuries should first determine if the problem is an overuse syndrome
or acute traumatic injury. As previously
mentioned, both types of conditions commonly occur to this area of the body. An
overuse injury is suggested when the etiol-

ogy of the injury is of gradual onset. This type of injury may begin as a nagging pain during activity or may only be apparent after a workout. On the other hand, an acute traumatic injury occurs suddenly. Questioning the athlete helps the athletic trainer to quickly distinguish between an acute injury and an overuse syndrome and also assists in determining the questions that should be asked to complete the evaluation.

To begin the questioning, ask the athlete to describe, as clearly as possible, the primary complaint or complaints. Allow the athlete enough time to thoroughly describe the manner in which the injury occurred, factors surrounding the disorder, and any symptoms associated with the injury. By allowing the athlete to talk freely about the incident, many questions will be answered. When the athlete is finished relating the chain of events surrounding the injury, ask pertinent questions to clarify the situation and complete a thorough history.

Overuse syndromes. The foot and leg are especially susceptible to overuse injury, particularly in activities requiring innumerable repetitions of the same action, such as running or jumping. It is not enough to merely treat the symptoms that result from an overuse injury because the athlete will continue to perform using the same mechanisms that produced the problems, thus causing the symptoms to reappear. The athletic trainer must attempt to recognize factors that may be causing the problem and implement appropriate treatment procedures to alleviate or improve conditions producing overuse syndromes. With overuse injuries the history is extremely important in attempting to determine possible causes or conditions. The history-taking process can be time-consuming in assessing overuse injuries, but its importance cannot be overemphasized because many conditions that contribute to an overuse injury can be recognized only by completing a careful history.

Overuse injuries may first be noticed as an inconvenience to the athlete. The area may be bothersome and painful only before or after athletic activities, but not during actual participation. These types of injuries are often ignored by the athlete until they become more serious and begin to affect performance. Overuse injuries may progress to a point at which the athlete's activity must be severely limited or discontinued. Therefore a thorough history should include how and when the symptoms first appeared. Question the athlete at length about all symptoms associated with the injury. When do the symptoms occur? Where are they located? How have they progressed and what activities decrease or increase the severity of these symptoms? Is the athlete ever symptom free?

During the early stages of an overuse injury, athletes will often treat themselves. These treatments may improve the athlete's condition, alleviating the symptoms or at least preventing them from getting worse. However, if the symptoms do become more severe and the athlete reports the overuse injury, the history should include the treatment procedures the athlete used to correct or alleviate the symptoms. Did any of the techniques used help or aggravate the condition?

Also question the athlete about any previous injuries to the area. If the current problem is a foot injury, ask about previous injuries to other components of the lower extremity. Has the athlete ever experienced a similar injury? If the area has been injured before, obtain as much information as possible about all previous injuries. What was the nature of the previous injury? Is the current injury an aggravation or recurrence of that injury? What treatment procedures were used? The more information gained pertaining to previous injuries, the better the athletic trainer can evaluate the nature and status of the current injury.

To complete the history of an overuse injury, the athletic trainer should ask questions about the athlete's training program and footwear and any recent changes in either. The training program includes many factors, such as training routines, strength and flexibility exercises, and playing surfaces. All of these can contribute to or cause an overuse syndrome, and the athletic trainer must consider the importance of each factor.

Training is essentially preparing the body to adapt to a stressful situation, in this case, an athletic activity. When more stress is placed on a body part than it is accustomed to tolerating, the symptoms of an overuse syndrome may begin. Overuse syndromes are often the result of errors in training methods, changes in training routines, or an overzealous training program. Therefore it is very important to question the athlete about his or her training methods. How long has the athlete been training? Has there been a dramatic change in the workout pattern, such as a rapid increase in mileage or speed? The body must adapt to increases in stress, and drastic changes may bring about overuse syndromes. Modern training methods impose tremendous stresses on the body. With these additional stresses, it is easy to understand why there has been an increase in overuse syndromes affecting the feet and legs of athletes involved in all sports activities.

In addition to the training routine, is the athlete doing any strength or flexibility exercises? Is weight training a part of the overall routine? If the athlete is on a strengthening program, is it designed to increase strength or endurance? Is the athlete overtraining certain muscle groups and causing a muscle imbalance? For example, distance runners tend to overdevelop their posterior muscles. This can result in a muscle imbalance between tightened calf and hamstring muscles and weakened anterior leg muscles. Also question the athlete about flexibility routines he or she may be following. Often it is helpful to ask the athlete to demonstrate how he or she is stretching. Lack of flexibility in the foot or ankle can be a factor in overuse injuries. Evaluating possible muscle imbalances and flexibility problems will be discussed in greater detail later in the assessment process.

Another important factor that can contribute to overuse syndromes is the surface or terrain on which the athlete has been training. Question the athlete concerning the types of surfaces used. Has training been on a very hard surface, such as cement or asphalt? Continuous training on hard surfaces can place tremendous stresses on the structures of the lower extremity. Has the athlete been working out on an indoor track with tight corners or banked curves? These conditions can place abnormal stress on the legs and contribute to overuse syndromes. Have there been any changes in surfaces or terrains? For example, has the athlete started running on hills after spending much time training on flat surfaces, or gone from a grass field to a hard court? Overuse injuries can be related to abrupt changes in surfaces or terrain, and proper training should include a gradual transition.

It is also important to question the athlete concerning footwear. Athletic footwear, having become as specific as the sports themselves, can help or hinder an athlete. Athletic shoes are made for a variety of surfaces, sports, and types of foot mechanics. There is no one best type of shoe for any athletic activity. A shoe that works well for one athlete may cause pain for another athlete involved in the same sport. For example, a shoe that is good for controlling a hypermobile foot may cause trouble in a high-arched, rigid foot. It is not our intent to go into detail about the advantages and disadvantages of the various types of shoes and the modifications that may be necessary for their use by certain athletes. However, the athletic trainer evaluating overuse injuries of the foot or leg must consider the shoes as a possible source of the problem. It is recommended that athletic trainers learn as much as possible about the various types of shoes. Answers to the following questions may indicate that the shoes have contributed to the overuse syndrome. Do the shoes fit the athlete correctly and comfortably? Has the athlete recently changed the type or brand of shoes? Is the athlete wearing new shoes? Are the old shoes in need of repair? Perhaps the athlete has allowed the shoes to wear down too much. For example, the more a shoe wears down along its outer edge, the more weight is placed on the outside of the foot during activity. Overuse injuries may be related to abnormal shoe wear. Is the athlete wearing shoes that were designed for the activity? For example, an athlete wearing shoes designed for tennis may develop problems if these shoes are worn for long distance running. An athlete training in a running shoe with a cushioned heel may develop symptoms on changing to racing spikes with no heel. Any change in footwear may place unaccustomed stresses on parts of the foot or leg and contribute to overuse injuries.

During the history portion of the assessment process, try to gain as much information as possible concerning the nature of the injury, the training history, and the athlete's shoes. This information, along with that gained during the physical examination that follows, will allow you to arrive at possible causes or contributing conditions for the overuse syndrome. Information is vital to planning treatment strategies designed to improve or eliminate overuse syndromes.

Acute traumatic injury. An acute traumatic injury to the foot, ankle, or leg will present an entirely different history to the athletic trainer than that of an overuse injury. The athlete will normally report that the injury occurred suddenly and will be able to describe a definite mechanism of injury. Encourage the athlete to describe in detail those events surrounding the traumatic injury and then question for information to complete the history. The information pertinent to this history can be divided into three main areas: (1) the mechanism of injury, (2) signs and symptoms related to the injury, and (3) any previous injuries to the same body area.

Ask the athlete to describe and demonstrate if possible the mechanism of injury. How did the injury occur? What activities was the athlete participating in at the time of the injury? Was the athlete running, jumping, cutting, or twisting? Was there a direct blow related to the injury? Did the ankle turn in or out? What was the position of the foot at the time of injury? Was an irregular surface involved, such as a hole in

the playing field or landing on another player's foot? The athletic trainer should gain as much information as possible in order to have an accurate impression of the mechanics involved in causing the injury.

Have the athlete describe as specifically as possible any signs and symptoms associated with the injury and their behavior since the injury occurred. Ask the athlete to detail the location of pain and any tender areas. What movements or activities increase the pain? Is there a loss of motion, function, or strength associated with the injury? Is there any swelling? How soon after the injury did the swelling occur? For example, rapid swelling in the **sinus tarsi** is usually a sign of at least a second-degree sprain of the anterior talofibular ligament. However, swelling is not directly related to the severity of injury. For example, a rapidly ballooning ankle may be a simple reflection of minimal ligament stretching with involvement of a blood vessel. Also question the athlete about any sensations associated with the injury. Did he or she hear or feel anything at the time of injury, such as a popping or snapping sensation? If the athlete reports a snap or pop at the time of injury, keep the possibility of a fracture in mind, but remember that a torn ligament can also cause these sensations. Does the athlete have the sensation of the foot or ankle giving way or being unstable? Listen to the athlete's description of all signs, symptoms, and sensations associated with the injury. This valuable information is necessary to determine the nature of the injury and the structures involved.

Question the athlete about any previous injuries to the foot, ankle, or leg. Has there been a similar injury or problem to this area of the body? Obtain as much information as possible about any previous injuries. Remember, the more information gained concerning previous injuries, the better the athletic trainer can evaluate the nature and status of the current injury.

Observation

Valuable information can be gained during the observation portion of the assessment

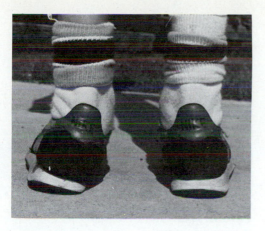

FIGURE 17-27
Evidence of pronated feet by observing an athlete's footwear.

process. The observation begins as soon as you see the injured athlete and continues throughout history, palpation, and stress segments of the injury evaluation. If the athlete is walking, notice his or her gait pattern. Does the athlete limp or seem to favor one leg? If the athlete is sitting or lying down, notice the alignment, contours, and position of the legs. Does either leg appear to be in an abnormal position? Is the athlete holding a certain area of the foot, ankle, or leg? Observe the athlete's attitude and behavior concerning the injured area. Assessing chronic overuse syndromes can be enhanced by observing the athlete's gait pattern and footwear (Figure 17-27). Does the athlete appear to have normal function or mechanics of both lower extremities? Do the shoes appear to be worn abnormally or unevenly? Always ask the athlete to show you his or her shoes when evaluating a chronic or overuse condition.

The foot and ankle are easily inspected. Shoes, socks, and any tape should be removed from the injured area. If the athlete is in considerable pain, attempt to calm and elicit his or her cooperation before removing any clothing. During this time, continue talking with the athlete and observe what you can.

Once shoes and socks are removed, inspect the injured area carefully. Look for any obvious deformities and signs of swelling.

Notice the appearance of the skin for any signs of trauma. Remember to always compare the injured area to the contralateral uninjured area, to note any differences in symmetry or contour.

If the injury to the foot, ankle, or leg is of an acute traumatic nature, you can proceed to the palpation portion of the assessment process. However, if the injury is an overuse syndrome, continue to inspect the injured area, as well as the entire lower extremity, in an attempt to recognize all possible contributing factors. A complete observation of this area of the body includes an examination of the athlete during non-weight bearing, weight bearing, and walking. In each of these situations, criteria discussed previously and considered normal for alignment, foot structure, and functional mechanics should be individually sought. All deviations from normal should be recognized and their possible contribution to overuse syndromes appreciated.

The athletic trainer should recognize signs about the feet which may indicate abnormal conditions. These include: excess callus formation, blisters, clawed toes, bunions, and corns. Each of these signs is an indication of adjustments being made in the feet as the result of abnormal stresses, faulty mechanics, or poorly fitting shoes.

Physical Examination

The physical examination portion of the assessment process is used to perform a more detailed examination of the musculoskeletal system. Depending upon what your impressions are up to this point in the assessment process, you may continue with palpation techniques, movement procedures, or neurological and circulatory evaluations. Not all these procedures will be used in any one athletic injury. Choose the specific tests or procedures that will assist in completing your assessment of the foot, ankle, or leg injury or condition.

Palpation

Palpation of the injured area is used to further identify specific structures involved in the injury. This is accomplished by accurately locating all areas of associated tenderness and swelling. The bones and ligaments composing the foot and ankle are easily accessible to palpation because most structures are subcutaneous. If the underlying anatomy is clearly understood, tenderness can be readily identified with those anatomic structures suspected of being injured. Palpation, combined with a careful history and observation, can be informative in identifying structures involved in the injury.

Palpation of the foot, ankle, and leg should be conducted with the area as relaxed as possible. This can be accomplished by having the athlete sit with both legs dangling over the edge of the table or sit back on the table with both legs supported. As with most athletic injuries, the integrity of the bony anatomy is usually evaluated first, followed by an assessment of damage to the soft tissues. Carefully palpate the bones and bony landmarks about the site of injury, noting any points of tenderness. If you elicit any pain or crepitation as you feel these bony areas, the suspicion of a possible fracture should be increased. Remember to begin palpation gently and increase pressure until you are satisfied that no fracture line pain or crepitation exists. Gently palpate the various ligaments and other soft tissues suspected of being injured, again noting specific areas of tenderness. Tenderness must be carefully outlined and precisely identified to accurately identify the underlying structures that may be damaged. The specific structures to be palpated will be determined by the information gained during the history and observation. Procedures used to palpate the various anatomic structures about the foot, ankle, and leg are discussed briefly in the following pages, as are the common athletic injuries that may be indicated by tenderness. Pay particular attention to the bony landmarks.

Toes. In palpating the injured toes of an athlete, it is important to locate the point tenderness precisely. The structures of the toes are very superficial, and it is usually

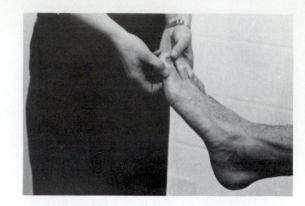

FIGURE 17-28
Palpating great toe.

easy to localize the pain. Notice whether the tenderness is located in one of the phalanges or primarily at a joint or articulation (Figure 17-28). This information, combined with the stress procedures described later, will allow you to distinguish between a fracture and a sprain of the toes.

Medial aspect of the foot and ankle. Along the medial aspect of the foot, you can palpate the head of the first metatarsal bone and the metatarsophalangeal joint (Figure 17-29, *A*). A sprained or jammed toe causes pain in this area. This is also the site of hallux valgus or bunion formation. The first metatarsal can be palpated along its entire shaft to the first metatarsocuneiform joint (Figure 17-29, *B*). This is the insertion of the tibialis anterior muscle. Continuing to palpate proximally, the next bony landmark is the navicular tubercle (Figure 17-29, *C*). Immediately proximal to the navicular bone is the talus, which is not readily palpable, and above that the medial malleolus. The medial malleolus is the major bony landmark on the medial ankle. Its entire surface should be thoroughly palpated. Pain elicited as you palpate the medial malleolus should raise your suspicion of a possible fracture. Tenderness elicited with palpation just inferior to the medial malleolus or along its edge may indicate a sprain to the deltoid ligament (Figure 17-29, *D*). The depression lying between the posterior aspect of the medial malleolus and the Achilles tendon contains

FIGURE 17-29
Palpating medial aspect of the foot and ankle: **A**, first metatarsophalangeal joint; **B**, metatarsocuneiform joint; **C**, navicular tubercle (under index finger); **D**, deltoid ligament just inferior the medial malleolus; and, **E**, flexor tendons lying posterior the medial malleolus.

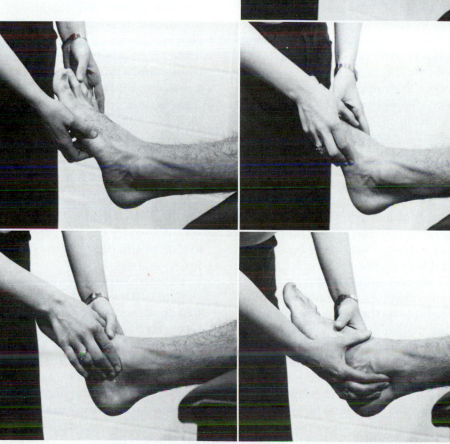

the tendons of the tibialis posterior, flexor digitorum longus, and flexor hallucis muscles, as well as the posterior tibial nerve and artery. Tenderness expressed in this area may indicate a strain of these muscle tendons or an inflammation of the synovial lining protecting them (Figure 17-29, *E*).

Lateral aspect of the foot and ankle. Along the lateral aspect of the foot, you can palpate the head of the fifth metatarsal bone and the metatarsophalangeal joint (Figure 17-30, *A*). This is the site of a **bunionette,** or tailor's bunion, which is a bunionlike enlargement of this joint caused by excessive friction or lateral pressure to this area. The fifth metatarsal can be palpated along the entire shaft to its flared base (styloid process) (Figure 17-30, *B*). The peroneus brevis muscle has its insertion on this process. Tenderness in this area may be caused by an avulsion of the tendon's insertion, fracture of the styloid process, or an inflamed bursa over the process. Proximal to the styloid process lies a bony depression in the cuboid containing the tendon of the peroneus longus muscle. Continued palpation proximally will bring you to the calcaneus. A bony landmark on the lateral calcaneus is the peroneal tubercle, which separates the peroneus brevis and longus tendons as they pass around the calcaneus. The peroneus brevis lies above the tubercle, and the peroneus longus lies below. These tendons are surrounded by synovium and held to the tubercle by a retinaculum. Tenderness identified by palpating the peroneal tubercle may indicate tenosynovitis. Just above the peroneal tubercle lies the lateral malleolus, which is the major bony landmark on the lateral ankle (Figure 17-30, *C*). The entire surface of the lateral malleolus should be palpated, and any pain caused by palpation should raise a suspicion of a possible fracture. The lateral collateral ligaments of the ankle attach to the lateral malleolus, and tenderness elicited on palpation of these ligaments is usually indicative of an inversion sprain. The anterior talofibular ligament is the ligament most commonly sprained. It is most easily palpated in the sinus tarsi (Figure 17-30, *D*).

This concavity just in front of the lateral malleolus is commonly filled with edema after an ankle sprain. The calcaneofibular ligament is palpable directly beneath the lateral malleolus (Figure 17-30, *E*), whereas the posterior talofibular ligament can be palpated from the posterior edge of the lateral malleolus (Figure 17-30, *F*).

Dorsal aspect of the foot. The dorsum of the foot is subcutaneous and easily palpated. You can feel the lengths of the second, third, and fourth metatarsals, as well as the metatarsophalangeal and tarsometatarsal joints (Figure 17-31, *A*). To palpate the main tendons on the dorsum of the foot, palpation should be combined with active or resistive motion. For example, to palpate the tibialis anterior tendon, ask the athlete to dorsiflex and invert the foot. The tendon should become prominent as it crosses the ankle joint and can be easily palpated to its insertion on the first cuneiform and metatarsal (Figure 17-31, *B*). The tendon of the extensor hallucis longus muscle can be more easily palpated when the great toe is actively extended. The tendons of the extensor digitorum longus muscle can be palpated when the toes are actively extended. The dorsalis pedis artery lies between the extensor hallucis longus tendon and the extensor digitorum longus tendon. The pulse of this artery is usually easy to detect and is used to evaluate circulation distal to the knee as previously described.

Plantar aspect of the foot. The plantar surface of the foot is usually more difficult to palpate because of the thickened skin, calluses, fascial bands, and pads of fat. To palpate the plantar surface, have the athlete sit back on a table with the leg extended and supported and the sole of the foot facing you. Each of the metatarsal heads can be palpated separately by squeezing them between your thumb and forefinger or palpating with your fingers on the dorsal surface (Figure 17-32, *A*). Pain beneath the metatarsal heads, especially the second and third, is referred to as **metatarsalgia.** This usually indicates abnormal pressure being applied to this area of the foot and can result from a variety of

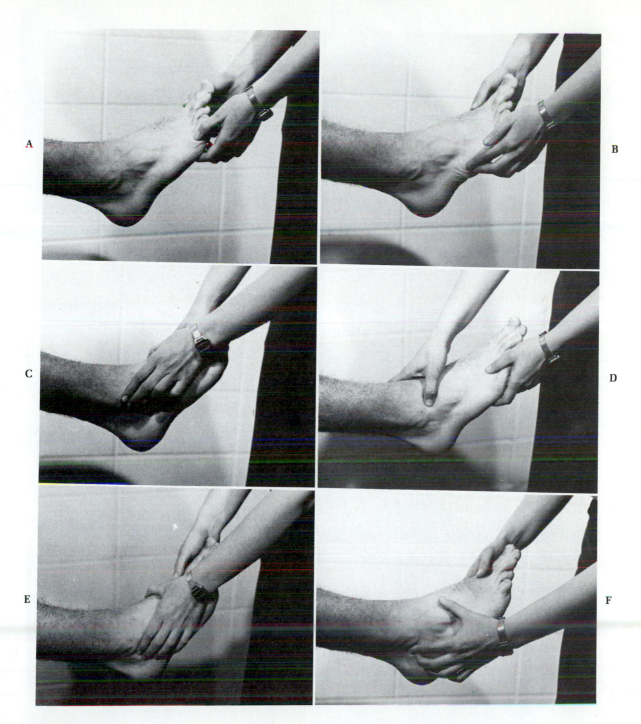

FIGURE 17-30
Palpating lateral aspect of the foot and ankle: **A**, fifth metatarsophalangeal joint; **B**, styloid
process of fifth metatarsal; **C**, lateral malleolus; **D**, talofibular ligament in the sinus tarsi; **E**,
calcaneofibular ligament; and **F**, posterior talofibular ligament.

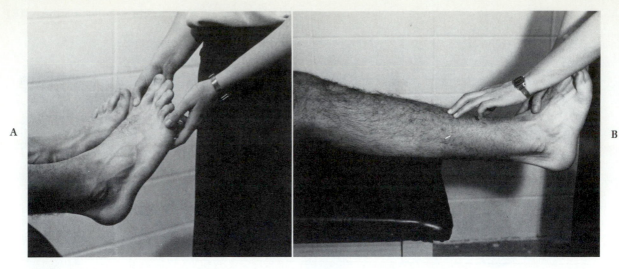

FIGURE 17-31
Palpating the dorsal aspect of the foot: **A**, first metatarsophalangeal joint and, **B**, anterior tibialis muscle and tendon.

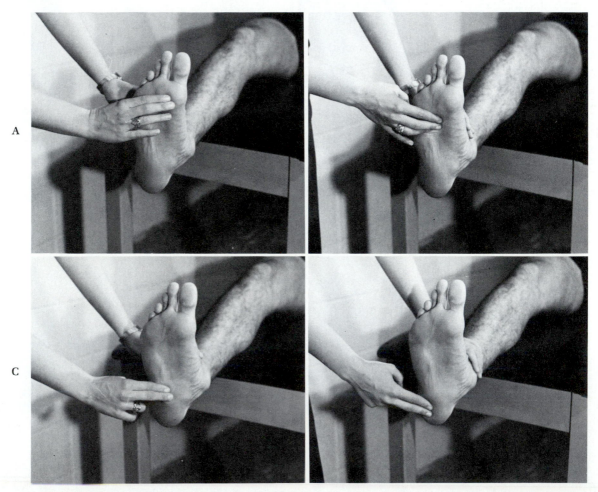

FIGURE 17-32
Palpating the plantar aspect of the foot: **A**, metatarsal heads; **B**, plantar aponeurosis along sole of the foot; **C**, proximal attachment of plantar aponeurosis; and, **D**, plantar aspect of calcaneus.

conditions. The transverse (metatarsal) arch of the foot is located directly behind the metatarsal heads, and pain in the area may indicate a fallen or weakened arch. Also, with increased pressure or abnormal stress, callosities may form under any of the metatarsal heads. Tenderness and swelling palpated between the metatarsal heads may indicate a neuroma in this space.

The plantar aponeurosis, or plantar fascia, can also be palpated along the sole of the foot (Figure 17-32, *B*). Point tenderness along these fibrous bands may indicate plantar fasciitis. Point tenderness is usually found at the proximal portion of the arch (Figure 17-32, *C*). A plantar fascia problem may be aggravated by a coexistent heel spur or bursitis. If either of these conditions is present, the point tenderness will be located directly over the medial process of the tuberosity of the calcaneus. An athlete suffering from a bruised heel will express pain during palpation of the plantar aspect of the calcaneus (Figure 17-32, *D*). Another test used to evaluate the integrity of the bones of the heel and ankle is percussion of the plantar surface of the heel. This impacts the calcaneus, talus, tibia, and fibula together. If the athlete expresses pain in one of these bones, you may suspect a fracture. Remember to percuss gently at first and increase intensity to the athlete's tolerance.

Posterior aspect of the leg. The deep posterior compartment of the leg contains the gastrocnemius and soleus muscles and their common tendon, the Achilles, which is attached to the calcaneus. With the athlete in a prone position, and the foot hanging free over the edge of the table, the gastrocnemius can be palpated along its entire course (Figure 17-33, *A*). Locate tender areas and areas of tightness or swelling, which may be associated with a strain or contusion. It is easier to detect swelling and compare symmetry by palpating both calves at the same time.

The Achilles tendon can be palpated from about the lower one third of the calf to the calcaneus (Figure 17-33, *B*). A strain of the Achilles tendon or an inflammation of the peritenon tissue causes pain on palpa-

tion of the involved area. Retrocalcaneal bursitis causes pain when the tissue just anterior to the Achilles tendon is palpated (Figure 17-33, *C*). If the Achilles tendon has been ruptured, there is often a palpable gap or defect. To further evaluate the continuity of the Achilles tendon, the **Thompson test** should be performed. This is accomplished with the athlete prone or kneeling, with the feet extended beyond the edge of the table. Squeeze both calves just below their widest circumference (Figure 17-33, *D*). The test is positive when the foot on the injured side fails to plantar flex or the motion is markedly diminished.

Lateral aspect of the leg. The lateral aspect of the leg includes the fibula and the lateral compartment containing the peroneal muscles. The fibula should be carefully palpated whenever a fracture is suspected (Figure 17-34, *A*). Locate any existing areas of tenderness. If tender, the fibula can then be stressed above or below the point tenderness to evaluate the integrity of the bone. This can be accomplished by gently lifting or pushing on the fibula away from the painful area (Figure 17-34, *B*). If pain is always expressed at the same site as the palpable tenderness during these maneuvers, the athlete should be treated as if he or she has a fractured fibula. If the bony integrity appears normal, the athlete has probably suffered a contusion at the site of the palpable tenderness.

The muscles within the lateral compartment can also be palpated. Depending on the mechanism of injury, tenderness expressed during palpation combined with pain on active and resistive eversion is used to recognize involvement of the peroneal musculature and the possibility of lateral compartment syndrome.

Anterior aspect of the leg. The anterior compartment of the leg contains the tibialis anterior, extensor hallucis longus, and extensor digitorum muscles. These muscles can be palpated along their entire course. It is easier to locate these muscles during mild resistance to the action in which each muscle is involved. For example, it is easiest to

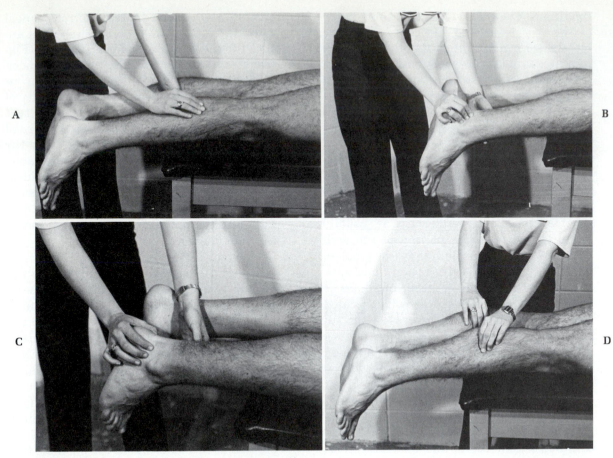

FIGURE 17-33
Palpating posterior aspect of leg: **A**, gastrocnemius muscle; **B**, Achilles tendon; **C**, test for retrocalcaneal bursitis; and, **D**, Thompson test.

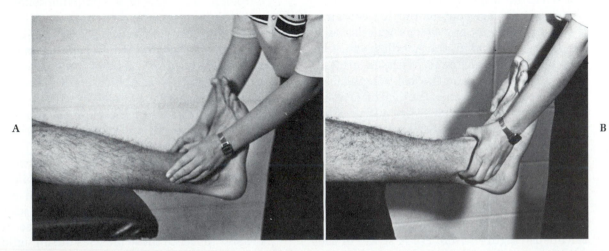

FIGURE 17-34
Palpating lateral aspect of leg: **A**, feeling distal fibula. **B**, Gently lifting the fibula.

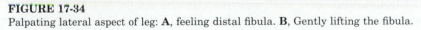

palpate the tibialis anterior during mild resistance to dorsiflexion and inversion, as previously explained. During this maneuver the tendon of the tibialis anterior can be easily identified and palpated. Knowing the area of point tenderness, the mechanism of injury, and the location of pain with active and resistive motion, you will be able to determine the involvement of these muscles. Remember the importance of early recognition in the development of anterior compartment syndrome and immediate referral if suspected.

Medial aspect of the leg. The medial aspect of the leg contains the subcutaneous anteromedial surface of the tibia called the shin. The entire length of this surface of the tibia is easily palpated. Pain expressed along either the anteromedial or anterolateral border of the tibia is commonly classified as "shin splints." Understanding the underlying anatomy allows you to determine which structures may be involved by identifying the areas of point tenderness.

Movement procedures

After history, observation, and palpation procedures, movement procedures are very helpful to complete the assessment process conducted by the athletic trainer. The precise maneuvers used depend on which joints and structures appear to be involved in the injury. Not all of the maneuvers described in this section will be used with any particular foot, ankle, or leg injury. The athletic trainer will select the appropriate maneuvers based on information gained during the assessment process up to this point.

Active movements. Active movements are performed to evaluate the range of motion (ROM) of the foot and ankle joints, as well as to begin testing the integrity of the muscles responsible for these motions. Ask the athlete to perform each movement through as great a ROM as possible and to express any sensations or feelings experienced during movement. Refer to Figure 17-35 to review normal ROMs for the foot and ankle. With foot and ankle motion, it may help to have the athlete perform active

movements with both extremities at the same time. This will provide you with an immediate reference for comparing the injured side to the uninjured side. Whenever an athlete expresses pain upon active movement, attempt to localize this pain as precisely as possible. For example, does the pain appear to be in a bone, at a joint, along a tendon, or in a muscle? Remember, pain located in contractile tissue should be further evaluated using resistive movements, whereas pain in noncontractile tissue should be further evaluated using passive movements. These procedures are described later.

To evaluate the active motion of the toes, instruct the athlete to flex and extend all the toes on both feet. Is the ROM limited or restricted on the injured side? Does the athlete express any pain, discomfort, or other sensations during these movements?

To evaluate subtalar motion, ask the athlete to invert and evert both feet. Does the ROM appear to be equal on both sides? It is more difficult to accurately evaluate active inversion and eversion than other motions about the foot and ankle. However, if there is a distinct and obvious difference between the motions on either side, further evaluations should be performed. What types of sensations are expressed by the athlete while performing these movements? Remember, pain or swelling associated with a sprained ankle may severely restrict active inversion and eversion.

To evaluate ankle motion, instruct the athlete to dorsiflex and plantar flex both feet. Again, does the ROM appear to be equal on both sides, and does the athlete express any pain during these movements? To specifically test for dorsiflexion, which is many times restricted, the following procedure should be performed. With the athlete sitting and the legs supported, passively move both feet until each foot is at a right angle to the leg. (Figure 17-36, *A*). Instruct the athlete to dorsiflex the feet, bringing both feet toward the knees (Figure 17-36, *B*). If the athlete has normal dorsiflexion, he or she should be able to dorsiflex the feet between 15 and 20 degrees. Often an athlete

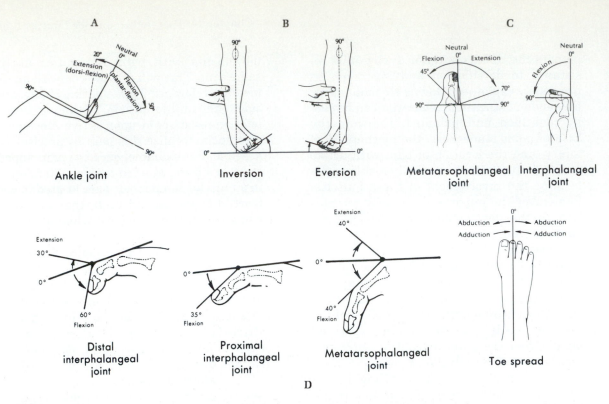

FIGURE 17-35
Active motion of the ankle, foot, and toes. **A**, Dorsiflexion and plantar flexion are measured in degrees from the right-angle neutral position or in percentages of motion as compared to the opposite ankle. **B**, Inversion and eversion are normally estimated in degrees or expressed in percentages as compared to the opposite foot. **C**, Flexion and extension of the great toe. **D**, ROM for the lateral four toes.

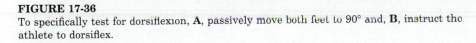

FIGURE 17-36
To specifically test for dorsiflexion, **A**, passively move both feet to 90° and, **B**, instruct the athlete to dorsiflex.

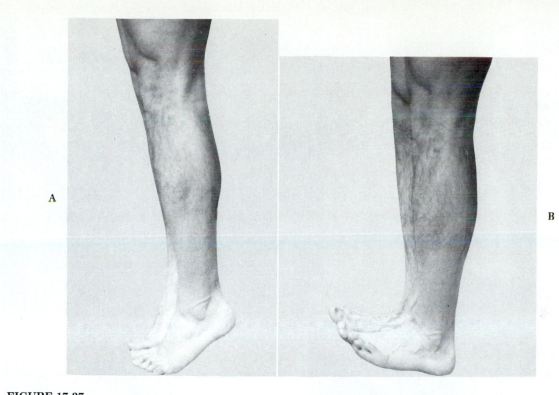

FIGURE 17-37
Checking ankle motion by instructing athlete to **A**, raise up on toes and, **B**, then on heels.

with an overuse syndrome, such as shin splints, will have little if any dorsiflexion. To determine if the lack of dorsiflexion is caused by tightness in the gastrocnemius or soleus muscles, perform the same procedures with the athlete sitting on the table with his or her legs hanging down. Flexing the knee relaxes the gastrocnemius and tests the flexibility of the soleus muscles. A stretching routine can then be initiated once the tight muscles are identified.

An alternate method of quickly checking ankle and foot motion is to have the athlete stand on his or her toes and then on the heels (Figure 17-37). This can be accomplished while you are evaluating the weight-bearing alignment described previously. Although these tests do not allow precise measurement of each motion, they do indicate functional abilities and provide a quick test. If the athlete is unable to perform these procedures, further evaluation is indicated.

Resistive movements. Resistive movements are used to further evaluate the integrity of the contractile tissues. Manual resistance applied against active motion can accurately identify specific painful areas, allowing one muscle to be differentiated from another. Resistive movements are also used to compare muscular strength between extremities. Resistive procedures are potentially the most informative maneuvers used in assessing muscle injuries. To accurately use resistive movements in the injury evaluation process, you must have a general understanding of the underlying muscular anatomy, as well as the movement for which each muscle is responsible.

It is important that you explain exactly what you want the athlete to do during resistive movements and how you are going to apply resistance. Because of the limited ROM in the foot and ankle, most resistive maneuvers are usually performed as an iso-

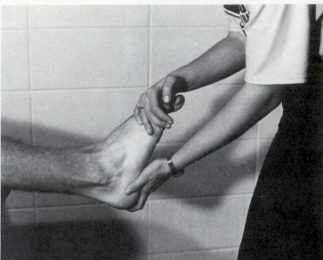

FIGURE 17-38
Applying manual resistance against the muscles in the anterior compartment: **A**, the anterior tibialis by dorsiflexion of the foot; **B**, the extensor hallucis longus by extension of the great toe; and, **C**, the extensor digitorum by extension of the other four toes.

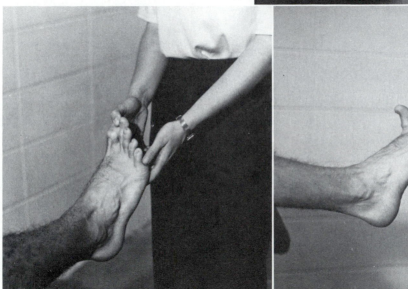

metric contraction. In other words, the athlete is instructed to perform a certain movement, and manual resistance is provided against that movement. The intensity of the resistance should be determined by the athlete's tolerance.

To evaluate the integrity of the tibialis anterior muscle, instruct the athlete to dorsiflex the foot as resistance is applied to the dorsal aspect of the foot (Figure 17-38, *A*). The tendon of the tibialis anterior should be visually and palpably prominent on the anterior aspect of the ankle. Palpate the mus-

cle as you perform this resistive maneuver.

The other two muscles in the anterior compartment are evaluated in a similar manner. The integrity of the extensor hallucis longus muscle is evaluated by applying resistance against extension or dorsiflexion of the great toe (Figure 17-38, *B*). The extensor digitorum longus muscle is evaluated by putting manual resistance against extension of the other four toes (Figure 17-38, *C*). The tendons of these muscles should become prominent on the dorsum of the foot.

The muscles in the lateral compartment,

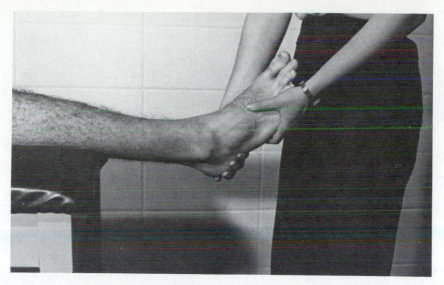

FIGURE 17-39
Applying manual resistance against the muscles in the lateral compartment by resisting eversion of the foot.

the peroneus longus and brevis, are evaluated simultaneously. Instruct the athlete to plantar flex and evert the foot. Resistance is then applied against the lateral aspect of the fifth metatarsal bone (Figure 17-39). The tendons of the peroneal muscles should become prominent as they pass around the lateral malleolus, run on either side of the peroneal tubercle, and continue to their respective insertions.

The three muscles in the deep posterior compartment, whose tendons pass around the medial malleolus, can also be individually tested. The flexor hallucis longus muscle is evaluated by applying resistance against flexion of the great toe (Figure 17-40, *A*). To manually test the integrity of the flexor digitorum longus muscle, resistance is applied to the plantar surface of the distal phalanges as the athlete attempts to flex the toes (Figure 17-40, *B*). The tibialis posterior is evaluated while resistance is applied against the medial aspect of the first metatarsal bone during plantar flexion and inversion (Figure 17-40, *C*). The tendon of this muscle should be prominent and palpable as it comes around the medial malleolus.

The gastrocnemius and soleus muscles

can be evaluated by applying resistance against plantar flexion. This is accomplished by applying resistance to the ball of the foot and instructing the athlete to plantar flex or point the toes as far as possible (Figure 17-41). As mentioned earlier, to isolate the soleus muscle, flex the knees during this maneuver. Remember, to compare the relative strengths of these muscles, or any of those discussed in this section, always repeat each of the resistive procedures on the uninjured foot.

Passive movements. Passive movements are maneuvers performed completely by the athletic trainer while the athlete relaxes the contractile tissues as much as possible. These procedures can be used to evaluate the ROM and the integrity of the noncontractile tissues about the foot and ankle. Remember, begin passive movements gently so as not to aggravate the injury or increase the pain and lose the athlete's cooperation. The intensity or force used with each passive maneuver can then be increased depending on the athlete's tolerance and the severity of the injury. It may also be beneficial to perform passive procedures on the uninjured side first, to elicit the athlete's

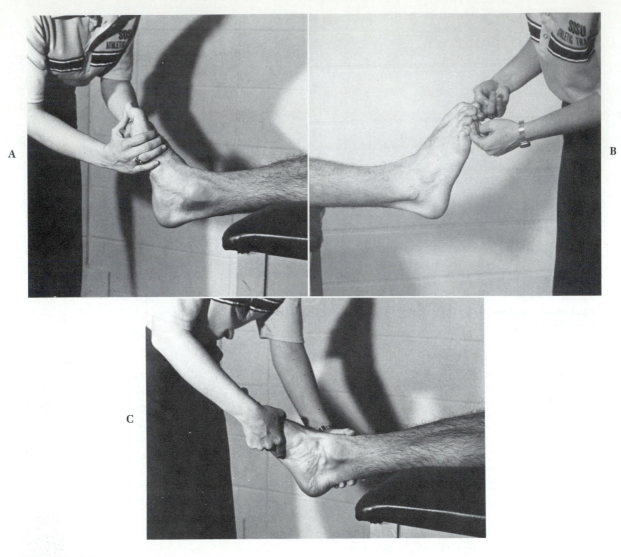

FIGURE 17-40
Applying manual resistance against the muscles in the deep posterior compartment: **A**, the
flexor hallucis longus by flexion of the great toe; **B**, the flexor digitorum longus by flexion of the
other four toes; and, **C**, the tibialis posterior by plantar flexion and inversion.

cooperation and provide you with a point of
reference.

Passive maneuvers can be used to evaluate the integrity of the bones in the foot. If
the symptoms indicate a possible fracture to
the phalanges or metatarsals, longitudinal
stress should be applied to these bones. This
can be accomplished by stabilizing the foot
with one hand and with the other hand applying stress directly along the long axis of
the bone or bones suspected of being frac-

tured (Figure 17-42). The stress should be
very gentle to begin with and then increased, depending on the athlete's tolerance. If the bone integrity is intact, there
should be no pain associated with this type
of a stress procedure. However, if a fracture
is present, the athlete will usually express
pain at the fracture site during longitudinal
stress.

To assess the integrity of the ligaments
supporting these bones, valgus and varus

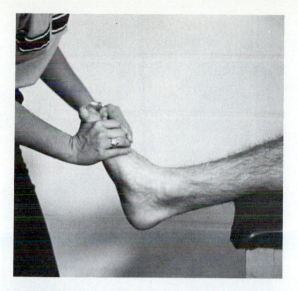

FIGURE 17-41
Applying manual resistance against the gastrocnemius and soleus muscles by resisting plantar flexion.

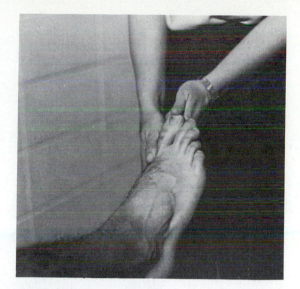

FIGURE 17-42
Applying a longitudinal compression stress to the great toe.

stresses should be applied. If the symptoms indicate a possible sprain of the supporting ligaments and the bony integrity appears intact, apply forces that will stress the ligaments. For example, to evaluate the integrity of the supporting structures around one of the interphalangeal or metatarsophalangeal joints, support the bone on either side of the joint and gently apply lateral force (Figure 17-43). Pain or instability with this type of a maneuver indicates a sprain of the supporting structures.

Passive ROM of the foot or ankle is often evaluated in conjunction with injuries to this area of the body. Remember to always compare the passive ROM on the injured side to the uninjured side. Each of the toes can be passively moved through a complete ROM. Dorsiflexion and plantar flexion of the ankle can be evaluated by passively moving both ankles through as great a ROM as possible. Remember, pain or swelling associated with an acute injury may greatly limit the motion available.

The passive motion available during inversion and eversion should be evaluated in conjunction with assessing the integrity of

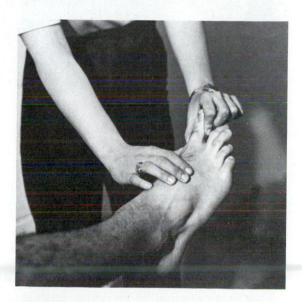

FIGURE 17-43
Applying a transverse (varus) stress to the metatarsophalangeal joint of the great toe.

the ligaments supporting the ankle. Stabilize the tibia with one hand and grip the foot with the other. Alternately invert and evert both feet (Figure 17-44). Locate any pain or instability associated with these move-

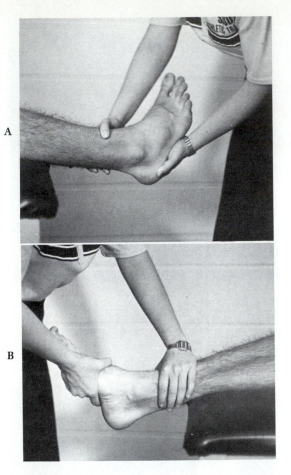

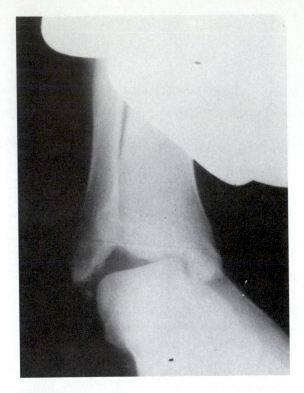

FIGURE 17-45
Stress radiograph of ankle. Note how the joint opens laterally under stress.

FIGURE 17-44
Passively **A**, inverting and **B**, everting the foot.

ments. Pain along the course of one of the lateral ligaments that increases with inversion suggests that the ligament is sprained. Pain expressed in one of the components of the deltoid ligament during eversion also suggests a ligament sprain. Compare the amount of inversion and eversion of both ankles in an attempt to recognize any instability. Unless there is obvious instability, it is often difficult to assess the degree of instability associated with a sprained ankle. Stress radiographs may be required to accurately measure the instability present at the ankle joint (Figure 17-45).

Another procedure that should always be performed on a suspected sprained ankle is the **anterior drawer test.** This tests the integrity of the anterior talofibular ligament, which is the ligament most commonly injured in the ankle. This procedure is performed with the injured ankle in a relaxed and slightly plantar flexed position. The athletic trainer stabilizes the lower leg by placing one hand on the anterior aspect of the tibia and grips the calcaneus in the palm of the other hand. The calcaneus is then lifted forward while the tibia is kept steady (Figure 17-46). If the anterior talofibular ligament is intact, there should be no anterior movement of the talus in relation to the tibia. If, however, the anterior talofibular ligament is ruptured, the drawer test will be positive and the talus will slide forward from under the tibia. You may feel a distinct "clunk" as the talus slides out and back again. Whenever this anterior drawer test is positive, the athlete should be referred to a physician.

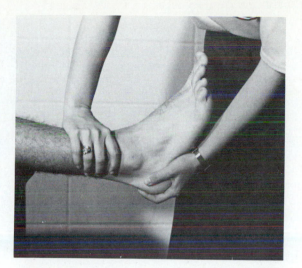

FIGURE 17-46
Anterior drawer test for ankle.

Functional movements. Functional movements can be very helpful in evaluating injuries to the foot, ankle and leg. This is especially true for the overuse syndromes because these injuries are often the result of functional problems. Some of the commonly used functional movements have been previously discussed, such as having the athlete bear weight, alternately rising on the toes and heels, and walking. Additional functional tests include asking the athlete to hop on the injured leg, jog, sprint, run figure-of-eight patterns, and perform cutting, starting, and stopping activities. These procedures are used to localize pain or instability and to recognize any functional factors that may be associated with the injury. Symptoms associated with an overuse injury are sometimes present only during activity, and these functional procedures may be necessary to reproduce the symptoms and assist in a comprehensive assessment.

Occasionally these same functional activities are used during the initial evaluation of an acute traumatic injury of the foot, ankle, or leg. This is particularly true when the assessment process completed to this point has produced few definitive signs and symptoms. The athlete may be asked to perform functional activities or replicate the mechanism of injury as closely as possible to

assist in identifying any structures that may be involved. Pain or instability may be demonstrated in this manner.

All restrictions placed on an athlete's participation are determined by the level of functional activity at which that athlete can perform. If the functional activities described can be performed without pain and disability, the athlete can return to full athletic activity. Functional movements should always be used on follow-up evaluations to determine at what level of activity the athlete can safely perform. As an athlete recovers from a foot, ankle, or leg injury, the intensity of functional activity should be increased according to the limits of pain and the ROM.

Neurological evaluations

Sensory functions. The athletic trainer should be aware of the basic sensory distribution of the various peripheral nerves and dermatomes in the leg and foot. Although dermatomes vary from one individual to the next, the primary dermatomes for this area of the body are L4, which covers the medial side of the leg and foot; L5, which covers the lateral side of the leg and the dorsum of the foot; S1, which covers the lateral side of the foot; and S2, which covers the posterior leg (Figure 17-47). Run your hand lightly over these surfaces and note any differences in sensations. Compare the sensations to the uninjured side if necessary.

Motor functions. Motor functions has been previously discussed under active movements. These procedures may occur early in the assessment process as you ask the athlete to perform each movement of the foot and ankle through as great a ROM as possible. The primary myotomes of the leg and foot are L4, tibialis anterior and extensor hallucis; L5, extensor hallucis and peroneals; S1, peroneals, gastrocnemius, and soleus; and S2, calf muscles and toe flexors.

Reflexes. The only reflex commonly checked in this region of the body is the Achilles tendon reflex, which is derived from the S1 nerve root. To test, have the athlete sit on the edge of a table with the legs hang-

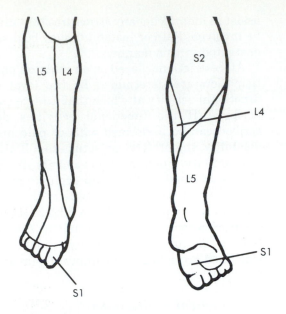

FIGURE 17-47
Dermatomes of the lower leg, ankle, and foot.

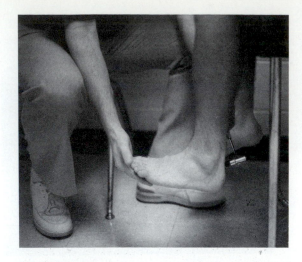

FIGURE 17-48
Test of the Achilles tendon reflex (S1).

ing freely. Dorsiflex the foot to put the tendon on slight stretch and tap the tendon (Figure 17-48). This should induce an involuntary plantar flexion of the foot. Remember to compare the reflex response bilaterally and note any differences between the two sides.

Circulatory evaluations

It is important to evaluate the adequacy of circulatory supply to the lower extremity with any major injury involving the lower extremity. Circulation can be evaluated by feeling for peripheral pulses, namely the dorsalis pedis on the dorsum of the foot and the posterior tibial behind the medial malleolus. Another method of evaluating circulation is to squeeze a small area of the athlete's foot or toe between your fingers to cause blanching, then release the pressure and observe how rapidly normal color returns. Immediate return indicates good arterial supply.

Evaluation of Findings

The foot, ankle, and leg are the most frequently injured areas of the body during ath-

letic activity. Because of the utilization of the lower extremities in most sports, tremendous amounts of physical stress and force are thrust on these portions of the body. Acute traumatic injuries to these structures are as prevalent as overuse syndromes, and both can result from or be influenced by a host of factors such as malalignments, structural abnormalities, faulty mechanics, improper training techniques, and footwear problems. An accurate and comprehensive assessment of an injury occurring to any segment of the lower extremity therefore should include an evaluation of all possible associated factors.

When to refer the athlete

Many injuries or conditions involving the foot, ankle, or leg can be accurately assessed and managed without medical referral. Other injuries to these structures require medical assistance for an accurate assessment and proper treatment. Occasionally these injuries must be referred to someone highly specialized in his or her diagnosis. The athletic trainer must continue therefore to develop assessment skills necessary to evaluate injuries involving these structures, to be able to recognize signs and symptoms that indicate the athlete should be referred

Athletic Injury Assessment Checklist: Foot, Ankle, and Leg Injuries

Secondary survey

———— History
———— Primary complaint
———— Mechanism of injury
———— Pain
———— Sensations
———— Previous injuries
———— Training program
———— Surface or terrain used for training
———— Footwear

———— Observation
———— Obvious deformity
———— Swelling
———— Contours
———— Alignment
———— Foot types
———— Pronated foot
———— Cavus foot
———— Morton's foot
———— Mechanics and functioning
———— Gait pattern
———— Abnormal conditions
———— Excess callus formation
———— Blisters
———— Clawed toes
———— Bunions
———— Corns
———— Footwear

———— Physical Examination

Palpation
———— Tenderness
———— Swelling
———— Deformity

Movement procedures
———— Active movements
———— ROM
———— Associated symptoms
———— Resistive movements
———— Pain
———— Strength
———— Passive movements
———— Bony integrity
———— Ligament integrity
———— ROM

Functional movements
———— Functional abilities

Neurological evaluations
———— Sensory functions
———— Motor functions
———— Reflexes

Circulatory evaluations
———— Pulses

When to Refer the Athlete . . .

Gross deformity

Suspected fracture or dislocation

Significant swelling

Significant pain, especially within the compartments of the leg

Persistent pain within the compartments of the leg

Decreased circulation, motor function, or sensations in the leg or foot

Significant loss of motion of the foot

Joint instability

Suspected malalignment or structural abnormalities

Any doubt regarding the severity or nature of the injury

---

for further diagnosis. See the box for a list of conditions that can be used to determine if medical referral is indicated.

REFERENCES

Alfred RH, Bergfeld JA: Diagnosis and management of stress fractures of the foot, *Phys Sportsmed* 15(8):83, 1987.

American Academy of Orthopaedic Surgeons: *Symposium on the foot and leg in running sports,* St. Louis, 1982, Mosby.

American Academy of Orthopaedic Surgeons: *Symposium on the foot and ankle,* St. Louis, 1983, Mosby.

DiManna DL, Buck PG: Chronic compartment syndrome in athletes: recognition and treatment, *Ath Train* 25(1):28, 1990.

Hamel R: Achilles tendon ruptures, *Phys Sportsmed* 20(9):189, 1992.

Henry JH: Soft tissue injuries of the foot, *Ath Train* 16(3):173, 1981.

Hoppenfeld S: *Physical examination of the spine and extremities,* New York, 1976, Appleton-Century-Crofts.

Katchis SD, Hershman EB: Broken nails to blistered heels: managing foot lesions in the office, *Phys Sportsmed* 21(5):95, 1993.

Latin RW, Kauth WO: Lower leg compartment syndromes, *Ath Train* 14(2):78, 1979.

Leach RE, Schepsis AA, Takai H: Achilles tendinitis: don't let it be an athlete's downfall, *Phys Sportsmed* 19(8):87, 1991.

Magee DJ: *Orthopedic physical assessment,* ed 2, Philadelphia, 1992, Saunders.

Meisterling RC: Recurrent lateral ankle sprains, *Phys Sportsmed* 21(3):123, 1993.

Nitz AJ and others: Nerve injury and grades II and III ankle sprains, *Am J Sports Med* 13(3):177, 1985.

O'Donoghue DH: *Treatment of injuries to athletes,* ed 4, Philadelphia, 1984, Saunders.

Rizzo TD: Plantar fasciitis: overcoming a nagging pain in the arch, *Phys Sportsmed* 19(4):129, 1991.

Sammarco GJ: Be alert for Jones fracture, *Phys Sportsmed* 20(6):101, 1992.

Seder JI: How I manage heel spur syndrome, *Phys Sportsmed* 15(2):83, 1987.

Shea MP, Manoli A: Recognizing talar dome lesions, *Phys Sportsmed* 21(3):109, 1993.

Stephens MM: Heel pain: shoes, exertion, and Haglund's deformity, *Phys Sportsmed* 20(4):87, 1992.

Subotnick SI: *Podiatric sports medicine,* Mount Kisco, 1975, Futura.

Taylor DC, Englehardt DL, Bassett FH: Syndesmosis sprains of the ankle: the influence of heterotopic ossification: *Am J Sports Med* 20(2):146, 1992.

Torg JS, editor: *Clinics in Sports Medicine: Symposium on, Ankle and foot problems in the athlete,* Vol I(1), 1982, Saunders.

Tropp H: Pronator muscle weakness in functional instability of the ankle joint, *Int J Sports Med* 7(5):291, 1986.

Whiteside JA, Andrews JR: On the field evaluation of common athletic injuries; part II: evaluation of the ankle and lower leg, *Sports Med Update* 5(4):11, 1990.

Williams JGP: Achilles tendon lesions in sport, *Sports Med* 3(2):114, 1986.

SUGGESTED READINGS

Ankle sprains: a round table, *Phys Sportsmed* 14(2):101, 1986.
Five specialists discuss types of ankle sprains, surgical versus nonsurgical treatment, tape versus brace for support, rehabilitation, and prevention.

Jones DC, James SL: Overuse injuries of the lower extremities: shin splints, iliotibial band friction syndrome, and exertional compartment syndromes, *Clin Sports Med* 6(2):273, 1987.
Discusses overuse injuries of the lower extremity including shin splints and chronic compartment syndromes. Etiology, diagnosis, and treatment are considered for each disorder.

Schon LC, Baxter DE, Clanton TO: Chronic exercise-induced leg pain in active people: more than just shin splints, *Phys Sportsmed* 20(1):100, 1992.
Discusses various conditions that should be considered when evaluating chronic leg pain in athletes.

Torg JS and others: Overuse injuries in sport: the foot, *Clin Sports Med* 6(2):291, 1987.
Discusses the clinical characteristics and treatment of overuse injuries of the foot. A consideration of orthotic devices is also provided.

Yocum LA, editor: *Clinics in Sports Medicine: Foot and ankle injuries,* 7(1), 1988, Saunders.
Presents an update of the common foot and ankle injuries in athletes. Many contributors discuss various topics such as biomechanics, epidemiology, diagnosis, treatment, and rehabilitation of injuries and conditions that can occur to this area of the body.

Wiley JP and others: A primary care perspective of chronic compartment syndrome of the leg, *Phys Sportsmed* 15(3):111, 1987.
Reviews chronic compartment syndrome of the leg and discusses symptoms, diagnosis, and treatment of this condition.

CHAPTER 18

Knee injuries

After you have completed this chapter, you should be able to:

- Identify the basic anatomy of the knee.
- Describe the common athletic injuries and conditions that may occur to each of the structures around the knee.
- List the signs and symptoms that may indicate the various chronic conditions and acute knee injuries.
- Describe the assessment process for an athlete suffering an injury to the knee.
- Explain the various manipulative procedures used to evaluate injuries and conditions of the knee.
- List the signs and symptoms that indicate an athlete suffering a knee injury should be referred to medical assistance.

The knee joint is often described as the largest and most complex joint in the human body. It is also one of the more superficial, more frequently injured, and more difficult to evaluate of the joints. The knee joint is the fulcrum of the body's longest lever and is subjected to tremendous torsional forces and loads during athletic activity. As a result, this vulnerable joint is the site of many athletic injuries.

ANATOMY OF THE KNEE

Begin your examination of the knee by reviewing the surface anatomy of the knee (Figure 18-1). Examination of the knee joint in an articulated skeleton makes it apparent that the bony components alone are not capable of providing the support required for weight bearing and athletic activity. The *tibiofemoral joint* is the largest in the body and is made up of the articulations between the vertically apposed ends (condyles) of the femur and tibia (Figure 18-2). The bones alone articulate in a precariously unstable way. It is the compensating reinforcement provided by the joint capsule, cartilages, ligaments, and numerous muscle tendons that provides the knee with the security and stability so essential for successful performance in athletic activity. The *patellofemoral joint* is between the patella and femoral condyles. This gliding type joint is frequently involved in conditions causing anterior knee pain. The third joint of the knee, the *superior tibiofibular* is the articulation between the head of the fibula and the tibia.

Movements

The knee is a hinge-type diarthrotic (freely movable) joint. As a uniaxial joint, movements of the knee are primarily restricted to flexion and extension. It is important to re-

FIGURE 18-1
Surface anatomy of the right knee from the **A**, lateral side and **B**, medial side.

A

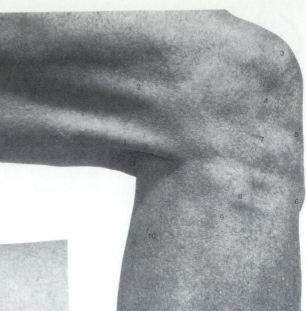

B

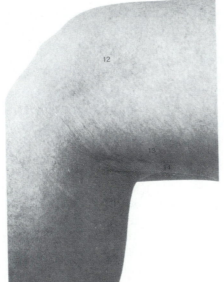

1	Biceps
2	Iliotibial tract
3	Patella
4	Margin of condyle of femur
5	Patellar ligament
6	Tuberosity of tibia
7	Margin of condyle of tibia
8	Head of fibula
9	Common peroneal nerve
10	Lateral head of gastrocnemius
11	Popliteal fossa
12	Vastus medialis
13	Semimembranosus
14	Semitendinosus

alize, however, that as a biologic joint the knee is not totally limited in its movement around a fixed axis, as is the pin of a door hinge. In addition to flexion and extension, some rotation of the knee is also possible, especially when the joint is flexed.

Full flexion occurs at about 130° and is limited by contact between the calf and the thigh. In the closed kinetic chain position of full extension, the knee is fixed and rigid. The rigidity results in part because the medial condyle of the tibia, which is larger than the lateral one, slides forward on the medial femoral condyle. This results in external (lateral) rotation of the tibia, which causes a firm "screwing" together of the opposing

bones. For flexion to occur, the fully extended knee must be "unscrewed." Thus slight internal (medial) rotation of the leg on the femur is the first step in flexion. This is brought about by contraction of the popliteus muscle, which is described later.

Structures

The anatomic components of the knee include the articular (joint) surfaces of the femur, tibia, and patella; the articular capsule lined with its synovial membrane comprising the synovial cavity; two cartilages called the medial and lateral menisci (singular, meniscus); the cruciate, collateral, and several other ligaments; and numerous

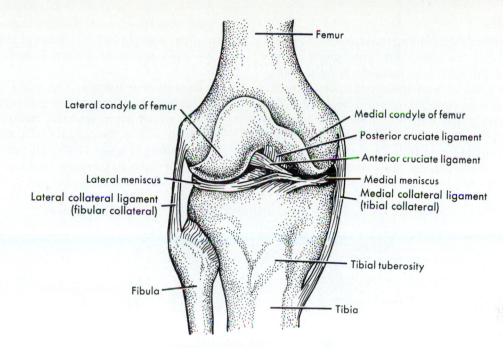

FIGURE 18-2
Right knee viewed from the front. Patella is removed.

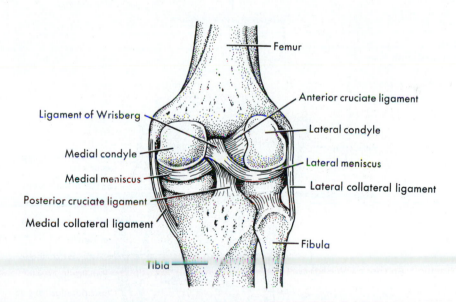

FIGURE 18-3
Right knee viewed from behind.

muscle tendons and bursae (Figures 18-2 to 18-5). Any combination of these structures may be injured during athletic activity.

Following is a brief description of the anatomic components of the knee. Because of the complexity of this body area, the common athletic injuries and conditions are discussed with each of these anatomic structures. The common mechanisms of injury and the frequent signs and symptoms denoting the various athletic injuries are also discussed.

Muscles

In addition to providing movement, the muscles about the knee contribute much in the way of support and stability for the joint. These muscles and their tendinous attachment are susceptible to injury because of the explosive muscular action required during most athletic activity (Figure 18-6). The most important muscles acting on the knee can be classified as the extensors (quadri-

ceps) and the flexors (hamstrings, gastrocnemius, and popliteus). Some of these muscles also serve as internal and external rotators of the tibia.

Extensor muscles. The main muscle of the extensor group is the quadriceps femoris, which comprises the rectus femoris, vastus medialis, vastus lateralis, and vastus intermedius (Figure 18-7). All four muscles converge into a common tendon that at-

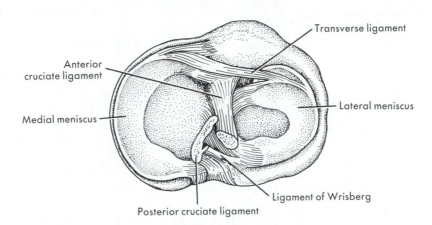

FIGURE 18-4
Right tibia viewed from above.

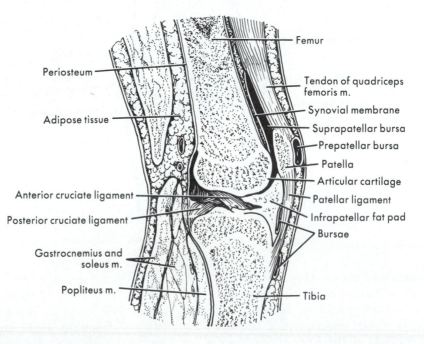

FIGURE 18-5
Sagittal section through the knee joint.

taches to the patella and then extends downward to insert into the tibial tuberosity. Collectively this unit is called the *quadriceps mechanism* or *extensor mechanism* and is the site of many athletic injuries. Injuries

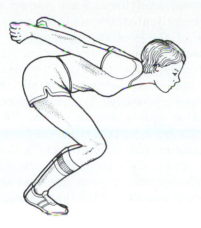

FIGURE 18-6
Possible mechanism of injury involving explosive muscular action.

can occur at any point along this mechanism at any time during explosive muscular activity or result from direct trauma. Overuse syndromes often involve components of the quadriceps mechanism.

A common site for strains or ruptures of the quadriceps mechanism is at the insertion point on the upper pole of the patella. Injuries of this type usually result from a sudden violent contraction of the musculature. Findings usually include tenderness and swelling at the insertion site, with pain when the quadriceps mechanism is subjected to stress. Additional strains involving the quadriceps are discussed in more detail in Chapter 19.

Flexor muscles. The flexor muscles of the knee include the hamstrings, sartorius, gracilis, gastrocnemius, and popliteus (Figure 18-7). The hamstrings are actually three muscles: the biceps femoris, the semimembranosus, and the semitendinosus. The bi-

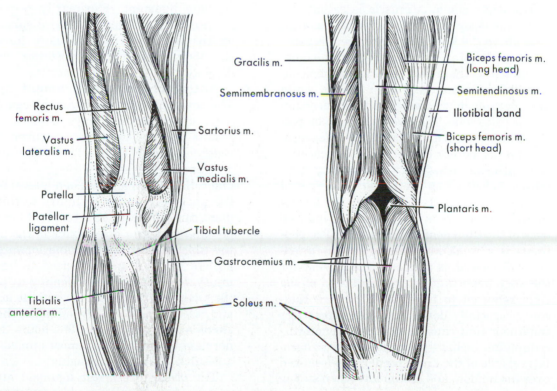

FIGURE 18-7
Muscles and structures about the knee joint.

ceps femoris, or lateral hamstring, is composed of two heads which attach to the head of the fibula. This muscle assists in stabilizing the posterior and lateral capsule and externally rotates the lower leg during knee flexion.

The semimembranosus attaches to the posterior side of the medial tibial condyle. It assists in stabilizing the medial and posterior capsular structures and internally rotates the tibia during knee flexion. The semitendinosus joins the sartorius and gracilis muscles to form a common tendon called the *pes anserinus*. Their attachment is on the medial aspect of the tibia (Figure 18-7), and they assist in medial stability along with the medial capsule and medial collateral ligament. These muscles also internally rotate the lower leg when the knee is flexed. Portions of this tendon are commonly transplanted during surgery to help correct anteromedial rotatory instability. Injuries involving the hamstring muscles are discussed in Chapter 19.

The gastrocnemius muscle is essentially a plantar flexor of the ankle but does originate above the knee and therefore has some effect on the joint. The two heads of the muscle attach to the medial and lateral epicondyles of the femur and then quickly unite and continue down the leg to their insertion on the calcaneus. The two heads can be palpated above the femoral condyles. They form the inferior border of the popliteal space.

✤ **Popliteus tendinitis.** The popliteus muscle is located on the posterior surface of the knee. It takes its origin from the lateral condyle of the femur and is inserted into the back of the tibia near its upper end. The popliteus is a weak knee flexor but, as previously discussed, is primarily responsible for the very important internal rotation of the tibia required to begin knee flexion. Running, especially down hills, can stress this tendinous unit causing popliteus tendinitis. Symptoms include pain along the posterolateral side of the knee, tenderness localized over the tendon, and discomfort when sitting cross-legged.

Cruciate ligaments

The cruciate ligaments are relatively short but strong, rounded bands that cross each other, forming an X within the joint capsule but are extrasynovial. They are located between the articular surfaces of the tibial and femoral condyles and are named according to their tibial attachments (Figure 18-4). The role of the cruciate ligaments is complex; however, their primary function is to provide anteroposterior stability. They also function to stabilize the knees from rotational stresses, excessive hyperextension, and abduction and adduction forces. These ligaments are most taut when the knee is in full extension, but some fibers of both cruciates are always tight throughout the full ROM.

The *anterior cruciate ligament* attaches to the anterior part of the tibia between its condyles, then crosses upward and backward to attach on the posterior aspect of the lateral condyle of the femur. When the knee is flexed 90°, this ligament is oriented almost parallel to the tibial plateau. The anterior cruciate ligament is primarily responsible for preventing anterior tibial displacement on the femur or, from a more functional standpoint, preventing posterior femoral displacement on a fixed lower leg.

✤ **Anterior cruciate ligament sprain.** The anterior cruciate ligament can be injured in a number of ways. Often an injury results from a twisting maneuver during weight bearing (Figure 18-8). The anterior cruciate is often injured along with the medial collateral as a result of a lateral blow to the knee (Figure 18-9). Injury to this ligament can also occur as a result of forced hyperextension or a direct blow to the back of the tibia that drives the tibia forward. The athlete with an anterior cruciate ligament injury will often describe feeling a "pop" in the knee, will be unable to continue activity, and will have a bloody effusion (**hemarthrosis**) within the first few hours. Loss of normal motion may be almost immediate as a result of this hemorrhaging.

The *posterior cruciate ligament* attaches posteriorly to the tibia and lateral meniscus, then crosses upward, forward, and inward to a fan-shaped line of attachment on the anterior aspect of the medial femoral condyle. This ligament is primarily responsible for preventing posterior tibial displacement on the femur or anterior femoral displacement on a fixed lower leg. The posterior cruciate is shorter than the anterior cruciate. With the knee in full extension, as in standing, the posterior cruciate ligament forms an angle of about 30° with the horizontal. This angle changes minimally during the first 90° of flexion, and the ligament remains taut throughout the full ROM. The posterior cruciate ligament appears to be located in the center of the joint and to function as the axis about which the knee moves, both in flexion-extension and rotation. Therefore it is the fundamental stabilizer of the knee. Experimental work has shown the posterior cruciate ligament to be twice as strong as the anterior cruciate or medial collateral ligaments, which may account for its not being injured as frequently.

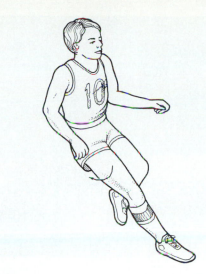

FIGURE 18-8
Possible mechanism of knee injury involving cutting, twisting, or turning activity during weight bearing on a fixed foot.

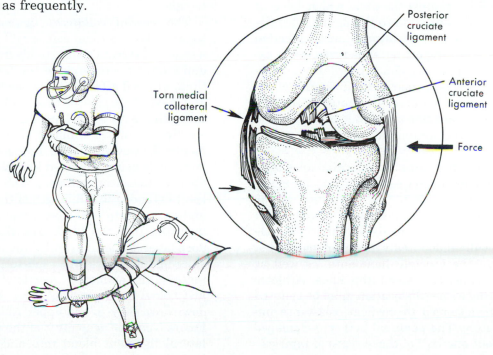

FIGURE 18-9
Classic knee injury occurring in football as a blow is delivered to the outside of the knee. Note on the insert the potential injury to the medial collateral and cruciate ligaments. The anterior cruciate ligament is more vulnerable to injury than the posterior cruciate.

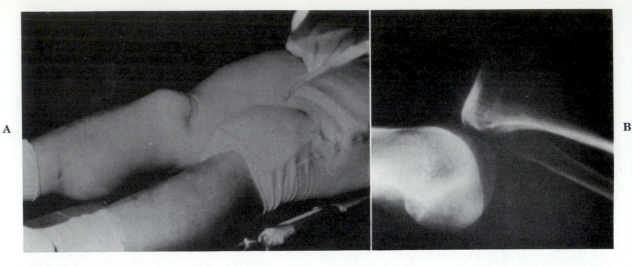

FIGURE 18-10
Dislocated knee. Note the obvious deformity of the knee, **A,** and on the X-ray, **B**.

❖ **Posterior cruciate ligament sprain.** The posterior cruciate may be injured by a direct force against the tibia, which drives it backward in relation to the femur. This ligament may also be injured, in conjunction with other supporting structures, from excessive hyperextension, hyperflexion, or abduction forces. A tear of the posterior cruciate ligament is often associated with such extensive capsular tears that extravasation prevents the accumulation of fluid within the joint.

❖ **Dislocated knee.** A dislocated knee is an infrequent but very serious orthopedic emergency (Figure 18-10). A disruption of the tibia-femoral relationship is discussed at this time because the dislocation of the knee joint will undoubtedly involved one if not both of the cruciate ligaments, as well as other structures about the knee. Athletes suffering a knee dislocation must be splinted and transported to medical assistance immediately. The popliteal artery is damaged in about one-half of these types of injuries.

Collateral ligaments

The collateral ligaments reinforce the joint capsule on the medial and lateral side. The primary purpose of the collateral ligaments is to provide lateral stability or to prevent abnormal movement of the knee from side to side.

The *medial collateral ligament* (sometimes called the tibial collateral ligament) is a strong, flat band that extends from the medial (adductor) tubercle of the femur to the tibia, where it attaches to the medial condyle and medial surface of the shaft. Anatomically, this 8 to 9 cm long ligament can be subdivided into a number of distinct segments. However, from a functional standpoint, it is usually divided into two layers of fibers—superficial and deep. The superficial layer extends the full length of the ligament and passes deep to the pes anserinus before inserting into the tibia. The fibers of the deep layer (sometimes called the medial capsular ligament) are much shorter. They originate on the adductor tubercle of the femur just below the superficial layer, but extend downward only to the upper tibial margin. Fibers from the deep layer of the medial collateral ligament blend into and fuse with both the joint capsule and medial meniscus. The primary function of the medial collateral ligament is to provide stability against valgus forces or to prevent abnormal movements to the inside. The ligament is tightest

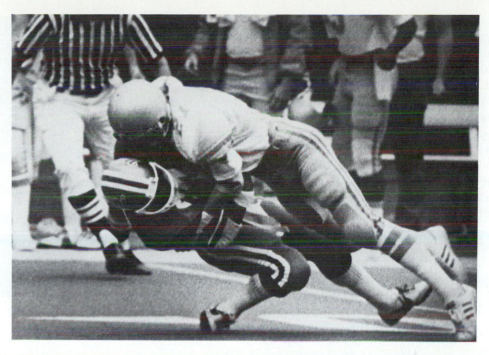

FIGURE 18-11
Mechanism of knee injury as the right knee is forced into valgus with external rotation of the tibia.

on complete extension; however, because it is a flat band, some of the fibers provide support throughout the ROM.

❖ **Medial collateral ligament sprain.** The medial collateral is the most frequently injured ligament in the knee. The most common cause of injury is a blow to the outside of the knee, which stresses the medial structures (Figure 18-9). Figure 18-11 shows another mechanism of knee injury as the joint is forced into valgus without a lateral blow. Because the superficial and deep layers are in effect anatomically separate structures, they often stretch or tear at different levels during injury. The medial collateral ligament can also be injured during rotational stress on the knee (Figure 18-8). This mechanism most commonly results in an injury to the femoral attachment of the medial collateral ligament.

Unhappy triad. A classic knee injury described by O'Donoghue is the "unhappy triad." This injury is a sprain of the medial collateral and anterior cruciate ligaments and damage to the medial meniscus. The

mechanism for this classic athletic injury is when the athlete receives a lateral blow to the knee with the foot fixed. A combination of valgus force and rotation of the leg places stress on the medial collateral ligament first. If this ligament tears or gives way, the force reaches the deep layer, which is attached to the medial meniscus. If the force continues, the anterior cruciate receives the stress and it too, may fail. This injury may stop at any point in this progression of events.

The *lateral collateral ligament* (sometimes called the fibular collateral ligament) is a rounded, pencil-like cord about 5 cm long. It passes from the lateral condyle of the femur to the head of the fibula just anterior to its apex. There is no attachment between the lateral meniscus and the lateral collateral ligament. The tendon of the biceps femoris muscle splits on either side of the ligament. Unlike its medial counterpart, the lateral collateral ligament is not a part of the joint capsule and plays a less significant role in joint stability. It is tight and contributes to stability mainly in extension of the knee; it becomes slack during flexion.

Much of the lateral support of the knee is provided by a structure called the **iliotibial band.** This structure is the distal attachment of the tensor fascia lata muscle, which originates at the iliac crest and posterior aspect of the sacrum. As it passes over the thigh in the region of the greater trochanter it condenses into a broad thick band of fascia called the iliotibial band. As it passes down the lateral aspect of the thigh it attaches indirectly to the distal femur just above the lateral condyle through an intramuscular septum. It then crosses the knee and inserts into the upper (proximal) end of the tibia at the *tubercle of Gerdy*. The iliotibial band is often considered to be the true lateral collateral ligament. It serves as a strong static stabilizer of the lateral side of the knee. There is no connection between the joint capsule and the fibular collateral ligament or iliotibial band. Portions of the iliotibial band are often transplanted during surgery to help correct rotatory instabilities of the knee.

✤   **Iliotibial band friction syndrome.** Iliotibial band friction syndrome is a condition frequently seen in runners. This is an inflammatory process or bursitis that develops deep to the iliotibial band as it crosses over the lateral femoral condyle during repetitive activity, such as running. The athlete suffering from this condition complains of pain or tenderness over the lateral femoral condyle. A test to assist in evaluating this condition is the **Noble Compression Test,** which is discussed later under palpation maneuvers.

Bursae

A **bursa** is a padlike sac or cavity found between tendon or ligament sheaths and bony prominences. This cavity is lined with synovial membrane and contains a small amount of synovial fluid that acts to reduce friction between two structures. Most bursae develop during fetal life. However, our body has the ability to develop new bursae in response to trauma or friction. These bursae are called **adventitious bursae.**

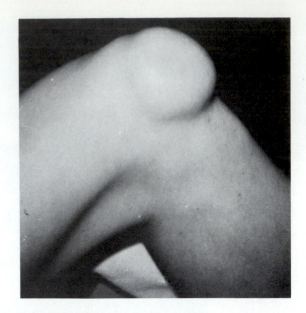

FIGURE 18-12
Prepatellar bursitis.

✤   **Bursitis.** Bursitis is an inflammation of a bursa. Bursae can become injured and inflamed as a result of direct trauma or constant friction between supporting structures. Around the knee joint there are at least 13 bursae; three or four anteriorly, four laterally, and four or five medially. Most of the bursae around the knee are not injured frequently.

✤   **Prepatellar bursitis.** The bursa most often injured in the knee is the prepatellar bursa, which lies between the front of the patella and the skin. This is the largest bursa in the knee and is usually injured by direct trauma. Historically it has been called *carpet layer's* or *housemaid's* knee. Prepatellar bursitis is a common problem in athletes who suffer repeated knee trauma, such as falling on the knee or getting hit on the patella. The condition is usually easy to evaluate because of the large amount of fluid between the skin and the patella (Figure 18-12).

✤   **Infrapatellar bursitis.** There are two infrapatellar bursae. The *superficial infrapatellar bursa* lies between the proximal patellar tendon and the skin, and the *deep infrapatellar bursa* lies between the distal patellar tendon and the tibia. These bursae are not injured as often as the prepatellar bursa. Infrapatellar bursitis can develop as a result of repetitive kneeling or repeated trauma over the patellar tendon. Frictional or overuse injuries may also cause deep infrapatellar bursitis. The symptoms may be very similar to patellar tendinitis or Osgood-Schlatter disease. Symptoms include pain deep in the patellar tendon just proximal to its insertion on the tibial tuberosity. Fluid accumulation in the bursa may cause the sac to bulge on either side of the patellar tendon.

✤ **Anserine bursitis.** The most common bursa affected by running is the anserine bursa. This lies between the pes anserine tendon insertion and the tibial attachment of the medial collateral ligament. Anserine bursitis is usually caused by constant friction or an external blow to the area. It is more common in athletes that have excessive pronation and valgus stress at the knee. The symptoms may be confused with an injury to the medial collateral ligament. However, it should be distinguishable during an assessment of the area.

✤ **Popliteal cyst.** Occasionally a swelling in the **popliteal** space on the posterior part of the knee may indicate a popliteal cyst, or **Baker's cyst.** This is normally a distension of the gastrocnemiosemimembranous bursa. However, these terms also apply to an inflammation and herniation of the synovial membrane in the popliteal region. Such a cyst appears as a large, soft, painless mass in the popliteal space. This bursa may communicate with the joint cavity, and the swelling may come and go. This type of bursitis may be the result of chronic trauma to the knee, internal derangement, recurring joint effusion, or simply asymptomatic swelling behind the knee.

Synovial cavity

The *synovial cavity* of the knee is the largest joint space in the body. The space surrounds the articulating bony condyles, extends upward behind the patella, and then communicates with the suprapatellar bursa (Figure 18-13). This large joint space extends three finger-breadths (4 to 6 cm) above the superior edge of the patella. The joint cavity also extends behind the posterior portion of each femoral condyle and under the tendon of the popliteus muscle. The knee joint cavity normally contains 1 to 3 ml of synovial fluid. In addition to providing lubrication for the joint surfaces, synovial fluid provides most of the nutrition for the articular cartilage. The articular cartilage and menisci rely on compressive forces during weight bearing to maintain a metabolic homeostasis. Immobilization or stress deprivation on synovial joints can have profound effects on a joint including, affecting the metabolic activity of cells, changing the normal color of the cartilage, and reducing the cartilage thickness. These effects add importance to the arguments for early mobilization of injured extremities. The volume of synovial fluid may be greatly increased as a result of an athletic injury that causes hemorrhage into the joint cavity or by inflammation of the synovial membrane (synovitis).

The synovial cavity is reinforced by a thin, strong articular capsule that surrounds the knee joint and is strengthened by several ligaments and muscle tendons. The patella is located in the tendon of the quadriceps femoris muscle and serves to replace a portion of the capsule in front. This joint capsule provides some stability for the knee in each direction and may be stretched or torn in injuries caused by abnormal motion, such as sprains.

✤ **Synovitis.** Synovitis is an inflammation of the synovial membrane. This condition can result from an infection, an injury such as a contusion of sprain, an irritation produced by damaged cartilage, or perhaps exposure. Synovitis of the knee increases the production of synovial fluid. This increased volume is called **joint effusion.** The contours of the joint will adapt to this increased fluid. This is a very important sign in evaluating injuries to the knee and is discussed in more detail later during the observation portion of this chapter. The volume capacity of the joint cavity is reduced when the knee is extended by compression of the gastrocnemius muscle against the posterior femoral condyles. In addition, when the knee is fully flexed, the quadriceps tendon compresses

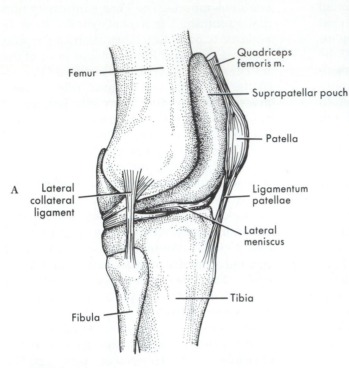

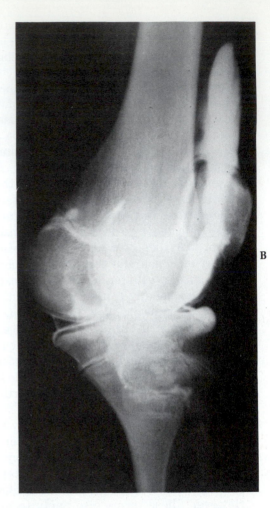

FIGURE 18-13
Synovial cavity. **A,** Diagram showing relationship of synovial joint space, suprapatellar pouch and related anatomical structures in the knee. **B,** Arthrogram of knee joint showing radiopagque dye in the joint cavity. Note that dye extends above level of patella, filling suprapatellar pouch.

the suprapatellar pouch, again reducing the capacity of the joint cavity. Therefore the athlete with a joint effusion will frequently hold the injured knee in 30° to 45° of flexion, at which point the volume of the joint cavity is the greatest; consequently the injured knee is less painful.

Menisci

The medial and lateral menisci are crescent-shaped pads of fibrocartilage attached to the flat top of the tibia. Because of their concavity, they form a shallow socket for the condyles of the femur. These semilunar cartilages enhance the total stability of the knee, assist in the control of normal knee motion, and provide shock absorption against compression forces between the tibia and femur.

The peripheral border of each meniscus is thick, convex, and attached to the inside capsule of the joint. The opposite border tapers to a thin, free edge.

The *medial meniscus* is larger and more oval or C-shaped in outline than the lateral meniscus. The medial cartilage is also more firmly fixed to the tibia and capsule than its lateral counterpart; as a result it is much more frequently injured than the lateral cartilage. Because of its attachments to the medial collateral ligament, the medial meniscus may also be injured in conjunction with a sprain of this ligament.

The *lateral meniscus* is smaller and more round or O-shaped. It is not as firmly attached to the tibia and is not connected to the lateral collateral ligament. Therefore the lateral meniscus has greater freedom of movement and is not injured nearly as often as is the medial cartilage.

❖ **Meniscal tear.** Meniscal tears are among the most common of all knee injuries. The menisci are frequently injured or torn as they become displaced, trapped, pinched, or crushed between the femoral condyles and the tibial plateaus. The damage sustained by the menisci varies, ranging from a very small tear along the periphery of the cartilage to a large longitudinal tear resulting in a displaced segment of the cartilage. This type of longitudinal tear is generally referred to as a *bucket handle* tear. The menisci are often injured by twisting activities during weight bearing but also can be damaged by direct blows to the knee or chronic trauma. Tears around the periphery of the meniscus or to the ligamentous attachments may heal because of the blood supply to this area. Tears involving the avascular body of the meniscus will not heal and usually result in persistent symptoms.

On initial evaluation it is often difficult to recognize a cartilage injury because symptoms may be limited or vague. Experienced athletic trainers stress the importance of a careful and accurate history concerning meniscal injuries. In many cases the suspicion of meniscal damage is made by history alone. Along with the mechanism of injury, the athlete may relate a popping or tearing sensation felt at the time of injury, followed by pain. Symptoms often occur as a result of synovial or capsular inflammatory changes associated with meniscal tears. With displacement of the torn meniscus, mechanical traction is placed on an area of the synovium, resulting in a localized synovitis at the joint line. Therefore, pain and swelling is usually localized along the medial or lateral joint line. The athlete may also complain that the knee "gives out" or buckles. Walking up and down stairs is frequently difficult, and squatting may be painful. The swelling associated with a damaged meniscus is usually caused by synovial irritation and occurs gradually over several hours. The maximum amount of swelling is frequently seen the day after a meniscus injury.

Two classic symptoms of meniscal injuries, which seldom occur with the initial injury, are *clicking* and *locking*. Clicking is an audible or palpable sensation often caused by a torn meniscal fragment rubbing against a femoral condyle. This clicking may become more evident with time as the torn edges of the injured cartilage harden. Locking is the mechanical blockage of the complete range of motion (ROM). This is usually caused by some type of internal derangement. The most common cause of locking of the knee results from a fragment of an injured meniscus becoming caught between the femoral condyle and tibial plateau, thus restricting complete extension. Athletic trainers must always be aware of pseudolocking, in which the athlete cannot complete the ROM and believes the knee is locked. This effect can be caused by hamstring spasms or swelling. If the athlete has normal ROM immediately after an injury and the loss of extension develops over a period of time, the restricted motion is probably caused by pseudolocking effect.

The acute symptoms of a meniscal injury may subside within a few days, only to recur when activity is resumed. The athletic trainer should suspect meniscus damage when indicated by history and recurrent episodes of effusion and disability. Various manipulative tests that place stress on each meniscus to assess its integrity are described later in this chapter.

Plica syndrome. Plicae are remnants of embryonic tissue that appear in the knee as folds or plications in the joint lining. Plicae are normally thin, elastic, pliable tissues. If subjected to acute or repetitive trauma, these tissues may become inflamed and edematous, making them inelastic. This can progress to thickening or fibrosis of the plica. This thickened band of scar tissue may cause binding or impingement in the knee. The medial plica is most often involved. Symptoms may include tenderness at the anteromedial femoral condyle and possibly an audible or palpable snap with active knee extension. This condition may exhibit symptoms similar to other knee maladies and may require referral for further diagnostic tests.

Discoid meniscus. A discoid meniscus is a round or disk shaped meniscus and is found in a small percent of the population. Individuals who become symptomatic from a discoid meniscus usually do so in the second decade of life. Symptoms include snapping, catching, and occasional swelling. If a discoid meniscus is torn, the symptoms are the same as a regular shaped meniscus.

Patella

The patella is a flat, triangular bone located in front of the knee joint. Its posterior surface articulates with the femur. It covers and protects the anterior aspect of the knee and increases the angle of pull, and therefore the leverage, of the quadriceps muscle. The posterior surface of the patella is divided by a ridge into two articular areas, or facets. The ridge articulates with a groove on the patellar surface of the femur.

Normally the patella is ossified from several centers. By 3 or 4 years of age they grow together or fuse to form a single center, which completes ossification about the age of puberty. In rare instances the ossification process results in two or three separate patellar components, or ossicles. This condition is called *bipartite* or *tripartite* patella. If it exists, the condition is almost always bilateral. This fact helps exclude the possibility of the condition being mistaken for a fracture.

There are a number of injuries or conditions that can involve the patella or structures around or connected to the patella. Some authorities refer to these various conditions as *patellofemoral dysfunction* while others use the term *anterior knee pain*. The primary symptom of each of these conditions is pain in the anterior knee, which is normally made worse by going up and down stairs, jumping, crouching, kneeling, quick stops and starts, and prolonged sitting. Pain is often relieved when the knee is fully extended.

✤ **Patellar dislocations.** The kneecap may fully dislocate (Figure 18-14) or, more commonly, sublux during activity. Movement is almost always lateral as the patella slides over the lateral femoral condyle. Recurrent

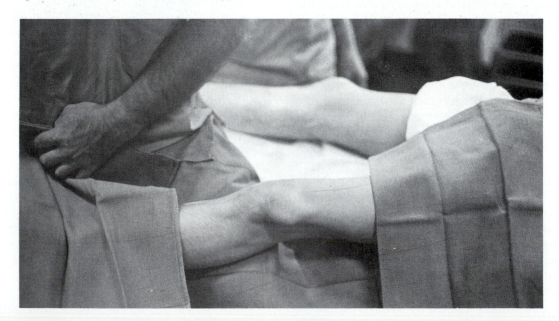

FIGURE 18-14
Dislocated patella.

dislocations or subluxations of the patella are usually associated with (1) congenital or (2) developmental deficiencies in the quadriceps mechanism. Congenital deficiencies include a shallow patellar groove, abnormal patella, a laterally displaced patellar tendon attachment (Q angle, which is described later), laxity of the patella, and genu valgum (knock-knees). Women are more prone to this problem because of their wider bony pelvic structure and internally angulated femurs. In both men and women displacement of the patella is most likely to occur with the knee flexed between 20 and 45 degrees. The dynamic forces of the quadriceps coupled with external rotation of the foot results in an increased Q angle. Developmental deficiencies have to do with the supporting muscles that guide the patella and influence the mechanics of knee motion. Underdevelopment of the vastus medialis muscle and atrophy secondary to other injuries or disuse are frequently associated with patellar dislocation.

It may be difficult to differentiate symptoms produced by recurrent subluxation of the kneecap because the symptoms are similar to other internal derangements of the knee. The athlete will frequently describe the knee as "giving way," popping, or catching. In addition, there will normally be tenderness on the medial or lateral edges of the patella, and the athlete will resist any attempt to move the kneecap. The apprehension test, which is described later during the palpation description, remains one of the most significant evaluative maneuvers to test a subluxating patella. Figure 18-15 is a radiograph taken using a "sunrise view" procedure that demonstrates subluxation and dislocation of the patella.

Acute dislocation of the patella can also occur with a direct blow against the medial aspect of the kneecap or a sudden valgus stress to the knee. Deformity is usually obvious, as the patella is displaced laterally and the knee held in slight flexion. Spontaneous reduction of an acute subluxation of the patella should be evidenced by the history and a positive apprehension test.

❖ **Patellar fractures.** The kneecap protects the anterior articular surface of the femur and increases the force of the quadriceps muscles. Patellar fractures do not occur often during athletic activity. The mechanism of injury is usually a significant

A   B

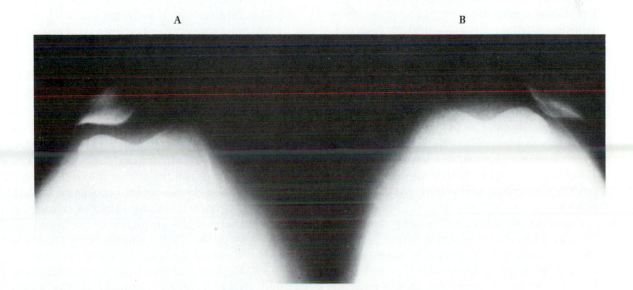

FIGURE 18-15
Sunrise view radiograph showing. **A,** patellar subluxation, and **B,** dislocation.

direct force or blow on the patella. A fractured patella is usually easy to recognize as the athlete has considerable pain and usually is unable to perform a straight leg raise. You may be able to palpate an indention in the patella.

❖ **Chondromalacia patellae.** Chondromalacia patellae is a degenerative process that results in a softening (degeneration) of the articular surface of the patella. The symptoms associated with chondromalacia of the patella are a common cause of knee pain in athletes. Chondromalacia is usually caused by an irritation of the patellar groove, with subsequent changes occurring in the cartilage on the posterior surface of the patella. There are many factors that may contribute to chondromalacia. It can be caused by direct trauma to the patella, malalignment and recurrent subluxations discussed previously, internal derangement, quadriceps muscle imbalance, increased Q angle, or abnormal anatomy of the patella or femoral groove. The symptoms of chondromalacia often include an insidious onset and progress slowly. The athlete will complain of pain arising from behind or beneath the kneecap, especially during activities that require flexion of the knee, such as climbing stairs, kneeling, and jumping or running. The athlete may also complain of the knee buckling during activity, a grating or grinding feeling with movement, an aching pain after vigorous exercise, or pain after sitting a prolonged time with the knees flexed. This is sometimes referred to as the *movie sign*. On evaluation of the knee, there is usually tenderness along the edges of the patella, especially under the medial facet and discomfort on compressing the kneecap into the femoral groove. The athlete may also exhibit swelling, crepitus, and a positive apprehension test.

❖ **Patellar tendinitis.** Patellar tendinitis (jumper's knee) is a condition found in many athletes involved in repetitive jumping activities. It is an inflammatory response to repeated stress or irritation at the patellar tendon insertion and it is normally characterized by pain localized at the distal pole of the patella; however, pain can also occur at the proximal pole of the patella. The athlete will complain of pain or discomfort during activity, which may become progressively worse with excessive quadriceps action. The athlete will usually experience aching after exercise, and occasionally swelling may occur. On examination of the knee, the athlete will have point tenderness with palpation at the tendon insertion and pain during resistive movements involving knee extension.

❖ **Patellar tendon ruptures.** Patellar tendon ruptures are uncommon in young athletes but the incidences increase with age. As more and more middle and older aged individuals participate in athletic activity, the incidences of patellar tendon ruptures will become more frequent. It is important in evaluating athletes with anterior knee pain to make sure they have an intact extensor mechanism.

❖ **Infrapatellar fat pad contusion.** The infrapatellar fat pad extends from the lower pole of the patella to the tibia, behind the patellar tendon. It acts as a dynamic shock absorber and a source of nutrition for the tendon. The fat pad can become irritated by chronic kneeling pressures or direct blows. Symptoms may include pain below the patellar tendon which is increased with knee extension, swelling in the area, and stiffness of knee movement.

Other athletic-related conditions of the knee

❖ **Osgood-Schlatter disease.** Osgood-Schlatter disease (traction apophysis) is probably the most common growth-related cause of knee pain in skeletally immature athletes. The condition results from repetitive traction on the tibial tuberosity apophysis. It occurs in young athletes when the attachment of the epiphysis of the tibial tuberosity to the shaft (diaphysis) of the bone is the weakest link in the extensor mechanism. Repeated stresses on the patellar tendon cause a minor avulsion of the tibial tuberosity, leading to an inflammatory reaction. Osgood-Schlatter disease is aggra-

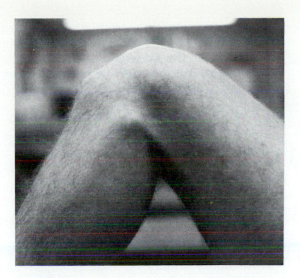

FIGURE 18-16
Note enlarged tibial tuberosity remaining as a result of Osgood-Schlatter syndrome.

vated by running, jumping, or kneeling. The young athlete will have anterior knee pain on active use of the quadriceps, which may limit normal activity. On evaluation the athlete may have local swelling, tenderness with direct pressure on the tuberosity, and pain on resistance to quadriceps action. Osgood-Schlatter disease is a self-limiting condition an athlete will eventually outgrow as the skeleton matures. However, an enlarged tibial tuberosity often remains (Figure 18-16). Normally, a conservative treatment plan consisting of modifying or restricting painful activities, flexibility exercises, and anti-inflammatory care will allow an athlete to continue athletic activity. Occasionally, symptoms may persist into adulthood.

❖ **Tibial tuberosity avulsion.** An avulsion or fracture of the tibial tuberosity is an uncommon injury. When it does occur, it most often affects boys between the ages of 12 to 16. It usually results from sudden flexion of the knee while the quadriceps are strongly contracted or during a violent active extension against resistance. High jumpers comprise the majority of athletes having an avulsion of the apophysis of the tibial tuberosity. These athletes may complain of pain in this region long before the

fracture occurs and are frequently treated for Osgood-Schlatter syndrome. Pain in the area of the tibial tuberosity in adolescent high jumpers and other high performance athletes should be carefully evaluated and monitored to prevent a complete avulsion fracture.

Sinding-Larsen-Johansson disease. Sinding-Larsen-Johansson disease resembles Osgood-Schlatter disease except that the pathology involves the proximal rather than the distal end of the patellar tendon. Athletes are generally younger than those with Osgood-Schlatter disease. The condition is caused by repetitive traction forces on the inferior patellar pole. Symptoms are similar to patellar tendinitis and it may take a radiograph to differentiate between the two.

❖ **Peroneal nerve contusion.** The peroneal nerve passes just below the head of the fibula, where it lies subcutaneously. A direct blow to this area can result in a contusion and injure the nerve, which is caught between the underlying bone and the force. The athlete may exhibit a localized pain from the contusion and a radiating pain to the anterior lateral leg musculature and dorsum of the foot. Numbness and tingling in the distribution of the nerve is also present. Normally the symptoms last only a few seconds or minutes, but in severe cases the hypoesthesia and weakness of the paroneals and dorsiflexors persist. The athlete may even develop a foot drop. Usually the contusion of the nerve is minor and symptoms subside within a day or two after the injury.

❖ **Chondral/osteochondral fractures.** Chondral fractures involve the articular cartilage, and osteochondral fractures involve the underlying bone and also the articular cartilage. These conditions can occur in other joints of the body but most commonly occur in the knee. These fractures result from acute trauma and are caused by direct stresses applied to the articular surfaces of the femur, tibia, or patella. The result may be an acute contusion to the articular surface with fissuring of the cartilage, which can be likened to the cracking of an egg shell. The fracture can be incomplete, so that no fragment is actually dislodged, or complete, with a loose piece of cartilage separated from the underlying bone to produce a loose body within the joint (Figure 8-23, *J*). These fractures may be difficult to evaluate or differentiate from cartilage injuries and may go completely unrecognized. If the fracture is complete and there are one or more cartilage fragments (commonly referred to as *joint mice*) within the joint, the symptoms may be similar to a meniscal injury. Fragments of this type may cause clicking, catching, or locking sensations.

✤ **Osteochondritis dissecans.** Osteochondritis dissecans is a condition of unknown cause in which a segment of subchondral bone undergoes avascular necrosis. The most common site for this condition is the lateral surface of the medial femoral condyle. It is believed that osteochondritis dissecans is the result of loss of circulation to the area, which may be the result of recurrent trauma. This may be initiated by a chondral or osteochondral fracture, a condition also difficult to evaluate. Symptoms may consist of pain, stiffness, and swelling that are made worse with activity. There may be a medial joint line tenderness and a limited ROM. Osteochondritis dissecans may also give rise to a loose body within the joint. These conditions should be suspected and the athlete referred to medical assistance when the athlete has persistent symptoms in an otherwise normal-appearing knee.

✤ **Epiphyseal injuries.** You should be suspicious with any skeletally immature athlete with acute knee trauma for the possibility of an epiphyseal injury. For example, the medial collateral ligament attaches on the epiphyseal portion of the femur and the metaphyseal portion of the tibia. This anatomically protects the proximal tibial epiphysis from stress while exposing the distal femoral epiphysis to external forces. An injury mechanism that would cause a medial collateral ligament (MCL) sprain in an adult may disrupt the distal femoral epiphyseal plate. It may be difficult to distinguish a lig-

amentous instability from an epiphyseal fracture. The tenderness should be predominantly over the growth plate. It is a good practice to refer for further medical attention any young athlete with instability or an acute hemarthrosis of the knee.

ATHLETIC INJURY ASSESSMENT PROCESS

All too often the evaluation of a knee injury begins in a haphazard or unstructured manner, and the athlete is seen for definitive diagnosis and treatment too late for an ideal result to be obtained. A careful, comprehensive, and systematic evaluation of every knee injury should be done promptly and completely so that an accurate assessment with definitive care can be achieved. It is not proper to simply rest an injured knee and then wait and hope for improvement to occur. An in-depth assessment must be made promptly if a knee injury is of any significance.

Secondary survey

Initial assessment of any knee injury must be performed promptly and competently by a person skilled in at least the techniques of a preliminary knee examination. If findings raise any questions as to the stability or function of the knee, it is imperative that the athlete be referred to someone who has expertise in knee injuries. It is the responsibility of the physician to make an absolute diagnosis of the knee injury and prescribe, in conjunction with the athletic trainer, a program of care and periodic assessment to evaluate the injury and subsequent recovery. By evaluating knee injuries in a careful, systematic manner, problems that arise from a neglected or poorly treated knee can be minimized.

The remainder of this chapter presents a common approach to evaluating an injured knee. Actual assessment procedures are described and explained. The examination of an injured knee should follow logical, sequential procedures designed to evaluate the various structures about the knee; however, each athletic trainer must develop his or her own techniques of evaluating a knee, which includes adding or deleting procedures depending on the pathology of the knee injury. All evaluative procedures discussed in this chapter will seldom if ever be used on any one knee injury. The procedures used with each injury will be determined by the information gained during the systematic assessment process.

History

The history is an extremely important aspect of knee evaluation. This phase of the assessment process helps distinguish between the acute, chronic, and overused knee injuries, as well as indicates which structures may be injured, and suggests which additional evaluative procedures should be used. The history should be completed as the first step in this assessment process and should include information concerning previous injuries, history of the present injury, and the postinjury course, if appropriate.

Previous injury. An important aspect of the history-gathering process is determining whether there has been any previous difficulty with the knee. If so, obtain as much information as possible about this previous injury, including the nature of the injury, the treatment, and the extent of rehabilitation. Had symptoms completely subsided before the onset of the present injury? Had full functional capabilities been regained? Was the knee weakened or susceptible to certain types of trauma because of earlier injuries? Are symptoms of the current injury similar to those of any previous injuries? All previous injuries should be documented, as should their postinjury course. If there has been surgery performed on the knee, it is essential to have accurate, detailed information as to the pathology, surgical procedures performed, and any evidence of injury to other structures at that time. In addition, it is important to inquire about any significant injuries to the opposite or uninjured knee, because they will be used as a baseline for comparison during the assessment.

Present injury. Next, question the athlete and develop a history of the present in-

jury. Was the onset gradual? There may not be a history of specific injury to the knee, but symptoms spontaneously arose during or after activity. This may reflect chronic or overuse conditions such as chondromalacia, tendinitis, or bursitis. Was the onset sudden? If the injury occurred as the result of direct trauma, ask the athlete to describe or demonstrate the mechanism of injury. It is important to detail the mechanism of injury because this can indicate which anatomic structures may have been injured. What types of stresses were applied to the knee? Was the athlete twisting so that rotation was involved in the injury? Did marked flexion or hyperextension occur at the time of injury? If the knee was hit, where was the blow delivered and what were the positions of the foot, knee, and hip at the time of injury? All these factors are extremely important to document when obtaining the current history. Take the time required to ask questions and listen attentively.

Common symptoms associated with knee injuries should be evaluated in some detail, as they will help in differentiating between various injuries. Have the athlete describe symptoms as specifically as possible. Ask for specifics concerning the nature and behavior of the symptoms. How long did these symptoms last, and were they constant, intermittent, or changing? First, is there pain, and if so, where? Localization of pain may help indicate the type of injury; however, in many knee injuries pain is poorly localized. This is especially true just after an acute injury. Is the pain constant or intermittent? Determine what types of activity produce the pain.

Is there swelling associated with the knee injury? The presence or absence of swelling within the knee is a very significant aspect of the history. When swelling occurs, it is important to determine how soon the swelling developed after the injury. Swelling that occurs in the first two hours after an injury usually indicates blood in the joint cavity (hemarthrosis). This condition is often associated with a more serious injury such as cruciate ligament involvement, patellar subluxation, osteochondral fracture, or a peripheral meniscal tear. Gradual swelling occurring over 12 to 24 hours suggests synovial irritation, which may accompany a more minor meniscal injury or ligament sprain. Swelling that occurs after activity and goes away with 1 or more days' rest may indicate an overuse process or an internal derangement of some kind. Absence of swelling may indicate a severe injury resulting in capsular tears and fluid extravasating into the soft tissues surrounding the knee joint.

Is there a loss of motion? If so, what type of motion loss? Is the athlete unable to extend or fully flex the knee, or are both extremes of motion limited? Loss of motion may be caused by pain, swelling, or protective muscle spasms around the knee, or may be the result of the knee locking, which prevents the athlete from fully extending the knee. Locking is a symptom associated with internal derangement of the knee and is usually caused by a loose body within the knee or a displaced fragment of a torn meniscus. Find out if the locking is intermittent or if the knee has been locked ever since the onset of the injury. Intermittent locking or catching suggests a loose body or dislodged fragment of meniscus that periodically becomes caught between the articular surfaces of the tibia and femur. Constant locking suggests a larger displaced bucket-handle tear of the meniscus.

In addition to questions concerning the symptoms associated with the injured knee, find out about any sensations the athlete has experienced. Did he or she feel or hear anything at the time of the injury, such as a popping, snapping, grinding, catching, or buckling sensation? Does the athlete complain of weakness in the injured knee? The feeling that the knee may give out during activity is another symptom that may be associated with internal derangement. These descriptions of sensations associated with a knee injury should never be ignored. Find out the athlete's impressions of the injury and use this information during the injury assessment.

Postinjury course. It is unfortunate that in many cases an injured knee is not evaluated immediately after the injury, the ideal time for assessment. In these instances, it is important to determine what has happened to the knee since the injury. Did the athlete continue activity without difficulty, developing soreness later, or did he or she have to stop activity immediately? Can the athlete walk, run, or climb stairs without pain or complications? Has there been any clicking, locking, or giving way of the knee? Has there been any change in the symptoms since the injury? What makes the symptoms better or worse? All these findings concerning postinjury should be carefully documented and later correlated with all data obtained as a result of the complete knee evaluation.

The information gained during the history portion of the assessment process is extremely important in selecting the appropriate evaluative procedures to be used in examining an injured knee. Knowing the mechanism of injury, the symptoms expressed by the athlete, and the conditions associated with the injury, coupled with an understanding of the anatomy of the area, will allow you to visualize those structures that may be injured and need to be evaluated.

Observation

The visual inspection of an injured knee begins as soon as you see the athlete. Watch the athlete's attitude about the injured knee and willingness to move and use the extremity. If the athlete walks on the injured knee, what is the gait pattern? Can the athlete bear full weight on the knee? Does the athlete limp? If so, how much? Does the athlete require assistance to walk?

As soon as possible, get the athlete to a place where clothing, equipment, and tape can be removed from both legs so that a complete inspection is possible and evaluation or assessment can continue. If possible, have the athlete stand with both feet together to observe the alignment and position of the knees. Terms used to describe any angulation between the tibia and femur are "valgus" and "varus." These terms refer to the body part distal to the joint in question. **Val-**

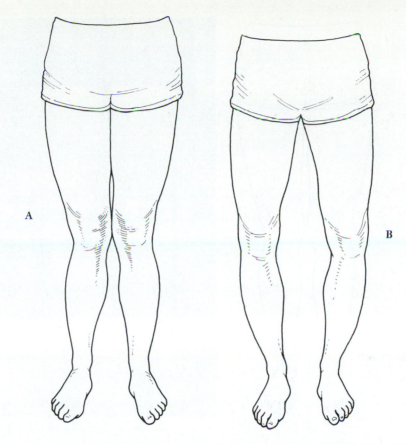

FIGURE 18-17
Valgus and varus angulation of the leg. **A,** Genu valgus, or knock-knee, and **B,** genu varus, or bowleg.

gus means an angulation outward, or away from the midline of the body, whereas **varus** indicates an angulation of the distal part toward the midline (Figure 18-17). An athlete with knock knee is said to have **genu valgum,** whereas an athlete with bowleg has **genu varum.** Women tend to have more valgus angle than men. View the extended knees from the side. Is there any evidence of hyperextension of the knees **(genu recurvatum)?** Women also tend to have more hyperextension than men. Remember, an athlete who has an injury may not be able to completely extend the knee. Compare the injured knee to the uninjured knee to note any difference in symmetry and alignment.

Observe the alignment of the patellae. Do they appear symmetric and level? Do the patellae face forward when the feet are pointed straight ahead or do they appear to face each other **(squinting patellae)** (Figure 18-18). A technique used to evaluate the position of the patellae is to measure the **Q angle.** The Q angle is formed by the intersection of a line from the anterior superior iliac spine to the midpatella and another line from the midpatella to the tibial tubercle (Figure 18-19). An angle of 15 degrees or less is considered normal. An angle greater than 20 degrees is considered excessive and may be associated with an unstable extensor mechanism and patellar instability.

Inspect the knee for any signs of trauma such as abrasions, contusions, or deformities, which may indicate areas of stress and give important clues as to the mechanism of injury. For example, a bruise on the outside of the knee indicates that the supporting

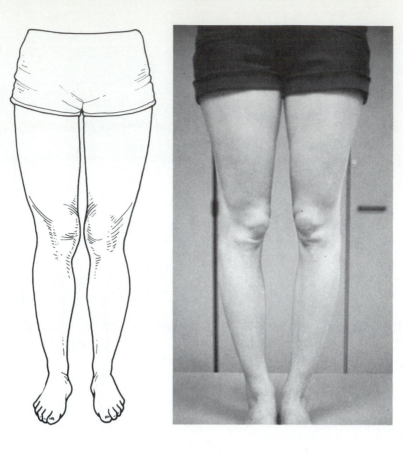

FIGURE 18-18
Squinting patellae.

structures on the inside of the knee may have been subjected to stress and injured by a blow to the outside of the knee. Therefore, the integrity of the supporting structures on the side of the knee opposite any signs of trauma should always be evaluated. Notice the contour of the legs. Are there signs of swelling? The swelling may be generalized over the entire area, which will mask the normal contour of the knee (Figure 18-20). As previously discussed, an athlete with marked effusion usually holds the knee in some degree of flexion rather than complete extension, because in flexion the volume of the joint capsule is greater. Localized swelling about the knee is normally at the site of the injury or over the bursae, such as over the patella (prepatellar bursitis), or under the patellar tendon (infrapatellar bursitis). Also look at the contours of the musculature

above the knee for any visible atrophy. Atrophy of the thigh will usually be present if the knee injury is a chronic problem. A convenient method to document atrophy is to measure thigh circumference at the same level in both legs; another method is to note the character of the muscle tone during maximal contraction of the quadriceps. Look specifically at the size and definition of the vastus medialis. It is the most superficial of the quadriceps muscles and the most sensitive to disuse. The involved leg may have noticeably decreased muscle size and definition.

Physical Examination

The physical examination portion of the assessment process is used to perform a more detailed investigation of the musculoskeletal system. Depending upon what your impressions are up to this point in the assessment

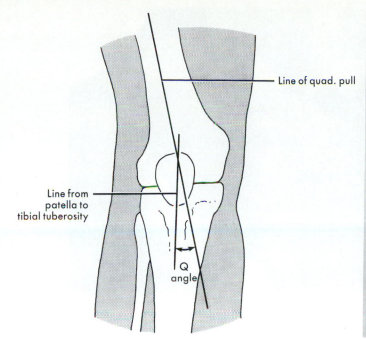

FIGURE 18-19
Q angle of the patella. An angle of 15° or less is considered normal.

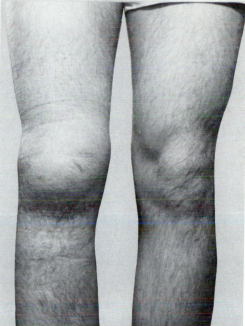

FIGURE 18-20
Example of generalized swelling of knee masking normal contours.

process, you may continue with palpation techniques, movement procedures, or neurological and circulatory evaluations. Not all these procedures will be used in any one athletic injury. Choose the specific tests or procedures that will assist in completing your assessment of the knee. Remember, physical examination is both a skill and an art, mastered only by study and experience.

Palpation

After completing the history and inspection of the knee, palpation can assist in locating specific structures involved in the injury. Remember, it is good practice to begin palpation away from the suspected area of injury. This promotes cooperation from the athlete. Take care not to overlook any unsuspected injuries. It is usually easier to palpate the knee when it is in a flexed position because the supporting structures are more relaxed and anatomic landmarks more distinct. However, certain palpation techniques require that the knee be extended.

Begin the palpation portion of a knee evaluation by localizing any pain or swelling. To localize pain, gently palpate various areas about the knee to elicit tenderness or pain. Tenderness is normally present, and swelling may be localized at the site of an injury. Evaluate any localized swelling by gently feeling for fluid that lies between the skin and the underlying structures. Swelling may also be within the knee joint capsule (effusion), or diffused outside the joint capsule. Diffuse swelling outside the knee joint usually indicates injuries to structures outside the joint capsule or an injury involving the capsule, allowing the fluid to escape from the knee joint into the surrounding soft tissue.

An athlete with marked effusion will usually demonstrate a **ballotable patella.** With the leg relaxed, push the patella downward and then release it quickly (Figure 18-21). The large amount of fluid under the patella will cause it to rebound or appear to be floating. In palpating for minor effusion,

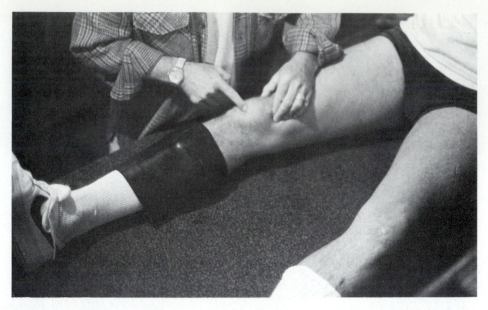

FIGURE 18-21
Ballotable patella.

gradually run one hand down the thigh, ending just above the kneecap to "milk" the suprapatellar pouch (Figure 18-22). Then feel for fluid on each side of the knee at the joint line. If there is fluid within the joint capsule, you will feel a fluid wave on one side of the joint as you push on the opposite side.

Careful palpation of all specific structures suspected of being involved in an injury can provide valuable assessment information. Procedures used to palpate the various structures about the knee, as well as the common injuries that may be indicated by tenderness expressed or swelling located during these procedures, are discussed below.

The patella is a good point of reference to begin palpating around the knee. The patella is best palpated with the leg in extension and the athlete relaxed. Prepatellar bursitis may be indicated by superficial swelling and tenderness over the kneecap. Place your fingers on either side of the kneecap and move it up, down, and from side to side to determine if tenderness exists. Push the kneecap against the femur as you repeat these same moves to evaluate the articulat-

ing surfaces of the patella and the trochlear grove of femur Figure 18-23. Pain on compression against the femur may indicate chondromalacia or a chondral fracture.

The **apprehension test** will indicate if the athlete has a patella that is prone to dislocation or subluxation. While palpating the patella, push it outward, attempting to dislocate it laterally (Figure 18-24). If the patella is not prone to dislocation and the extensor mechanism is stable, there will be no reaction or pain. However, if the extensor mechanism is weakened from a previous subluxation or dislocation injury, the athlete will become apprehensive about lateral movement of the patella. This test can be performed with the knee extended, as well as flexed about 20° to 30°.

Palpate just above the patella in the extensor mechanism and on up into the quadriceps muscles. Feel both thighs at the same time to compare the symmetry and definition of the quadriceps. Note any defects that indicate tears or ruptures. Tenderness in the muscle indicates a possible strain and should be evaluated further by resistive stress. Also palpate the lower end of the pa-

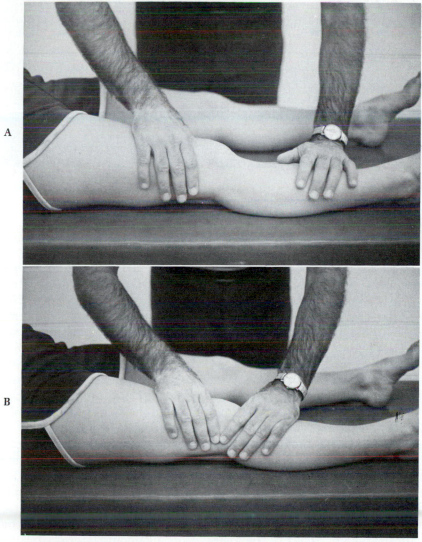

FIGURE 18-22
Palpating for effusion in the knee joint. **A,** Milking down suprapatellar pouch; **B,** feeling for
fluid wave.

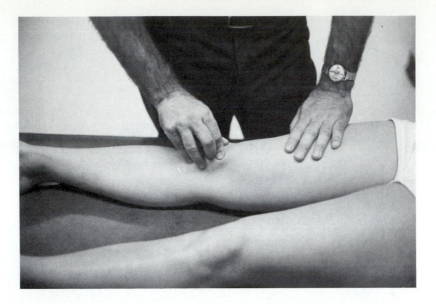

FIGURE 18-23
Evaluating the articulating surfaces of the patella and the trochlear groove of the femur by pushing the patella against trochlear groove.

tella and the point of attachment of the patellar tendon. Local swelling and tenderness here indicates patellar tendinitis, or jumper's knee. To assess this injury, "wing" the patella by pushing down on the upper end of the kneecap with one hand, then palpate the inferior pole using the index finger of your other hand (Figure 18-25, *A*).

Continue palpation along the length of the patellar tendon for any defects, swelling, and tenderness. Swelling and tenderness below the patellar tendon may be infrapatellar bursitis. Remember, the insertion of the patellar tendon at the tibial tuberosity is the site for Osgood-Schlatter syndrome in young athletes, which will produce point tenderness on palpation.

To palpate the medial aspect of the knee, begin at the joint line for orientation. This is easily located by having the knee flexed and feeling for the soft depression just inside the patellar tendon (Figure 18-25, *B*). The joint line is between the upper edge of the tibial condyle, called the tibial plateau, and femoral condyle above. You can follow this line between the femur and tibia all the way around to the back of the joint. Tenderness

along this line may indicate an injury to the medial collateral ligament, medial capsule, or medial meniscus. Next gently palpate along the course of the medial collateral ligament between the proximal attachment on the adductor tubercle to the distal insertion below the pes anserinus. Tenderness at the proximal portion of the adductor tubercle may indicate an avulsion of the attachment of the vastus medialis, often associated with patellar dislocation.

To palpate the lateral aspect of the knee, begin at the front soft depression just lateral to the patellar tendon (Figure 18-26, *A*) and palpate along the lateral joint line. Tenderness along the joint line in this area may indicate an injury to the lateral collateral ligament, lateral capsule, or lateral meniscus. The lateral collateral ligament is more distinguishable than the medial collateral. To augment the palpation of this ligament, have the athlete place the foot of the injured extremity on top of the uninjured knee (Figure 18-26, *B*). This relaxes the iliotibial band and stretches the lateral collateral ligament, making it easy to palpate along its entire length. The tubercle of Gerdy, which is the

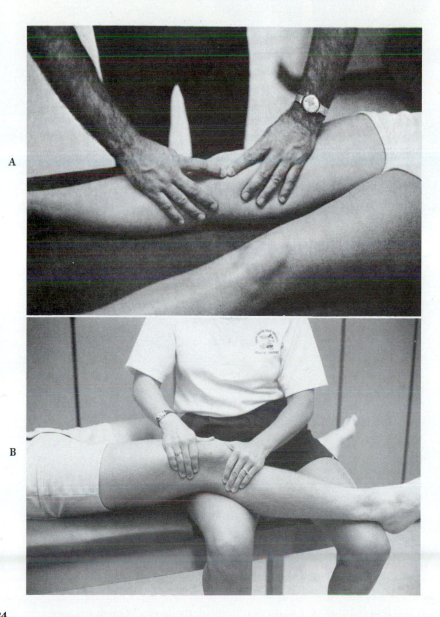

FIGURE 18-24
Apprehension test for possible subluxation of the patella. **A,** Knee extended and, **B,** knee flexed about 20°.

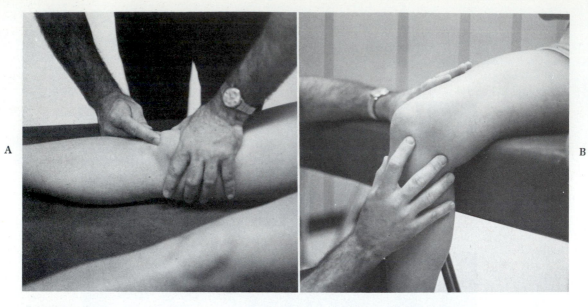

FIGURE 18-25
Palpating for **A,** patellar tendinitis and, **B,** medial joint line.

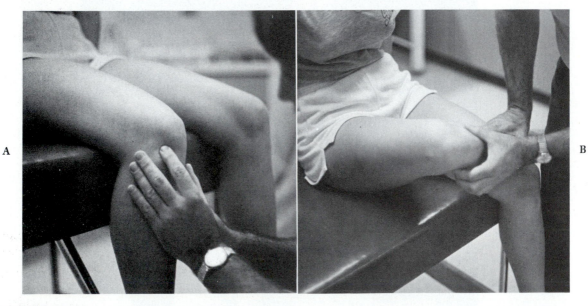

FIGURE 18-26
Palpating lateral aspect of the knee. **A,** Lateral joint line and, **B,** lateral collateral ligament.

attachment for the iliotibial band, can be felt anterior to the head of the fibula.

Tenderness over the lateral femoral condyle may indicate the athlete has an *iliotibial band friction syndrome*. The Noble Compression Test can assist in determining whether this syndrome exists. With the athlete lying supine and the knee flexed to 90°, apply pressure with your thumb to the lateral femoral epicondyle and maintain this

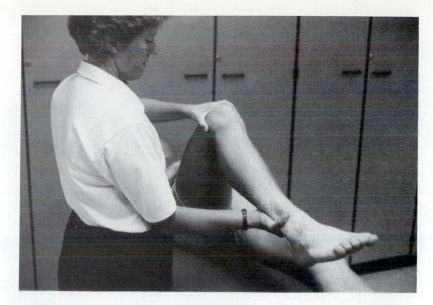

FIGURE 18-27
Noble Compression Test to evaluate for an iliotibial-band friction syndrome. With the knee flexed 90°, apply pressure with your thumb to the lateral femoral epicondyle. Maintain pressure as the athlete slowly extends the knee. A positive test is indicated if the athlete expresses pain as the iliotibial band slides over the epicondyle at about 30° of flexion.

pressure as the athlete slowly extends his or her knee (Figure 18-27). If this condition is present, pain will be produced as the iliotibial band slides over the epicondyle at about 30° of flexion. The athlete will often relate that this is the same pain that accompanies activity.

Another test that should be performed if iliotibial band friction syndrome is suspected, is **Ober's test.** This test assesses tensor fasciae latae and iliotibial band tightness. The athlete should be lying on a side with the lower leg flexed at the hip and knee for stability. Passively abduct and extend the athlete's upper leg so that the iliotibial band passes over the greater trochanter of the femur (Figure 18-28). Then slowly lower the upper limb. If any iliotibial band shortening or tightness is present, the hip will remain abducted and not fall to the table. The knee of the upper leg can be either flexed or extended. Remember, the iliotibial band has a greater stretch placed on it when the knee is extended. An athlete exhibiting a positive Ober's test should be placed on an exercise program to stretch the iliotibial band.

In the posterior aspect of the knee, palpate the lateral and medial hamstring insertions. Feel along these tendons (Figure 18-29, *A*) for any defects or tenderness that may indicate a strain. It is easier to palpate the hamstring tendons during resistive flexion of the knee. The two heads of the gastrocnemius muscle are also palpable at their origin just above the femoral condyles when the athlete flexes the knee against resistance. These are not as distinguishable as the hamstring tendons. The popliteal space can be palpated between the hamstring tendons and the heads of the gastrocnemius muscle. A swelling in this area may indicate a popliteal or Baker's cyst. This area is easier to palpate when the athlete's knee is extended (Figure 18-29, *B*).

In addition to palpating for tenderness and swelling, note any additional indicators of injury. Feel for any change in skin temperature. A noticeable increase in peripheral skin temperature about the knee indicates

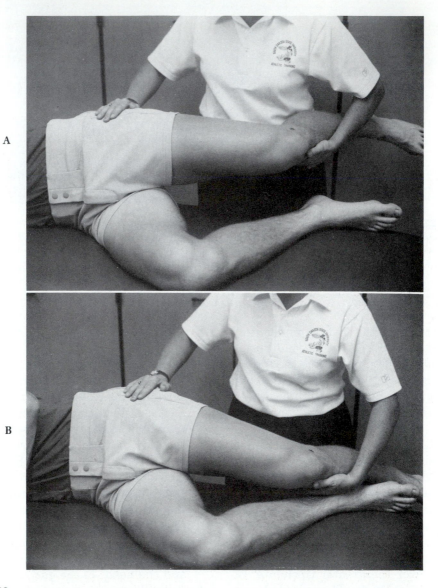

FIGURE 18-28

Ober's test to assess iliotibial band tightness. **A,** With the athlete sidelying, passively abduct and extend the athelete's upper leg. **B,** Slowly lower the leg. If there is an iliotibial band tightness or shortening, the hip will remain abducted.

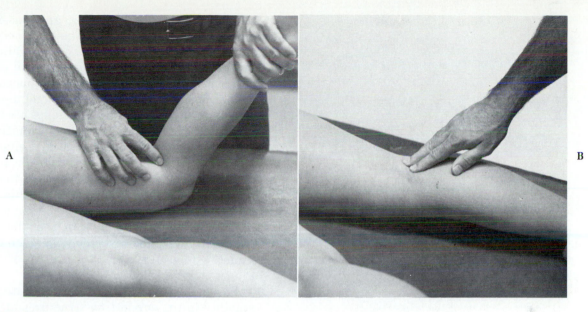

FIGURE 18-29
Palpating the posterior aspect of the knee. **A,** Hamstring tendons and, **B,** popliteal space.

an inflammatory process. A noticeable decrease in peripheral skin temperature below the knee may indicate that the injury has compromised blood flow. Changes in skin texture (smooth or tight skin) may signal early edema before actual swelling is evident.

Movement procedures

Movement procedures should not be attempted until the history, observation, and palpation steps in the assessment are completed and you have some indication of the nature of the injury. This section will discuss the more common stress maneuvers that can be used to examine an injured knee. Not all of these procedures will be used on any one knee; the athletic trainer must select the appropriate maneuvers based on information obtained during the initial steps of the assessment sequence.

Before performing any of the manipulative tests, make sure the athlete is as relaxed as possible. It is easier to perform many of these stressful procedures with the athlete lying down. Relaxation is more apt to occur if you talk to the athlete and explain what you are going to do. Performing stress tests on the uninvolved knee first will demonstrate to the athlete what the tests are like and give you a bilateral comparison. Always remember to begin any stress procedures gently and carefully.

Active movements. Active movements should be performed first to evaluate the integrity of the contractile elements and discover any limitation of motion. Ask the athlete to flex and extend each knee (Figure 18-30). Is there limitation of motion? Most knee injuries are associated with a temporary lack of complete flexion. However, a lack of complete extension is usually a more significant sign and requires further evaluation. The lack of extension can be caused by swelling, muscle spasms, or locking. Does the athlete complain of any pain during active motion? If so, where? If pain appears to be in the muscles, tendons, or musculotendinous junctions, further evaluation of these contractile tissues using resistive movements should follow.

Resistive movements. Resistive movements are used to further evaluate the integrity of contractile tissues. Manual resist-

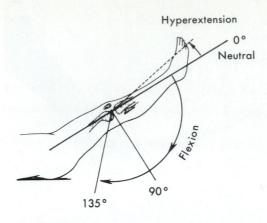

FIGURE 18-30
Active motion of the knee. Flexion is measured in degress from the zero starting position, which is an extended straight leg with the athlete either prone or supine. Hyperextension is measured with degrees opposite the zero starting point.

ance against knee extension, or asking the athlete to hold the knee in extension, while attempting to force the knee into flexion (Figure 18-31, *A*), will allow you to assess the integrity of the extensor mechanism. Manual resistance against flexion, or asking the athlete to hold the knee in some degree of flexion while attempting to force the knee into extension (Figure 18-31, *B*), will allow you to assess the integrity of the flexor musculature. Pain with any resistive maneuvers is an indication of an injury to contractile tissue. For example, pain expressed on resistance to flexion coupled with previously identified point tenderness in the hamstring musculature indicates a strain in the hamstrings.

Passive movements. Passive movements are used to evaluate the integrity of the noncontractile tissues about the knee. All passive movements should be performed with the contractile units as relaxed as possible, which can be very difficult with an acute knee injury. If the athlete contracts the muscles about the injured knee, or if the muscles are in spasms during passive tests, accurate results are hard to achieve. The athletic trainer must reassure and calm the injured athlete to get him or her as relaxed

as possible before initiating any passive stress tests or maneuvers. The time necessary for completing the history, observation, and palpation portion of the assessment process can greatly assist in attaining this goal. Proper positioning of the athlete and use of proper passive stress test techniques are important to ensure an accurate evaluation. The athlete should remain relaxed. Remember, all passive maneuvers should be performed gently to begin with, so as not to aggravate the injury and lose the athlete's cooperation. The intensity of force used with each of these maneuvers can then be increased on repeated tests, depending on the athlete's tolerance and the severity of the injury.

Passive procedures are used to locate instability in the supporting structures about the knee and to evaluate the degree of any laxity that may be present. Passive maneuvers are potentially the most informative procedures used in the assessment of knee injuries. Unfortunately, these maneuvers are also the most difficult to perform and are often subject to misinterpretation. Assessing joint instability is especially difficult for those persons first learning to perform passive stress tests. It takes much practice for anyone to become skilled in using these procedures. All stress tests should be performed consistently in order to develop skill in comparing the findings in any knee injury with those observed in previous injuries. If tests are performed differently each time, the evaluation will often be inaccurate and the findings inconsistent. Each athletic trainer must develop his or her own expertise in evaluating knee injuries and continue to refine the necessary techniques based on experience and knowledge. A discussion of various passive stress tests that can be used to evaluate knee injuries and provide a basis for developing an individualized knee evaluation process follows.

Instability of ligamentous structures is determined by comparing the degree of separation, or movement, of the injured knee with that of the uninjured knee. The importance of constant comparison of the injured

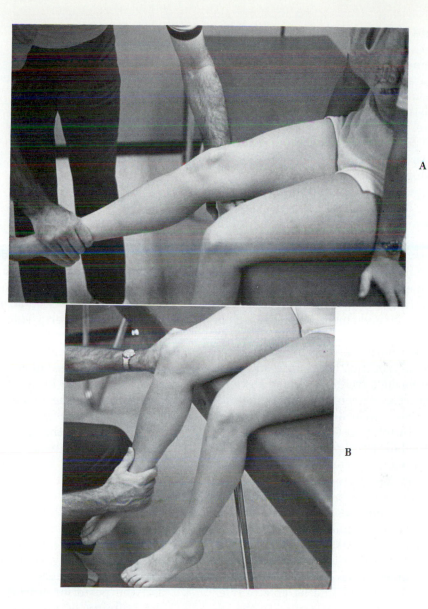

FIGURE 18-31
Manual resistance against, **A,** knee extension to assess integrity of quadriceps and **B,** knee flexion to assess integrity of hamstrings.

knee with the uninjured knee cannot be overemphasized. Instability, or the difference in movement between both knees, is normally rated according to the following scale: 0 indicates no difference in movement or separation; 1+, a mild instability, indicates the difference in separation between the injured knee and the uninjured knee is less than 0.5 cm; 2+, a moderate instability, indicates a difference of 0.5 to 1 cm; and 3+, a severe instability, indicates more than 1 cm difference between the two knees (see Figures 18-33 and 18-36). Remember that a negative test does not necessarily mean the supporting structures are intact. There are several factors that may prevent a passive stress test from being positive even when the ligament is ruptured. As already mentioned, muscle spasm, improper positioning, and improper techniques may compromise an accurate assessment. Joint effusion, meniscal tear, incomplete ligament tears, and the combined support of secondary ligaments can also interfere with an accurate test. In addition, the forces applied manually by the athletic trainer during an evaluation are very small compared to the amount of force placed on the knee during activity. An athlete may complain of instability during activity that cannot be demonstrated by passive evaluation techniques.

Stability and support of the knee joint involves many ligamentous and capsular structures that restrain abnormal motion. The primary support in one direction is provided by one or two ligaments, whereas other ligaments provide less important secondary restraints. Most knee injuries of any consequence involve more than one structure. Seldom is there an isolated ligament rupture. Therefore there are many possible laxities or instabilities that can result from injuries to various combinations of the supporting structures about the knee. Instabilities are named according to the movement of the tibia in relation to the femur and are listed in the box. Straight instabilities refer to abnormal motion in one plane around one axis. Rotatory instabilities refer to abnormal motion in two or more planes around two or more axes. It is not the responsibility of the athletic trainer to evaluate precisely each instability that may exist. However, anyone responsible for evaluating an injured knee should be able to recognize instabilities when they are present and be able to refer the athlete to a physician skilled in the examination and care of knee injuries.

Medial (valgus) instability is evaluated by applying stress to those structures that support the medial side of the knee. The test most commonly used is called the **abduction or valgus stress test.** The athlete should be in a supine position with both legs supported by a table or the ground to assist with relaxation and to avoid muscle contractions. Having the athlete in a supine position places the hips in relative extension, which helps relax the hamstrings. During the actual test, it may be advantageous to

---

Instabilities of the Knee

Straight instabilities

Medial
Lateral
Anterior
Posterior

Rotatory instabilities

Anteromedial
Anterolateral
Posterolateral
Combinations

---

lower the leg over the side of the table so that the thigh remains supported in an effort to keep the thigh muscles relaxed. To perform the abduction stress test, place one hand on the lateral side of the knee and place the other hand above the ankle. Then gently apply lateral stress against the ankle, and medial stress (valgus or abduction force) against the knee in an attempt to open the knee joint on the inside. Repeat the test, gradually increasing the stress up to the point of pain. In this manner, the maximum instability can usually be demonstrated without evoking muscle spasms. Look for any separation or laxity at the medial joint line. The abduction stress test should first be performed with the knee in complete extension and then in about 30 degrees of flexion (Figure 18-32). Medial laxity in complete extension usually reflects a more serious knee injury because the posterior capsule and the posterior cruciate ligament add to the stability of the knee when the leg is straight. Testing the knee in 30 degrees of flexion slackens the posterior capsule and posterior cruciate ligament, which places more stress on the medial collateral ligament and medial capsule. Laxity or pain reflects an injury to these structures. Figure 18-33 represents the rating scale for medial instability.

Lateral (varus) instability, instability of those structures supporting the outside or lateral aspect of the knee, is evaluated by means of the **adduction or varus stress test.** As shown in Figure 18-34, the hand

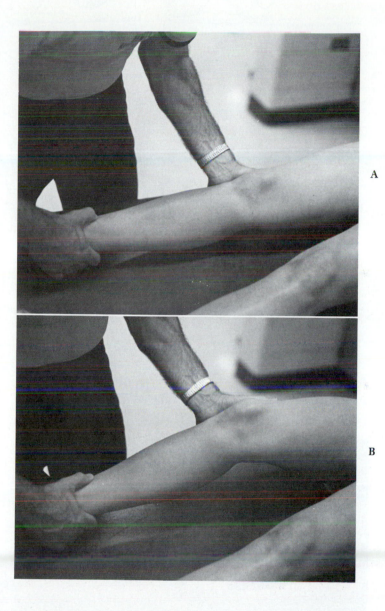

FIGURE 18-32
Abduction stress test to assess integrity of structures that support the medial side of the knee,
A, in complete extension and, **B,** in approximately 30° of flexion.

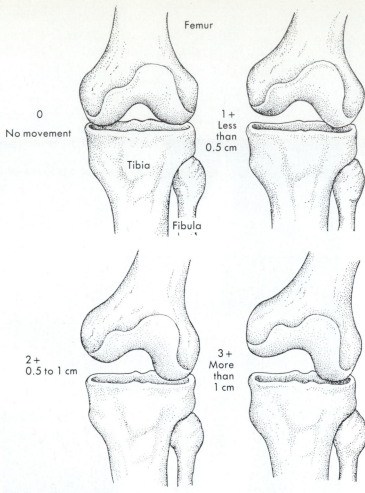

Femur

0
No movement

1+
Less
than
0.5 cm

Tibia

Fibula

2+
0.5 to 1 cm

3+
More
than
1 cm

FIGURE 18-33
Medial instability rating scale.

Anterior view of left knee

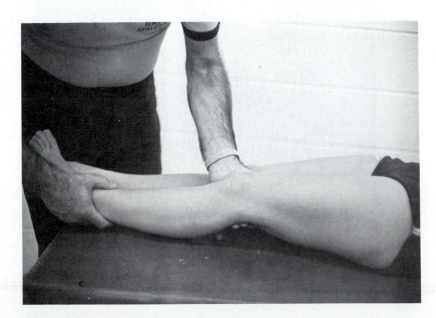

FIGURE 18-34
Adduction stress test to assess integrity of structures that support lateral side of knee.

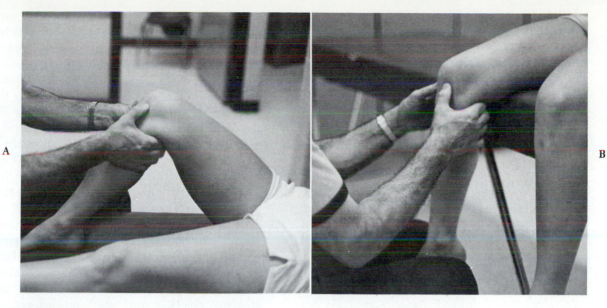

FIGURE 18-35
Anterior drawer test to assess anterior stability. **A,** Knee flexed to 90° and foot flat on table; **B,**
athlete sitting with knee hanging over edge of table and foot supported.

position is reversed from the abduction test so that one hand is placed on the inside of the knee and the other above the ankle. Medial stress is applied against the ankle and lateral stress (varus or adduction force) against the knee in an attempt to open the knee joint on the outside. Look for any separation or laxity at the lateral joint line. Instability present in complete extension again indicates a more severe injury. The structures that may be involved include the lateral collateral ligament, the lateral capsule, and possibly the cruciate ligaments. Instability noted on flexion of the knee, but not in complete extension, suggests that a rotatory instability exists. Rotatory instabilities are discussed later.

Anterior instability can be evaluated in several ways. The most commonly used method is called the **anterior drawer test.** This test is best performed with the athlete in a comfortable, relaxed, supine position. The hip is flexed approximately 45 degrees, and the knee about 80 to 90 degrees, with the foot resting flat on the table (Figure 18-35, *A*). The foot should be in a neutral position, facing straight ahead. Sit on the ath-

lete's foot to stabilize it and cup your hands around the upper tibia, with your thumbs on the medial and lateral joint lines. Some athletic trainers prefer to perform the anterior drawer test with the athlete sitting and the knee hanging over the edge of the table (Figure 18-35, *B*). The foot is then stabilized between the knees of the examiner and raised slightly to reduce the effects of gravity. If the foot is not supported while tension is applied to the ligaments, the test is much more difficult to evaluate. Palpate the hamstring tendons with your fingers to make sure the muscles are relaxed. Gently pull the tibia forward. A slow, steady pull is more effective than a jerk, which can cause pain. If the tibia slides forward under the femur, a positive anterior drawer sign is present. Figure 18-36 illustrates the rating scale for anterior instability. Instability indicates an injury involving the anterior cruciate ligament and possibly the joint capsule or the medial collateral ligament. Any instability noted should be evaluated for rotatory instability, which will be explained later.

Another test used to evaluate anterior instability is **Lachman's test,** which is nor-

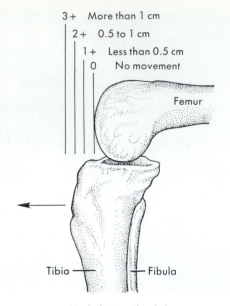

3+   More than 1 cm
2+   0.5 to 1 cm
1+   Less than 0.5 cm
0   No movement

Femur

Tibia   Fibula

Medial view of right knee

FIGURE 18-36
Anterior instability rating scale.

mally more reliable than the anterior drawer test. It is particularly useful when muscle relaxation is a problem, because the hamstrings and the iliotibial band have little effect on the outcome. When the knee is flexed 90 degrees, as with the anterior drawer test, the hamstrings directly oppose forward movement of the tibia. If the athlete contracts the hamstrings, or if the muscles are in spasm, there may not be any abnormal movement even though an instability exists.

Lachman's test is performed with the athlete supine on the table and the knee flexed 10 to 15 degrees. The femur is stabilized with one hand while the other grasps the upper tibia with the thumb along the joint line, as shown in Figure 18-37, *A*. When an athlete's leg is too large or the evaluator's hands too small to grasp the tibia in one hand, the tibia can be held between the arm and the chest of the evaluator as shown in Figure 18-37, *B*. The tibia is then lifted forward and any instability noted.

Posterior instability is usually evaluated in conjunction with the anterior insta-

bility tests. It is presented separately only for instructional purposes. The **posterior drawer test** or Lachman's test is used to evaluate posterior instability. Positioning the athlete is the same as for anterior instability, except now the force applied to the tibia is directed backward, or posteriorly. An important point to remember before evaluating an athlete for posterior instability is the starting position of both knees. Whenever there is increased instability of any kind after an injury, the neutral or starting position becomes more difficult to define. This is especially true for the posterior cruciate ligament when the athlete is supine. Compare normal lateral contours with both knees flexed 90 degrees and the feet flat on the table. If posterior instability exists, the starting position may shift posteriorly because of gravity, and there will be a backward sag, or concave appearance, on the injured side when compared to the uninjured side. The results of posterior stress applied to the tibia in this abnormal starting position may be interpreted as negative, whereas anterior stress applied would bring this tibia to its normal position and may be falsely interpreted as a positive anterior drawer sign. When the lateral contours are normal at the start of a test and a positive posterior drawer sign (Lachman's sign) occurs, an injury to the posterior cruciate ligament has probably occurred.

Rotatory instabilities are abnormal anteroposterior movements combined with inward or outward rotation of the tibia. Tests for these rotatory instabilities are among the most complex procedures to perform and interpret. They are used to assist in completing a more thorough examination of an injured knee. The most common rotatory instabilities are anteromedial and anterolateral. Posterolateral rotatory instability has also been described. This is an injury caused by a tear of the **arcuate complex,** which consists of the arcuate ligament, the popliteal tendon, the lateral collateral ligament, and the posterior third of the capsular ligament. Some authorities have described a posteromedial rotatory instability. However,

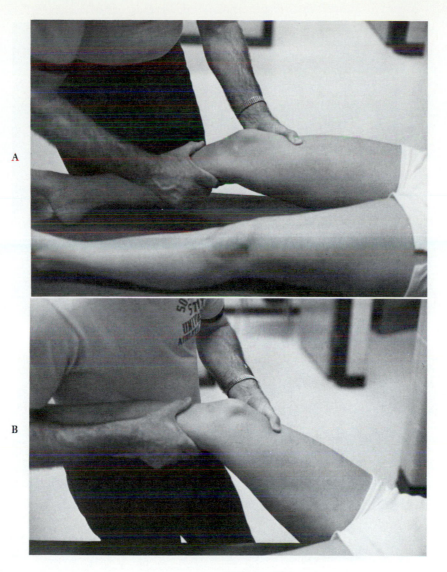

FIGURE 18-37
Lachman's test to assess anterior stability. **A,** Leg held in hand; **B,** leg held between arm and body of trainer.

others believe that this type of instability does not occur if the posterior cruciate ligament is intact, because the tightening of the posterior cruciate ligament that accompanies inward rotation would prevent such instability. If the posterior cruciate ligament is ruptured, the athlete would then demonstrate a straight posterior instability. The two most common combinations of rotatory instabilities are (1) anterolateral and posterolateral rotatory instability and (2) an-

terolateral and anteromedial rotatory instability. The basics of the more common rotatory tests are presented in this text for general knowledge and for those more highly skilled in knee evaluations.

Rotatory instability should be evaluated initially in conjunction with the anterior and posterior drawer tests. Whenever a drawer test is positive and instability is noticed or felt, it is important to observe the movement of the tibia in relation to the femur. Watch

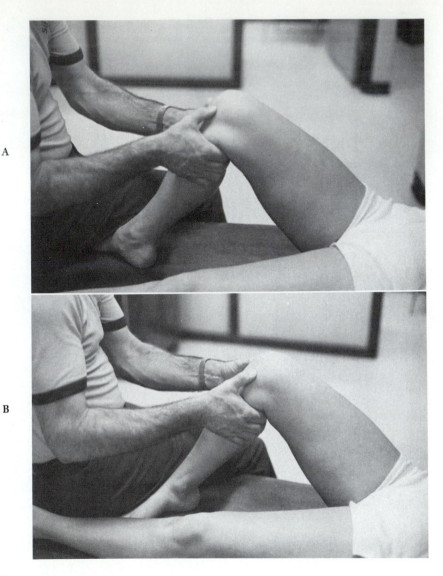

FIGURE 18-38
Anterior drawer test for rotatory instability. **A,** Anteromedial test with athlete's leg outwardly rotated; **B,** anterolateral test with athlete's leg inwardly rotated.

and feel the medial and lateral tibial plateaus at the anterior joint line. Rotatory instability is indicated whenever both plateaus do not move equally. Does one of the tibial plateaus displace more anteriorly than the other during the anterior drawer test? For example, anteromedial rotatory instability is recognized by observing that the medial tibial plateau has a greater displacement forward than the lateral plateau during the anterior drawer test.

To test for **anteromedial rotatory instability,** repeat the anterior drawer test with the athlete's tibia in outward rotation (Figure 18-38, *A*). When the tibia is outwardly rotated, the cruciate ligaments unwind from each other and more stress is applied to the medial structures such as the medial capsule and the medial collateral ligament. Anteromedial rotatory instability is indicated if the medial tibial plateau rotates and displaces anteriorly from beneath the medial femoral condyle.

To test for **anterolateral rotatory instability,** which occurs more frequently, repeat the anterior drawer test with the tibia inwardly rotated (Figure 18-38, *B*). The cruciate ligaments are tightened as the tibia is inwardly rotated. Additional stress is placed on the posterolateral capsule, the iliotibial band, and lateral collateral ligament. Anterolateral rotatory instability is indicated if the lateral tibial plateau rotates and displaces anteriorly from beneath the lateral femoral condyle.

There are additional tests used to evaluate anterolateral rotatory instability of the knee. Normally these tests are not used on an acute knee injury because of pain, swelling, or protective muscle spasms. They may be used on follow-up assessments or under anesthesia to evaluate the presence of anterolateral rotatory instability. These tests, if positive, involve subluxation and relocation of the anterolateral aspect of the tibial condyle from under the lateral femoral condyle at approximately 30 to 40 degrees of flexion.

The **lateral pivot shift test** (MacIntosh) begins with the athlete supine and the muscles relaxed. The injured leg is lifted from the table and supported by the examiner as the tibia is inwardly rotated. One hand grasps the lateral side of the upper tibia at the level of the fibular head and lifts the knee into slight flexion while applying a valgus force (Figure 18-39, *A*). If positive, this produces a subluxation of the lateral aspect of the tibial condyle. Flexion of the knee is continued maintaining the valgus thrust. As the knee passes into 30 to 40 degrees of flexion, the lateral femoral condyle spontaneously reduces with a "jump" or "thud" as a result of the tension of the iliotibial band on the anterior lateral tubercle of the tibia (Figure 18-39, *B*). This subluxation-reduction phenomenon may be reversed. This procedure begins with the hip in 45 degrees of flexion, the knee in 90 degrees of flexion, a valgus force at the knee, and the tibia inwardly rotated. The leg is then extended, and, if the test is positive, a "jerk" occurs when there is subluxation of the condyle at

about 30 to 40 degrees and another "snap" or "pop" when relocation occurs as the knee is extended further. This is referred to as the **jerk test** (Hughston).

The **Slocum test** is a modification of the lateral pivot shift test that begins with the athlete lying on the uninjured side. The bottom leg is flexed at the hip and knee so that the medial side of the foot of the injured leg rests on the examining table free of contact with the uninjured extremity. The pelvis and torso are then rotated posteriorly and fixed at a point where the weight of the lower extremity is borne on the heel of the injured leg (Figure 18-40, *A*). Place your hands on the lateral aspect of the injured leg, one hand below the knee with the thumb overlying the fibular head and the index finger palpating the anterolateral aspect of the joint line to determine the tibiofemoral relationship. The other hand embraces the lateral side of the distal femur with the thumb over the posterior lateral femoral condyle. With equal pressure on the lateral femoral condyle and fibular head, the knee is pushed gently forward into flexion (Figure 18-40, *B*). When anterolateral rotatory instability is present, a reduction phenomenon is felt as the knee passes into 30 to 40 degrees of flexion. This may occur as a sudden, palpable and occasionally audible repositioning.

The presence of an audible click or sudden jump as these maneuvers are performed is usually indicative of anterolateral rotatory instability. However, there are conditions, such as a torn meniscus, which may give a false positive test. These procedures are normally used by athletic trainers more highly skilled in evaluating knee injuries.

Posterolateral rotatory instability occurs when the lateral tibial plateau displaces backward in relation to the lateral femoral condyle. The resulting instability can be recognized by two specific tests: the posterolateral drawer test and the external rotational recurvatum test. The posterolateral drawer sign is only positive when the posterior drawer test is performed with the tibia in external rotation. This same test would be negative with the tibia internally

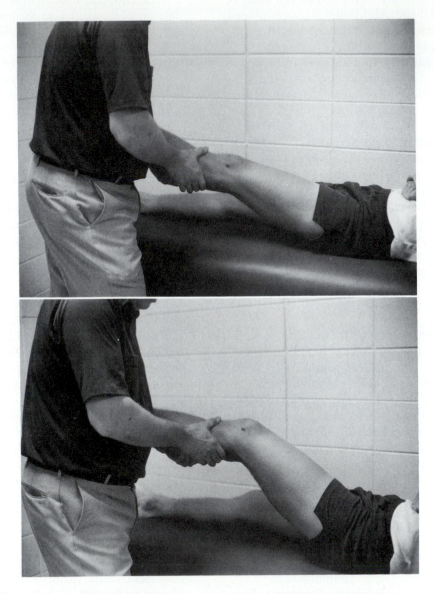

FIGURE 18-39
Lateral pivot shift test. **A,** Leg extended with inward rotation of the tibia and valgus stress at the knee; **B,** knee flexed to approximately 30°. If this test is positive, there will be a subluxation and reduction of the lateral aspect of the tibial condyle.

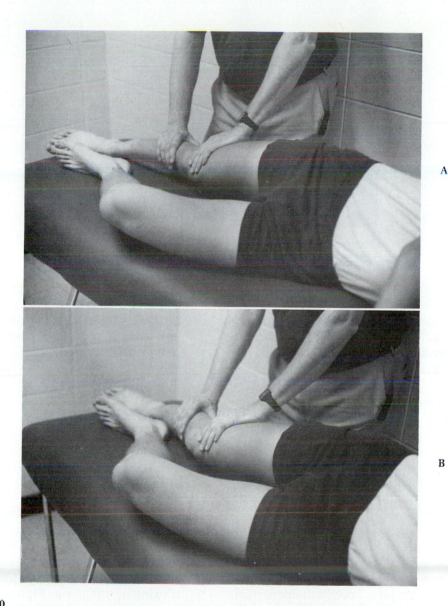

FIGURE 18-40
Slocum anterolateral rotatory instability test. **A,** Athlete lying on the uninjured side with the medial side of the foot on the injured leg resting on the table. **B,** The knee is pushed gently forward into flexion. The test is positive when a reduction phenomenon is felt as the knee passes into 30° to 40° of flexion.

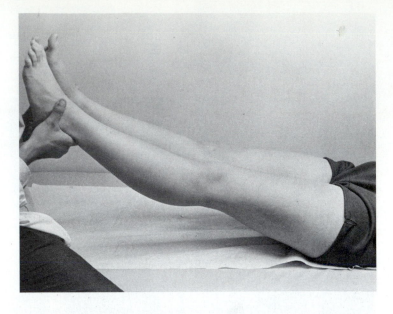

FIGURE 18-41
External rotational recurvatum test for posterolateral rotatory instability. The test is positive if the tibia shows excessive hyperextension and external rotation.

rotated because of an intact posterior cruciate ligament. The **external rotational recurvatum test** is performed with both legs extended and the feet held by the heels (Figure 18-41). The test is positive if the tibia shows excessive hyperextension and external rotation.

Meniscus tests. There are also passive stress tests that can be performed to assist in detecting an injury to a meniscus. Point tenderness along the joint line, especially in the absence of a positive abduction or adduction stress test, may indicate an injury to the meniscus. If so, further evaluation should be performed. With the presence of significant ligament instabilities, it may be extremely difficult to recognize an associated meniscus injury. Specific meniscal tests need not be performed at this time, and the athlete should be treated for the ligament laxity. The torn meniscus may then be recognized on further diagnostic tests by the physician or picked up on repeated evaluations by the athletic trainer.

All of the meniscal tests are founded on the same mechanical basis: attempting to trap, pinch, or displace the injured meniscus

between the articular surfaces of the femur and tibia by performing various circumduction or rotatory maneuvers. The torn meniscus may cause pain or a clicking, grinding, or snapping sensation during these procedures.

The **McMurray test** is performed with the athlete supine and the hip and knee flexed maximally. Hold the athlete's heel in one hand and palpate the medial and lateral joint lines with the thumb and index finger of the other hand (Figure 18-42, *A*). Inwardly and outwardly rotate the tibia with the hand holding the heel to loosen the knee joint and ensure that the athlete is relaxed. With the tibia in outward rotation, extend the leg passively while feeling and listening for any clicking or snapping (Figure 18-42, *B*). This maneuver will evaluate the integrity of the medial meniscus. To test the lateral meniscus, repeat the test with the tibia in inward rotation during extension.

The McMurray test is most effective for evaluation of the posterior half of a meniscus because this procedure does not place as much pressure on the anterior half of a meniscus. You may also apply a valgus or varus

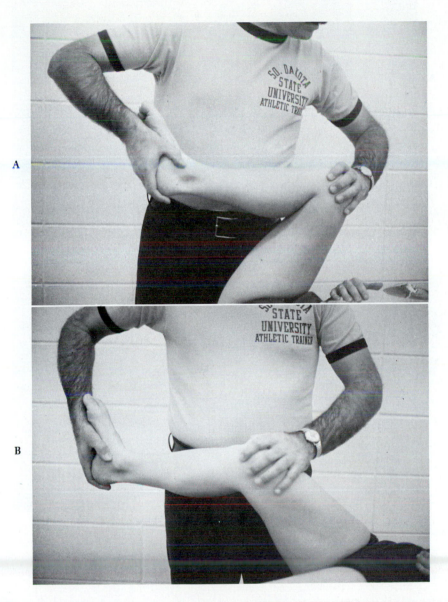

FIGURE 18-42

McMurray test to test the integrity of the menisci. **A,** Hip and knee flexed while palpating the joint lines; **B,** as the leg is passively extended the tibia is rotated and valgus or varus force is applied to the knee.

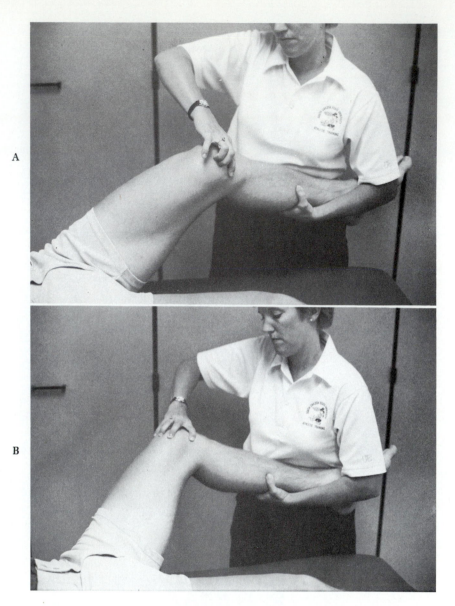

FIGURE 18-43
Medial-lateral grind test to evaluate the integrity of the menisci. **A,** With the athlete supine,
hold the injured leg as you palpate the joint lines. **B,** A circular motion is produced at the knee
by applying valgus and varus stresses as the knee is passively flexed to 45° and extended.

force to the knee during this maneuver in an
attempt to distract or trap the damaged cartilage. The McMurray test requires knee
flexion, which is frequently impossible after
an acute injury.

The **medial-lateral grind test** can be
performed in many acute knee injuries.
With the athlete supine, firmly hold his or
her leg with one hand or between your arm
and chest as indicated in Figure 18-43, *A*.
Place the index finger and thumb of the opposite hand over the medial and lateral joint
lines. Apply a valgus stress as the knee is
flexed to 45° and a varus stress as it is extended (Figure 18-43, *B*). This produces a
circular motion of the knee. Repeat this test

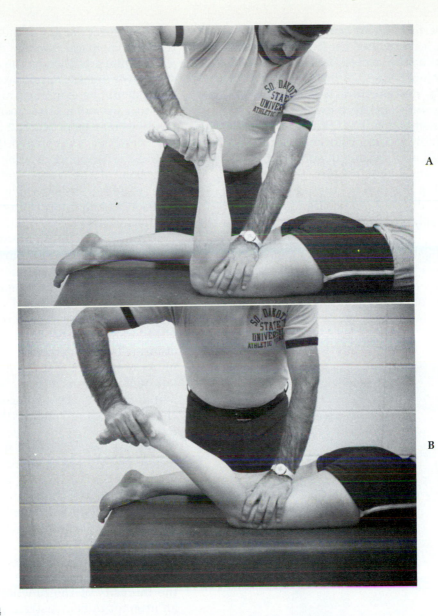

A

B

FIGURE 18-44
Apley's compression test for assessment of meniscal integrity. **A,** With the knee flexed to 90°
apply pressure on the heel while rotating the tibia; **B,** maintain compression as the leg is
passively extended.

applying progressively more stress. A torn
meniscus may produce a grinding sensation,
as well as joint line pain. The advantage of
this test over the McMurray test is that the
knee only has to be flexed about 45 degrees.

Another test that can be used in an attempt to evaluate a torn meniscus is **Apley's
compression test.** Have the athlete lie
prone with the injured knee flexed to 90 de-

grees. Apply pressure on the heel in an attempt to compress the articular surfaces of
the tibia and femur while rotating the tibia
(Figure 18-44, *A*). While continuing to maintain compression, extend the leg in an attempt to elicit pain as the meniscus becomes
entrapped between the articular surfaces
(Figure 18-44, *B*). Pain or clicking may indicate an injured meniscus. This may be dif-

ficult to perform on an acute knee injury because the accuracy of the test depends on relaxation of the athlete and the ability to flex the injured knee.

Apley's distraction test can be performed to differentiate between a meniscal and ligamentous injury. Stabilize the athlete's thigh by putting your knee on the back of the thigh and pulling up on the leg to distract the knee joint (Figure 18-45). While maintaining traction on the leg, rotate the tibia inwardly and outwardly to stress the medial and lateral ligaments while reducing pressure on the menisci. If the athlete has suffered ligamentous injury, this maneuver should elicit pain. If the athlete has suffered only a meniscal injury, this maneuver should not elicit any additional pain.

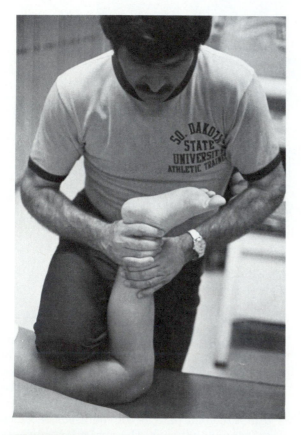

FIGURE 18-45
Apley's distraction test to differentiate between meniscal and ligamentous injury.

The accuracy of any of these manipulative tests for meniscal damage depends on subjective interpretation by the athletic trainer. Whenever a positive test occurs, the normal knee should be examined in the same manner to rule out a false positive test. False positives may be produced by patellofemoral abnormalities, snapping of the medial hamstrings, or trapping of a lax normal meniscus. Accurate assessment of meniscal damage requires considerable experience in performing and interpreting the various manipulative tests.

Functional movements. Functional movements are used primarily to determine when an injured athlete can safely return to activity. However, functional tests can also be used during the initial assessment process in an attempt to localize pain or instability. There will be times when the evaluation will not demonstrate a significant injury or problem with the knee, yet the athlete will continue to complain of pain and instability. In these instances the evaluation should continue and include functional tests.

One method of using a functional test is to ask the athlete to reproduce the injury-producing event as closely as possible to assist in identifying those structures that may be involved. Pain or instability may be demonstrated in this manner when passive tests are negative.

Ask the athlete to squat, bounce up and down, or duck walk. Continue to increase the intensity of the functional activities in an attempt to demonstrate pain or instability. Have the athlete run at various speeds, run figure eights, and perform cutting, starting, stopping, and jumping maneuvers. Running up and down a slope or stairs places a high demand on the knees. The inability to perform these functional activities, or pain associated with them, may assist in identifying injuries or conditions requiring further diagnostic tests.

Neurological evaluations

Sensory functions. With any significant injury to the knee it is important to evaluate the cutaneous distribution of the various nerve roots and dermatomes. In fact, following a major injury to the knee, evaluating the neurological and circulatory status of the leg may be the first assessment procedures performed. To test for altered sensations after a knee injury, run your fingers gently over all aspects of the thigh, knee, and leg. Note any differences in sensations. Remember to compare the sensations to the uninjured side. A more detailed evaluation of the cutaneous distribution of the leg and foot is presented in Chapter 17 and the thigh is discussed in Chapter 19.

Motor functions. Motor functions were discussed under active movements. These procedures may occur early in the assessment process as you ask the athlete to move

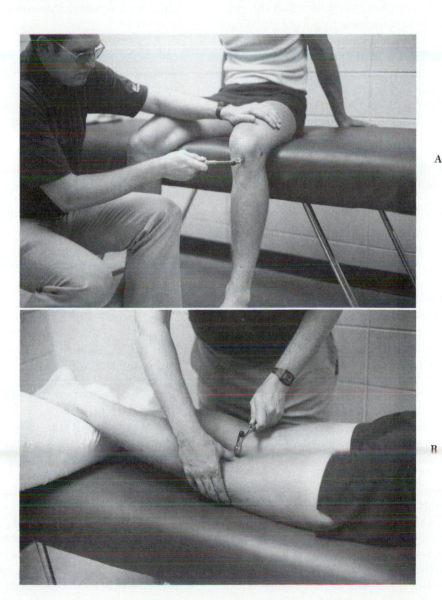

FIGURE 18-46
Test of the, **A,** patellar reflex (L_3 and L_4) and, **B,** medial hamstring reflex (L_5).

the foot, ankle, and knee through as great a ROM as possible. The myotomes of the leg and foot are discussed in Chapter 17 and those of the thigh are discussed in Chapter 19.

Reflexes. Two reflexes about the knee can be checked for differences between the injured and uninjured sides. The patellar reflex (L3 and L4) can be tested by having the athlete sit on the edge of the training table with both legs hanging freely or sit with one leg crossed over the other knee. Tap the patellar tendon just inferior to the patella (Figure 18-46, *A*). The normal response is extension or kicking out of the leg. The medial hamstring reflex (L5) can be tested by having the athlete lying prone with the knee slightly flexed. Place your thumb over the hamstring tendons (semitendinosus and semimembranosus) and tap the thumbnail to elicit the reflex (Figure 18-46, *B*). Compare the reflex responses bilaterally and note any differences between the two sides.

Circulatory evaluations

It is important to evaluate the adequacy of circulatory supply to the lower extremity with any major injury involving the knee. Evaluate the circulation below an injured knee by feeling for a pulse. Whenever ligamentous injuries are of significant severity, consideration must be given to the possibility of vascular injury. The popliteal (behind the knee), posterior tibial, or dorsalis pedis pulses may be used to evaluate the circulation below the knee. Absence of a pulse below the knee after a significant injury indicates an immediate need for referral of the athlete to a physician or medical facility.

Evaluation of Findings

The nature and severity of knee injuries can be extremely difficult to accurately evaluate. A significant knee injury is usually quite easy to recognize and identify. However, less serious knee injuries present the athletic trainer with a difficult and challenging task. The following questions must be considered

---

When to Refer the Athlete ...
Gross deformity
Significant swelling and especially an early hemarthrosis
Loss of motion
Joint instability
Significant pain
Dislocated patella
Abnormal sensations such as clicking, popping, grating, or weakness
Locked knee or excessively limited motion
Any doubt regarding the severity or nature of the injury

---

when evaluating an injured knee. How seriously injured is the knee? Should the athlete be referred for further diagnosis? When can the athlete safely return to activity? Often these are not easy questions to answer. The degree of success in answering these questions and accurately evaluating knee injuries is directly related to the level of skill and experience of the person performing the assessment. This chapter has presented basic evaluation procedures and techniques, as well as guidelines to assist athletic trainers in assessing knee injuries.

When to refer the athlete

Not all knee injuries require referral to a physician or medical facility. Some injured knees, providing they are accurately evaluated, can be properly cared for without seeking additional medical assistance. However, because of the complexity of the joint and the importance of early care, injuries involving the knee frequently require referral and further assistance for an accurate assessment. There are guidelines that can assist in determining if a knee injury is significant and if referral or further assessment is indicated. The list of conditions or findings in the "When to Refer the Athlete . . ." box indicate the athlete should be withheld from further activity until an accurate assessment of the knee is completed and the cause of the condition has been determined.

Athletic Injury Assessment Checklist: Knee Injuries

Secondary survey

_____ History

_____ Previous injury

_____ Nature

_____ Treatment

_____ Extent of rehabilitation

_____ Similar symptoms

_____ Surgery

_____ Present injury

_____ Onset

_____ Mechanism of injury

_____ Pain

_____ Swelling

_____ Loss of motion

_____ Locking

_____ Sensations

_____ Postinjury

_____ Continued activity

_____ Symptoms

_____ Sensations

_____ Observations

_____ Bear weight

_____ Limp

_____ Alignment

_____ Q angle

_____ Signs of trauma

_____ Swelling

_____ Atrophy

_____ Physical examination

Palpation

_____ Tenderness

_____ Swelling

_____ Effusion

_____ Apprehension test

_____ Skin temperature and texture

Movement procedures

_____ Active movements

_____ ROM

_____ Pain

_____ Resistive movements

_____ Pain

_____ Strength

_____ Passive movements

_____ Pain

_____ Instability

_____ Medial—Abduction stress

_____ Lateral—Adduction stress

_____ Anterior

_____ Drawer test

_____ Lachman's test

_____ Posterior

_____ Drawer test

_____ Lachman's test

_____ Anteromedial rotatory

_____ Drawer test (tibia externally rotated)

_____ Anterolateral rotatory

_____ Drawer test (tibia internally rotated)

_____ Lateral pivot shift

_____ Jerk test

_____ Slocum test

_____ Posterolateral rotatory

_____ Posterior drawer test (tibia externally rotated)

_____ External rotational recurvatum test

_____ Meniscal test

_____ McMurray test

_____ Medial-lateral grind test

_____ Apley's compression test

_____ Apley's distraction test

_____ Functional movements

_____ Replicate mechanism of injury

_____ Functional activities

_____ Jogging

_____ Running

_____ Figure of eights

_____ Cutting

_____ Jumping

_____ Starting and stopping

_____ Squatting

_____ Bouncing up and down

_____ Duck walking

_____ Running up and down a slope or stairs

Neurologic evaluations

_____ Sensory functions

_____ Motor functions

_____ Reflexes

Circulatory evaluations

_____ Pulses

REFERENCES

American Academy of Orthopaedic Surgeons: *Athletic training and sports medicine,* ed 2, Park Ridge, 1991, The Academy.

Anderson SJ: Acute knee injuries in young athletes, *Phys Sportsmed* 19(11):69, 1991.

Anderson SJ: Overuse knee injuries in young athletes, *Phys Sportsmed* 19(12):69, 1991.

Arnheim DD, Prentice WE: *Principles of athletic training,* ed 8, St. Louis, 1993, Mosby.

Aronen JG and others: Practical, conservative management of iliotibial band syndrome, *Phys Sportsmed* 21(6):59, 1993.

Bowyer BL: Patellofemoral dysfunction and overuse syndromes, *J Back Musculoskel Rehabil* 2(1):23, 1992.

Clancy WJ, Wilk KE: Medial collateral ligament of the knee, Part II: mechanism of injury & clinical exam, *Sports Med Update* 5(3):12, 1990.

Draper DO: A comparison of stress tests used to evaluate the anterior cruciate ligament, *Phys Sportsmed* 18(1):89, 1990.

Eisele SA: A precise approach to anterior knee pain: more accurate diagnoses and specific treatment programs, *Phys Sportsmed* 19(6):127, 1991.

Ferretti A: Epidemiology of jumper's knee, *Sports Med* 3(4):289, 1986.

Hoppenfeld S: *Physical examination of the spine and extremities,* New York, 1976, Appleton-Century-Crofts.

Israeli A and others: Stress fracture of the tibial tuberosity in a high jumper: case report, *Int J Sports Med* 5(6):299, 1984.

Jensen K: Manual laxity tests for anterior cruciate ligament injuries, *J Orthop Sports Phys Ther* 11(10):474, 1990.

Kannus P and others: Injuries to the posterior cruciate ligament of the knee, *Sports Med* 12(2):110, 1991.

Magee DJ: *Orthopedic physical assessment,* ed 2, Philadelphia, 1987, Saunders.

Mannherz RE: Stress injuries of the extensor mechanism, *Sports Med Update* 4(3):7, 1989.

Nicholas JA, Hershman WB, editors: *The lower extremity and spine in sports medicine:* Volume I and II, St. Louis, 1986, Mosby.

Nilsson S: Overuse knee injuries in runners, *Int J Sports Med* 5(S):145, 1984.

O'Donoghue DH: *Treatment of injuries to athletes,* ed 4, Philadelphia, 1984, Saunders.

Roland GC, Beagley MJ, Cawley PW: Conservative treatment of inflamed knee bursae, *Phys Sportsmed* 20(2):67, 1992.

Steiner ME, Grana WA: The young athlete's knee: recent advances, *Clin Sports Med* 7(3):527, 1988.

Sutker AN, and others: Iliotibial band syndrome in distance runners, *Sports Med* 2(6):447, 1985.

Tegner Y and others: A performance test to monitor rehabilitation and evaluate anterior cruciate ligament injuries, *Am J Sports Med* 14(2):156, 1986.

Zuelzer WA: Meniscal injuries, *J Back Musculoskel Rehabil* 2(1):32, 1992.

SUGGESTED READINGS

Altchek DW: Diagnosing acute knee injuries: the office exam, *Phys Sportsmed* 21(7):85, 1993.
Discusses a systematic method for evaluating acute knee injuries.

Anderson AF, Lipscomb AB: Clinical diagnosis of meniscal tears: description of a new manipulative test, *Am J Sports Med* 14(4):291, 1986.
Compares the clinical diagnosis of meniscal tears using the McMurray test and the medial-lateral grind test. The medial-lateral grind test had a significantly lower number of false positives and was recommended as an adjunct test to improve diagnostic accuracy.

Hughston JC and others: Classification of knee ligament instabilities; Part I. The medial compartment and cruciate ligaments. Part II. The lateral compartment, *J Bone Joint Surg* 58A(2):159, 1976.
Classic article that presents the standardized terminology and classification of knee ligament instabilities used most often today.

Johnson RJ: The anterior cruciate: a dilemma in sports medicine, *Int J Sports Med* 3:71, 1982.
Presents an extensive review of the literature concerning the natural history, diagnosis, and treatment of anterior cruciate injury.

Larson RL, Singer KM, editors, The knee, *Clin Sports Med* 4(2), 1985.
Devoted to knee injuries. Contributors discuss various topics related to conditions and injuries to this area of the body.

Noble HB and others: Diagnosis and treatment of iliotibial band tightness in runners, *Phys Sportsmed* 10(4):67, 1982.
Discusses the assessment and management of iliotibial band friction syndrome.

CHAPTER 19

Thigh and hip injuries

After you have completed this chapter, you should be able to:

- Identify the basic anatomy of the thigh and hip.
- Describe the common athletic injuries that may occur to the thigh and hip.
- Describe the assessment process for an athlete suffering an injury to the thigh or hip.
- List the signs and symptoms that would indicate an athlete suffering a thigh or hip injury should be referred to medical assistance.

The thigh and hip present contrasting characteristics in relation to the incidence of athletic injuries. The thigh muscles are subjected to extreme stresses during most athletic activity and are very vulnerable to impact forces, especially during contact sports. As a result of these factors, the thigh is among those areas of the body more commonly injured during athletics. The hip, on the other hand, is one of the strongest and most stable joints in the body; athletic injuries to this joint are relatively uncommon. However, athletic injuries occurring to the thigh and hip are similar in that most injuries involve the musculotendinous unit.

ANATOMY OF THE THIGH AND HIP

It is important to re-emphasize that the study of assessment procedures should always begin with a careful review of appropriate regional anatomy. The major skeletal components of the thigh and hip are reviewed in Figure 19-1. It is particularly important to note the anatomic landmarks on the femur and bony pelvis. Such bony prominences provide for the attachment of major muscles and also serve as palpation reference points during the assessment process.

The femur, the long single bone of the thigh, is surrounded by thick musculature. The proximal rounded end of the femur (head) articulates with the innominate bone to form the hip joint. The head of the femur is attached to the body of the bone by a neck that projects medially at an angle. Where the neck joins the body there is a large protuberance, the greater trochanter, which projects upward. On the posteromedial side of the neck is the lesser trochanter. The distal end of the femur was previously discussed in conjunction with the knee.

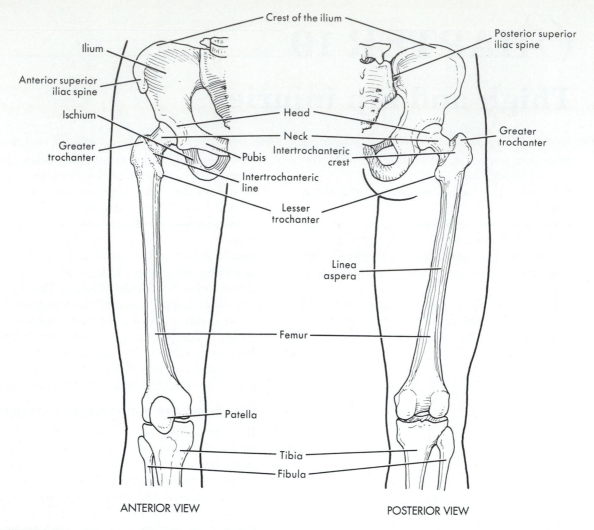

FIGURE 19-1
Major skeletal components of the thigh and hip.

Hip Joint

The hip joint, made up of the head of the femur and the acetabulum, is perhaps the best example of a diarthrodial ball-and-socket joint in the body. Like the shoulder joint, the hip is multiaxial. The hip, however, is modified in several ways to increase its stability. As a result of these modifications, the hip is less mobile than the shoulder and has less freedom of movement. The articulation of the hip occurs between the cup-shaped acetabulum of the innominate or pelvic bone and the smooth, globular head of the femur (Figure 19-2). The depth of the acetabulum is increased by a triangular rim of fibrocartilage called the **acetabular labrum,** which forms an incomplete ring around the margin of the socket. The labrum actually turns into the acetabular cavity and embraces the head of the femur. The stability of the hip is largely the result of the shape of the head of the femur and the deep acetabular socket into which the femoral head fits. Stability is also affected by the powerful and dense ligaments, especially those located in front of the joint.

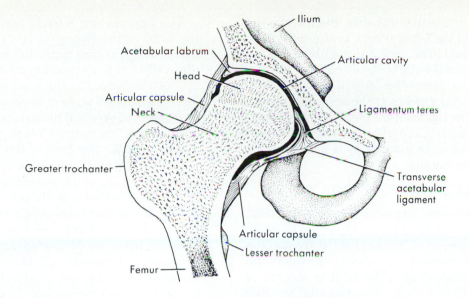

FIGURE 19-2
Frontal section through the hip joint.

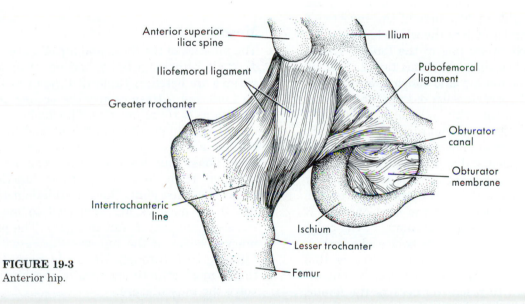

FIGURE 19-3
Anterior hip.

Articular (Fibrous) Capsule

The articular, or fibrous, capsule that encloses the hip joint is quite dense and very strong. The capsule is attached above to the bony margin of the acetabulum and to the acetabular labrum. The thickest part of the capsule is located at the anterosuperior aspect of the joint and provides the greatest resistance in the standing position. On the femur, the capsule is attached to the junction between the neck and trochanters and to the intertrochanteric line (Figure 19-3). The articular capsule is strengthened by the iliofemoral, ischiofemoral, and pubofemoral ligaments. The coarse exterior of the capsule is covered by numerous muscles and is separated in front from the psoas major by a bursa, which may communicate with the joint space.

The synovial membrane of the hip joint

lines the articular capsule and covers the portion of the femoral neck contained within the capsule. The synovial membrane is reflected over the rim of the acetabular labrum above and covers the fat pad near the inferior exit of the socket at the acetabular notch below. The ligamentum teres, which permits blood vessels and nerves to pass to the head of the femur, is covered by a sheath of synovial membrane.

Ligaments

The *iliofemoral ligament* is a strong, thick, inverted Y-shaped ligament (also known as the Y ligament of Bigelow) at the front of the hip that merges with and strengthens the joint capsule (Figure 19-3). It is shorter in women than in men. Functionally, the iliofemoral ligament is the most important hip ligament. The stem of the inverted Y is attached to the anterior inferior iliac spine. The two divergent bands of the inverted Y fan out and attach to the whole length of the intertrochanteric line of the femur. The iliofemoral ligament becomes taut in full extension of the hip and helps prevent inadvertent hyperextension of the trunk (falling over backward) while standing. It is the iliofemoral ligament that allows us to remain in an erect position without continuous muscular exertion and subsequent fatigue.

The *pubofemoral ligament* is a triangular band of fibers that strengthens the medial and inferior portion of the joint capsule. It arises from the superior ramus of the pubic portion of the innominate bone and a portion of the acetabular rim. Note in Figure 19-3 that fibers in the apex of the ligament extend down to reach the neck of the femur, where they blend with the lower medial fibers of the iliofemoral ligament. The pubofemoral ligament is tight in extension and also limits abduction of the hip.

The triangular *ischiofemoral ligament* lies on the posterior aspect of the joint capsule. It extends from the ischium of the innominate bone below and behind the capsule to the trochanteric fossa of the femur. It is the ischiofemoral ligament and posterior part of the fibrous capsule that help limit medial rotation of the hip.

The *ligamentum teres* is the ligament to the head of the femur. It is a short (about 3.5 cm long), strong band that extends from the wall of the acetabulum to a roughened depression *(fovea)* on the head of the femur. The ligamentum teres is completely covered by a sleeve of synovial membrane and serves as a bridge permitting blood vessels and nerves to enter the head of the femur. This ligament becomes taut in adduction of the femur, when the thigh is semiflexed, and relaxed when the limb is abducted.

The acetabular labrum is a triangular or horseshoe-shaped ridge of cartilage that is deficient below at the *acetabular notch*. The transverse ligament of the acetabulum bridges this notch and completes the circular ring around the socket. In crossing the acetabular notch the ligament creates an opening (foramen) through which blood vessels and nerves can enter the joint space.

Muscles

The muscles of the thigh and hip (Figure 19-4), their primary actions, and nerve innervations are listed in Table 19-1. Refer to Tables 5-9 and 5-10 to review the origins and insertions of these muscles. The major muscles of the thigh, the quadriceps and hamstrings, are illustrated in Figures 19-5 and 19-6. These muscles were also discussed in Chapter 18 in relation to their function about the knee joint. During athletic activity, these muscles are subjected to many stresses that may result in injury. The primary muscles of the hip are illustrated in Figures 19-7 through 19-10. As with the thigh, most athletic injuries of the hip involve the musculature.

Movements

The hip joint allows flexion, extension, abduction, adduction, rotation, and circumduction. As a multiaxial joint the hip permits flexion and extension through a transverse axis, adduction through an anteroposterior axis, and medial and lateral rotation through a vertical axis. Refer to Figure 19-11 for the normal ROMs at the hip.

Text continued on p. 519.

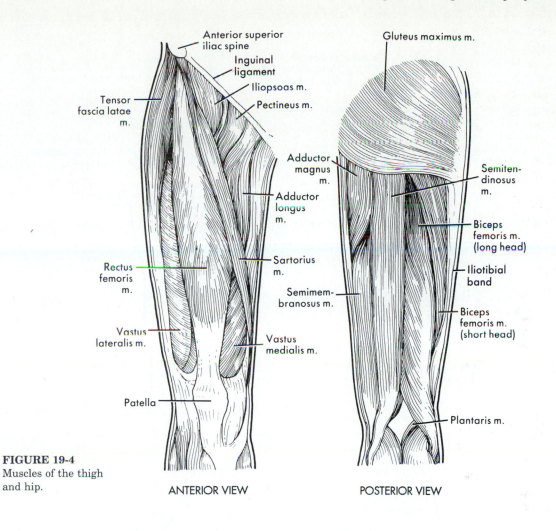

FIGURE 19-4
Muscles of the thigh
and hip.

TABLE 19-1

Muscles of the Thigh and Hip

Muscle	Nerve	Segmental innervation	Primary action(s)
Gluteus medius	Superior gluteal	L_4-S_1	Abduction and internal rotation of hip
Gluteus minimus	Superior gluteal	L_4-S_1	Abduction and internal rotation of hip
Tensor fascia latae	Superior gluteal	L_4-S_1	Flexion and internal rotation of hip
Gluteus maximus	Inferior gluteal	L_5-S_2	Extension and adduction of hip
Iliopsoas	Femoral	L_2-L_4	Flexion of hip
Sartorius	Femoral	L_2, L_3	Flexion and rotation of hip & knee
Quadriceps	Femoral	L_2-L_4	Extension of knee
Pectineus	Obturator	L_2, L_3	Adduction and flexion of hip
Adductor longus	Obturator	L_2, L_3	Adduction and flexion of hip
Adductor brevis	Obturator	L_3, L_4	Adduction and flexion of hip
Adductor magnus	Obturator	L_3, L_4	Adduction and flexion of hip
Gracilis	Obturator	L_3, L_4	Adduction of hip and flexion of knee
Hamstrings	Sciatic	L_5-S_2	Extension of hip and flexion of knee
Biceps femoris (short head)	Sciatic	L_5, S_1	Flexion of knee

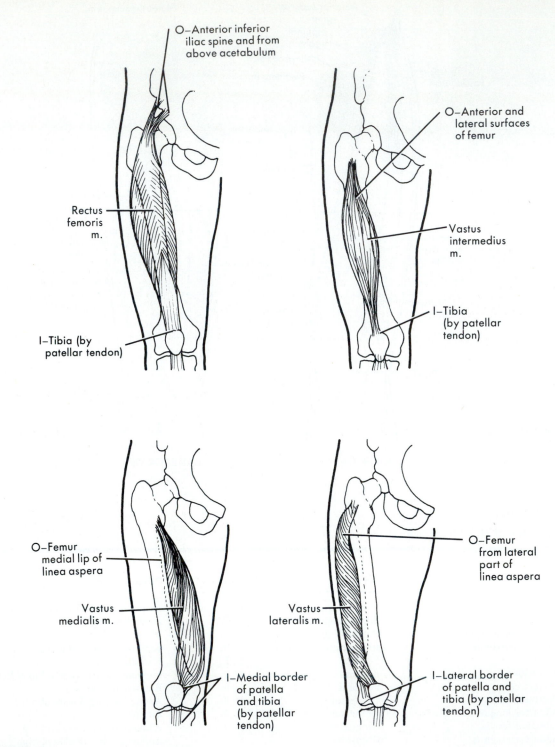

FIGURE 19-5
Quadriceps femoris group of thigh muscles.

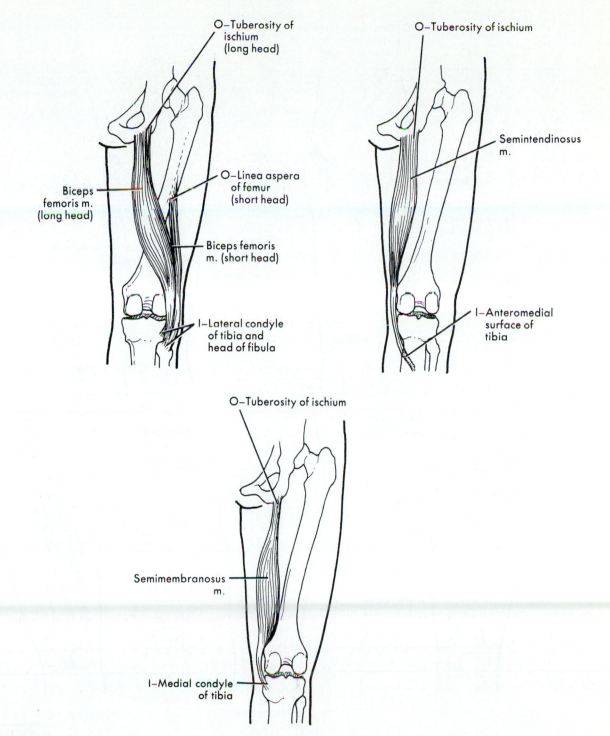

FIGURE 19-6
Hamstring group of thigh muscles.

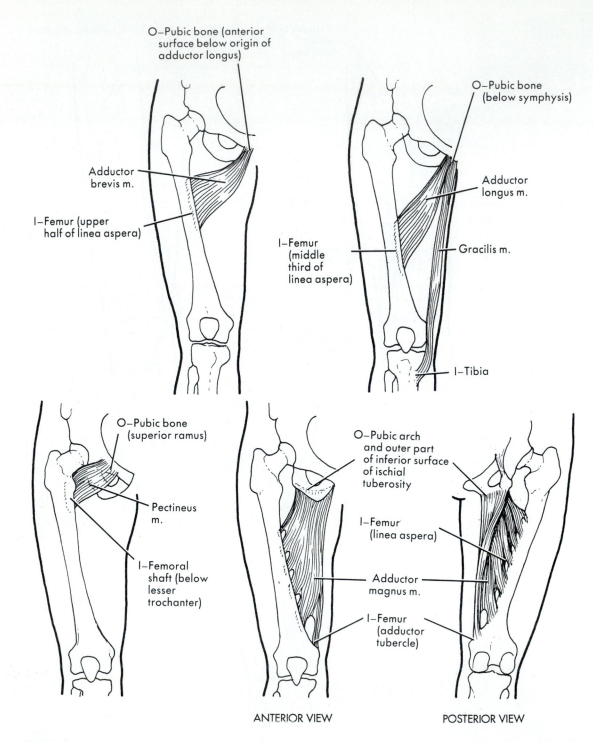

FIGURE 19-7
Muscles that adduct the hip.

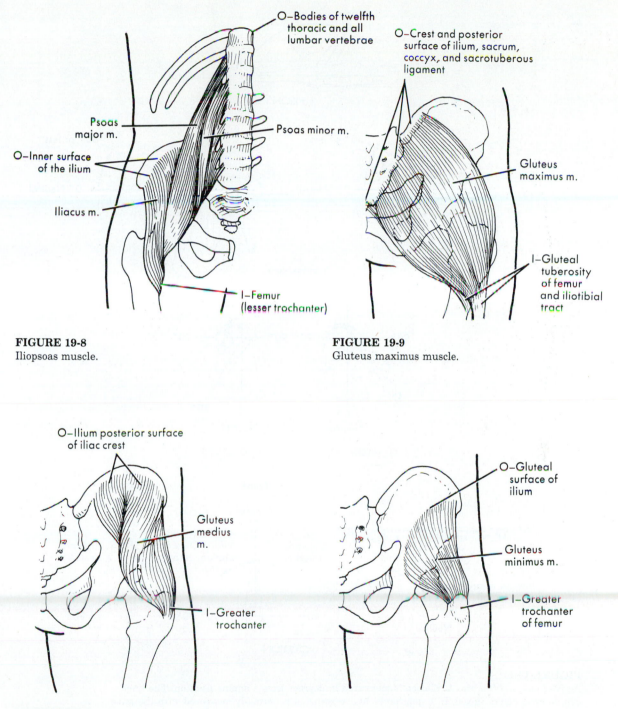

FIGURE 19-8
Iliopsoas muscle.

FIGURE 19-9
Gluteus maximus muscle.

FIGURE 19-10
Muscles that abduct the hip.

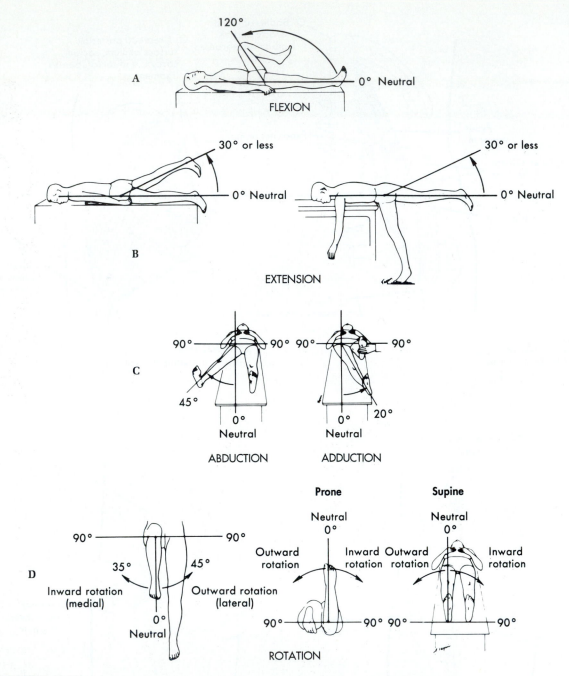

FIGURE 19-11

Active motion of the hip. **A,** Flexion is measured in degrees from a supine position. The knee can be extended or flexed. **B,** Extension or hyperextension is normally measured with the knee extended. **C,** Abduction can be measured in a supine or sidelying position; adduction is best measured with the athlete lying supine. **D,** Inward and outward rotation can be evaluated in a supine or prone position.

Forward movement about a transverse axis (flexion) is limited to about 90° when the knee is extended because of tension of the hamstrings. With the knee flexed, the range of motion (ROM) in flexion at the hip is very free (about 120° to 130°), limited only by contact between the thigh and abdomen. Extension of the hip is limited to about 30° (hyperextension) by the iliofemoral and pubofemoral ligaments.

Adduction and abduction of the hip are movements about an anteroposterior axis. Adduction, movement towards the midline, is limited by the opposite limb and by the ischiofemoral ligament and the ligamentum teres. With one leg crossed over the other, the athlete should be able to achieve about 20° of additional adduction. Abduction, movement away from the midline, is a relatively free movement to about 45° and is limited by the pubofemoral ligament, the medial portion of the iliofemoral ligament, and by tension of the adductor muscles.

Lateral and medial rotation of the hip are movements that occur about a longitudinal axis. Lateral or outward rotation turns the anterior surface of the thigh laterally. Lateral rotation of the hip is a powerful movement and is free through about 45°. It is limited by tension of the front of the capsule and by the lateral band of the iliofemoral ligament. Medial or inward rotation, the weakest movement at the hip, is possible through approximately 35°. It is limited by tension on the posterior fibers of the joint capsule.

INJURIES TO THE THIGH AND HIP
Contusions
❖ **Quadriceps contusion.** Common thigh injuries are contusions to the anterior thigh, or quadriceps muscle group that occur as the result of a direct blow (Figure 19-12). This type of injury, often called a *charley horse,* occurs frequently during contact activities. Symptoms of a contusion may range from mild tenderness with little restriction of motion to marked pain, swelling, and disability. A potentially serious assessment problem with thigh contusions is delayed or silent bleeding within the injured muscle that may

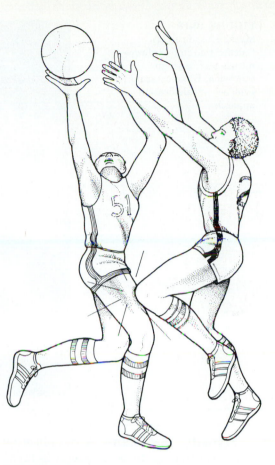

FIGURE 19-12
Quadriceps muscle contusion caused by a direct blow.

continue for varying periods of time. In these cases the full extent of the injury may not be recognized for 12 to 24 hours. Frequently the athlete will continue activity during this time, and only after re-evaluation the following day will the severity of the injury be recognized. The signs and symptoms of a muscle contusion will depend on the severity and location of the injury, but usually there are varying degrees of pain, tenderness, swelling, and restricted motion or function. The signs and symptoms associated with thick-muscle injuries are often less localized than in other more subcutaneous areas of the body. As with thigh strain, the signs and symptoms of a thigh contusion are intensified by active and resistive motion.

FIGURE 19-13
Myositis ossificans.**A,** Calcification in quardiceps muscle after a thigh contusion; **B,** no external evidence of calcification apparent.

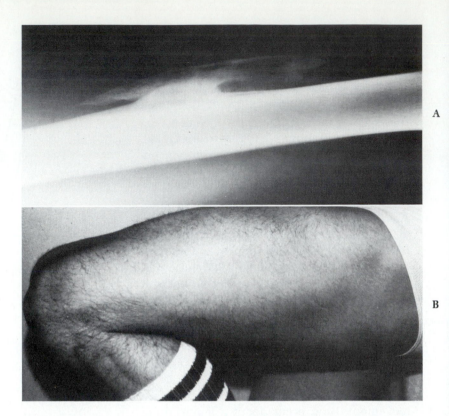

A

B

❖   **Myositis ossificans.** A complication of thigh contusions to be aware of is myositis ossificans, which was described in Chapter 8. Myositis ossificans can occur anywhere in the body but more frequently involves the quadriceps. The bony deposits may occur as a separate piece or pieces of bone lying entirely within the muscle or by direct attachment to the femur. Remember that the tissue involved is not the muscle, but rather the connective tissue of the fascia and its intramuscular extensions. This complication seldom develops as a result of a single injury; it is more likely to occur after chronic irritation, such as continued use of the injured quadriceps or repeated trauma to the thigh. Whatever the reason, the hematoma fails to resolve, resulting in myositis ossificans (Figure 19-13). It is important for the athletic trainer to recognize the possibility of myositis ossificans after a severe thigh contusion or repeated bruising. This condition should always be suspected if hematoma formation does not promptly resolve

and pain, a palpable mass within the muscle, and loss of motion persists for 2 to 3 weeks. When this occurs, the athlete should be withheld from activity until symptoms subside. It is important that athletes suffering from severe thigh contusions be evaluated frequently.

❖   **Iliac crest contusion.** The massive hip area is vulnerable to direct blows, which result in contusions. One of the more common contusions is to the iliac crest, commonly called a **hip pointer.** The iliac crest extends from the anterior superior iliac spine to the posterior superior iliac spine. This crest is the most subcutaneous area of the hip and is especially susceptible to injury during contact sports. A contusion to the iliac crest can involve the hip muscles that originate along its outer border or the abdominal muscles that insert along its upper and inner border. Figure 19-14 illustrates ecchymosis resulting from a hip contusion. The hip and abdominal muscles can also be strained or avulsed along their attachment to the iliac crest.

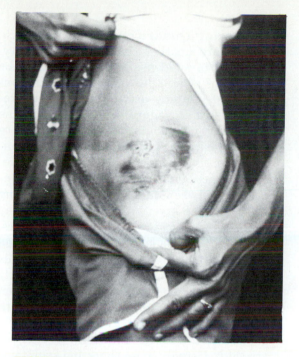

FIGURE 19-14
Ecchymosis resulting from a hip contusion.

This may result from forced lateral flexion during contraction of these muscles. The athletic trainer can usually determine if the injury is primarily a contusion or if the muscular attachments are strained by careful scrutiny of active movements during the assessment process. If the injury is primarily a bruise, active movements of the hip should not increase the pain dramatically. However, if the injury is a strain involving the muscle attachments, active movements utilizing the involved muscle will significantly increase the pain. Look for voluntary guarding by the athlete. For example, active hip abduction resulting in increased pain below the crest of the ilium may indicate a strain to the gluteus medius muscle. It may be difficult to determine the severity of injuries about the crest of the ilium, and the athlete is normally treated symptomatically, that is, kept inactive until the symptoms subside or referred to a physician if the symptoms persist or are of a severe nature.

❖   **Trochanteric bursitis.** Another area of the hip region vulnerable to contusions lies over the greater trochanter of the femur. The bony trochanter is covered only by the trochanteric bursa and tensor fascia latae muscle. The function of the bursa is to lessen friction as the tensor fascia latae slides over the trochanter during movement. A direct blow to the trochanter may result in a contusion of the muscle or lead to trochanteric bursitis. Friction within the bursa caused by the tensor fascia latae muscle constantly gliding over the trochanter can also result in bursitis. Palpating the greater trochanter will cause pain with both a contusion and trochanteric bursitis. However, if the bursa is inflamed, movements forcing the tensor fascia latae muscle over the trochanter will cause pain. Chronic trochanteric bursitis with thickening of the bursal walls can cause a condition known as a **snapping hip.** As the tensor fascia latae slides back and forth over the trochanteric bursa, an audible and palpable snap will occur. This condition is more common in women because they have a wider pelvis and a more prominent trochanter.

❖   **Ischial bursitis.** Ischial bursitis can result from a direct blow to the ischial bursa such as being kicked or falling on the ischial tuberosity. Another possible cause can be sitting for a prolonged period of time, especially with the legs crossed or on a hard surface. This condition has been referred to as *bench-warmer's bursitis*. Symptoms would include tenderness over the ischial bursa.

❖   **Iliopectineal bursitis.** The iliopectineal bursa lies between the iliopsoas tendon and the iliopectineal eminence on the pelvic bone. Repetitive irritation can cause iliopectineal bursitis that may be seen as an acute pain in the anterior aspect of the hip. The athlete is more comfortable in flexion and external rotation of the hip and stressing the iliopsoas muscle accentuates the discomfort.

Thigh compartment syndrome. Acute thigh compartment syndrome is a rare but limb-threatening condition that can result when an athlete sustains a serious thigh contusion. There are three major compartments in the thigh: the anterior contains the quadriceps muscles and the femoral artery and nerve; the medial contains the adductor muscles and the cutaneous branch of the obturator nerve; and the posterior contains the hamstrings and the sciatic nerve. These compartments are larger than those in the leg, allow more room for muscle expansion after injury, and the large muscles can disseminate traumatic forces more widely than those of the leg. Therefore, the thigh is less vulnerable to compartment syndromes. It is believed that compartment syndrome is more common in athletes who have marked muscle hypertrophy. When a thigh compartment syndrome does occur, the symptoms include significant pain, thigh distension, decreased knee ROM, neurovascular impairment, and elevated compartment pressures. Pain is exacerbated by passive stretching of the involved muscles. It is important to recognize this injury so the athlete can receive prompt treatment.

Strains

✤ **Hamstring\Quadriceps strain.** Muscle strains are another common thigh injury. The type of sudden violent contractions or stretching of muscles associated with running and jumping activities frequently results in strains (Figure 19-15, *A*). Conditions which may contribute to muscle strains are lack of flexibility, fatigue, inadequate warmup, muscle weaknesses, deficiency in the reciprocal action of opposing muscles, or imbalance between quadriceps and hamstring strength. The severity of thigh strains may range from muscle cramps to complete tears, or ruptures. The hamstrings are strained more frequently than the quadriceps. This type of injury tends to recur and frequently becomes a chronic problem. The signs and symptoms most commonly associated with thigh strains are pain, tenderness, muscle spasm, and loss of function, motion, or strength. Usually these signs and symptoms

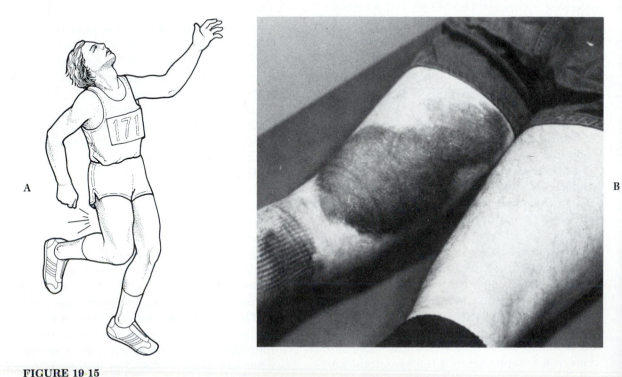

FIGURE 19-15
Muscle strain. **A,** Runner suddenly straining a hamstring muscle as a result of a violent contraction. **B,** Ecchymosis 5 days after a hamstring strain.

are intensified by both active and resistive motion. In moderate to severe strains, the athlete often experiences a pop or snap in the musculature, with immediate pain and loss of function. There may be a palpable gap within the torn fibers or a lump resulting from the contraction of ruptured muscle tissue or hematoma. Ecchymosis may appear a few days after the injury as blood collects under the skin (Figure 19-15, *B*). Strains of the quadriceps are prone to occur in fatigued, injured, or incompletely rehabilitated quadriceps muscles which are placed under ballistic or explosive demands.

Of the muscles about the hip, those in the groin are injured most frequently during athletic activity and can be very debilitating. The groin includes the body area lying between the thigh and abdominal wall. The muscles in this region consist of the hip adductors (Figure 19-7) and flexors (Figure 19-8). Groin muscle strains are common in all athletic activities that involve running, especially those characterized by sudden bursts of speed requiring explosive or almost violent types of muscular contractions. Injuries to groin muscles may also be caused by sudden, unexpected overstretching of the muscles, as well as by forced extension or abduction during muscle contraction. In case of injury the athlete may report feeling a sudden twinge or tearing sensation in the groin. In other instances, initial symptoms may be mild and the athlete may not notice or report the injury until after activity is completed. The signs and symptoms of a groin strain are similar to those of other muscle strains. To determine which muscles are involved and the severity of the injury, the athletic trainer must use active and resistive movement tests during the assessment process.

The other muscles about the hip are not strained nearly as often or as severely as those in the groin. However, these muscles can be strained by the same mechanisms responsible for thigh and groin muscle injuries. In most cases signs and symptoms will also be similar to those described for thigh and groin strains. The athletic trainer must be familiar with the various active and resistive assessment procedures used to determine specific muscle injury. These procedures are also used to evaluate the functional integrity of individual muscles.

❖ **Piriformis syndrome.** Piriformis syndrome is a condition of tension pain in the pelvic floor. Repetitive muscular stresses to the pelvis during athletics or frequent increases of the inner abdominal pressure can cause irritation and pain in the muscles and fascia of the pelvic floor. The piriformis muscle runs from the anterior sacrum to the medial aspect of the greater trochanter and is frequently involved in this type of pain. Symptoms include back and leg pain and a heavy feeling in the pelvis. A tight piriformis muscle can also compress the sciatic nerve and cause localized tenderness in the buttock area between the ischium and the greater trochanter. Possible mild involvement of the nerve roots and tingling may be encountered.

Sprains

❖ **Hip sprain.** Any of the supporting ligaments of the hip joint may become stretched or torn as a result of some type of violent movement that forces the hip to exceed the normal ROM in any direction. Hip sprains, however, are uncommon and seldom serious. When they do occur, the athlete may express pain in the hip at the limits of motion restricted by the sprained ligament. In addition, pain may be expressed during circumduction of the hip. If the pain is severe enough, the athlete may be unable to circumduct the hip.

An athlete may suffer from traumatic synovitis of the hip caused by either a direct blow to the greater trochanter or a sprain. However, it is difficult to recognize effusion of the hip joint or actually identify a distention of the joint capsule. Traumatic synovitis should be suspected in an athlete with an undiagnosed painful hip, a limp, complaints of general soreness in the hip during movement, and pain during palpation over the greater trochanter.

❖ **Avascular necrosis.** A possible complication of synovitis is avascular necrosis of the femoral head. This is especially true in preadolescent athletes. In this condition the hip joint is filled with an excess of synovial fluid as the result of the inflammatory process. The pressure from this increased synovial fluid may occlude the blood supply to the femoral head. Young athletes complaining of continued or severe pain in the hip should be carefully evaluated and referred to a physician for assessment of avascular changes. Another possible cause of avascular necrosis is a hip dislocation or subluxation that interferes with the blood supply to the femoral head. When the blood supply is compromised, some of the cells may die and the tissue may become nonviable.

✤ **Osteitis pubis.** Osteitis pubis is an inflammation of the pubic bones in the region of the symphysis. It can be caused by excessive or repetitive stresses to the symphysis during vigorous athletic activities, such as running, jumping, and kicking. Symptoms include the gradual onset of localized pain in the region of the pubis, which may extend to the groin or lower abdomen. Kicking, sprinting, jumping, stretching, climbing stairs, or sudden changes in direction can aggravate the symptoms. Often there is loss of range of motion of one or both hips and pain on adductor muscle stretch.

Dislocations

✤ **Hip dislocation.** Dislocations of the hip as the result of athletic activity are rare. A hip dislocation normally occurs only after a violent force is directed along the femur when the hip is flexed. With this type of injury, the athlete has severe pain and is totally disabled immediately. Because the hip usually dislocates posteriorly, the athlete normally assumes a characteristic position of flexion, adduction, and internal rotation of the hip. The greater trochanter appears quite prominent, and the knee of the dislocated extremity rests on the uninvolved extremity. If the hip dislocates anteriorly, the hip is held in abduction, external rotation, and slight flexion. The femoral head may be palpable anteriorly and the greater trochanter is less

prominent. A hip dislocation is easily recognized and requires medical attention immediately. The primary danger or complication of a hip dislocation is the possibility of damage to the blood supply to the head of the femur.

Even a partial dislocation or subluxation may interrupt the blood supply to the head and neck of the femur. If this happens, *avascular necrosis* can occur, which is death of the bone cells due to a deficient blood supply. This can lead to further cartilage degeneration. It is important to recognize this potential problem early. Any athlete who has limited motion of the hip and pain on weight bearing should be referred for further diagnostic examinations.

Fractures

✤ **Femur fracture.** Fractures to the femur as the result of athletic activity occur infrequently. The neck of the femur in young athletes is very resilient and rarely fractures. If the femoral neck is fractured by a violent force, the athlete usually assumes a characteristic position of external rotation and abduction of the thigh and exhibits shortening of the involved extremity and severe pain. This type of injury should be readily recognized and the athlete should be referred to medical attention.

Fractures to the shaft of the femur also occur infrequently during athletic activity. When they do occur, it is normally the result of a tremendous force, such as a violent direct blow, or excessive rotatory stress. Most of the time during a traumatic episode, the ankle, leg, or knee will give way before the femur fractures. When the femur is fractured, disability or loss of function is usually immediate, accompanied by a significant amount of pain. Because of the strength of the musculature surrounding the femur, bony displacement, causing an overriding of the bone fragments, may occur. This can cause a shortened limb on the fractured side. Additional signs and symptoms may include deformity or abnormal rotation of the thigh, swelling of the soft tissues, and shock. Athletes with fractured femurs should be immediately immobilized and referred to medical attention. Fracturing the shaft of the femur is a very serious injury that can be associated with life-threatening blood loss.

❖ **Pelvic fractures.** Fractures of the pelvis are not frequent athletic injuries. These fractures are more common in high-energy accidents such as those involving a vehicle or a snowmobile, or in hang gliding, or equestrian accidents. In addition to a history of a high-energy accident, pelvic fractures are associated with pain, swelling, and difficulty in weight-bearing.

❖ **Stress fractures.** Stress fractures of the pelvis and femur are relatively uncommon. Stress fractures of the pelvis are more common in women and usually occur at the junction of the ischium and the inferior pubic ramus. Symptoms often include pain in the perineal (pelvic floor) or groin area, increased with adduction and weight bearing. Stress fractures to the femur are more likely to occur to the neck of the femur rather than the shaft. The primary symptom is pain. Initially the pain may be related to stress and relieved by rest, but may become constant. Pain may be referred to the knee. There may also be some deep tenderness of the anterior aspect of the hip, slight limitation of motion, and discomfort in the extremes of movement. Unexplained pelvic of thigh pain, even with negative X-rays, should be watched closely for the possibility of a stress fracture.

❖ **Apophysitis.** The same mechanisms of injury that cause muscle strains in the adult athlete may cause avulsion of the apophysis in pediatric and adolescent athletes. These injuries are associated with separation of the cartilaginous tendon attachment from the bone before this junction is ossified. Several large muscle groups (such as the abdominals, iliopsoas, hip adductors, and hamstrings) insert or originate from about the innominate bone. In young athletes, these muscle attachments are particularly susceptible to avulsion injuries during sudden or violent muscle contractions. These attachments may completely avulse or only partially separate. Assessment is established clinically by palpating for tenderness and by

eliciting pain with the appropriate resistive movements. Because the amount of displacement is generally minimal, satisfactory healing can be expected with proper management.

❖ **Epiphyseal fractures.** In adolescent athletes, the epiphyses about the proximal femur may be fractured or separated. This can occur to the greater trochanteric epiphysis, in which part of the greater trochanter is completely or incompletely avulsed. Another area of epiphyseal plate fracture occurs to the capital femoral epiphysis in the head of the femur. This may occur in an adolescent athlete with an nonfused capital femoral epiphysis. The signs and symptoms associated with this type of an injury normally resemble those of a hip dislocation.

❖ **Slipped capital femoral epiphysis.** A slipped capital femoral epiphysis is not a true athletic injury. However, activity may exacerbate the symptoms in a predisposed athlete and the condition will present itself during athletics. Displacement or slippage of the femoral head on the femoral neck occurs as a result of a growth disturbance in the capital femoral epiphysis. This condition can be caused by apparently minor trauma as there is an existing mechanical weakening of the area. Frequently, pain associated with this type of condition is in the groin but may be referred to the knee or anterior thigh. There will also be pain and limitation to hip movements. A slipped capital femoral epiphysis occurs in preadolescent or adolescent athletes. Be highly suspicious of a young athlete complaining of groin, hip, or knee pain without an obvious cause. These athletes should be referred to a physician. Diagnosis of a slipped capital femoral epiphysis is made from radiographic examinations.

ATHLETIC INJURY ASSESSMENT PROCESS

Secondary survey ━━━━━━

Evaluation of a majority of athletic injuries involving the thigh or hip consists of identifying the injured muscle or muscles and assessing the degree of severity. Athletic injuries to the thigh occur frequently and are a source of obvious concern. This commonly injured area is often inadequately or poorly evaluated. Less painful thigh injuries are often ignored by both athlete and trainer, and athletic participation continues. Quite frequently, injuries may not be apparent to the athlete or reported until after activity, and often the significance of the injury is not known for 12 to 24 hours after the incident. In addition, many athletic trainers tend to push an athlete back into activity too quickly after a seemingly minor bruise or pull to the thigh muscles. All of these factors can lead to additional damage, increase the severity of the original injury, and promote chronic thigh injury problems.

History

The history phase of the assessment process will quickly determine if the injury is chronic or acute. Many thigh injuries have a high incidence of becoming chronic problems. Therefore question the athlete carefully concerning any previous injuries to the thigh or hip to determine if the current complaint is an aggravation or recurrence of a previous injury. If the area has been injured before, obtain as much information as possible about the nature of previous injuries, the treatment procedures used, and the extent of rehabilitation. Details are important. Are symptoms of the current injury similar to those of any previous injuries? Had symptoms completely subsided and full function been restored before the onset of the present injury? The more information gained concerning previous injuries, the better the evaluation will be of the nature and severity of the current problem. This type of information is also useful in establishing a treatment and rehabilitation program, if required.

Next question the athlete concerning the present injury. Was the onset gradual? Unfortunately, many thigh and hip injuries are not reported immediately. Injured athletes will often tolerate increasing soreness or tightness until, with continued activity, the symptoms become progressively worse and function is impaired. Only when the level of performance declines, or obvious symptoms such as limping or favoring an extremity are noted, is the injury reported and assessment initiated. Attempt to find out what has happened and how the symptoms have progressed since the athlete first noticed the injury. If the onset is sudden, the athlete will normally relate a sudden sharp pain and immediate loss of some functional ability. Have the athlete describe or demonstrate the mechanism of injury. Was there a direct blow delivered to the area, or did the injury result from forceful contraction or overstretching? This type of information is important in evaluating the nature of the injury and can indicate which anatomic structures may be involved.

Have the athlete describe any signs and symptoms associated with an injury to the thigh or hip as specifically as possible. Localization of pain is important. It is also important to determine when signs and symptoms occurred, if there has been any change, and what movements or motions affect them. The remainder of this section discusses the signs and symptoms that must be considered when evaluating thigh and hip injuries.

Ask the athlete to specifically locate and describe the pain. Are there any movements or activities that cause the pain to increase? This information will assist in identifying the structures involved and the actual extent of physical damage. It will also help differentiate among various injury types.

Is there a loss of motion, function, or strength associated with the thigh or hip injury? Loss in these three areas is normally caused by pain associated with the injury, swelling, or protective muscle spasms. Question the athlete about these areas because, later in the assessment process, each will be evaluated in more detail.

Also question the athlete about other sensations associated with the injury. Did he or she hear or feel anything at the time of injury, such as a popping or snapping sensation? When the injury results from a sudden explosive contraction of a muscle, the athlete may express the feeling of being kicked or hit at the time of injury. Ask if there are feelings of tightness or tension in the thigh, which may indicate swelling or muscle spasms. The athlete's descriptions of any sensations associated with the injury, as well as his or her impressions concerning the injury itself, should never be ignored. They often yield valuable information.

Observation

Observation begins as soon as you see the injured athlete. If the athlete is lying on the field or court, notice the alignment of the legs. Does the injured leg appear to be in an abnormal position? Is the athlete holding or rubbing a certain area of the hip or thigh? As you approach the injured athlete, notice his or her attitude and behavior concerning the injured area. If the athlete is moving around, notice the gait pattern. Does the athlete walk with a limp, favor the thigh or hip, or appear to have normal function at the hip and knee joints?

To conduct a complete inspection and continue the evaluation process, clothing and equipment should be removed from the thigh and hip area. Try to avoid causing any unnecessary embarrassment or discomfort.

In most cases it is not necessary to remove the athlete's shorts or underwear. The individual should be sitting or lying with both legs supported in an attempt to relax the muscles.

Carefully inspect the thigh and hip area for obvious signs of injury (Figure 19-16). Are there any signs of trauma, such as abrasions or contusions? Notice and compare the contours of both legs. Is there any sign of swelling, abnormal bumps, gaps, or loss of muscle definition or symmetry? Ask the athlete to contract both quadriceps muscles to compare the character of the muscle tone. Note any differences.

If you want to further evaluate the alignment of the lower extremity, have the athlete stand with his or her feet together and visually check the alignment from the front, back, and side. Look for any obvious malalignments, structural faults, or leg length discrepancies. This area of assessment was covered in detail in Chapter 17; refer to this segment of the text for a review of lower extremity alignment. Use the **Trendelenburg test** to assess the stability of the hip and the ability of the hip abductors to stabilize the pelvis on the femur. Ask the athlete to stand on one leg. Normally the pelvis on the op-

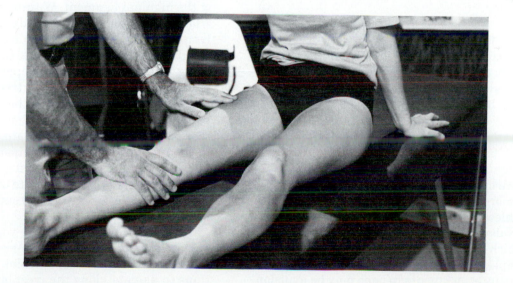

FIGURE 19-16
Inspecting the thigh and hip area for obvious signs of injury.

posite side should rise slightly. This indicates that the gluteus medius muscle on the supported side is functioning properly. However, if the pelvis on the unsupported side drops, a weak gluteus medius muscle or an unstable hip on the affected side is indicated. This is a positive **Trendelenburg sign.** An individual who has a weakened gluteus medius muscle will often exhibit a **Trendelenburg** or **abductor gait** when they walk. This is an exaggerated shift of the trunk toward the stance leg in an attempt to maintain the center of gravity closer to the base of support.

Physical Examination

The physical examination portion of the assessment process is used to perform a variety of procedures or maneuvers to complete a more detailed examination of the musculoskeletal system. Depending upon what your conception of the injury is up to this point in the assessment process, you may continue with any of the following techniques. Choose the specific tests or procedures that will assist in completing your assessment of the thigh and hip injury. Remember, if you have a significant injury, you may want to start your assessment with an evaluation of the neurovascular status of the leg.

Palpation

Palpation can further identify specific structures involved in the injury and locate pain and swelling. Palpation should be conducted with both legs supported and the muscles as relaxed as possible. If the muscles are relaxed you have a better opportunity to feel any palpable masses or deficits within the thigh and will be able to recognize the presence of localized muscle spasms. This is also a more comfortable position for the injured athlete. Because most thigh and hip injuries involve muscles, it is important to determine which area of the muscle is injured. For example, injuries involving the muscle or tendinous attachments to bone may be avulsion injuries and may require further evaluation or referral.

When the injury is on the anterior aspect of the thigh or hip, the athlete should be supine. The quadriceps muscle unit can then be palpated along its entire course. Locate areas of point tenderness and feel for any masses that may indicate bleeding or swelling. If the injury is severe, you may be able to palpate a gap in the muscle definition, which may indicate a rupture of muscle fibers. Always remember to compare any palpable lumps or deficits with the uninjured leg to note differences or similarities. This can be accomplished by observing and palpating both thighs at the same time to compare symmetry.

Palpate the groin area to locate point tenderness associated with a groin strain or related injury. Palpation is most effective when the heel of the injured leg is resting on the knee or shin of the uninjured leg (Figure 19-17). This position places the hip in flexion, abduction, and external rotation. Palpate the femoral triangle, the boundaries of which are the inguinal ligament (superiorly), the sartorius muscle (laterally), and the adductor longus muscle (medially). Palpate along the inguinal ligament from the anterior superior iliac spine to the pelvic tubercles (symphysis pubis). A swollen psoas bursa may be palpable about the midpoint of the inguinal ligament. Within the femoral triangle, you may want to palpate swollen lymph glands if infection is suspected. You should also be able to locate the femoral pulse. The femoral artery lies approximately in the center of the femoral triangle. The femoral nerve lies laterally to the artery and the femoral vein lies medial, but neither of these structures is easily palpated. Muscles in the groin are difficult to palpate individually, and resistive movements, described later in this chapter, are used to distinguish specific muscle or muscle group involvement.

While the athlete is supine, you can also palpate the bony rim of the pelvis. Begin at the anterior superior iliac spine and continue to palpate along the crest of the ilium (Figure 19-18). Remember, tenderness directly over the anterior superior iliac spine,

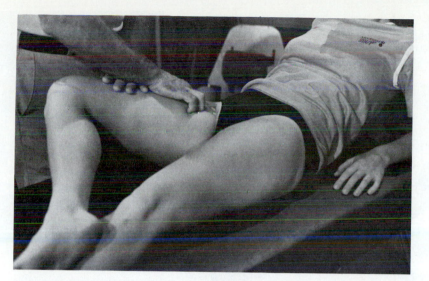

FIGURE 19-17
Palpating the groin musculature.

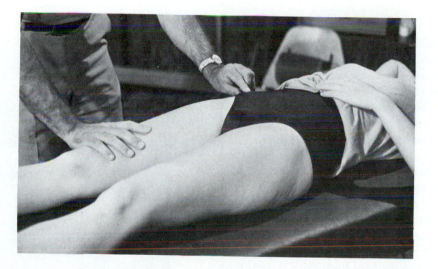

FIGURE 19-18
Palpating the anterior superior iliac spine.

especially in an adolescent athlete, may indicate an avulsion fracture. The iliac crest is subcutaneous and can be easily palpated along its entire length. Figure 19-19 illustrates palpation along the iliac crest following a direct blow to the area. It is easier to palpate the posterior portion of the iliac crest, as well as the posterior superior iliac spine, with the athlete lying on the uninjured side.

To palpate for injuries on the posterior aspect of the thigh or hip, the athlete should be lying prone. In this position, the hamstrings can be palpated along their entire course. Remember, it is easier to feel the hamstring insertions during mild resistance

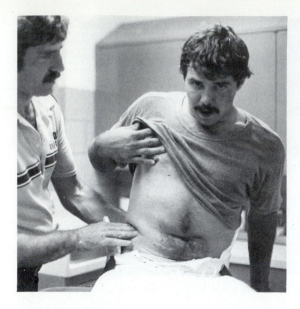

FIGURE 19-19
Palpating the iliac crest.

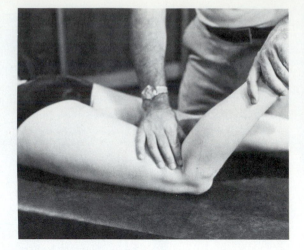

FIGURE 19-20
Palpating hamstring insertions.

to knee flexion (Figure 19-20). Proceed to locate areas of tenderness, as well as any palpable masses or deficits. Palpation can be continued to the origin of the hamstrings on the ischial tuberosity. If the injury involves the ischial tuberosity, the area can also be easily palpated with the athlete in the sidelying position. Tenderness directly over the ischial tuberosity may indicate ischial bursitis or possibly an avulsion fracture.

To place an injured athlete in a sidelying position, have him or her turn on to the uninjured side and bring the knee of the injured leg up toward the chest. In this position the posterior hip, including the gluteus maximus and gluteus medius, can easily be palpated. The greater trochanter of the femur can also be felt in this position (Figure 19-21). Tenderness directly over the greater trochanter may be indicative of trochanteric bursitis or a localized contusion.

Movement procedures

Because most athletic injuries to the thigh and hip involve the musculotendinous unit, the stress maneuvers used to evaluate the integrity of contractile elements are extremely important. Complete assessment of

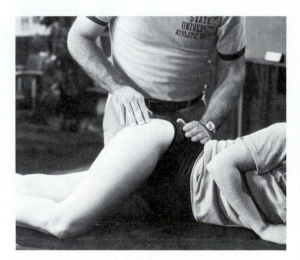

FIGURE 19-21
Palpating the greater trochanter.

injuries to the thigh and hip requires accurate interpretation of active, resistive, and functional movement tests. Correct interpretation of the results of these tests depends on a knowledge of the muscles involved and the types of movement each muscle or muscle group produces. An understanding of functional anatomy is essential

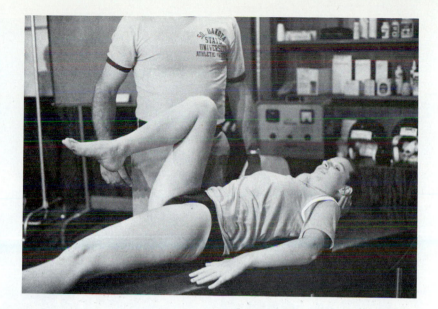

FIGURE 19-22
Athlete actively flexing hip and knee in a supine position.

for correct interpretation of stress procedures. Review the major muscles or muscle groups in this area and the movements produced by each.

Active movements. Evaluation of active movements at the hip and knee joints is extremely useful in assessing ROM. It is important to recognize any pain or discomfort with each movement. Instruct the athlete to perform each movement through as great an ROM as possible and to express any sensations or feelings he or she may experience. Refer to Figure 19-11 to review normal ROMs.

In the supine position, instruct the athlete to alternately pull each knee up to the chest (Figure 19-22). This movement permits evaluation of both hip and knee flexion at the same time. Compare the motion of the injured leg to that of the uninjured leg. Is the ROM limited or restricted? Does the athlete express any pain, discomfort, or other sensations during these movements? Evaluation of hip flexion with the knee extended is another active movement performed with the athlete in the supine position. This movement will give some indication of hamstring muscle flexibility. Remember to compare both sides.

To adequately evaluate the active range of movement of the knee joint, instruct the athlete to lie in the prone position and flex each knee, bringing the heel as close to the buttock as possible (Figure 19-23, *A*). Again, compare the ROM in each knee and ask the athlete to describe any pain or discomfort. The prone position is also used to evaluate hip extension. Instruct the athlete to lift each leg as high as possible, keeping the knee extended and fixed (Figure 19-23, *B*).

To evaluate active abduction of the hip, have the athlete lie on his or her uninjured side and raise the injured leg as high as possible (Figure 19-24) with the knee extended. To compare ROM, have the athlete switch sides and complete the same movement with the uninjured leg.

Resistive movements. Resistive movements are used to further evaluate the integrity of contractile tissues. Manual resistance against active motion can accurately identify specific painful areas, allowing one muscle to be differentiated from another. Resistive movements are also used to compare muscular strength between extremities. Resistive procedures are potentially the most informative maneuvers used in assessing muscle injuries, and the knowledge

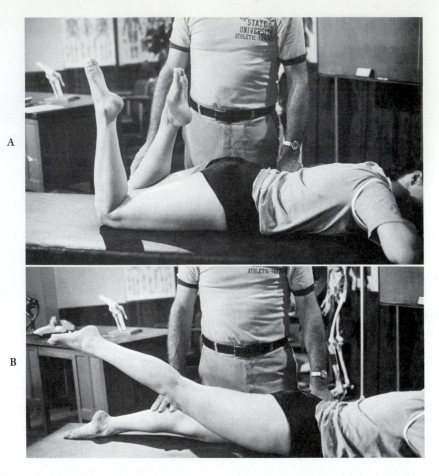

FIGURE 19-23
Active motion in a prone position. **A,** Knee flexion and, **B,** hip extension.

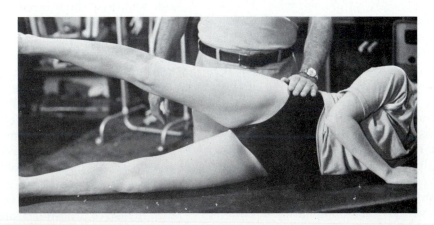

FIGURE 19-24
Athlete actively abducting the hip in a sidelying position.

gained during this part of the evaluation will indicate which muscles are involved.

When performing resistive movements, it is important that you explain exactly what you want the athlete to do, as well as how and what you are going to do in applying resistance. The procedures can be performed with the uninjured side first to make sure the athlete understands. The exercises should be controlled and limited by the athlete's tolerance. Resistance should initially be applied gently and the intensity increased according to the athlete's tolerance. If you begin the procedure using too much force or pressure, you may cause additional pain and discomfort, lose the athlete's cooperation, and possibly cause further damage.

When applying resistance, there should be just enough resistance against the movement to allow the athlete to complete the full ROM. Some resistive procedures call for an isometric exercise. In these cases the athlete is instructed to hold a certain position while resistance is applied. These maneuvers are probably less effective because the muscle is evaluated in only one position or length. Therefore whenever isometric resistive exercises are used, the involved joint should be placed in various positions to evaluate the muscles at different functional lengths.

To evaluate the integrity of the quadriceps, instruct the athlete, in a sitting position with the legs hanging over the side or edge of a table, to extend the knee as you apply resistance against the anterior aspect of the ankle (Figure 19-25, *A*). An alternate method is to apply an isometric resistance against extension, or attempt to flex the knee while the athlete is instructed to keep the knee straight and fixed, as described in Chapter 16.

To evaluate the integrity of the hamstrings, instruct the athlete to flex the knee as resistance is applied against the back of the ankle (Figure 19-25, *B*). An alternate method is to instruct the athlete to hold the knee in various degrees of flexion as you attempt to straighten the leg. Resistance can also be applied against the hamstrings with the athlete lying prone with instructions to flex the knee while resistance is applied to the back of the ankle.

The integrity of the hip flexors is easiest to evaluate in the sitting position. Instruct the athlete to bring the knee up toward his or her chest while resistance is applied on top of the knee (Figure 19-26, *A*). Again,

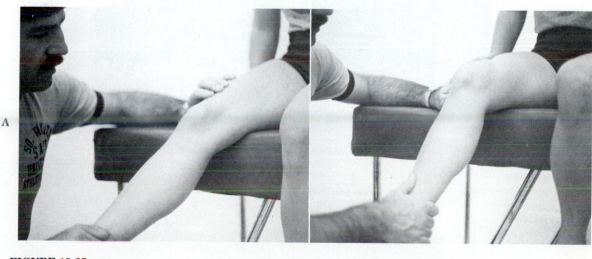

FIGURE 19-25
Applying resistance, to, **A,** knee extension to assist in evaluating integrity of the quadriceps and, **B,** to knee flexion to assist in evaluating integrity of the hamstrings.

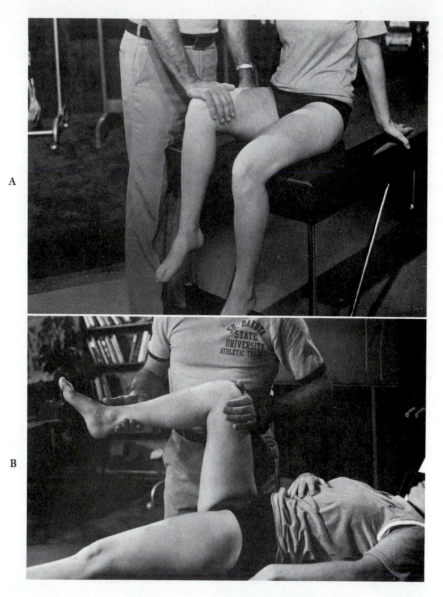

FIGURE 19-26
Applying resistance to hip flexion, **A,** in a sitting position and, **B,** in a supine position.

apply just enough resistance to allow slow movement. Resistance can also be applied against hip flexion while the athlete is lying supine, as described previously during active movements (Figure 19-26, *B*).

To evaluate the integrity of hip adductors, ask the athlete to bring both legs together while resistance is applied against the medial side of both knees (Figure 19-27). The hip abductors can be tested by instructing the athlete to spread both legs while resistance is applied against the lateral aspect of both knees (Figure 19-28). Both of these procedures can be performed with the athlete supine or in a sitting position.

An alternate method of testing the abductors and adductors is to have the athlete, in a sidelying position on the uninjured side, raise the leg upward while resistance is placed against the lateral aspect of the knee (Figure 19-29). If you are evaluating a hip pointer, pay particular attention to the exact location of pain caused by this movement. To test the hip adductors, have the athlete bring the legs together while resistance is applied to the medial aspect of both knees (Figure 19-30).

To evaluate the integrity of the hip extensors, instruct the athlete to lie in the prone position, and lift the leg as high as possible while resistance is applied against the posterior aspect of the thigh (Figure 19-31). To decrease the action of the hamstrings, have the athlete flex the knee during hip extension. Be sure that motion is taking place at the hip joint by stabilizing the pelvis. Occasionally an athlete will raise the pelvis using the lower back muscles in an attempt to substitute this motion for hip extension.

Passive movements. Passive movements are seldom necessary in evaluating thigh or hip injuries. However, sacroiliac and lumbosacral injuries may be associated with the hip. These injuries, and the pelvis, are discussed in Chapter 16. Occasionally, the ROM of the knee or hip is evaluated passively. These procedures involve the same positioning as described during active movements. The athlete is instructed to relax the muscles, and all motion is performed by the

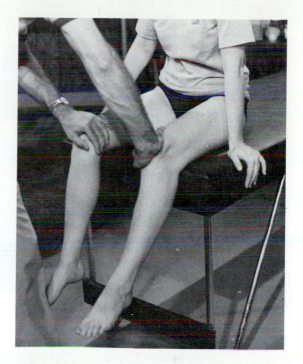

FIGURE 19-27
Applying resistance to hip adductors.

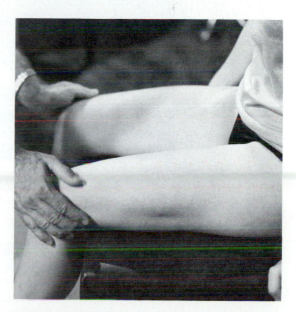

FIGURE 19-28
Applying resistance to hip abduction in a sitting position.

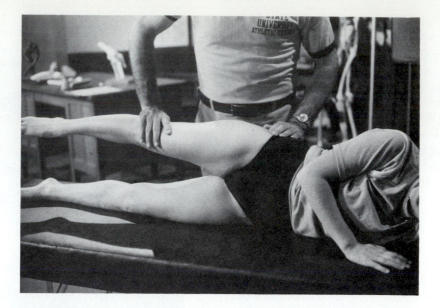

FIGURE 19-29
Applying resistance to hip abduction in a sidelying position.

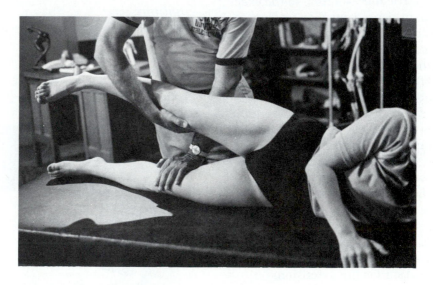

FIGURE 19-30
Applying resistance to hip abduction in a sidelying position.

athletic trainer. Caution must be exercised in performing these procedures because the tolerance level is no longer controlled by the athlete and additional damage could result.

Another passive procedure that may accompany hip injuries is the Ober's test. This test is used to evaluate tightness in the iliotibial band, especially when an iliotibial band friction syndrome or trochanteric bursitis is suspected. The Ober's test is described in the previous chapter and illustrated in Figure 18-28.

Functional movements. Functional movements are used to determine when an

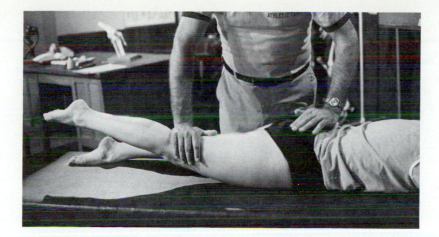

FIGURE 19-31
Applying resistance to hip extension in a prone position.

athlete with a thigh or hip injury can return
to full activity. As an athlete recovers from
a thigh or hip injury, information obtained
from functional exercises becomes increasingly important on each re-evaluation. The
intensity of functional activities should be
continually increased within the pain tolerance level and ROM limits. Limited athletic
activities can be performed until functional
performance of activities is at or near optimum capacity.

Neurological evaluations

Sensory functions. The athletic trainer
should be aware of the basic sensory distribution of the normal dermatomes, as well as
the cutaneous distribution of the various peripheral nerves in the thigh. The dermatomes in the thigh are L1, which lies immediately below the inguinal ligament and
covers the upper anterior position of the
thigh, L2 which supplies the lateral and anterior midthigh, and L3, which consists of an
oblique band immediately above the patella.
Posterior sensation of the thigh is supplied
by S2, which extends from the gluteal crease
to beyond the popliteal fossa (Figure 19-32).
Run your relaxed hands and fingers over the
pelvis and thigh anteriorly, posteriorly, and
laterally. Note any differences in sensations
and compare to the uninjured side.
  Motor functions. Motor functions have

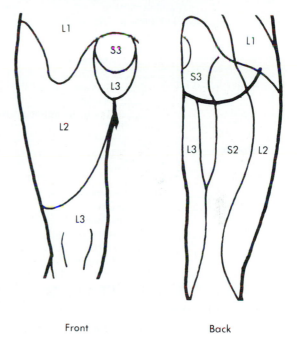

Front   Back

FIGURE 19-32
Dermatomes of the thigh and hip.

been discussed under active movements.
These procedures may occur early in the assessment process as you ask the athlete to
perform each movement of the knee and hip
through as great a ROM as possible. The primary myotomes of the thigh and hip are L1
hip adduction, L2 and L3 hip flexion and

Athletic Injury Assessment Checklist: Thigh and Hip Injuries

Secondary survey

_____ History
_____ Previous injuries
_____ Nature
_____ Treatment
_____ Rehabilitation
_____ Present injury
_____ Onset
_____ Sudden
_____ Gradual
_____ Mechanism of injury
_____ Signs and symptoms
_____ Pain
_____ Motion
_____ Function
_____ Strength
_____ Observation
_____ Gait pattern
_____ Function
_____ Alignment
_____ Signs of trauma
_____ Abrasions
_____ Contusions
_____ Contours
_____ Swelling
_____ Muscle definition or symmetry
_____ Physical examination

Palpation

_____ Tenderness
_____ Swelling
_____ Masses or deficits
_____ Muscle spasms
_____ Muscle involved
_____ Anterior thigh
_____ Groin
_____ Pelvic area
_____ Posterior thigh
_____ Posterior hip

Movement procedures

_____ Active movements
_____ ROM
_____ Pain
_____ Resistive movements
_____ Pain
_____ Strength
_____ Passive movements
_____ ROM
_____ Functional movements
_____ Functional activities

Neurological evaluations

_____ Sensory functions
_____ Motor functions

Circulatory evaluations

_____ Pulses

knee extension, L4 knee extension, L5 hip abduction and knee flexion, and S1 hip extension and knee flexion.

Reflexes. There are no reflexes about the hip that can be easily evaluated. Reflexes that are normally checked in the lower extremity are discussed in the previous two chapters.

Circulatory evaluations

As discussed in the previous two chapters, it is important to evaluate the adequacy of circulatory supply to the lower extremity with any major injury. With any significant injury to the thigh or hip, evaluate the circulation at or below the knee by feeling for a pulse. The popliteal (behind the knee), posterior tibial, or dorsalis pedis pulses may be used to evaluate the circulation. Absence of a pulse below the knee after a significant injury indicates an immediate need for referral of the athlete to a physician or medical facility.

Evaluation of Findings

Severe injuries, such as fractures of the femur or hip dislocations, are uncommon in athletic activities. These types of injuries can usually be identified readily, do not require extensive evaluative skills, and need immediate medical attention. Remember, young athletes may injure their epiphyseal plates or growth centers. These types of conditions must be recognized and the athletes referred to medical attention to avoid complications.

Most injuries involving the thigh and hip will require at least some of the preceding evaluative techniques for an accurate assessment. The responsibility of the athletic trainer is to determine which skeletal component, muscle, or muscle group is involved, as well as the severity of the injury. The athlete should be withheld from activity as long as he or she has a limited ROM or pain with exercise. Thigh and hip injuries require almost daily evaluation in order to monitor progress and decide when the athlete can return to full activity. Once an athlete demonstrates full pain-free function of the injured area, he or she may return to activity.

When to Refer the Athlete ...

Gross deformity or swelling
Significant loss of motion
Severe disability
Noticeable and palpable deficit in the muscle or tendon
Tenderness palpated at the bony attachments
Continued or severe pain in the hip
Thigh or hip injury that does not respond to treatment within 2 to 3 weeks
Any doubt regarding the severity or nature of the injury

When to refer the athlete

Many injuries to the thigh or hip may not require medical attention. Providing an accurate assessment has been made and standard guidelines are followed as to when an athlete can return to activity, many thigh or hip injuries can be cared for by the athletic trainer. Although severe injuries are uncommon, serious complications can arise from an improperly recognized and managed injury. Always keep a high index of suspicion when evaluating preadolescent and adolescent athletes. The criteria listed in the "When to Refer the Athlete ..." box can be used to determine if further medical attention is indicated.

REFERENCES

Arnheim DD, Prentice WE: *Principles of athletic training,* ed 8, St. Louis, 1993, Mosby.

Estwanik JJ, Sloane B, Rosenberg MA: Groin strain and other possible causes of groin pain, *Phys Sportsmed* 18(2):54, 1990.

Fricker PA, Taunton JE, Ammann W: Osteitis pubis in athletes: infection, inflammation or injury?, *Sports Med* 12(4):266, 1991.

Gallaspy JB: Evaluation of groin injuries, *Sports Med Update* 5(2):25, 1990.

Hoppenfeld S: *Physical examination of the spine and extremities,* New York, 1976, Appleton-Century-Crofts.

Kuland DN: *The injured athlete,* Philadelphia, 1982, Lippincott.

Magee DJ: *Orthopedic physical assessment,* ed 2, Philadelphia, 1992, Saunders.

Novak PJ, Bach BR, Schwartz JC: Diagnosing acute thigh compartment syndrome, *Phys Sportsmed* 20(11):100, 1992.

O'Donoghue DH: *Treatment of injuries to athletes,* ed 4, Philadelphia, 1984, Saunders.

Parris HG, Sallis RE, Anderson DV: Traumatic hip dislocation: reducing complications, *Phys Sportsmed* 21(5):67, 1993.

Post M: *Physical examination of the musculoskeletal system,* Chicago, 1987, Year Book Medical.

Rich BS, McKeag D: When sciatica is not disk disease: detecting pirifirmis syndrome in active patients, *Phys Sportsmed* 20(10):105, 1992.

Sothmayd W, Hoffman M: *Sports health, the complete book of athletic injuries,* New York, 1981, Quick Fox.

SUGGESTED READINGS

Agre JC: Hamstring injuries, proposed aetiological factors, prevention, and treatment, *Sports Med* 2(1):21, 1985. *Discusses many factors concerning hamstring injuries, including anatomy, biomechanics of running, etiology, and treatment.*

Combs JA: Myositis ossificans traumatica, pathogenesis and management, *Ath Train* 22(3):193, 1987. *Reviews the recent research conducted on myositis ossificans and discusses treatment of this condition.*

Lindenberg G and others: Iliotibial band friction syndrome in runners, *Phys Sportsmed* 12(5):118, 1984. *Thirty-six distance runners suffering from iliotibial band friction syndrome were treated and observed for at least 1 year. Several etiological factors were identified, and conservative treatments for most cases were suggested.*

Martinez SF, Steingard MA, Steingard PM: Thigh compartment syndrome: a limb-threatening emergency, *Phys Sportsmed* 21(3):94, 1993.
Discusses acute and chronic thigh compartment syndrome and the importance of early diagnosis.

Smith RL and others: A survey of overuse and traumatic hip and pelvic injuries in athletes, *Phys Sportsmed* 13(10):131, 1985.
Analyzes different factors involved in hip and pelvic injuries.

Waters PM, Millis MB: Hip and pelvis injuries in the young athlete, *Clin Sports Med* 7(3):513, 1988.
Discusses the common hip and pelvic injuries occurring in the young athlete and the management of these injuries.

Whiteside JA, Andrews JR: On the field evaluation of common athletic injuries: Part IV: evaluation of the thigh and hip, *Sports Med Update* 6(2):17, 1991.
Discusses a variety of athletic injuries and conditions that can occur to the thigh and hip.

UNIT VI

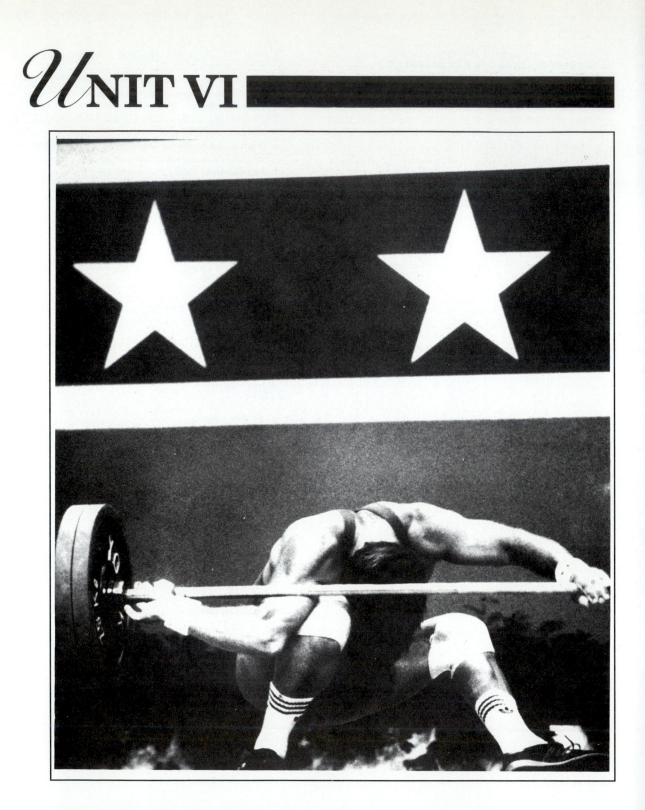

Athletic Injuries of the Upper Extremities

The final unit of this text is concerned with athletic injuries or conditions involving the upper extremities. The upper extremities play a vital role in athletic activity and present a unique assessment challenge to the athletic trainer. Injuries to the upper extremities seldom involve a single anatomic structure or affect an isolated functional ability. As a result, complete and accurate assessment of injuries in this complex, highly mobile, and relatively unstable area will tax the skill and expertise of even the most seasoned athletic trainer. Upper extremity injuries occur less frequently than injuries to the knee, ankle, and foot. The result is a reduced frequency of assessment in this area compared to the high incidence of evaluations performed on the lower extremity area. Because of the importance of the upper extremities in athletic activity, athletic trainers, and especially students of athletic training, must devote considerable time and effort to develop or retain proficiency in evaluation procedures. Practice and frequent review of skills is essential.

20   Shoulder injuries
21   Elbow and forearm injuries
22   Hand and wrist injuries

CHAPTER 20

Shoulder injuries

After you have completed this chapter, you should be able to:
- Identify the basic anatomy of the shoulder complex.
- Identify the common athletic injuries that may occur to each of the structures about the shoulder.
- Describe the assessment process for an athlete suffering an injury to the shoulder.
- Explain the various manipulative procedures used to evaluate injuries and conditions about the shoulder.
- List the signs and symptoms that would indicate an athlete suffering a shoulder injury should be referred to medical assistance.

The shoulder is more than simply the juncture of the arm and torso or the articulation between the humerus and the glenoid cavity. The shoulder encompasses all of the intricate arm-trunk mechanisms, including the elaborate anatomic and functional interrelationships between the thorax, clavicle, scapula, and humerus. This area is usually referred to as the shoulder girdle or complex. Each area or portion comprising the shoulder girdle plays an important role in the coordinated movements of the arm. Each of these areas must function properly, both separately and as a unit, for the shoulder complex to function smoothly. Because of the synchronous movements required for normal shoulder function, an athletic injury to any one area of the shoulder may cause impaired function of all areas. Therefore, to perform a comprehensive assessment of shoulder injuries, athletic trainers must possess a sound knowledge of the functional anatomy of the shoulder girdle and an understanding of its complex movements.

ANATOMY OF THE SHOULDER

To become proficient in the assessment of injuries to the shoulder and related areas, reviewing the anatomic structures is required. Begin by reviewing the surface anatomy in Figure 20-1. The major skeletal components of the shoulder are reviewed in Figure 20-2. Pay particular attention to the bony landmarks. Understanding the complexities of the sternoclavicular, acromioclavicular, and glenohumeral joints, the bony components, and associated ligaments and muscles is particularly important. In addition to the anatomy of the shoulder complex, a brief summary of common athletic injuries and conditions, along with mechanisms of

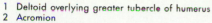

1 Deltoid overlying greater tubercle of humerus
2 Acromion
3 Acromioclavicular joint
4 Acromial end of clavicle
5 Trapezius
6 Supraclavicular fossa
7 Infraclavicular fossa
8 Upper margin of pectoralis major
9 Anterior margin of deltoid
10 Deltopectoral groove and cephalic vein
11 Lower margin of pectoralis major
12 Serratus anterior
13 Biceps
14 Areola
15 Nipple

A

B

FIGURE 20-1
Surface anatomy of the right shoulder. **A,** Anterior
view and, **B,** posterior view.

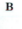

1 Trapezius
2 Acromial end of clavicle
3 Acromioclavicular joint
4 Acromion
5 Deltoid
6 Level of axillary nerve behind humerus
7 Triceps
8 Latissimus dorsi
9 Inferior angle of scapula
10 Teres major
11 Infraspinatus
12 Spine of scapula
13 Vertebral border of scapula

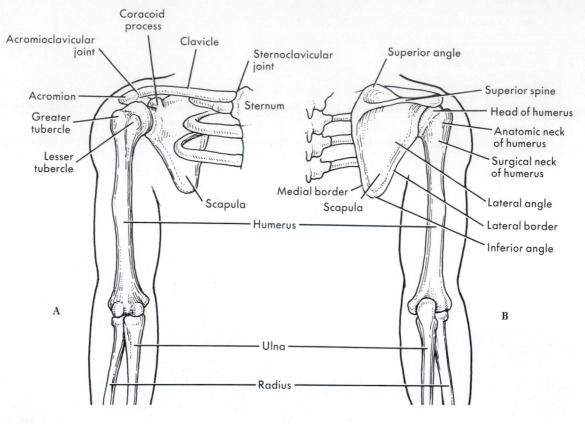

FIGURE 20-2
Skeletal components for right shoulder and arm. **A,** Anterior view and, **B,** posterior view.

injury is discussed in order to provide the athletic trainer with greater insight during the evaluation process.

Sternoclavicular Joint

The sternoclavicular joint is composed of the sternal end of the clavicle, the cartilage of the first rib, and the uppermost portion, or manubrium, of the sternum. The joint is surrounded by a loose articular capsule that is lined with a synovial membrane and attached to the margins of the articulating bones. This articular capsule is reinforced by the anterior and posterior *sternoclavicular ligaments*. An important accessory ligament that plays a role in limiting clavicular movements is the *costoclavicular ligament*. This dense band of fibers passes upward from the first rib to attach to the lower surface of the sternal end of the clavicle.

The thick *interclavicular ligament* (Figure 20-3) strengthens the superior aspect of the joint capsule. It stretches from clavicle to clavicle across the upper surface of the capsule, where it attaches to the suprasternal, or jugular, notch. Comparative anatomists often compare this ligamentous band to the wishbone of a bird. It plays an important role in stabilizing both the right and left sternoclavicular joints. The sternoclavicular joint space is divided into two synovial cavities by a flat, circular articular disc of fibrocartilage. When the shoulder is elevated or depressed, the clavicle moves on the articular disc, which exerts a cushioning effect to the forces that are transmitted from the upper extremity.

Athletic injuries to the sternoclavicular joint occur infrequently. However, this synovial joint is critically important because it

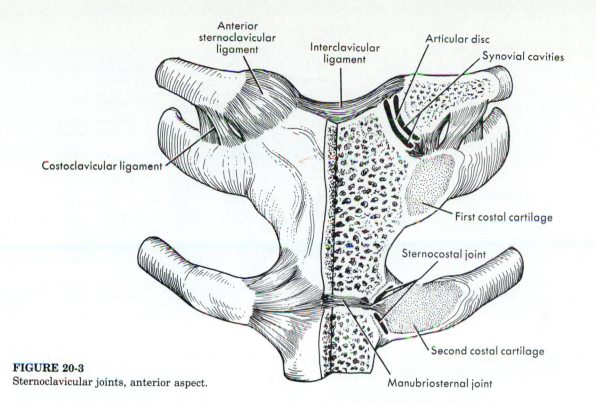

FIGURE 20-3
Sternoclavicular joints, anterior aspect.

is the only bony attachment between the upper limb and the axial skeleton. The articulation between the clavicle and sternum is actually the pivot point about which movements of the shoulder as a whole occur.

Acromioclavicular Joint

The acromioclavicular joint is the articulation between the lateral end of the clavicle and the medial margin of the **acromion** process of the scapula (Figure 20-4). This small synovial joint permits a limited amount of rotation and numerous gliding movements. The long axis of the joint lies in an antero-posterior direction. The placement of the clavicle is normally higher than the acromion at the point of articulation; as a result, a slope exists between the surfaces, which tends to predispose displacement of the acromion downward and under the clavicle when a blow is delivered to the tip of the shoulder.

The articular surfaces of the joint are covered with fibrocartilage. In addition, a wedge-shaped articular disc of shock-absorbing cartilage is found in the joint space.

The disc does not, however, divide the space into two separate synovial cavities as in the sternoclavicular joint. A synovial membrane lines the relatively loose-fitting articular capsule, which completely surrounds the joint. The capsule is strengthened by the short *acromioclavicular ligament* extending between the lateral tip of the clavicle and the adjoining portion of the acromion over the superior aspect of the joint. The joint capsule and acromioclavicular ligament play only a minor role in holding the clavicle and scapula together. However, because they are richly supplied by sensory nerves, an injury to these structures is painful.

The *coracoclavicular ligament* plays the most important role in preventing separation of the clavicle from the scapula. This very strong ligament is divided into two components, the *trapezoid* and *conoid* ligaments. The flat, quadrilateral trapezoid ligament passes upward and laterally (in front) from coracoid process to the clavicle. The triangular conoid ligament passes downward and medially (behind) from the clavicle to the

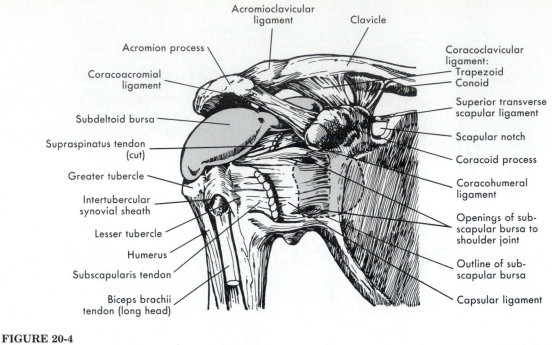

FIGURE 20-4
Right shoulder joint, anterior aspect.

base of the coracoid process. The conoid portion of the ligament restrains backward movement of the scapula, whereas the trapezoid portion prevents excessive forward displacement. If the coracoclavicular ligament is torn, displacing forces acting on the shoulder can cause the acromion to be forced down and away from the clavicle.

Glenohumeral Joint

The shoulder (glenohumeral) joint is a synovial (diarthrotic) joint of the ball-and-socket variety (Figure 20-4). Recall from Chapter 4 that ball-and-socket type diarthroses are multiaxial joints that have two or more axes of rotation and permit movement in three or more planes. The shoulder, our most mobile joint, allows all types of movement and has three axes around which these actions occur: transverse (flexion and extension), anteroposterior (abduction and adduction), and vertical (medial and lateral rotation). The components of the shoulder joint include the large head of the humerus and the much smaller adjacent glenoidal

surface of the scapula, the glenoid labrum, the fibrous articular capsule lined with synovial membrane, and the coracohumeral, glenohumeral, transverse, and coracoacromial ligaments.

The disparity in size between the large and nearly hemispheric head of the humerus and the much smaller and shallow glenoid cavity of the scapula is of great clinical significance to the athletic trainer. Because the head of the humerus is over two times larger than the shallow glenoid concavity that receives it, only about one-quarter of the articular surface of the humeral head is in contact with the fossa in any given position of the joint. This anatomic fact helps explain the inherent instability of the shoulder joint. The stability and function of the shoulder are so interrelated, many problems of the shoulder are related to instability. The glenohumeral joint is particularly vulnerable because of the tremendous stresses that athletic activity places on its stabilizing mechanisms. The static stabilizers of the shoulder are the ligaments, joint capsule, and glenoid

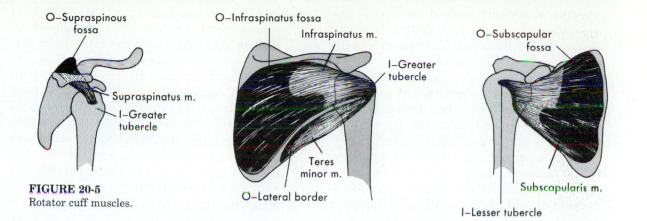

FIGURE 20-5
Rotator cuff muscles.

labrum. The dynamic stabilizers are the rotator cuff and adjacent muscles.

The *glenoid labrum* is a triangular ring of fibrocartilage attached to the margin of the glenoid cavity. Although the labrum helps deepen the concavity, its stabilizing effect on the joint is minimal. This ring of fibrocartilage can split or tear, giving rise to loose pieces within the joint that may cause catching, clicking, or locking with movement of the shoulder. Disruption of the glenoid labrum is a common lesion in recurrently dislocating shoulders. Anterior labrum damage is usually associated with an injury in which the shoulder is forcefully abducted, extended, and outwardly rotated. Posterior labrum damage is usually associated with an injury in which a force is applied to the humerus in the direction of its longitudinal axis while the shoulder is in 90° of flexion. Athletes are generally able to state whether the symptoms are anterior or posterior and relate them to certain positions or activities. Athletes may describe their shoulders as weak, loose, "slipping out of place," or catching. A painful click or discomfort is due to either the humeral head subluxing out of the confines of the glenoid fossa or the torn labrum fragment moving between the opposing articular surfaces.

A thin articular capsule surrounds the shoulder joint. It is attached above to the edge of the glenoid fossa and below to the anatomic neck of the humerus. The capsule is extremely loose and does not function to keep the articulating bones of the joint in contact. This fact is obviously correlated with the great ROM possible at this articulation. The tendons of the supraspinatus, infraspinatus, teres minor, and subscapularis muscles (called the SITS muscles) all blend with and strengthen the articular capsule. They fuse with the capsule near its distal margin. The musculotendinous cuff resulting from the blending of these muscle tendons with the fibrous joint capsule is called the **rotator cuff** because these muscles are also important in rotation at the shoulder. The supraspinatus is primarily an abductor of the arm. The infraspinatus and teres minor muscles are external rotators attached to the greater tuberosity. The subscapularis is an internal rotator attached to the lesser tuberosity. The rotator cuff provides the necessary strength to help prevent anterior, superior, and posterior displacement of the humeral head during most types of activity. Review the placement and points of attachment of these muscles in Figure 20-5.

A unique relationship exists between the articular capsule of the shoulder joint, the tendon of the long head of the biceps muscle, and the synovial lining of the capsule. The tendon is within the substance of the capsule (intracapsular) but outside the actual joint cavity. The tendon invaginates the lining of the cavity until it is surrounded by the synovial membrane. The membrane then fuses over the tendon and encloses it in a tubular sheath, which surrounds it during its passage through the bicipital (intertubercular) groove of the humerus. The transverse ligament of the joint creates a canal for the tendon by bridging the groove between the greater and lesser tubercles. The distal segment of this ligament then arches over the tendon as it emerges from the capsule. The result is a continuous tubular sheath of synovial membrane that covers the long head of the biceps tendon from its point of origin and is continuous above with the general synovial lining of the joint and extends distally to the surgical neck of the humerus. It is important to understand that fusion of the synovial membrane "tube" around the tendon prevents infectious material, which can migrate along the surface of the tendon, from gaining access to the true joint space unless the membrane ruptures. This fact explains how a case of tenosynovitis can seemingly pass through the shoulder without infecting the joint space.

The *coracohumeral ligament* is a broad band that strengthens the upper portion of the joint capsule. Fibers from this ligament blend with the tendon of the supraspinatus muscle. As the name implies, it extends from the coracoid process of the scapula to the humerus.

The *glenohumeral ligament* is actually a strengthening band within the joint capsule that can be separated into three components: the superior, middle, and inferior glenohumeral ligaments. All three extend from the anterior glenoid margin and radiate into the anterior wall of the capsule.

The *coracoacromial ligament* is actually a ligament of the scapula; however, it is often described as a component of the shoulder joint and classified as an accessory ligament of this joint. It is a strong triangular band that is attached to the entire length of the lateral border of the coracoid process and to the tip of the acromion. Together with the acromion and coracoid process this ligament forms an arch above the head of the humerus and helps to protect the joint. It is in contact with the deltoid muscle above and the infraspinatus muscle below. The subdeltoid bursa lies wedged between this liga-

ment and the superior surface of the joint capsule below and the deltoid muscle above (Figure 20-4). Although the interior, or cavity, of this bursa may occasionally be connected with or open directly into the joint space, it usually does not. There are several additional bursae associated with muscles around the shoulder in addition to the subdeltoid. A bursa that does communicate with the joint space occurs deep to the subscapularis muscle. There is a bursa between the joint capsule and the infraspinatus muscle, whereas others are found between the coracoid process and the capsule, behind the coracobrachialis muscle, between the tendon of the subscapularis and the capsule, and one in front of and another behind the tendon of the latissimus dorsi muscle.

Any of these bursae can become inflamed and painful as a result of overuse or trauma to the area. The subdeltoid bursa is the most often affected. As it becomes aggravated, normally from friction, its lining often thickens, thus increasing pressure and in some cases creating a fold in the lining. This causes rough movement and possibly a snap as the humerus moves. Symptoms include tenderness just distal to the acromion and pain on active motion of the shoulder, especially abduction and rotation. This can accompany an impingement syndrome, which is described later.

Total motion of the shoulder is the sum of motion at two areas: the glenohumeral joint and the gliding of the scapula on the thorax (scapulothoracic). The scapula may not move much during the initial movements of shoulder flexion or abduction. However, once the arm gets above a certain degree of movement, the humerus and scapula move continuously and synchronously at approximately a 2:1 ratio. This has been described as the *scapulohumeral rhythm.*

Shoulder Muscles

The principle muscles of importance in moving the shoulder joint and their actions and innervations are listed in Table 20-1. Points of attachment and relationships between individual muscles in the shoulder girdle or joint are shown in Figures 20-5 to 20-13.

TABLE 20-1

Muscles of the Shoulder

Muscle	Nerve	Segmental innervation	Primary action(s)
Trapezius	Accessory	Cranial XI	Retract and upward rotate scapula (upper fibers—elevate and lower fibers—depress)
Levator scapulae	C_3 and C_4 nerve roots		Elevate and downward rotate scapula
Rhomboids	Dorsal scapular	C_5	Retract, elevate, and downward rotate scapula
Serratus anterior	Long thoracic	C_5-C_7	Depress, protract, and upward rotate scapula
Supraspinatus	Suprascapular	C_5, C_6	Abduct arm
Infraspinatus	Suprascapular	C_5, C_6	Outward rotate arm
Teres minor	Axillary	C_5, C_6	Outward rotate arm
Subscapularis	Subscapular	C_5, C_6	Inward rotate arm
Teres major	Subscapular	C_5, C_6	Extend and inward rotate arm
Deltoid	Axillary	C_5, C_6	Middle fibers—abduct arm Anterior fibers—flex and inward rotate arm Posterior fibers—extend and outward rotate arm
Pectoralis major (upper fibers)	Lateral pectoral	C_5-C_7	Adduct, flex, and inward rotate arm
Pectoralis major (lower fibers)	Medial pectoral	C_8, T_1	Adduct, extend, and inward rotate arm
Pectoralis minor	Medial pectoral	C_8, T_1	Depress scapula
Latissimus dorsi	Thoracodorsal	C_6-C_8	Adduct, extend, and inward rotate arm
Biceps	Musculocutaneous	C_5, C_6	Flexion of arm
Coracobrachialis	Musculocutaneous	C_5-C_7	Flexion and adduct arm
Triceps	Radial	C_5-C_8	Extend arm

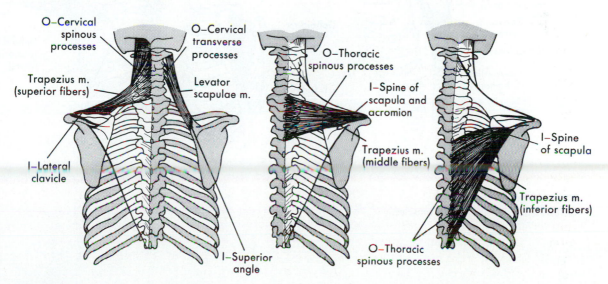

FIGURE 20-6
Trapezius and levator scapulae muscles.

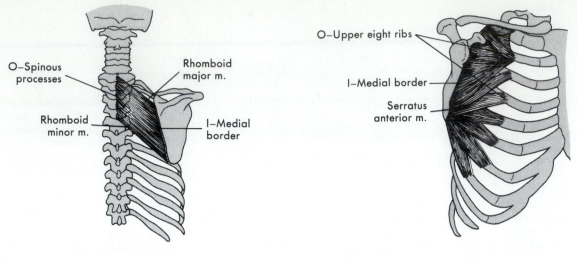

FIGURE 20-7
Rhomboid major and minor muscles.

FIGURE 20-8
Serratus anterior muscle.

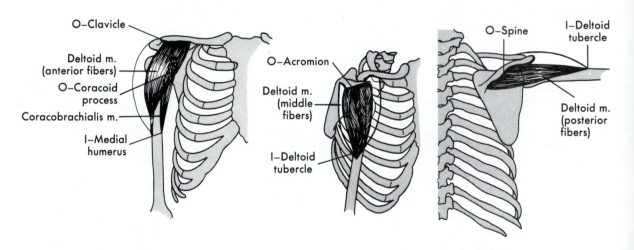

FIGURE 20-9
Deltoid and coracobrachialis muscles.

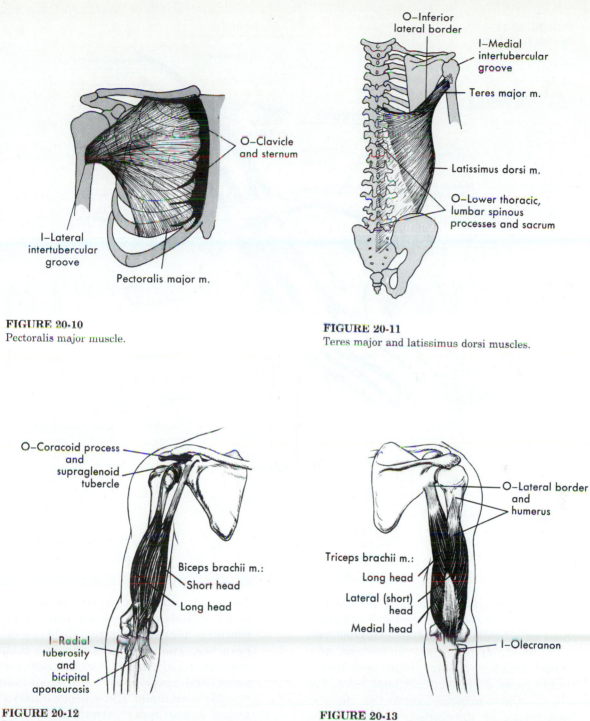

FIGURE 20-10
Pectoralis major muscle.

O—Inferior
lateral border

I—Medial
intertubercular
groove

Teres major m.

Latissimus dorsi m.

O—Lower thoracic,
lumbar spinous
processes and sacrum

O—Clavicle
and sternum

I—Lateral
intertubercular
groove

Pectoralis major m.

FIGURE 20-11
Teres major and latissimus dorsi muscles.

O—Coracoid process
and
supraglenoid
tubercle

Biceps brachii m.:

Short head

Long head

I—Radial
tuberosity
and
bicipital
aponeurosis

FIGURE 20-12
Biceps brachii muscle.

O—Lateral border
and
humerus

Triceps brachii m.:

Long head

Lateral (short)
head

Medial head

I—Olecranon

FIGURE 20-13
Triceps brachii muscle.

FIGURE 20-14
The brachial plexus.

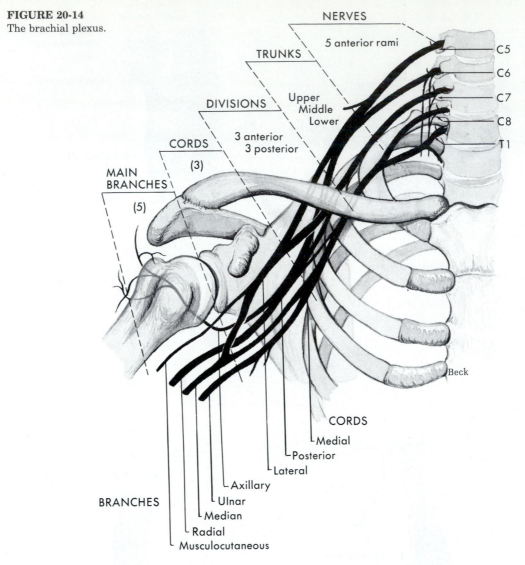

NERVES

5 anterior rami

TRUNKS

Upper
Middle
Lower

DIVISIONS

3 anterior
3 posterior

CORDS

(3)

MAIN
BRANCHES

(5)

C5
C6
C7
C8
T1

Beck

CORDS

Medial
Posterior
Lateral

Axillary
Ulnar
Median
Radial
Musculocutaneous

BRANCHES

Remember, if the position of the upper extremity is markedly changed or if the arm is held in a flexed, rotated, or extended position, points of reference change and additional muscles assume important and in many cases differing functional roles. Further, other muscles serve as fixators, synergists, or antagonists in the various movements. A detailed explanation of the complex array of specialized movements possible at the shoulder girdle and joint is beyond the scope of this text. Interested students should refer to specialized texts in kinesiology and biomechanics.

Brachial Plexus

The most important nerves involved in the axilla and shoulder are components of the brachial plexus (Figure 20-14) and its branches. The brachial plexus is a complex network consisting of nerves, trunks, divisions, and main branches that ultimately provide both motor and sensory innervation to the entire upper extremity. Pressure to this nerve plexus or its accompanying blood vessels can produce serious injury.

Anatomic Relationships

The principal anatomic structures in relation to the shoulder joint and articular cap-

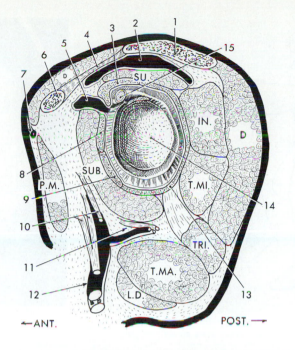

FIGURE 20-15

Relations of the left shoulder joint; *D* deltoid, (*SU.*) supraspinatus, (*IN.*) infraspinatus, (*P.M.*) pectoralis major, (*SUB.*) subscapularis (*T.MI.*) teres minor, (*T.MA.*) teres major, (*TRI.*) long head of triceps brachii, (*L.D.*) latissimus dorsi, (*1*) acromion, (*2*) subcromial bursa, (*3*) superior glenohumeral ligament, (*4*) coracoacromial ligament, (*5*) subscapular bursa, (*6*) coracoid process of scapula, (*7*) cephalic vein, (*8*) middle glenohumeral ligaments, (*9*) inferior glenohumeral ligament, (*10*) parts of brachial plexus and its branches, (*11*) axillary nerve and posterior humeral circumflex vessels traversing quadrilateral space, (*12*) axillary vessels, (*13*) capsular ligament, (*14*) glenoid cavity, and (*15*) biceps tendon and synovial sheaths.

sule are illustrated in Figure 20-15. They are, above, subacromial bursa, supraspinatus muscle, acromion and coracoacromial ligament; in front, subscapular bursa and subscapularis muscle; behind, teres minor muscle, infraspinatus muscle and its bursa; below, long head of the triceps brachii muscle, teres major muscle, and the inferior portion of the subscapularis muscle. Note how the supraspinatus, infraspinatus, teres minor, and subscapularis muscles serve to support the joint and help hold the articular surfaces of the joint against one another.

INJURIES TO THE SHOULDER

A variety of athletic injuries can occur to the shoulder joint. Because of the extensive motion available and the inherent instability of the shoulder joint, this area of the body is very vulnerable to acute athletic injuries and chronic overuse conditions. The mechanisms causing most injuries to the shoulder are direct trauma, indirect trauma, or throwing movements. Direct trauma occurs because the shoulder is the portion of the anatomy best suited for forcible ramming, such as tackling in football or checking in ice hockey. This exposes the shoulder to direct contact. Athletes who are falling or being tackled may also land on their shoulder, which can result in direct trauma to the shoulder complex. Indirect trauma can occur as injurious forces are transmitted to the shoulder joint or the entire shoulder complex through the humerus as the result of direct trauma to the hand or elbow. Examples of indirect trauma to the shoulder girdle are athletes landing on an outstretched

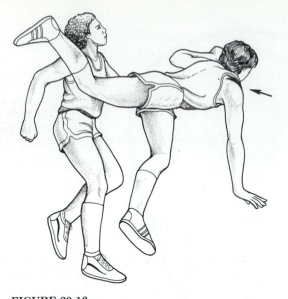

FIGURE 20-16
Mechanism of injury to shoulder complex. Injurious forces are transferred to shoulder area as athlete falls on an outstretched arm.

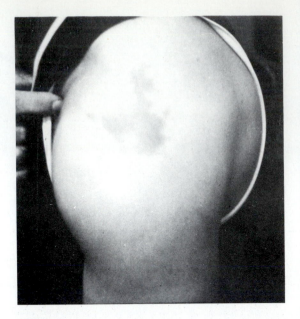

FIGURE 20-17
Contusion injury. Note discoloration over tip of the shoulder (shoulder pointer).

hand or the point of a flexed elbow (Figure 20-16). Participants in all athletic activity are subject to falls that can cause an indirect insult to the shoulder. Attempts to break a fall frequently result in indirect shoulder trauma. Athletic injuries also occur frequently as a result of throwing movements. This includes all sports requiring throwing or swinging motions of the shoulder. Injuries resulting from any of these mechanisms can be acute, including contusions, sprains, strains, dislocations, and occasionally fractures and chronic conditions. The athletic trainer must also consider the accessory structures that support the shoulder (that is, muscles that stabilize the scapula) when evaluating the shoulder complex because injury to any of these structures will influence ROM.

Contusions

The most common contusion about the shoulder is to the tip of the shoulder or acromion process (Figure 20-17). This is commonly called a **shoulder pointer.** A shoulder pointer implies a contusion with no ligamentous involvement. With this injury, the athletic trainer must be concerned with a more serious injury to the acromioclavicular joint. Accurately locate areas of tenderness and carefully examine the area to determine if there is any involvement of the acromioclavicular joint. The deltoid muscle is also susceptible to direct blows, which can result in contusions to the area. A possible complication of repeated contusions to the region of the deltoid attachment on the lateral humerus is a painful periostitis, which can develop into an irritative **exostosis** or spur formation sometimes referred to as a

✦ **blocker's spur.**

Contusions to the shaft of the clavicle can occur during athletic activity as this bone is subcutaneous and subject to direct trauma to the area. Clavicular contusions will cause tenderness and swelling at the site of injury but normally little increase in pain with shoulder motion.

Strains

A common injury about the shoulder joint is some type of muscular or musculotendinous strain. The glenohumeral joint relies on the surrounding musculature for most of its stability, as well as its motion and power. Therefore the muscles and musculotendinous structures are involved in many types of athletic injuries. Various mechanisms can produce injuries to the musculotendinous units, including overstretching, violent contractions, and repetitive use.

Strains about the shoulder are especially common in athletic activities that require the arm to propel an object, such as pitching, or to overcome a resistance, such as in swimming. During racquet sports the shoulder serves as the fulcrum for the arm, and major stresses are placed on the elbow and forearm. However, significant and often injurious forces are also placed on the shoulder joint. Each sport presents its own problems or situations for the shoulder, and the responses to stress vary in intensity and location. The nature of shoulder strains is influenced by many things, such as the age and maturity of the athlete; the type and weight of the object being propelled; the type of delivery; the presence of weakness, fatigue, or incoordination; fibrous scarring or degenerative changes from previous injuries; and microtrauma from repetitive activity. All of these factors must be considered during the assessment of shoulder injuries.

In evaluating an injury to the many muscles that attach and function about the shoulder, attempt to locate as precisely as possible the area of local tenderness and correlate this information with pain elicited on active contraction or passive stretching of the involved muscle. Because most muscles about the shoulder function during more than one movement, a basic knowledge of the functional anatomy of the area is necessary to isolate each muscle suspected of being injured. Evaluation techniques for the muscles most frequently injured are discussed in the assessment portion of this chapter.

✤   **Rotator cuff strains.** Injuries involving the rotator cuff muscles are difficult to detect and isolate because these muscles, which reinforce the joint capsule, lie deep in the shoulder. Any of the mechanisms previously described can cause an injury to these muscles; however, when they occur in young athletes the problem is normally the result of direct trauma. As an athlete becomes older, he or she is more susceptible to rotator cuff injuries resulting from repeated stress. Repetitive use of the shoulder can result in microscopic damage to the rotator cuff muscles. A great deal of difficulty may be encountered in assessing these soft tissue lesions. Bursitis, tendinitis, partial rotator cuff tears, loose pieces of fibrocartilage, and calcific deposits are all capable of producing similar signs and symptoms.

✤   **Biceps strain.** Another relatively common strain in the shoulder occurs to the long head of the biceps tendon. This is especially true in athletes who are skiing, throwing overhand, or playing tennis. As previously discussed, the long head of the biceps tendon lies in a tubular sheath as it passes through the bicipital groove. Repetitive motion of the shoulder causes this tendon to slide up and down through the tunnel. The irritation of constant motion can cause an inflammatory

✤   reaction. This **bicipital tenosynovitis** causes tenderness along the bicipital groove and pain on active and resistive contraction or passive stretching of the biceps.

✤   **Dislocation\subluxation of the biceps tendon.** Dislocation or partial dislocation (subluxation) of the biceps tendon from its tunnel may occur with limited rupture or tears of the transverse ligament or the rotator cuff, especially the subscapularis tendon. In these cases, arm movement that involves external rotation of the humerus will cause sudden pain and a locking sensation accompanied by an audible click in the shoulder. The athletic trainer will usually be able to feel displacement or crepitus by applying finger pressure over the bicipital groove during external rotation of the humerus. Repeated or recurrent subluxation or dislocation requires surgical repair. Occasionally the biceps tendon ruptures as a result of degeneration caused by chronic tendinitis. The onset is normally sudden, with the athlete experiencing a sharp snap followed by pain and weakness of the arm. The evaluation is easily made by observing the abnormally large bulging muscle mass in the arm. Acute ruptures of the biceps tendon are more common in weight lifters and gymnasts.

❖ **Rupture to the long head of the biceps.** The long head of the biceps tendon is intimately involved with the rotator cuff. It lies between the subscapularis and supraspinatus muscles and attaches to the superior glenoid labrum. Tears can occur in conjunction with subacromial impingement syndrome. When a tear occurs to the biceps tendon within the joint, the tendon may not slide in the bicipital groove and allow the familiar deformity of contraction of the muscle belly. Symptoms of this type of rupture of the biceps tendon may be indistinguishable from impingement syndrome. When the biceps tendon ruptures outside the joint, it normally occurs in or near the bicipital groove between the tuberosities of the humeral head. This type of tear can occur as the result of impingement of the tendon on the underside of the acromion and is usually evidenced by the characteristic prominence of the muscle belly. In addition there is usually a measurable loss of elbow flexion and supination.

❖ **Impingement syndrome.** A very common injury involving the soft tissues of the shoulder comprising the subacromial space, it is normally referred to as an impingement syndrome. Other terms that describe these conditions are supraspinatus syndrome, bursitis, rotator cuff impingement, painful arc syndrome, and internal derangement of the subacromial joint. Impingement syndromes often produce progressive degenerative changes to the affected structures. Often it begins as a tendinitis especially involving the supraspinatus or biceps tendons. This produces some edema and hemorrhage which is often referred to as Stage 1. In Stage 2 there is thickening and fibrosis of the soft tissue structures; Stage 3 involves rotator cuff tears, biceps tendon ruptures, and bony changes. As time progresses, the subdeltoid bursa becomes secondarily in-

❖ volved **(subdeltoid bursitis).** Swelling and thickening of the bursa in the confined space lead to further impingement. If this process is allowed to continue, progressive wearing and attrition occurs within the tendons, resulting in micro tears and partial tears of the rotator cuff. In advanced stages of shoulder impingement, the acromioclavicular joint can be involved as a result of painful degenerative changes, including osteophytes, along the undersurface of this joint.

Activities involving repetitive use of the arm above the horizontal level, such as throwing, playing tennis, or swimming **(swimmer's shoulder)**, may produce this overuse syndrome. The most significant symptom of impingement is pain about the acromion, often described as "deep" within the shoulder. Initially the pain may be a dull ache about the shoulder after strenuous activity and often at night. This pain may progress to discomfort during activity and eventually affects performance. Athletes may restrict movements and refrain from particular maneuvers that cause the impingement. Physical findings include palpable tenderness over the greater tuberosity at the supraspinatus insertion, palpable tenderness along the anterior edge of the acromion, a painful arc of abduction between 60° to 120°, and positive impingement signs during passive procedures (explained later).

Sprains

❖ **Acromioclavicular sprain.** The most common sprains about the shoulder complex are to the acromioclavicular joint. They generally occur as a result of a blow to the tip of the shoulder or falling on an outstretched arm. The most common mechanism of injury occurs when the athlete falls onto the point of the shoulder or receives a direct blow to the tip of the shoulder. The acromion may be driven downward. During a sudden unexpected fall, an athlete may land on an outstretched hand or flexed elbow, which transmits force directly to the shoulder girdle and can drive the acromion backward and away from the clavicle. Either of these mechanisms can cause a sprain to the supporting ligaments, an injury commonly called a **shoulder separation.**

Sprains to the acromioclavicular joint are graded according to the degree of severity. A mild (first-degree) sprain is stretching or slight tearing of the ligament fibers. There is normally tenderness directly over the joint, mild swelling, and little or no disability of the shoulder. A moderate (second-degree) sprain is a partial disruption of the supporting ligaments. Such injuries will have pain and tenderness directly over and around the joint, local swelling, and an increase in pain on forced motion. This is accomplished by pulling downward or pushing upward on the arm in an attempt to separate the clavicle from the acromion, thereby applying stress to the supporting ligaments. A moderate sprain may or may not exhibit upward displacement of the clavicle. A severe (third-degree) sprain involves total disruption of one or more of the supporting ligaments. The athlete will generally exhibit varying degrees of tenderness, swelling, instability, and an increase in pain with any effort to stress the joint. The space between the acromion and clavicle may be widened and the coracoclavicular ligaments torn. When this occurs there is a characteristic upward riding of the clavicle (Figure 20-18). This sign becomes more obvious when weight or downward traction is applied to the arm. A third-degree sprain of the acro-

mioclavicular joint will often exhibit a **piano key sign;** that is, the clavicle can be pushed down but will spring back up when pressure is released. An upward riding of the clavicle in relation to the acromion has traditionally been called a **knocked-down shoulder.** Complete acromioclavicular dislocations may require surgical intervention.

Complications that may accompany acromioclavicular sprains include pain, disability, and a decrease in shoulder range of motion (ROM). Degenerative changes often develop in this joint. Persons may have activity-limiting symptoms years later as a result of apparently "minor" injuries. The lateral end of the clavicle may remain prominent, but this is often painless and may not interfere with shoulder function.

❖ **Glenohumeral sprain.** The ligaments and capsule about the glenohumeral joint contribute minimally to the stability of the shoulder joint. Therefore sprains of the shoulder joint seldom occur unless there is a subluxation or dislocation which is discussed later.

❖ **Sternoclavicular sprain.** The most common injuries to the sternoclavicular joint are sprains. These result when force is directed along the long axis of the clavicle toward the sternal end and stress is applied to the sternoclavicular and costoclavicular ligaments. When these supporting ligaments are stretched significantly or torn, the

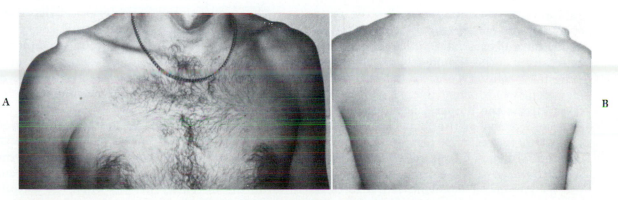

A   B

FIGURE 20-18
Severe sprain of the right acromioclavicular joint exhibiting elevation of the clavicle. **A,** Anterior view and, **B,** posterior view.

sternal end of the clavicle may sublux or dislocate. Dislocation of the sternoclavicular joint is almost always in an anterior direction, so that the sternal end of the clavicle passes forward. The anterior sternoclavicular ligament is torn by the stress, and the clavicle passes upward to lie in the suprasternal notch. In a complete anterior dislocation, the costoclavicular ligament is ruptured, making reduction difficult. This injury commonly results in tenderness, swelling, and a visible prominence at the sternoclavicular joint. Discomfort and a limited range of shoulder motion are usually present.

A posterior subluxation or dislocation of the sternoclavicular joint, although rare, is potentially much more serious than an anterior dislocation. With a posterior dislocation, the posterior sternoclavicular ligament is ruptured and the clavicle may compress the anterior structures of the neck. This may lead to dyspnea if the trachea is compressed. A posterior dislocation can also compress or rupture the innominate vein as it passes directly behind the sternoclavicular joint.

Dislocations

❖ **Glenohumeral dislocation.** Because of its inherent instability, the shoulder joint has the highest incidence of dislocation of any major joint in the body and accounts for one-half of all dislocations. Shoulder dislocations are classified depending on the location of the head of the humerus. The anterior, or subcoracoid, dislocation is by far the most common. The mechanism of injury is forced abduction and external rotation. The athlete generally has the shoulder in an abducted, externally rotated position and receives a blow somewhere along the extremity. This force directs the humeral head toward the anterior portion of the joint capsule. This forward progression is checked by the coracoacromial ligament and diverted down toward the area of the capsule supported by the glenohumeral ligament. If the force is sufficient, the capsule and ligaments surrender and allow the humeral head to slip out of the glenoid fossa to lodge between the rim

of the glenoid and coronoid process. A dislocated shoulder that remains displaced will usually be readily recognized, because there is normally an associated deformity and the athlete is unable to produce or resist any movement of the arm. If the force is insufficient to cause a complete dislocation, the humeral head may sublux and then relocate, causing a sprain of the anterior capsule and supporting ligaments. The history of the injury then becomes more important. The athlete will often relate that the arm was forced into external rotation and abduction and he or she felt the humerus "slip out of place." This will be accompanied by pain in the anterior aspect of the joint, which is increased by any attempt to abduct and externally rotate the arm. The abduction and external rotation is the basis for the apprehension test described later.

❖ A complication of anterior shoulder dislocations is **axillary nerve injury.** The axillary nerve can be contused, stretched, and possibly torn resulting in a temporary or permanent loss of function. The athlete may have loss of sensation over the lateral aspect of the shoulder and decreased function of the deltoid muscle.

A less common form of shoulder dislocation is a posterior dislocation. The mechanism involves a posteriorly directed force against a flexed humerus. The humeral head slides posteriorly past the glenoid and posterior capsule to lodge against the rotator cuff musculature. Because of the tension of this musculature, posterior dislocations have a high incidence of spontaneous relocation, which makes the evaluation difficult. Symptoms are those of a strain or sprain of the posterior structures and an increase in pain when replicating the mechanism of injury.

Another seldom encountered dislocation is an inferior dislocation in which the head of the humerus lies inferior to the lip of the glenoid. This type of dislocation can occur during forced abduction, when the capsule and supporting ligaments are torn and allow the humeral head to slip below the glenoid rim. An inferior dislocation that remains displaced may cause a **luxatio erecta,** in which the arm stands straight above the head and the athlete is unable to bring it down. An inferior subluxation will cause the arm to be held at the side because any attempt to abduct it will cause the athlete to feel as if the arm will slip out of place.

Dislocations of the shoulder have a high incidence of recurrence without a period of immobilization and a vigorous rehabilitation program. When a shoulder is not rehabilitated sufficiently after a dislocation, this joint is very susceptible to repeated episodes. Each successive dislocation requires less force to drive the humeral head out of the glenoid and also causes it to reduce more easily. Recurrent episodes can develop into a condition in which the shoulder will dislocate during abduction and external rotation without much additional trauma. This demonstrates the importance of early recognition and proper rehabilitation of all shoulder dislocations.

Fractures

Fractures about the shoulder joint are not common in athletic activity, with the exception of the clavicle. Fractures to the glenohumeral area are often associated with subluxations or dislocations and appear as avulsion fractures of the rotator cuff tendons, supporting ligaments, or capsular attachments. This is a sound reason to refer all athletes with first-time shoulder dislocations to a physician for probable radiographic evaluation. In young athletes fractures may be through the proximal epiphysis.

❖ **Clavicle fracture.** The clavicle is frequently fractured during athletic activity. This is especially true in preadolescent and adolescent athletes. In older athletes, ligament injuries to the sternoclavicular or acromioclavicular joints are more likely than fractures. Most fractured clavicles in young athletes are of the greenstick type. These can be difficult to detect because there may be no evident displacement of bone fragments or resulting angulation. Athletic trainers should suspect a greenstick fracture

whenever there is tenderness directly over the shaft of the clavicle in a young athlete who has suffered trauma to the shoulder. Although the clavicle is fractured more frequently than any other major long bone in the body, serious complications are rare. The break is usually at the junction of the middle and outer thirds of the bone or where the clavicle changes direction. In older athletes, the medial fragment is normally pulled upward by the contractions of the sternocleidomastoid and trapezius muscles, whereas the lateral portion is displaced downward by the contraction of the pectoralis major muscle and the weight of the arm (Figure 20-19).

❖ **Humerus fracture.** Occasionally an athlete may suffer a fracture of the surgical neck of the humerus instead of a dislocation. This type of injury most often is the result of a fall on an outstretched arm. Depending on the tensile strength of the bone and surrounding ligaments, younger athletes tend to dislocate while older individuals are prone to fracture. Fractures to the humeral shaft most often result from a direct blow to the arm. Occasionally, severe twisting of the arm or a fall on an outstretched hand can produce this type of fracture (Figure 20-20). Humeral fractures should be readily recognized as there will be localized pain, swelling, and all movements restricted. Deformity and crepitus may also be present over the fracture site. The most common complication of humerus shaft fractures is **radial**
❖ **nerve injury.** The radial nerve winds around the posterior aspect of the humerus. If this nerve is involved in the injury, the athlete may complain of numbness and tingling extending down the forearm and dorsum of the wrist. The wrist extensors may be weak, with the athlete exhibiting a wrist drop. A neurovascular exam should always be performed early in the assessment process following a possible shoulder dislocation or humerus fracture.

❖ **Proximal humerus epiphyseal fracture.** A fracture or separation of the proximal humeral epiphysis is an uncommon injury. However, the mechanisms that may cause a shoulder to dislocate or sublux in

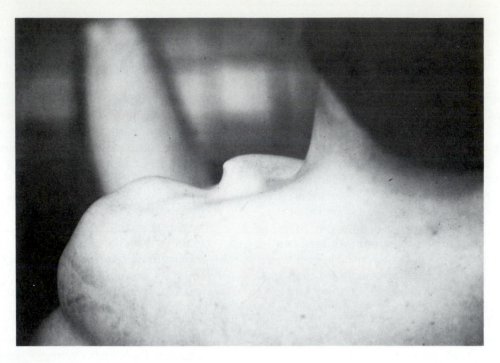

FIGURE 20-19
Complete fracture of the clavicle as viewed from behind. Note the elevated medial fragment.

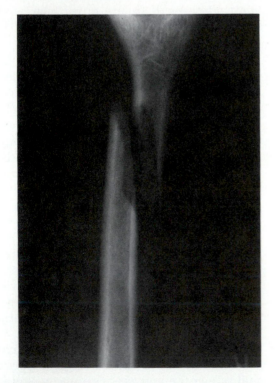

FIGURE 20-20
X-ray showing fracture of the shaft of the humerus caused by pitching a baseball.

adults, can lead to a proximal humerus epiphyseal fracture in a young athlete because the joint capsule is stronger than the epiphyseal plate. Symptoms include a swollen and very tender proximal humerus. The athlete will probably be supporting the injured arm against the trunk by the opposite extremity.

Other Conditions of the Shoulder

Adhesive capsulitis. An athletic trainer must be alert to the development of adhesive capsulitis. This condition is often referred to as a "frozen shoulder." It is an inflammation about the rotator cuff and capsular area that can result in dense adhesions and capsular contracture causing restriction of motion and pain. The exact cause remains unknown. The onset of symptoms are often insidious with gradual increase in pain and decrease in motion. It can develop because an athlete protects a painful shoulder by limiting movement. In some cases it may develop if the joint is immobilized after a serious injury. The main feature of adhesive capsulitis is lack of passive ROM, especially rotation and abduction. If the athletic trainer cannot move an athlete's shoulder passively through a normal ROM after the recovery period, adhesive capsulitis should be suspected and steps taken to correct the situation.

Brachial plexus injuries. Injuries to the brachial plexus normally involve the cervical spine, but the symptoms are exhibited in the shoulder and upper extremity. When an athlete's neck is violently forced into rotation or lateral flexion, especially while the opposite shoulder is depressed, considerable tension can be placed on the nerve branches of the brachial plexus. Occasionally part of the brachial plexus is compressed between the clavicle and first rib. Both of these mechanisms can result in transitory paralysis of the arm, with numbness or a burning sensation radiating down the arm and sometimes into the hand. This normally disappears in a matter of seconds to a few minutes. Occasionally recovery may take days. An injury to the brachial plexus is frequently called a "pinched nerve," "burner," "hot shot," or "stinger." Occasionally a persistent disability may result from this type of injury. Athletes experiencing repeated episodes of brachial plexus injuries or who complain of weakness or numbness in the arm that persists for an hour or more after the injury should be carefully evaluated and referred to a physician for a neurologic examination.

Thoracic outlet syndrome. Thoracic outlet syndrome is a group of symptoms resulting from compression of the thoracic neurovascular bundle, which includes the brachial plexus and subclavian artery and vein. This neurovascular bundle emerges from the thorax through an outlet or triangle formed by the scalene muscles and the first rib. Any changes in the relationship between these anatomic components that tends to narrow the outlet may cause a variety of symptoms, which is known as thoracic outlet syndrome. Many etiologies have been described as contributing to this condition, such as hypertrophy of one of the sca-

lene muscles, shape of the first rib, scar tissue formation around the nerve roots, cervical ribs, excess callus formation as a result of a fractured clavicle, and hyperabduction or stretching of the brachial plexus.

Clinical manifestations are often complex and varied depending on which components of the neurovascular bundle are compressed. Nerve symptoms are present in 95% of the cases, and vascular symptoms are present in only 5% to 10%. Symptoms attributed to neural compression include (1) aching pain across the shoulder; (2) pain in the side of the neck, often accompanied with pain down the arm; and (3) a sensation of weakness, heaviness, and easy fatigability when using the arm, especially above shoulder height. Weakness for fine movements of the hand may be noted. Other characteristics include numbness and tingling, particularly along an ulnar nerve distribution. Additional symptoms that are normally attributed to vascular compression include deep aching, cold sensitivity, pallor, swelling, and temperature changes in the skin.

Athletes exhibiting thoracic outlet syndrome often have a history of trauma to the head, neck, or shoulder area. However, this condition can also result from muscular and bony abnormalities. Excessive use of the extremity can be a cause of persistent symptoms. Evaluation of thoracic outlet syndrome is made on the basis of characteristic symptoms during the clinical history with attempted reproduction of these symptoms during the assessment process. The most useful physical finding is reproduction of the symptoms on hyperabduction and outward rotation of the arm. Additional shoulder girdle stress maneuvers are described later in this chapter.

ATHLETIC INJURY ASSESSMENT PROCESS

The shoulder girdle is the most frequently injured area of the upper extremity. This complex is very vulnerable to acute athletic injuries and chronic overuse conditions because it serves as the attachment and fulcrum for upper extremity action and is the portion of anatomy best suited for forcible ramming or butting. Although the glenohumeral joint has an extensive ROM, it is relatively unstable compared to other major joints of the body. A wide variety of athletic injuries to the shoulder complex result from direct or indirect trauma, as well as from activities requiring throwing movements. To complete a comprehensive assessment of injuries involving the shoulder girdle, athletic trainers must take many factors into consideration, such as: (1) unique anatomic features, (2) intricate functional characteristics, (3) various mechanisms of injury, and (4) associated signs and symptoms. A meticulous and systematic examination is often necessary to identify the anatomic structures involved and to determine the nature and severity of the injury. The initial assessment process is designed to generate a comprehensive data base for use in further evaluation, treatment, and rehabilitation programs.

Secondary survey

The evaluation procedures used to assess shoulder injuries will initially depend on the position and status of the athlete at the time the injury is recognized or reported. Your initial observations and judgment will normally determine the direction in which you should proceed with the secondary survey. Most athletes with a shoulder injury will be sitting, standing, or moving around. It is unusual for an athlete with an isolated shoulder injury to remain lying on the field or court unless the injury is a dislocation or fracture. It is possible that an athlete involved in an injury, especially some type of collision, can sustain an injury to the head or neck, as well as the shoulder. Whenever an athlete remains down after incurring what appears to be a shoulder injury, your suspicion level should remain high. Carefully check for a more serious injury to the head or neck or additional involvement such as internal thoracic injuries. Injuries to the head or neck must be ruled out before evaluating the shoulder.

Another important consideration is the adequacy and integrity of circulation and neurologic pathways distal to a shoulder injury. These evaluative procedures may be completed first in the assessment process. Circulation is assessed by feeling for distal pulses, usually the radial. Neurologic involvement can be evaluated by checking skin sensations over the shoulder and arm and evaluating active motion of the shoulder and upper extremity as a whole. Remember, when a serious injury or circulatory or neurologic involvement is recognized, it is not necessary to continue with the assessment procedures. Emergency care, referral, or carefully supervised transportation techniques should be instituted as indicated.

The specific assessment procedures used in evaluating shoulder injuries will vary depending upon the injured athlete's signs and symptoms revealed during the process.

History

A comprehensive shoulder examination begins with a careful review of the history relevant to the shoulder injury (Figure 20-21). Questioning should quickly determine if the injury is an acute or a chronic problem. Many shoulder injuries are recurrent con-

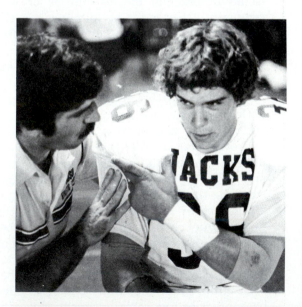

FIGURE 20-21
Obtaining the history of a shoulder injury.

ditions or chronic overuse syndromes. If the area has been injured before, obtain as much information about the previous injury as possible. Question the athlete about the nature of previous injuries, the treatment procedures used, and the extent of rehabilitation. Had symptoms completely subsided and full function been restored before the onset of the current injury? Are symptoms of the current injury similar to those of any previous injuries? The more information gained concerning previous injuries, the better you can evaluate the nature and severity of the current problem.

Question the athlete concerning the present injury. When did the onset of symptoms occur? Chronic overuse syndromes normally begin slowly and insidiously with a low-grade ache. Symptoms gradually increase as the athlete continues to use and stress the shoulder. What has happened to the symptoms since the athlete first noticed the injury? If the onset is sudden, the athlete will usually relate a traumatic episode. Have the athlete describe the mechanism of injury in detail. Was there a direct blow delivered to the shoulder? What was the angle of the impact? Attempt to determine the amount of force at impact. Did the direct blow involve the side of the head or neck? Did the athlete fall and land on the shoulder or an outstretched arm? What was the position of the arm at the time of injury? Was the arm forced beyond normal limits? Did the injury result from a forceful muscular contraction? Obtain as much information as possible concerning the mechanism of injury because this knowledge is important in determining the nature of the injury and the structures involved.

Have the athlete describe the symptoms associated with the injury in as much detail as possible. Where is the pain? Ask the athlete to locate the pain or tender areas as precisely as possible and describe the characteristics of the pain. Is the pain sharply localized or dull and diffused? Is there any pain radiating down the arm? Are there any activities or movements that cause the pain to increase or decrease? Ask if there are any activities or movements that are difficult or impossible for the athlete to initiate. Is the pain severe enough to wake the athlete or prevent him or her from sleeping? Occasionally pain will be present only during certain movements or at a particular point in the ROM. Ask the athlete to demonstrate the motion or movements that aggravate the shoulder. Remember, the shoulder is a classic area for referred and radiating pain. Therefore the chest, upper abdomen, neck, or spine may have to be carefully examined to determine if the pain is being referred or radiated to the shoulder.

Question the athlete about any other sensations associated with the injury. Did he or she hear or feel anything at the time of injury, such as a popping or snapping sensation? Does the athlete feel any tightness, tension, locking, or swelling associated with the injury? Is there or has there been any clicking or crepitation? Does the athlete complain of any numbness, burning, weakness or tingling in the upper extremity? Ask the athlete to describe his or her impressions concerning the injury and integrate this information into the assessment. If an athlete says a bone is broken or the shoulder is dislocated, believe it and proceed with the evaluation as if this is the problem until it is proved otherwise.

Observation

The statement "look before you touch" is one of the cardinal rules of assessment. The impact of your visual observations on the formal assessment process will diminish once you begin using other senses. It is important therefore that your initial assessment observations begin before you touch or even talk to the injured athlete. First note the overall position or posture of the athlete and the alignment of the upper extremities. Is the athlete moving or using the injured extremity? Is he or she holding, supporting, or favoring any area of the shoulder or arm? Does the shoulder or arm appear to be in an abnormal position, which may indicate a dislocation or fracture? Does the arm appear to be hanging limp at the athlete's side, which

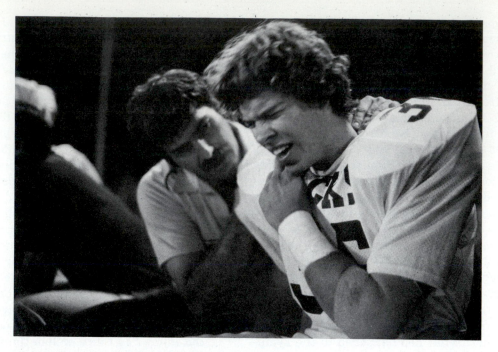

FIGURE 20-22
Initial palpation of shoulder under protective equipment.

reflects the athlete's reluctance to move the arm? Always remember to observe the athlete's face. Does he or she appear to be uncomfortable or in a great deal of pain?

Often, especially in contact sports, the injured shoulder will be covered with protective equipment and clothing. Do not disturb the shoulder girdle by removing the uniform and equipment until you are relatively sure of the nature and severity of the injury. Uniforms and protective equipment can be cut off as previously described, but in most cases the early stages of the assessment procedures can continue with the equipment in place. Palpation techniques are used at this time to further evaluate the injured shoulder. Gently slide your hand under the uniform or protective equipment to feel the entire shoulder complex (Figure 20-22). Being firm but gentle, palpate the shoulder to locate any pain, tenderness, or deformity. Continue questioning the athlete in a soft reassuring voice and watch his or her face to note any discomfort or reactions. In this manner a preliminary evaluation of the in-

jury can be performed without removing the uniform and causing unnecessary movements of the shoulder. Remember to palpate the uninjured shoulder and to compare symmetry. Of course, should a significant injury be found, the uniform and equipment can be cut off or the athlete referred to a physician or medical facility with the apparel left in place. Once you are relatively sure no serious injury exists, you can assist the athlete in removing the uniform and equipment and continue with a more thorough evaluation. Clothing and equipment should be removed from the uninjured extremity first and then slid off the involved side to prevent needless movement of the injured extremity. As the athlete disrobes, notice the shoulder movement. Does he or she favor the injured side? Look for any signs that may indicate neurologic involvement, such as paralysis or weakness.

Once clothing and equipment have been removed, observe the overall posture, muscular development, and alignment of both shoulders with the athlete standing or sit-

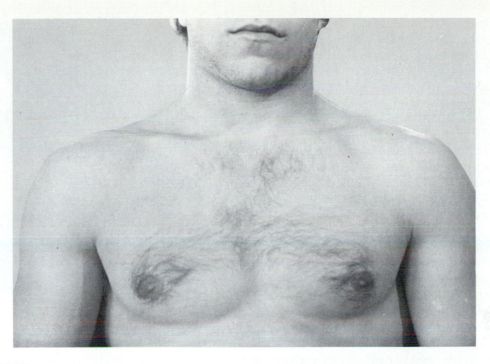

FIGURE 20-23
Comparing symmetry and appearance of both shoulders. Note the prominence of the distal clavicle on the right side (second-degree acromioclavicular separation).

ting and the arms at the sides. Compare the symmetry and appearance of the upper extremities from the anterior, as well as the posterior, position (Figure 20-23). Note the contours. Are there any signs of deformities, marked swelling, or definite atrophy of the muscles surrounding the shoulder girdle? Occasionally with a chronic condition there will be associated atrophy of muscle groups. Carefully inspect the injured shoulder for signs of trauma, such as abrasions or contusions. These signs can indicate what types of forces have been applied to the athlete's body and help establish the mechanism of injury.

Physical Examination

The physical examination portion of the assessment process is used to perform a more detailed investigation of the musculoskeletal system. Depending upon what your impressions are up to this point in the assessment process, you may continue with palpation techniques, movement procedures, or neu-

rological and circulatory evaluations. Not all these procedures will be used in any one athletic injury. Choose the specific tests or procedures that will assist in completing your assessment of the shoulder. Remember, physical examination is both a skill and an art, mastered only by study and experience.

Palpation

Thorough palpation techniques can be extremely beneficial in the assessment of athletic injuries of the shoulder. Palpation is used to investigate or confirm those findings or suspicions formulated during the history and observation procedures. The shoulder girdle is usually easily accessible to palpation because most of the structures are subcutaneous. However, palpation techniques may be more difficult in the overweight or highly muscular athlete. If the underlying anatomy is clearly understood, tenderness can normally be readily associated with those anatomic structures suspected of being injured.

Palpation of the shoulder girdle should be conducted with the area as relaxed as possible. Normally this is accomplished by having the athlete sit on a table or stand with the arms in a comfortable and relaxed position. The shoulder can also be palpated with the athlete supine and the arms supported by the table, ground, or floor. This position should be used if the athlete is uncomfortable in an upright position or possibly suffering from the effects of shock. The initial structures to be palpated will be determined by the suspicions raised during the preceding phases of the assessment process. Remember, palpation techniques should be performed gently. Always begin away from the suspected area of injury to promote cooperation from the athlete. Palpate both the injured and uninjured sides.

Bony anatomy. The integrity of the bony anatomy is normally evaluated first, followed by the assessment of any damage to the soft tissues. Carefully palpate the bones and bony landmarks about the suspected site of injury, noting any points of tenderness or crepitation. Palpate the various muscles and other soft tissue structures suspected of being involved in the injury, again noting specific areas of tenderness. Tenderness must be carefully localized and precisely identified in an attempt to accurately recognize the underlying structures that may be damaged. In the following paragraphs, the procedures used to palpate the various anatomic structures about the shoulder girdle are discussed briefly. In addition, the common athletic injuries that may be indicated by the physical signs noted during the assessment are reviewed.

The clavicle is a good point of reference to begin palpating the shoulder because it is subcutaneous along its entire length. It is generally easier to palpate both clavicles simultaneously to note any differences in symmetry. Begin by placing your hands medially to feel the sternoclavicular joint (Figure 20-24). This easily palpated joint is not commonly injured in athletic activity. A sprain of the sternoclavicular joint can be recognized by pain and point tenderness at this

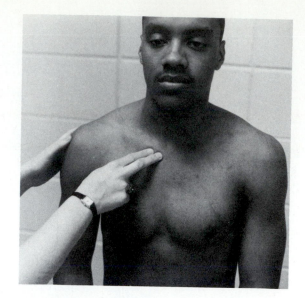

FIGURE 20-24
Palpating the sternoclavicular joint.

articulation, and depending on the severity, there may be varying degrees of visible and palpable deformity. The sternal end of the clavicle will normally be displaced forward and upward in a second or third degree sprain. Although rare, remember that posterior displacement of the clavicle or manubrium of the sternum can compress the trachea and occlude the airway. Displacement can occur with traumatic movements of the sternal portion of the clavicle or by a direct blow to the upper chest.

The anterior and superior surfaces of the clavicle can be palpated throughout its length. Slowly palpate this smooth S-shaped bone from its distal to proximal end, noting any tenderness, swelling, crepitation, or disruption of continuity. Fractures of the clavicle, one of the more frequent fractures in athletics, can normally be recognized by careful palpation. There may be no deformity associated with a clavicular fracture in a young athlete, because it is usually the greenstick type of fracture. Once an area of point tenderness is located along the clavicle, the possibility of a fracture should be considered. In the absence of deformity, an area of point tenderness can be further eval-

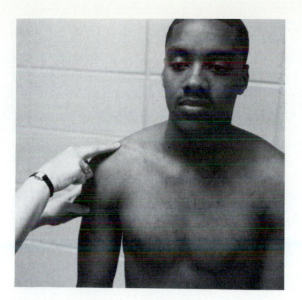

FIGURE 20-25
Palpating the acromioclavicular joint.

uated by applying stress to the clavicle away from the site of pain. Move away from the tender area an inch or two and very gently apply mild pressure to the clavicle. Remember to inform the athlete that you are going to press gently and to tell you if the procedure increases the pain. If this maneuver causes additional pain at the original site of tenderness, the athlete should be treated as if he or she has a fracture.

Continue palpating distally to the lateral end of the clavicle where it articulates with the acromion to form the acromioclavicular joint (Figure 20-25), a frequently injured joint in the shoulder girdle. Tenderness expressed in this area indicates an injury to the acromioclavicular joint. The lateral end of the clavicle normally rides just slightly higher than the acromion. If the clavicle on the injured side is abnormally higher than the acromion when compared to the uninjured side, a second- or third-degree sprain of this joint should be suspected. A third-degree sprain will normally exhibit gross deformity, with the distal end of the clavicle being quite prominent. This type of injury should be readily recognized. Keep in mind that this athlete may have suffered a pre-

vious injury to the acromioclavicular joint, and the clavicle could have been higher before the current injury. Press down on the distal end of the clavicle. Is there an increase in pain? Is there an increase in mobility of the clavicle in its relationship to the acromion? Compare any hypermobility to the uninjured side. Remember, a second-degree sprain or partial separation will be indicated by increased tenderness and hypermobility of the acromioclavicular joint.

The acromion process of the scapula can be palpated at the tip of the shoulder. This flared projection is the lateral end of the scapular spine. Athletes landing on the tip of the shoulder may bruise this area; such an injury is commonly referred to as a "shoulder pointer."

The spine of the scapula is a sharp subcutaneous ridge running diagonally across the posterior surface of the shoulder blade. It can usually be palpated along its entire length (Figure 20-26, *A*). Athletic injuries seldom occur to the scapular spine, but it is a good point of reference for palpating soft tissue structures about the scapula. The borders of the scapula can also be readily felt. Palpate along the vertebral or medial borders of both scapulae (Figure 20-26, *B*) from the superior to the inferior angles. Normally the vertebral borders lie approximately 2 inches from the spinous processes of the thoracic vertebrae, and palpating both simultaneously can assist in determining if one of the scapulae is carried forward. The vertebral border is also the point of reference for the muscles attached along its length. From the inferior angle of the scapula, the lateral or axillary border can be palpated for a short distance before it is covered with muscles.

The head of the humerus can be palpated laterally and inferiorly to the acromion process. Although this area is covered by the deltoid muscle, careful palpation will reveal the greater and lesser tuberosities bordering the bicipital groove. The greater tuberosity forms the lateral border of the bicipital groove, whereas the lesser tuberosity comprises the medial lip. These structures are more easily recognized if the arm is rotated

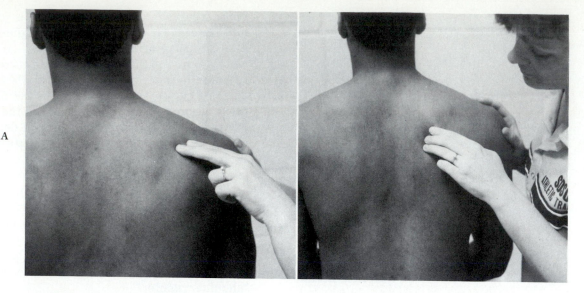

FIGURE 20-26
Palpating the scapula: **A,** spine and, **B,** vertebral border.

during palpation. With the humerus externally rotated, the bicipital groove and lesser tuberosity are in a more exposed position (Figure 20-27, *A*). With internal rotation, the greater tuberosity becomes more prominent and easier to feel (Figure 20-27, *B*). The long head of the biceps tendon lies in the bicipital groove, and point tenderness or crepitus in this area may indicate tenosynovitis or tendon subluxation. Palpation maneuvers of the bicipital groove should be performed gently so as not to cause unnecessary pain in the area, causing the athlete to become tense.

Two other bony landmarks that may be palpated in the shoulder girdle and serve as reference points are the deltoid tuberosity and the coracoid process of the scapula. The deltoid tuberosity is a V-shaped, roughened area midway down the lateral surface of the shaft of the humerus where the deltoid muscle inserts (Figure 20-28, *A*). This is the site for the possible development of a blocker's spur. The coracoid process lies about 1 inch below the clavicle and may be felt in the groove between the deltoid and pectoralis major muscles. Because this structure lies beneath muscle, firm pressure is necessary

to feel the tip of the coracoid process (Figure 20-28, *B*).

Soft tissue anatomy. The majority of soft tissue structures about the shoulder girdle can be palpated to evaluate their involvement in an athletic injury. Knowledge of the underlying anatomy combined with careful palpation techniques provide the athletic trainer the opportunity to recognize any areas of tenderness, swelling, or anatomic inconsistencies. This information, combined with various stress procedures, is valuable in assessing soft tissue injuries. Although palpation of bony and soft tissue structures is discussed separately, they are normally performed in conjunction with one another during a shoulder assessment.

The prominent muscles of the shoulder girdle can be palpated individually. Anteriorly, the pectoralis major muscle can be palpated from its origins on the chest wall and clavicle to its insertion on the greater tuberosity of the humerus. This muscle forms the anterior wall of the axilla when the arm is abducted (Figure 20-29).

The deltoid muscle covers the lateral aspect of the shoulder, and each of the three portions can be easily palpated. This muscle

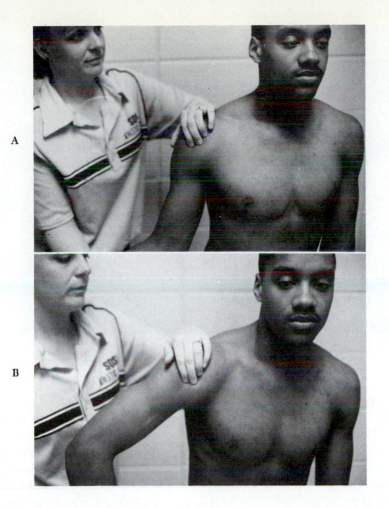

FIGURE 20-27
Palpating, **A,** the bicipital groove during external rotation of the arm and, **B,** the greater tuberosity during internal rotation of the arm.

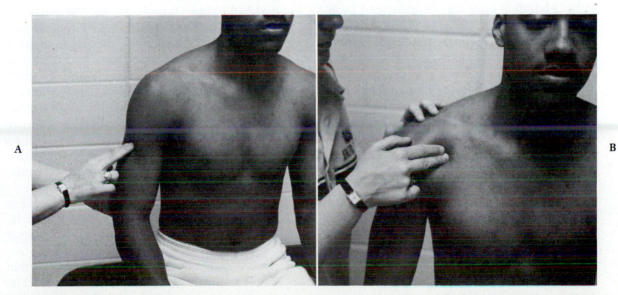

FIGURE 20-28
Palpating, **A,** the deltoid tuberosity and, **B,** the corcoid process.

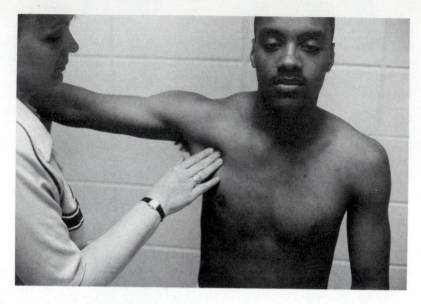

FIGURE 20-29
Palpating the pectoralis major muscle.

must be carefully palpated, as it covers several structures that are often involved in athletic injuries; thus tenderness elicited by touch may be common to one of several different structures. For example, tenderness over the bicipital groove may indicate a tenosynovitis of the biceps tendon or an injury to the deltoid muscle. Tenderness deep to the deltoid muscle is also frequently associated with subdeltoid bursitis or rotator cuff problems.

The large subdeltoid (subacromial) bursa, wedged between the superior surface of the joint capsule and the inferior surface of the deltoid muscle, may be tender to touch just below the edge of the acromion process if bursitis is present. Passively hyperextending the arm exposes a greater portion of the bursa, as well as the insertion of the supraspinatus muscle, from beneath the acromion process. Palpate just below the anterior border of the acromion. Tenderness elicited during this maneuver may indicate an injury to the rotator cuff or bursitis. To distinguish between these conditions, passive techniques described later must be employed.

Several muscles on the posterior surface of the shoulder girdle can be palpated. The most superficial and readily felt of these is the trapezius, which originates on the occipital bone and the cervical and thoracic spinous processes and inserts on the scapular spine, acromion, and clavicle. The superior portion of the trapezius is frequently involved in neck strains, which may be recognized by point tenderness and increased pain on active and resistive motion. The latissimus dorsi muscle forms the posterior border of the axilla and can be readily palpated when the arm is abducted, making this muscle more prominent and easier to locate (Figure 20-30). Additional muscles can be palpated on the posterior surface of the shoulder; however, they are not subcutaneous or readily distinguishable and are seldom involved in athletic injury. When these muscles are strained, they are identified by local tenderness and pain when the particular muscle is contracted.

The major muscles of the upper arm are occasionally injured as the result of athletic activity. Palpate the biceps on the anterior aspect of the humerus (Figure 20-31, *A*). This muscle becomes more prominent when the elbow is flexed. Finding the tendon of the long head of the biceps as it lies in the bicip-

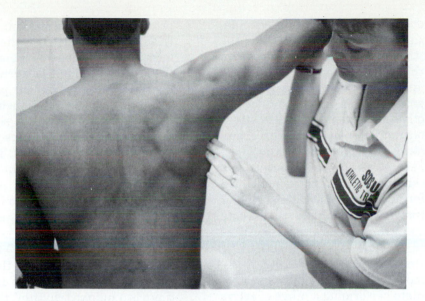

FIGURE 20-30
Palpating the latissimus dorsi muscle.

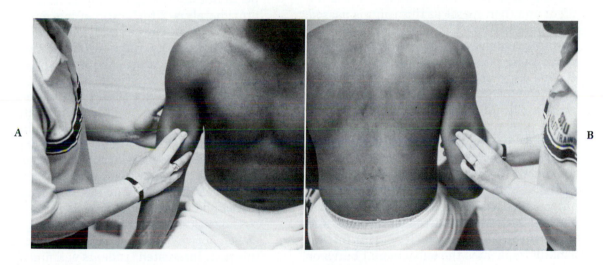

FIGURE 20-31
Palpating major muscles of the upper arm; **A,** biceps and, **B,** triceps.

ital groove has already been discussed. The triceps can be palpated on the posterior surface of the humerus (Figure 20-31, *B*).

Movement procedures

Movement procedures are often used to facilitate the assessment of athletic injuries occurring to the shoulder girdle, especially those involving the glenohumeral joint. The stability of this highly mobile joint is almost totally dependent on combined muscular and ligamentous structures. Because of the anatomic characteristics of this area, a comprehensive examination of the shoulder will normally include a progressive series of functional tests.

Active movements. Active movements are performed to evaluate the relationships between movements of the clavicle, scapula, and humerus, to determine the ROM of the entire arm-trunk mechanism, and to begin assessing the integrity of the contractile units. It is important to remember, because of the anatomic features of the shoulder girdle, that active movements will also stress some noncontractile structures. For example, the acromioclavicular and sternoclavicular joints are stressed during active motions of the shoulder. Active movements can best be performed with the athlete sitting or standing. Instruct the athlete to execute each movement through as great a ROM as possible and to express any sensations or symptoms that are experienced.

A phenomenon to keep in mind as you observe an athlete performing a range of active movements is a **painful arc.** This is pain that is absent at the beginning of the ROM but develops near the midrange of a movement and then ceases as this point is passed. This pain is caused by a tender tissue being painfully squeezed when passing a certain point during the ROM. A painful arc is best evoked by active movements and appears most commonly in shoulder injuries; however, a painful arc can be recognized in injuries involving other joints. This phenomenon may appear only during the upward or downward movement of the arm or during movement in both directions. A painful arc at the shoulder normally indicates an impingement syndrome, as tender tissue is pinched between the acromion process and one of the humeral tuberosities. This finding usually implicates the subacromial bursa or the supraspinatus tendon.

When evaluating active motion always remember that the shoulder girdle functions in complex movement patterns. For example, to abduct the arm to 180°, an athlete must also elevate the shoulder girdle, upwardly rotate the scapula, and outwardly rotate the arm. Without this combination of movements, an athlete could not abduct the arm through a normal ROM. Although it is not necessary in every case to separately evaluate motions available at each joint in the shoulder girdle, such observations can

provide useful information. In most cases it is sufficient to instruct the athlete to perform active motions of the arm and observe the gross movement patterns. While observing these gross movement patterns, look for similarity in the relationship and ratio of movements between the scapula, clavicle, and humerus on both sides of the body. For example, during the first 30° of abduction the scapula will move on the trunk to a point of maximum stability. It is interesting to note that arm abduction to this point can be accomplished without the use of the deltoid muscle. Movement can occur simply by "shrugging the shoulders," that is, by moving the scapula and fixing the glenohumeral joint. However, from 30° to 180° of abduction there is a unique "rhythm" that normally exists between movements of the scapula and humerus. Kinesiologists often refer to a "scapulohumeral rhythm" that results in approximately a 2 to 1 ratio of movement between the humerus and scapula during abduction. Look for this ratio of movement as the athlete abducts the arm beyond 30°. For every 30° of additional abduction, 20° of movement normally occurs at the glenohumeral joint and 10° results from rotation of the scapula on the trunk. It may be helpful to place your hand on the inferior angle of the scapula and assess its movement during arm movements. In cases of acute paralysis of the deltoid muscle, abduction beyond 30° (accomplished by scapular movement) is impossible. Detailed explanations of arm-trunk movement rhythms are beyond the scope of this text. Interested students will find ample information in most advanced kinesiology texts.

Ask the athlete to flex and extend the arm through as great a ROM as possible (Figure 20-32, *A*). Normally an athlete should be able to flex the arm 180°, bringing the arm up even with the ear, and backward extension or hyperextending the arm approximately 60°. Can the athlete complete a normal ROM? Was the motion comfortable without any complaints of pain or weakness? Is the motion available in both shoulders equal? Ask the athlete to flex both arms at

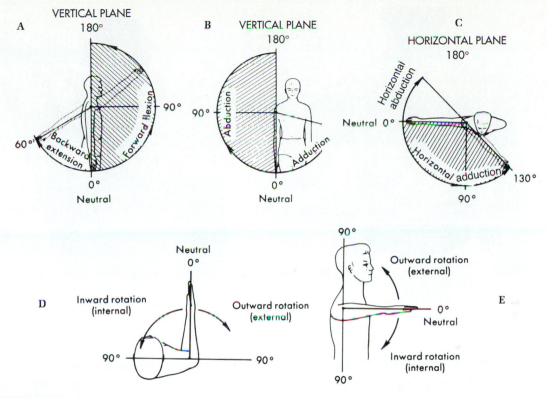

FIGURE 20-32
Range of motion of the shoulder. **A,** Flexion and extension; **B,** abduction and adduction; **C,** horizontal abduction and adduction; **D,** inward and outward rotation with the arm at the side of the body, and, **E,** inward and outward rotation with the arm abducted to 90°.

the same time to provide a bilateral comparison.

In evaluating shoulder abduction and adduction, an athlete can normally abduct the arm 180° and adduct the arm approximately 45° across the front of the body (Figure 20-32, *B*). Can the athlete perform these motions? Is the ROM equal on both sides? Does the athlete express any pain or weakness? Determine the site of any pain elicited with this active motion. Horizontal abduction and adduction can also be evaluated as the athlete moves the arm in the horizontal plane (Figure 20-32, *C*).

Rotation of the humerus is essential for normal elevation of the upper extremity. Internal and external rotation of the arm can be evaluated with the arm at the side and the elbow flexed to 90° (Figure 20-32, *D*). Keeping the arm next to the body, instruct

the athlete to rotate the arm outward and inward. Normally an athlete should be able to outwardly rotate the arm about 45° and inwardly rotate until the forearm touches the body. Rotation can also be tested with the arm in 90° of abduction and the elbow in 90° of flexion (see Figure 20-32, *E*). Instruct the athlete to rotate the arm up and down and compare to the uninjured side. Rotation in this position normally has less range than with the arm at the side of the body. The rotator cuff muscles together with the pectoralis major and latissimus dorsi muscles aid in arm rotation.

A quick and easy method to evaluate active ROM in the shoulder is the **Apley scratch test.** The athlete is instructed to place each hand in two different places to determine the active ROM of the shoulder while you compare bilaterally. Ask the ath-

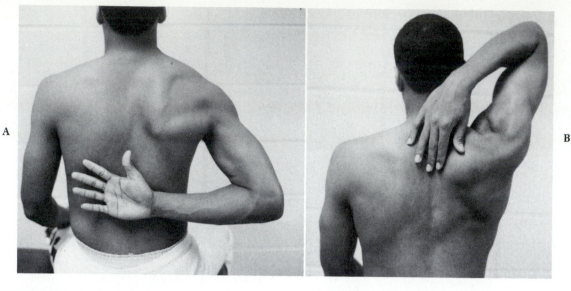

FIGURE 20-33
Apley scratch test. **A,** Athlete reaching behind back; **B,** athlete reaching behind head and down the back.

lete to reach behind his or her back as high as possible (Figure 20-33, *A*). Notice the distance the fingertips reach in relation to the scapula or thoracic spine. This movement involves inward rotation and adduction of the shoulder. Then have the athlete reach behind the head and down the back as far as possible (Figure 20-33, *B*). Again note the distance the fingertips can reach. This involves outward rotation and abduction. Can the athlete complete these maneuvers or reach as far with the injured side as the uninjured? Was there any limitation of motion, weakness, or pain expressed?

A special test used to evaluate the status of the supraspinatus muscle is the **drop arm test.** Instruct the athlete to abduct the arm past 90° and then slowly lower it to the side (Figure 20-34). A positive test is indicated if the athlete is unable to return the arm to the side slowly or has pain when attempting the movement. If there is a tear in the supraspinatus muscle, the arm will often drop to the side from a position of about 90° abduction because of weakness or pain. If the athlete can hold the arm in 90° abduction, a gentle tap or manual resistance against the forearm may cause the arm to

fall. Another position to evaluate the supraspinatus muscle is the **empty can position.** The arm is horizontally abducted 30 degrees with the arm internally rotated and the thumb pointing downward. Ask the athlete to hold this position or apply a downward force. If there is a tear in the supraspinatus muscle, the arm will again drop because of weakness or pain.

Depending on the injury suspected, additional active motion tests can be used to evaluate scapulothoracic movements specifically. Scapular elevation and rotation is accomplished by asking the athlete to shrug both shoulders (Figure 20-35, *A*). Scapular protraction and retraction is evaluated by having the athlete bring both shoulders forward and then backward as far as possible (Figure 20-35, *B* and *C*). Note any pain, weakness, or limitation of motion between the shoulders. Watch for any winging of the scapula, which may indicate a weakness of the serratus anterior muscle. Remember, performing these motions also puts mild stress on the sternoclavicular and acromioclavicular joints and may be used to assess their integrity when moving the arm is too painful.

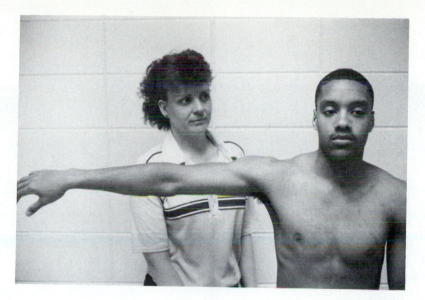

FIGURE 20-34
Drop arm test to evaluate status of the supraspinatus muscle. Athlete abducts arm past 90°
and then slowly lowers it to the side. A positive test is indicated if athlete is unable to return
arm slowly to the side or has pain attempting the movement.

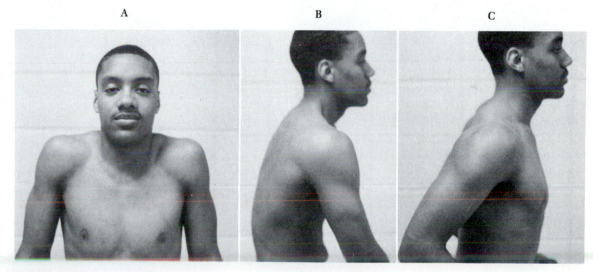

A   B   C

FIGURE 20-35
Active scapulothoracic movements. **A,** Elevation; **B,** protraction; and **C,** retraction.

Resistive movements. Following the evaluation of the active ROM, resistance can be applied against these same movements to further assess the integrity of the contractile units. Whenever a muscle injury is suspected or indicated, resistive movements can assist in identifying specific tender areas, as well as assessing and comparing muscular strengths. Once again, manual isometric resistance can be applied in various positions throughout the ROM. Resistive movements can be performed with the athlete sitting, standing, or lying down. Remember, because shoulder motions are complex patterns, sev-

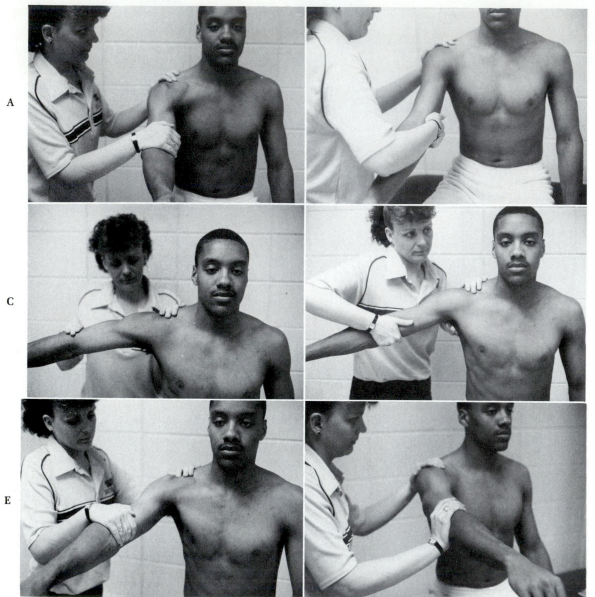

FIGURE 20-36
Applying manual resistance against shoulder motion; **A,** flexion; **B,** extension; **C,** abduction;
D, adduction; **E,** horizontal adduction; and **F,** horizontal abduction.

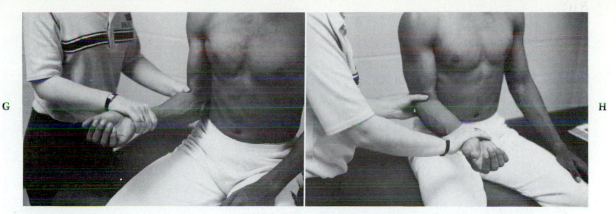

G

H

FIGURE 20-36, cont'd.
G, inward rotation; and, **H,** outward rotation.

eral muscles are being evaluated with each movement. For example, resistance against shoulder flexion may also cause pain in muscles responsible for shoulder elevation or upward rotation of the scapula. To be effective in assessment the athletic trainer must possess a sound knowledge of functional shoulder anatomy.

To apply resistance against shoulder flexion, place one hand on the athlete's shoulder for stability and the other just proximal and anterior to the elbow (Figure 20-36, *A*). The stabilizing hand can also palpate the muscles primarily responsible for the action throughout each movement. Instruct the athlete to flex the shoulder or move the arm forward and up as you apply resistance. Gradually increase your resistance until you can determine the maximum resistance the athlete can overcome. To reduce the effects of the biceps muscle, have the athlete flex the elbow.

Those muscles involved with shoulder extension can be stressed by applying resistance to the posterior distal portion of the humerus (Figure 20-36, *B*). This test should follow the evaluation of shoulder flexion without interruption. Moving your resistive hand from the anterior surface of the athlete's arm to the posterior surface will ensure a smooth transition from testing flexion to extension.

Shoulder abduction and adduction can also be evaluated during the same cycle of motion. Again place one hand on the point of the shoulder to stabilize the shoulder girdle and to palpate the involved muscles. To test shoulder abduction, place the other hand on the distal and lateral aspect of the humerus (Figure 20-36, *C*). Instruct the athlete to abduct the arm, lifting it away from the side of the body. To test shoulder adduction, move your resistance hand to the medial side of the humerus and apply resistance as the athlete adducts the arm (Figure 20-36, *D*).

Horizontal adduction and abduction are additional motions commonly evaluated using resistive techniques. For horizontal adduction, begin with the arm abducted to 90° and apply resistance on the medial side of the arm proximal to the elbow (Figure 20-36, *E*). Instruct the athlete to bring his or her arm straight across the chest. Moving your resistive hand to the posterior surface of the arm, ask the athlete to move the arm straight back to test horizontal abduction (Figure 20-36, *F*).

Inward the outward rotation are normally tested with the arm at the side of the body and elbow flexed to 90°. Stabilize the flexed elbow to the body to ensure the athlete does not substitute abduction for rotation. Instruct the athlete to outwardly and inwardly rotate the arm as you apply resistance at the athlete's wrist with the other hand (Figure 20-36, *G* and *H*)

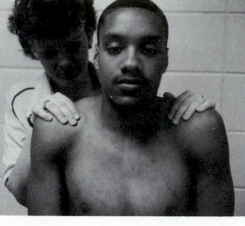

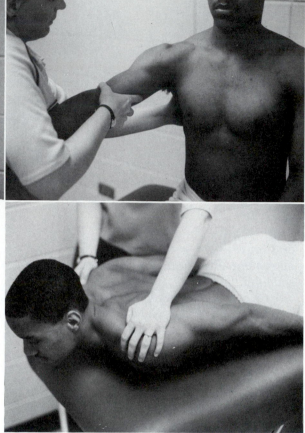

A

B

C

FIGURE 20-37
Applying manual resistance against scapulothoracid movements. **A,** Shoulder elevation; **B,** shoulder protraction; **C,** shoulder retraction.

Resistance can also be applied to scapulothoracic movements. Resist scapular elevation by placing your hands on each shoulder and pressing down as the athlete shrugs both shoulders (Figure 20-37, *A*). Normally an athlete can still shrug his or her shoulders against your maximum resistance. Scapular protraction and retraction are best evaluated unilaterally so the thorax can be stabilized to prevent substitute motions. With the athlete sitting and the shoulder flexed to 90°, place one hand along the spine to stabilize the thorax and apply resistance to protraction with the other (Figure 20-37, *B*). Note any winging of the scapula. Winging may also be demonstrated when an athlete performs a pushup or pushes against a wall (Figure 20-38).

Scapular retraction is probably best performed with the athlete lying in a prone position. Resistance is applied to the lateral angle of the scapula as the athlete lifts the shoulder or brings the shoulder blades together (Figure 20-37, *C*).

Special resistive tests are used to evaluate specific anatomic structures when an injury is suspected. One such maneuver is called the **Yergason test.** This test determines if the tendon of the long head of the biceps is stable in the bicipital groove or if a

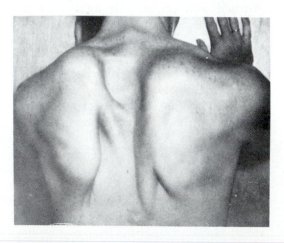

FIGURE 20-38
Winging of the left scapula.

tenosynovitis exists. Have the athlete flex the elbow on the involved side to 90°. Support the elbow with one hand and grasp the athlete's wrist with the other. Instruct the athlete to maintain this position as you attempt to extend the elbow and outwardly rotate the arm (Figure 20-39). This places stress on the biceps tendon and will normally produce pain in the bicipital groove if there is a tenosynovitis. A painful snap along the bicipital groove may be caused by subluxation of the tendon because of a tear of the transverse humeral ligament. If the tendon is not injured or involved in an injury, this test will produce no discomfort in the bicipital groove.

Passive movements. Passive movements are often used to facilitate the assessment of shoulder injuries. The specific maneuvers used depend on the type of injury suspected or indicated by the evaluation up to this point.

Occasionally, the ROM of the shoulder will be evaluated passively. In order to obtain the most useful information, the shoulder must be relaxed during these maneuvers. It is best to have the athlete lying down and in a comfortable position. Passive ROM may be especially informative when active motion appears limited. Is motion limited by pain or muscular weakness or restricted by a frozen shoulder syndrome? Athletes exhibiting restricted active motion but a normal ROM when the contractile units are relaxed probably have muscular involvement resulting in pain and weakness. Passive ROM procedures must be performed *cautiously* so as not to cause further damage.

Passive movements are also used to evaluate impingement syndromes of the shoulder. Remember, these conditions are caused as soft tissue structures are impinged (squeezed) between the unyielding coracoacromial arch and the greater tuberosity of the humerus. Two procedures are commonly used in an attempt to reproduce the symptoms associated with an impingement syndrome. One is to passively bring the arm into complete flexion, driving the greater tuberosity against the anteroinferior surface of

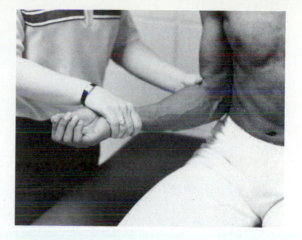

FIGURE 20-39
Yergason test to evaluate stability of the tendon of long head of the biceps. With the elbow held in a 90° flexed position, attempt to extend the elbow and outwardly rotate the arm as the athlete resists.

the acromion (Figure 20-40, *A*). This will compress the irritated tissues and is frequently positive in impingement. This test is also known as the **impingement sign.** An alternate method to test for an impingement is to forcibly rotate the proximal humerus inwardly when the arm is flexed 90° (Figure 20-40, *B*). This maneuver drives the greater tuberosity under the coracoacromial ligament, which may reproduce the impingement pain. This procedure is also known as the **Hawkins-Kennedy Impingement Test.**

Passive procedures can also be used to assess the integrity of the articulations of the shoulder girdle. These procedures are used to assess the severity of the injury and should not be attempted until you are relatively sure of the nature of the injury. Passive maneuvers should be performed gently to begin with, so as not to aggravate the injury and lose the athlete's cooperation. The force used with each of these maneuvers can then be increased, depending on the athlete's tolerance and the severity of the injury.

To passively stress the sternoclavicular and acromioclavicular joints, attempt to

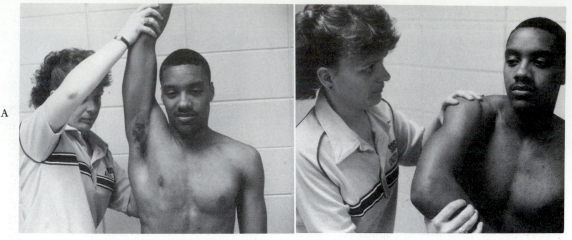

FIGURE 20-40

To evaluate the presence of an impingement syndrome: **A,** forcibly flex the arm to drive the greater tuberosity against the anteroinferior surface of the acromion and, **B,** forced inward rotation of the proximal humerus with the arm flexed to 90° to drive the greater tuberosity under the coracoacromial ligament.

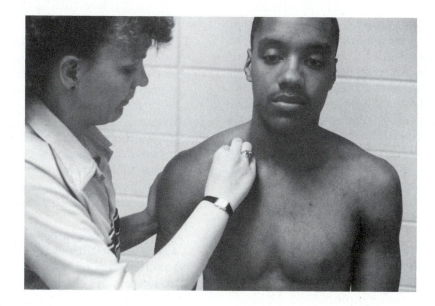

FIGURE 20-41

Applying passive stress to the clavicle to evaluate the strenoclavicular and acromioclavicular joints.

manually move the clavicle. This can be accomplished by grasping the clavicle between the thumb and fingers and attempting to move it up and down or simply pressing down (Figure 20-41). An alternative method of passively stressing the acromioclavicular joint is to place your hands over the shoulder, the heel of one hand on the clavicle and the other on the scapular spine. Then squeeze the heels of the hands together (Figure 20-42, *A*). This causes a shearing movement, especially at the acromioclavicular

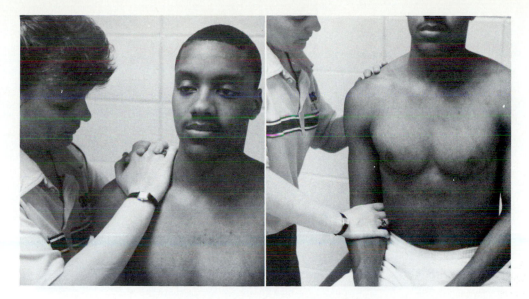

A   B

FIGURE 20-42
Passively stressing the acromioclavicular joint by, **A,** squeezing the clavicle toward the scapula and, **B,** pulling down on the arm to stress the joint.

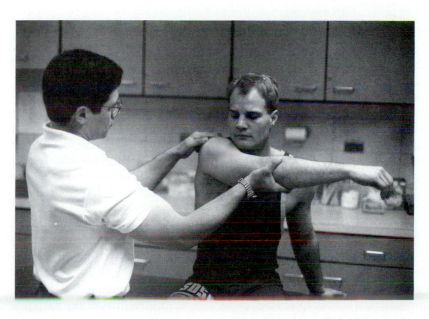

FIGURE 20-43
Crossover maneuver to stress the acromioclavicular joint.

joint, and may elicit abnormal mobility or pain. Another procedure that may be used to stress the acromioclavicular joint is to attempt to separate the acromion and clavicle by pulling down on the arm (Figure 20-42, *B*). Pain and mobility may be increased by this maneuver if the athlete has suffered a partial separation. Another passive test (or active, if the athlete does it) for assessment of abnormalities within either the acromioclavicular or sternoclavicular joint is to bring the abducted arm across the front of the body, thus compressing both of these joints (Figure 20-43). This is known as the

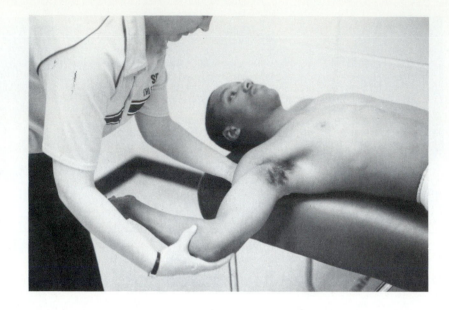

FIGURE 20-44
Apprehension test to evalaute status of anterior stability for the glenohumeral joint.

crossover maneuver and the presence of superior pain or discomfort may confirm an injury to the acromioclavicular joint.

To passively evaluate the integrity of the glenohumeral joint, the athletic trainer commonly uses *apprehension tests*. To test for anterior shoulder instability, have the athlete in a supine position so the muscles about the shoulder are as relaxed as possible. Passively move the arm to 90° of abduction and then gently outwardly rotate (Figure 20-44). This puts the glenohumeral joint in a compromising position; if there is a history of subluxations or dislocations, the athlete will normally express apprehension in this position and resist any further motion.

If the apprehension test is tolerated, pressure may be applied to the posterior aspect of the shoulder, pushing the humeral head anteriorly. If the pain and apprehension is increased with this forward force (anterior translation), a posterior translation force is applied to the humeral head. This is called a **relocation test.** If this results in a decrease of pain and apprehension, the athlete is likely to have some anterior instability of the glenohumeral joint. During these apprehension tests, the humeral head may actually sublux if the athlete has a chronic subluxation of the shoulder. The athlete may also relate that this is how it felt when the shoulder was previously injured.

To test for posterior shoulder instability, move the arm to 90° flexion and inwardly rotate the shoulder. Apply a posterior force at the elbow and note any apprehension. A positive test is indicative of a posterior instability.

Inferior instability may be demonstrated by pulling down the relaxed arm, as was previously illustrated in Figure 20-42, *B*. Note any inferior migration of the humeral head or apprehension. If there is a "hollowing out" or dimpling of the skin just distal to the acromion, this is a positive test for inferior instability. This is called a **sulcus sign.**

Another procedure used to evaluate shoulder stability is the **glenohumeral translation test**. With the athlete sitting or lying supine, use one hand to stabilize the scapula and the other to grasp the humeral head. The athlete must be relaxed. Apply anterior and posterior force to the humeral head and attempt to recognize the degree of glenohumeral translation. Translation up to 50% of the humeral head diameter is considered normal.

Although there is no single test that can establish a positive assessment, there are several passive procedures that are commonly used to assist in evaluating a possible thoracic outlet syndrome. Probably the most reliable is the reproduction of symptoms on hyperabduction and outward rotation of the arm. This maneuver compresses the brachial plexus against the scalene muscles and may reproduce symptoms if the outlet is narrowed.

Another commonly used test for thoracic outlet syndrome is the **Adson maneuver,** which involves feeling the radial pulse as you passively abduct, extend, and outwardly rotate the arm (Figure 20-45). Instruct the athlete to take a deep breath while extending and turning his or her head toward the involved side. If there is compression of the subclavian artery, you will feel a marked diminution or absence of the radial pulse. A positive Adson's sign may indicate a thoracic outlet syndrome, although a positive test has also been found in healthy individuals.

Functional movements. Functional movements or activities can be very beneficial to the comprehensive assessment of shoulder injuries. Because many injuries involving the shoulder result from repetitive throwing or swinging activities, those same activities may be required to replicate the injury-causing movements and demonstrate the signs and symptoms associated with the injury. Occasionally, this is the only type of activity that will reproduce the signs and symptoms. The action of throwing or swinging involves complex, coordinated movements, and athletic trainers must possess a fundamental knowledge of these important skills to accurately assess associated injuries.

When the assessment process completed to this point has produced few definitive signs and symptoms, functional activities can be very helpful in evaluation. Instruct the athlete to perform functional activities of the shoulder that are required for his or

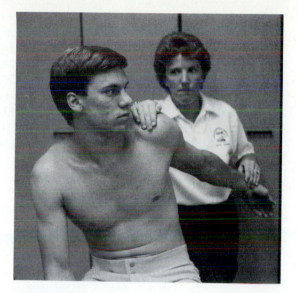

FIGURE 20-45
Adson maneuver, which involves feeling for the radial pulse as you passively abduct, extend, and outwardly rotate the arm.

her particular sport. These activities will vary greatly, depending on the sport, the equipment used, the age and maturity of the athlete, any history of previous injuries, or the presence of weakness, fatigue, or incoordination of motion. Swinging activities are in many ways similar to the throwing motion. Can the athlete perform the activity normally and without pain or other symptoms? During which phase of the motion are signs and symptoms expressed? Correlating the precise location of pain with the specific function will greatly assist in identifying the anatomic structures involved in the injury.

Functional movements are always used to determine when an athlete can return to activity. As an athlete recovers from a shoulder injury, functional activities become increasingly important on each re-evaluation. Keep accurate and dated records of each evaluation. The intensity of functional movements should be progressively increased within the limits of pain and ROM.

Neurological evaluations

Sensory functions. The athletic trainer should be aware of the basic sensory distribution of the normal dermatomes and the cutaneous distribution of the various peripheral nerves about the shoulder complex. The dermatomes about the shoulder are C4, which supplies the top of the shoulder; C5, the lateral arm; C6, the anterior and posterior arm; C7, the posterior lateral arm; T1, the medial arm; and T2, the axilla (Figure 20-46). Run your relaxed hands and fingers over these surfaces, note any differences in sensations, and compare the sensations to the uninjured shoulder.

Motor functions. Motor functions have been previously discussed under active movements. These procedures may occur early in the assessment process as you ask the athlete to perform each movement of the shoulder through as great a ROM as possible. The primary myotomes of the shoulder are C3 and C4, trapezius; C5 and C6, biceps, Pectoralis major, and deltoid; and C7 and C8, triceps and latissimus dorsi.

Reflexes. The reflexes that are commonly checked in the shoulder region are the biceps (C5 to C6) and triceps (C7). The biceps tendon reflex is checked with the athlete's arm flexed at the elbow and supported so that the muscle is relaxed. Place your thumb over the biceps tendon and strike the thumb with a reflex hammer with a slight downward thrust to augment the tendon stretch (Figure 20-47, *A*). The normal response is flexion at the elbow. To test the triceps reflex, tap the triceps tendon with the reflex hammer (Figure 20-47, *B*). The normal response is extension of the forearm or straightening.

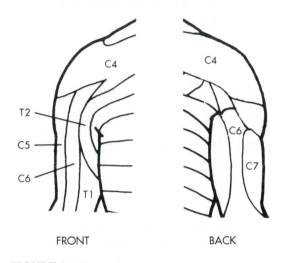

FIGURE 20-46
Dermatomes of the shoulder and upper arm.

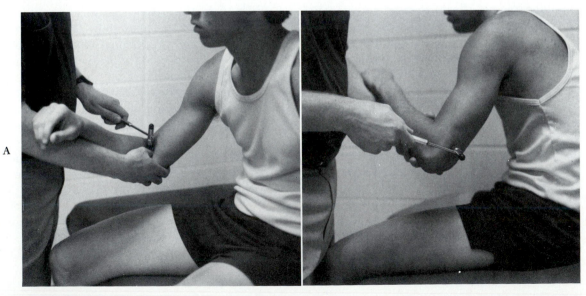

FIGURE 20-47
Test of the, **A,** biceps reflex (C5, C6) and, **B,** triceps reflex (C7).

Circulatory evaluations

It is important to evaluate the adequacy of circulatory supply to the upper extremity with any major injury involving the upper extremity. Circulation can be evaluated by feeling for peripheral pulses, namely the radial at the wrist or the brachial at the elbow.

Evaluation of Findings

The shoulder is one of the most frequently injured areas of the upper extremity. The extensive ROM and the inherent instability of the shoulder joint make this area of the body vulnerable to acute athletic injuries, as well as chronic overuse conditions. Because of the complex movement patterns of the shoulder girdle, an injury to one segment can involve the others; in addition, many different shoulder structures can be involved in a single injury. The nature and severity of shoulder injuries can therefore be extremely difficult to accurately assess.

This chapter has presented basic evaluative procedures used to isolate the various structures about the shoulder to either implicate or rule out their involvement following injury. All of these procedures will not be applicable to any one shoulder injury. Whenever a serious injury is indicated or suspected, the athlete should be promptly referred to a physician. In the interim, the arm should be maintained in a position that provides optimum comfort and supported by the use of a pillow or sling. The athlete should be withheld from full activity as long as he or she has a limited ROM or pain with exercise. Shoulder injuries require frequent re-evaluations to monitor progress and determine when the athlete can return to activity.

When to refer the athlete

Because of the complexity of this body area and the importance of early care, many shoulder injuries should be evaluated by a physician. Conditions or findings that can be used to determine if medical referral is indicated are listed in the "When to Refer the Athlete . . ." box on page 588.

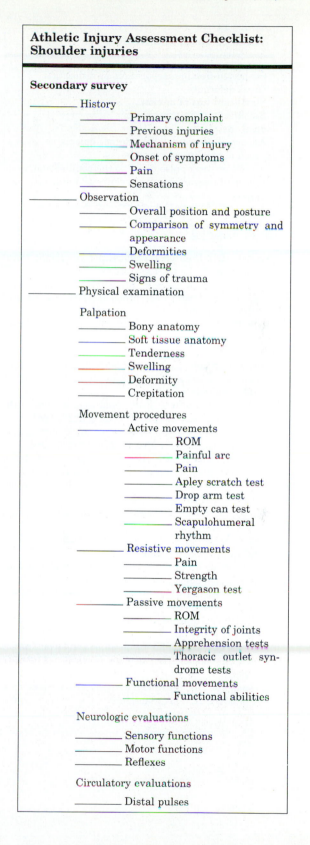

Athletic Injury Assessment Checklist: Shoulder injuries

Secondary survey

———— History
  ———— Primary complaint
  ———— Previous injuries
  ———— Mechanism of injury
  ———— Onset of symptoms
  ———— Pain
  ———— Sensations
———— Observation
  ———— Overall position and posture
  ———— Comparison of symmetry and appearance
  ———— Deformities
  ———— Swelling
  ———— Signs of trauma
———— Physical examination

Palpation
  ———— Bony anatomy
  ———— Soft tissue anatomy
  ———— Tenderness
  ———— Swelling
  ———— Deformity
  ———— Crepitation

Movement procedures
  ———— Active movements
    ———— ROM
    ———— Painful arc
    ———— Pain
    ———— Apley scratch test
    ———— Drop arm test
    ———— Empty can test
    ———— Scapulohumeral rhythm
  ———— Resistive movements
    ———— Pain
    ———— Strength
    ———— Yergason test
  ———— Passive movements
    ———— ROM
    ———— Integrity of joints
    ———— Apprehension tests
    ———— Thoracic outlet syndrome tests
  ———— Functional movements
    ———— Functional abilities

Neurologic evaluations
  ———— Sensory functions
  ———— Motor functions
  ———— Reflexes

Circulatory evaluations
  ———— Distal pulses

When to Refer the Athlete . . .

Suspected fracture, separation, or dislocation
Gross deformity
Significant loss of motion
Significant or continued pain
Joint instability
Abnormal sensations that do not quickly go away, such as weakness or numbness
Absent or weak pulse distal to the point of injury
Any doubt regarding the severity or nature of the injury

REFERENCES

Arnheim DD, Prentice WE: *Principles of athletic training,* ed 8, St. Louis, 1993, Mosby.

Bach BR, Novak PJ: Chronic acromioclavicular joint pain: an overlooked problem, *Phys Sportsmed* 21(1):63, 1993.

Bach BR, VanFleet TA, Novak PJ: Acromioclavicular injuries: controversies in treatment, *Phys Sportsmed* 20(12):87, 1992.

Jobe FW, editor: *Clinics in Sports Medicine: Symposium on injuries to the shoulder in the athlete,* Vol 2, 1983, Saunders.

Davies GJ and others: Functional examination of the shoulder girdle, *Phys Sportsmed* 9(6):82, 1981.

Gallaspy JB, Poole WH: Evaluation of the acromioclavicular joint, *Sports Med Update* 4(3):28, 1989.

Grana WA and others: How I manage acute anterior shoulder dislocations, *Phys Sportsmed* 15(4):88, 1987.

Harrelson GL: Evaluation of brachial plexus injuries, *Sports Med Update* 4(2):3, 1989.

Henry JH: How I manage dislocated shoulder, *Phys Sportsmed* 12(9):65, 1984.

Magee DJ: *Orthopedic physical assessment,* ed 2, Philadelphia, 1992, Saunders.

McMaster WC: Painful shoulder in swimmers: a diagnostic challenge, *Phys Sportsmed* 14(12):108, 1986.

Neviaser TJ: Adhesive capsulitis, *Orthop Clin North Am* 18(3):439, 1987.

Neviaser JS: Injuries of the clavicle and its articulations, *Orthop Clin North Am* 11(2):233, 1980.

Neviaser RJ: Anatomic considerations and examination of the shoulder, *Orthop Clin North Am* 11(2):187, 1980.

O'Donoghue DH: *Treatment of injuries to athletes,* ed 4, Philadelphia, 1984, Saunders.

Poole WH, Gallaspy JB: Swimmer's shoulder: anatomy, cause, evaluation, treatment, *Sports Med Update* 6(1):3, 1991.

Sallis RE, Jones K, Knopp W: Burners: offensive strategy for an underreported injury, *Phys Sportsmed* 20(11):47, 1992.

Sartoris DJ: Diagnosing shoulder pain: what's the best imaging approach, *Phys Sportsmed* 20(9):151, 1992.

Strauss MB and others: The shrugged-off shoulder: a comparison of patients with recurrent shoulder subluxations and dislocations, *Phys Sportsmed* 11(3):85, 1983.

Zarins B and others: *Injuries to the throwing arm,* Philadelphia, 1985, Saunders.

SUGGESTED READINGS

Aronen JG: Anterior shoulder dislocations in sports, *Sports Med* 3:224, 1986.
Discusses the diagnosis, treatment, and rehabilitation of anterior shoulder dislocations.

Capistrant TD: Thoracic outlet syndrome in cervical strain injury, *Minn Med* 69:13, 1986.
Reviews the current criteria for diagnosis of thoracic outlet syndrome and recommends a direct treatment approach for this condition.

Hawkins RJ, Abrams JS: Impingement syndrome in the absence of rotator cuff tear (stage 1 and 2), *Orthop Clin North Am* 18(3):373, 1987.
Two orthopedic surgeons discuss the pathology, diagnosis, and management of impingement syndromes.

McMaster WC: Anterior glenoid labrum damage: a painful lesion in swimmers, *Am J Sports Med* 14(5):383, 1986.
Describes the functional instability problem of glenoid labrum damage in the swimmer, as well as its diagnosis and management.

Nicholas JA, Hershman EB, editors: *The upper extremity in sports medicine,* St. Louis, 1990, Mosby.
An excellent text by many contributors discussing the various upper extremity injuries and conditions.

Pappas AM and others: Symptomatic shoulder instability due to lesions of the glenoid labrum, *Am J Sports Med* 11(5):279, 1983.
Discusses glenoid labrum lesions, including various etiological factors, diagnosis, and management procedures.

$\mathscr{C}$HAPTER 21

Elbow and forearm injuries

After you have completed this chapter, you should be able to:

- Identify the basic anatomy of the elbow and forearm.
- Discuss the common athletic injuries that may occur to the elbow and forearm.
- Describe the assessment process for an athlete suffering an injury to the elbow or forearm.
- Discuss the various manipulative procedures used to evaluate injuries and conditions about the elbow.
- List the signs and symptoms that indicate an athlete with an elbow or forearm injury should be referred to medical assistance.

The elbow and forearm are important functional links between the shoulder and the intricate mechanisms of the hand. The elbow joint is the central link in the upper extremity kinetic chain and allows the arm to flex and extend. The articulations between the radius and ulna permit the forearm to rotate, that is, pronate and supinate. In addition, all the **extrinsic** muscles of the hand originate about the elbow or forearm. Therefore the ability to perform athletic skills involving the upper extremities is dependent on the integrity of the bones, ligaments, and muscles of the elbow and forearm.

ANATOMY OF THE ELBOW

The elbow is sometimes described as "three joints in one capsule." One joint exists between the humerus and ulna, a second between the humerus and radius, and a third between the proximal ends of the ulna and radius. These components of the elbow share a common articular capsule, and their joint spaces are continuous. Although movements at the elbow joint proper should not be confused with those that occur at the superior radioulnar joint, it would be unwise from a functional standpoint for the athletic trainer to only consider one and not the others when assessing an elbow injury.

The elbow joint is often subdivided into two points of articulation: (1) the humeroulnar, between the trochlea of the humerus and the ulna, and (2) the humeroradial, between the capitulum of the humerus and the radius.

Begin your review of elbow anatomy by examining the surface markings in Figure 21-1. Review the bony anatomy in Figure 21-2. Identify the four bony projections on the distal end of the humerus—the medial and lateral epicondyles, the capitulum, and the

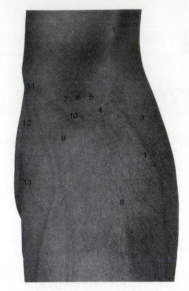

A

1	Cephalic vein
2	Lateral epicondyle
3	Brachioradialis
4	Median cephalic vein
5	Biceps tendon
6	Brachial artery
7	Median nerve
8	Median forearm vein
9	Pronator teres
10	Median basilic vein
11	Basilic vein
12	Medial epicondyle
13	Lateral cutaneous nerve of forearm
14	Medial cutaneous nerve of forearm
15	Median cubital vein
16	Brachialis
17	Radial artery
18	Bicipital aponeurosis
19	Nerve to pronator teres
20	A muscular artery
21	Medial intermuscular septum
22	Medial head of triceps

1	Triceps
2	Medial epicondyle of humerus
3	Ulnar nerve
4	Olecranon of ulna
5	Margin of olecranon bursa
6	Flexor carpi ulnaris
7	Posterior border of ulna
8	Anconeus
9	Extensor muscle
10	Head of radius
11	Capitulum of humerus
12	Lateral epicondyle of humerus
13	Extensor carpi radialis longus
14	Brachioradialis

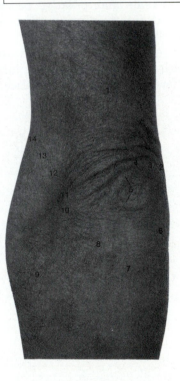

B

FIGURE 21-1
Surface anatomy of the left elbow. **A,** Anterior view and, **B,** posterior view.

trochlea—and two depressions—the olecranon and coronoid fossae. The epicondyles and their supracondylar ridges can be palpated as rough projections on both the medial and lateral sides of the distal humerus. These bony prominences are the points of attachment for the shared tendons called the common flexor and extensor tendons of the forearm, which are frequent sites of athletic related injuries. The capitulum and the trochlea are located just distal to the lateral and medial epicondyles of the humerus, respectively. The capitulum is a rounded knob that articulates with the head of the radius, whereas the trochlea is a pulley or spool-

shaped projection that fits into the trochlear notch of the ulna.

In the anatomic position the ulna is located on the medial (little finger) side and the radius on the lateral (thumb) side of the forearm. In this position both bones are approximately parallel and the forearm and hand are said to be in supination. The palm

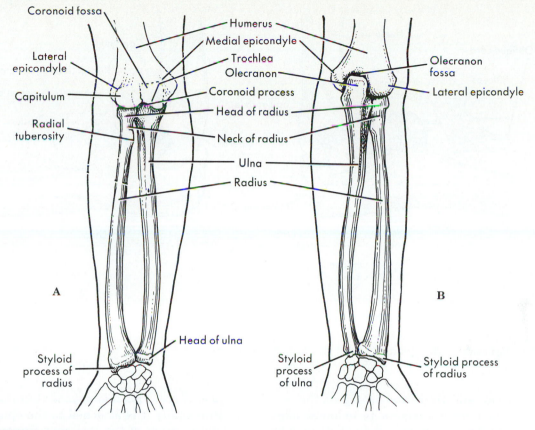

FIGURE 21-2
Bony anatomy of the elbow and forearm. **A,** Anterior view and, **B,** posterior view.

of the hand is turned forward (anteriorly) when the forearm is supinated. In the position of pronation the palm is turned backward (posteriorly) as the radius crosses in front of the ulna.

The upper (proximal) end of the ulna is easily identified by a large concavity called the semilunar (trochlear) notch. As indicated previously, this notch serves as a point for articulation with the trochlea of the humerus. This deep notch lies between two bony projections, the large proximal and posteriorly projecting **olecranon process** and the less massive, distal and anteriorly projecting coronoid process. These processes are the points of attachment for the triceps brachii and the brachialis, respectively. Just below the notch on the lateral side of the coronoid process is a small concave depression, the radial notch, which receives the head of the radius. During pronation and su-

pination of the forearm the head of the radius rotates within this notch.

The proximal end of the radius has three prominent bony features: a round head, which has a smooth, slightly concave upper surface; a narrow neck; and just below the neck, on the ulnar (medial) side of the body, the radial tuberosity, which is the insertion of the biceps brachii.

Articular Capsule and Collateral Ligaments

The elbow joint proper and the superior radioulnar joint share a common fibrous articular capsule and have a continuous joint space. The capsule is lined by a synovial membrane that reflects onto the bones of the joint and attaches to the edges of the articulating surfaces. This capsule is thin and rather loose on the anterior and posterior surfaces of the joint to permit flexion and

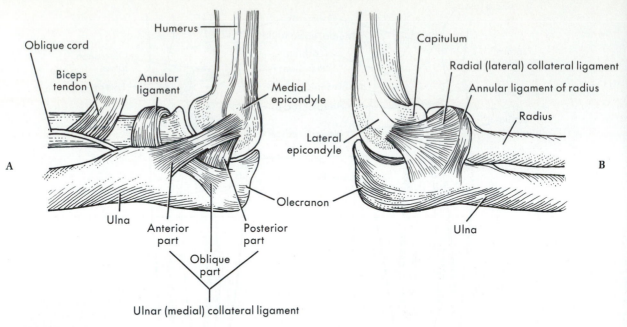

FIGURE 21-3
Major ligaments of elbow joint. **A,** Medial view and, **B,** lateral view.

extension, and thick and strong on the medial and lateral surfaces to enhance joint stability. The capsule is subdivided into four ligaments, the ulnar (medial) collateral ligament, the radial (lateral) collateral ligament, the anterior ligament, and the posterior ligament (Figure 21-3).

The *ulnar (medial) collateral ligament* consists of three bands passing between the medial epicondyle and the medial edge of the trochlear notch. The oblique portion of the ligament helps to deepen the socket for articulation of the trochlea of the humerus. The anterior part of the ligament becomes taut in extension and the weak, fan-shaped posterior portion becomes taut in flexion. The ulnar nerve lies on this ligament as it passes behind the medial epicondyle into the forearm. The strong fan-shaped *radial (lateral) collateral ligament* extends from the outer surface of the lateral epicondyle of the humerus to the outer edge of the annular ligament. The thin *anterior ligament* is attached to the medial epicondyle and to the humerus above the coronoid fossa. The distal portion of this ligament is continuous with the collateral ligaments. The medially

placed *posterior ligament* is thin and weak. Proximally it is attached to the epicondyles and margins of the olecranon fossa; distally it is attached to the olecranon process of the ulna.

Synovial Membrane and Subcutaneous Bursae

The synovial membrane that lines the articular capsule of the elbow is extensive. It projects into the recesses of the common joint space and extends into both the coronoid and olecranon fossae. A redundant fold of synovial membrane also extends under the annular ligament (Figure 21-4). This fold provides a cushion for rotation of the head of the radius during pronation and supination of the forearm.

Pads of fat are often found between the synovial membrane and fibrous capsule over or near the articular fossae. The largest of these fatty accumulations lies over the olecranon fossa. It is pressed into the fossa during extension by the tendon of the triceps.

The subtendinous olecranon bursa is located between the tendon of the triceps, the outer, or posterior, surface of the olecranon

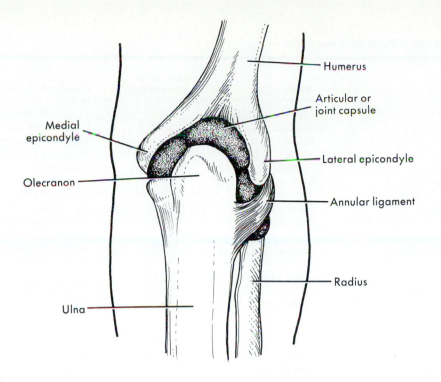

FIGURE 21-4
Elbow joint, posterior view. Note the fold of synovial membrane passing below the annular
ligament.

process, and the skin. It is most frequently
found just proximal to (above) the insertion
of the triceps tendon. The olecranon is the
most commonly injured bursa of the elbow,
as is discussed later in this chapter. Numerous other subcutaneous bursae are also
found (inconsistently) over the medial and
lateral epicondyles of the humerus.

Elbow Muscles and Movements

The principle muscles of the elbow and forearm are listed in Table 21-1. Some of the
more important muscles of this area of the
upper extremity and their points of attachments are illustrated in Figures 21-5 to 21-
10.

The reciprocally concave-to-convex articular surface between the trochlea of the humerus and the wrench-like upper end of the
ulna permits only flexion and extension. The
result is a typical uniaxial, or hinge-type,
joint. Flexion is produced primarily by the
biceps, brachialis, and brachioradialis muscles. In addition, in strongly resisted flexion,
muscles arising from the medial epicondyle

of the humerus act as weak accessory flexors. During flexion, the coronoid fossa on the
anterior surface of the humerus receives the
coronoid process of the ulna. The degree of
flexion that is permitted varies between persons and is limited by contact of soft tissues
between the forearm and arm. The prime
mover in elbow extension is the triceps muscle (Figure 21-6). The tiny anconeus muscle
arising from the lateral epicondyle and attaching to the ulna may act as a weak accessory extensor. The olecranon fossa, a depression on the posterior surface of the
humerus just above the trochlea, receives
the olecranon process of the ulna during extension of the forearm. Extension is limited
by actual contact of the olecranon with the
floor of the olecranon fossa.

When considered as a total functional
unit, the elbow complex permits not only
flexion and extension but also supination
and pronation of the forearm and hand.
These movements are possible because of
the uniaxial pivot-type articulation between
the head of the radius and the ulna, called

TABLE 21-1

Muscles of the Elbow and Forearm

Muscle	Nerve	Segmental innervation	Primary action(s)
Biceps	Musculocutaneous	C_5, C_6	Flexion at elbow and supination
Brachialis	Musculocutaneous	C_5, C_6	Flexion at elbow
Triceps	Radial	C_5, C_8	Extension at elbow
Anconeus	Radial	C_6, C_7	Extension at elbow
Pronator teres	Median	C_5, C_7	Pronation
Pronator quadratus	Median	C_7-T_1	Pronation
Flexor carpi radialis	Median	C_6, C_7	Flexion at wrist
Palmaris longus	Median	C_7, C_8	Flexion at wrist
Flexor digitorum superficialis	Median	C_7-T_1	Flexion of middle phalanges of digits
Flexor pollicis longus	Median	C_7-T_1	Flexion of distal phalanx of thumb
Flexor digitorum profundus	Median (radial)	C_8, T_1	Flexion of distal phalanges
	Ulnar (ulnar)	C_8, T_1	
Flexor carpi ulnaris	Ulnar	C_8, T_1	Flexion at wrist
Brachioradialis	Radial	C_5, C_6	Flexion at elbow
Extensor carpi radialis longus & brevis	Radial	C_6, C_7	Extension at wrist
Extensor carpi ulnaris	Radial	C_6-C_8	Extension at wrist
Supinator	Radial	C_5, C_6	Supination
Extensor digitorum	Radial	C_6-C_8	Extension of all joints of digits II–V
Extensor digiti minimi	Radial	C_6-C_8	Extension of all joints of digit V
Extensor indicis	Radial	C_7, C_8	Extension of all joints of digit II
Extensor pollicis longus	Radial	C_7, C_8	Extension and adduction of thumb
Extensor pollicis brevis	Radial	C_6, C_7	Extension of proximal phalanx of thumb
Abductor pollicis longus	Radial	C_6, C_7	Extension and abduction of thumb

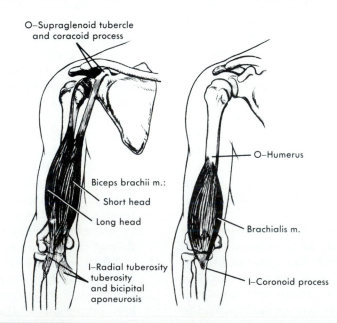

FIGURE 21-5
Biceps brachii and brachialis muscles.

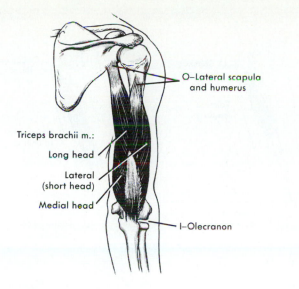

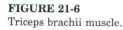

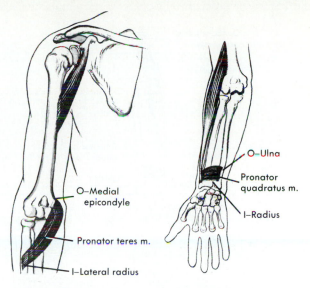

FIGURE 21-6
Triceps brachii muscle.

FIGURE 21-7
Pronator teres and pronator quadratus muscles.

the superior radioulnar joint. The superior radioulnar joint is supported by a strong *annular ligament* that encircles the head of the radius and forms a collar, holding it in close contact with the articular surface (radial notch) of the ulna. Pronation and supination movements produce rotation of the forearm along its long axis, with the radius "crossing over" the ulna. Pronation is produced primarily by the pronator teres and pronator quadratus muscles (Figure 21-7) and supination by the biceps and supinator muscles (Figure 21-8).

Muscles of the Forearm

The muscles of the forearm can be divided into flexor (Figure 21-9) and extensor (Figure 21-10) groups and act on the elbow, wrist, and digits. The flexor muscles arise in large part from the medial epicondyle from a shared tendon called the *common flexor tendon*. Muscles involved in pronation also originate in this area. The flexor and pronator muscles occupy the medial border and anterior surface of the forearm. The extensor muscles arise in large part from the lateral epicondyle from a shared tendon called the *common extensor tendon*. Muscles involved in supination also originate in this area. The extensor and supinator muscles

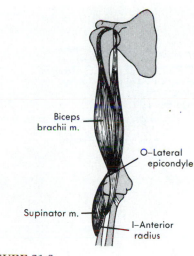

FIGURE 21-8
Supinator muscle.

occupy the lateral border and posterior surface of the forearm. In the upper part of the forearm, the flexor and extensor muscles form fleshy masses below the medial and lateral epicondyles. The hollow triangular area lying just distal to the elbow joint and formed between these two muscle masses is called the *cubital fossa*. The muscle mass of the forearm rapidly tapers off towards the wrist, where the long tendons of these muscles continue into the hand.

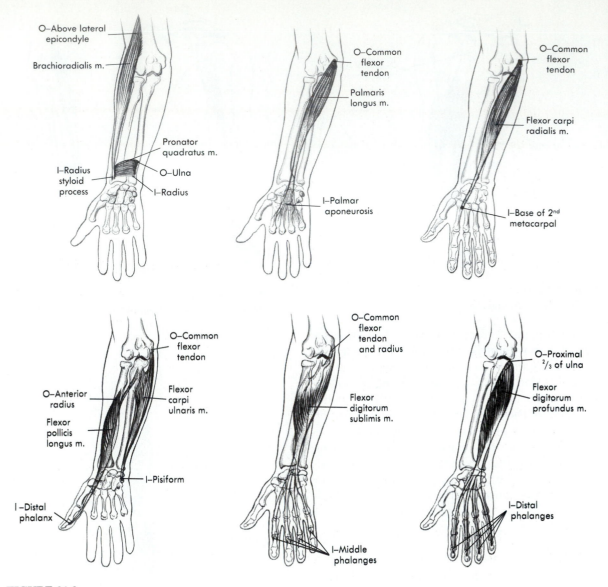

FIGURE 21-9
Some muscles of the anterior aspect of the right forearm.

Interosseous Membrane

The interosseous membrane is a strong fibrous sheet of connective tissue that connects the shafts of the radius and ulna. Its fibers run downward and medially from radius to ulna.

The proximal (superior) end of the ulna is heavy and firmly articulated at the elbow, whereas the radius is strong and broadened at the wrist. Therefore, for practical purposes, the athletic trainer should think of the ulna as the distal extension of the humerus, which is associated with elbow strength and motion, and the radius as an upward, or proximal, extension of the hand, which is associated with motions of the hand and wrist.

Forces placed against the hand must be transmitted from the radius to the ulna and then to the humerus. When this occurs, the radius is forced superiorly and the ulna inferiorly. The arrangement of fibers in the in-

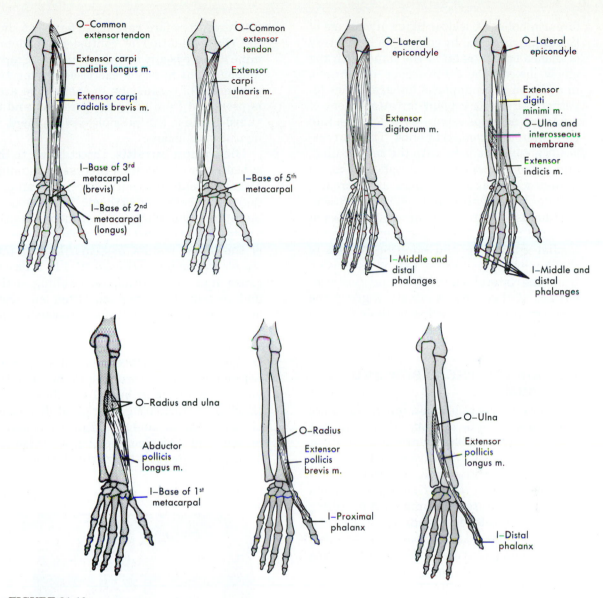

FIGURE 21-10
Some muscles of the posterior aspect of the right forearm.

terosseous membrane transmits to the ulna, and then to the humerus, forces acting upward through the hand. The membrane also prevents displacement that these forces would otherwise create between ulna and radius.

An understanding of the direction of fibers in the interosseous membrane (downward and medially from radius to ulna) explains the difficulty and forearm pain often associated with carrying or lifting, such as deadlifting a heavy weight. In this type of activity the weight is pulling the two forearm bones apart, and the interosseous membrane is constructed so that it can provide only very limited help in preventing displacement. Heavy loads can be carried more easily on the palm of the hand with the elbow flexed, as a powerlifter holds a weighted bar during a squat lift or deep knee bend. In this position the interosseous membrane helps prevent displacement of the forearm bones. A waiter takes advantage of this same principal by carrying a heavy tray of dishes on the palm of the hand with the elbow flexed. The interosseous membrane, in addition to binding the forearm bones together, serves as a point for attachment of muscles and helps separate the forearm into two anatomic compartments. The interosseous membrane joins with the radius, ulna, and a strong aponeurotic-like sheet of fascia (antebrachial fascia) to separate the forearm into dorsal (extensor) and volar (flexor) compartments. The result is an anatomic separation of the flexor muscles arising from the medial epicondyle and anterior surface of the forearm from those extensors arising from the lateral epicondyle and posterior surface of this area. Anatomists group the forearm muscles according to their location in either the dorsal (extensor) or volar (flexor) compartment.

INJURIES TO THE ELBOW AND FOREARM

Injuries involving the elbow and forearm are common in athletic activity. Many different types of force and stress are applied about the elbow during the various activities involved in different sports. A variety of athletic injuries can result from direct trauma to the area, indirect trauma such as falling on an outstretched hand, or acute and chronic stresses associated with throwing and swinging activities. These mechanisms of injury can result in contusions, sprains, strains, dislocations, fractures and nerve involvement.

Contusions

Contusions are common injuries to this area of the body and may involve the muscles of the forearm or the subcutaneous bony prominences of the elbow. An athlete's forearms absorb the brunt of many impacts during athletic activity, especially during contact sports. Direct blows to these muscular areas can result in bruising and subsequent bleeding, producing stiffness during function and active range of motion (ROM). The direct blow that causes the contusion may also be responsible for additional trauma such as a

fracture; therefore care must be taken during the evaluation of contusions to determine if there is any additional injury. Proper management must be exercised during the treatment of contusions to ensure the area is protected from additional trauma and to guard against the possible development of myositis ossificans.

✤ **Olecranon bursitis.** Direct blows to the subcutaneous olecranon process of the ulna can also result in a contusion which can produce an acute hemorrhagic bursitis or a more common chronic olecranon bursitis. Acute bursitis occurs when a blow to the tip of the elbow results in hemorrhaging into the olecranon bursa (Figure 21-11). This can cause immediate dramatic swelling, pain, and restriction of motion. Often an acute olecranon bursitis will spontaneously subside. Improper initial care and repeated irritation of this area may allow this condition to develop into a chronic bursitis. Chronic trauma or repeated bruising to the tip of the elbow can result in bursal membrane irritation and thickening, a gradual distention of the bursal sac, and the formation of excess bursal fluid. The olecranon bursa is also one of the more frequently infected bursae. This

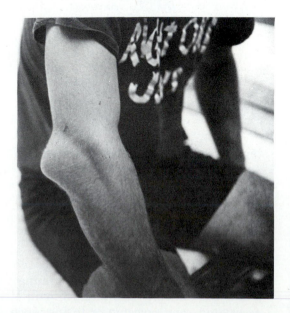

FIGURE 21-11
Acute olecranon bursitis.

is partially a result of the frequency of abrasions occurring over the tip of the elbow.

❖ **Ulnar nerve contusion.** An injury that almost everyone has suffered at one time or another is a blow or contusion to the ulnar nerve. As this nerve passes behind the medial epicondyle of the humerus, it lies subcutaneously in a groove and passes through the *cubital tunnel*. The relative lack of bony protection in this area make the ulnar nerve vulnerable to trauma. A direct blow to this area may cause immediate pain and burning sensations shooting down the ulnar side of the forearm to the ring and little fingers. This paresthesia, commonly referred to as hitting the "crazy bone," is normally transient and disappears in a few minutes depending upon the severity of the blow. Pain and numbness may persist for a period of time. Sometimes there is an associated weakness of the interossei muscles as well as the flexors of the ring and little fingers. Occasionally the ulnar nerve can be subluxed from its groove or involved in an entrapment syndrome, which is discussed later.

Strains

Strains to the muscular and musculotendinous structures about the elbow are common athletic injuries. These normally occur as a result of tremendous stresses being placed on the elbow joint, especially in sports requiring throwing or swinging motions. Strains are divided into acute and chronic types. Acute strains occur when a sudden overload is applied to the contractile units of the elbow joint. The resulting injury is a strain to muscles, musculotendinous junctions, or points of tendinous attachment in the area. The most common areas for acute strains are the common flexor tendon around the medial epicondyle and the common extensor tendon over the lateral epicondyle. There may also be an avulsion of muscle with a fragment of bone present. The biceps or triceps muscular unit may also be strained and occasionally the tendon of one of these muscles is ruptured. The symptoms of an acute strain to the musculature supporting the elbow include the history of an incident of sudden excessive overload followed by tenderness over the involved area and pain on function or resisted motion. If the injury results in a rupture of a tendon, there may also be a palpable gap, a bunching of the injured muscle, and a loss of efficient function of the involved muscle (Figure 21-12).

Chronic strains can occur about the elbow

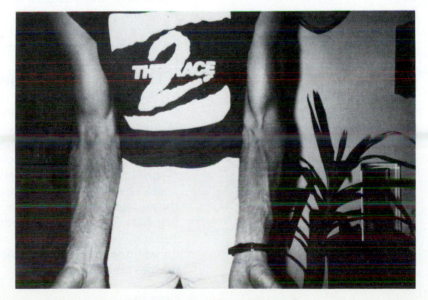

FIGURE 21-12
Biceps tendon rupture. Note absence of tendon on right side as athlete applies equal flexion forces.

as the result of continued overuse of a musculotendinous unit, with ultimate failure or impairment of function. Overuse, especially in sports requiring throwing or swinging, may cause irritation of the muscle fibers, resulting in microscopic tears of the contractile unit. Continued trauma to this area can develop into overuse syndromes and chronic degenerative processes. The process is one of progressive attritional wear and tear.

❖ **Epicondylitis.** Chronic strains commonly occur in the region of the medial and lateral epicondyles of the humerus, depending on the muscle groups irritated. For example, overuse of the wrist flexor-pronator muscles may cause symptoms over the medial epicondyle, whereas chronic irritation of the wrist extensor-supinator muscles may result in symptoms over the lateral epicondyle (Figure 21-13). These overuse conditions or chronic strains are usually caused by repeated overload of the musculotendinous units attaching to one of the epicondyles. Additional factors which may influence epicondylitis include faulty techniques or mechanics, weak muscle groups, and inappropriate

equipment. Names are frequently given to this overuse condition, depending on the athletic activity engaged in at the time of its development. For example, "tennis elbow" is a name commonly given to pain on the lateral side of the elbow because it frequently occurs in tennis players. However, tennis players can develop pain on the medial epicondyle, depending upon which muscle groups are irritated or overloaded. "Pitcher's elbow," "golfers elbow," "bowlers elbow," and "javelin thrower's elbow" are other names given to elbow epicondylitis that develops because of the sport in which the athlete is involved. "Little league elbow" is an inclusive term used to describe elbow lesions that result from the repetitive act of throwing by immature athletes. This term may encompass a variety of conditions within the elbow, such as epicondylitis or an injury to the epiphysis of the medial epicondyle of the humerus. This epiphysis is normally the last epiphyseal center to close around the elbow and one of the weakest. The symptoms may be of acute or gradual onset. When the onset is sudden, the injury is more likely to involve an avulsion of the epicondyle. Acute pain and tenderness over the epicondyle indicates that an immature athlete should be referred to a physician for further assessment. More commonly, little league elbow is a chronic condition, and the symptoms are usually those of persistent discomfort and stiffness about the elbow and are aggravated by use of the arm.

Early and accurate recognition is very important in the proper care of these overuse conditions. Initial symptoms of chronic strains are local tenderness over the involved epicondyle or common tendon, pain on use of the involved muscles, and perhaps swelling. Resisted wrist motion often reproduces the pain. Without proper treatment, these conditions may develop into prolonged degenerative changes resulting in chronic epicondylitis, contractures of the elbow, reduced function, and possible rupture of the muscle tendon unit.

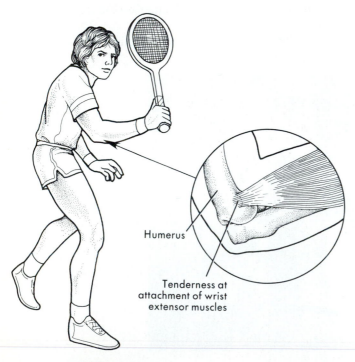

Humerus

Tenderness at
attachment of wrist
extensor muscles

FIGURE 21-13
Mechanism of injury that may result in tennis elbow (chronic irritation of the extensor-supinator muscles).

❖ **Sprains**

Sprains of the elbow joint are moderately common in athletic activity. Because of the configuration of the ulna in the trochlear notch, this is a relatively stable joint. Injuries involving the ligamentous system of the elbow most commonly result from forced hyperextension or valgus/varus forces. Athletes may describe a "click" or "pop" along with sharp pain at the time of injury. In addition to tenderness at the site of injury, there is normally localized swelling and pain on any attempt to reproduce the mechanism of injury. Pain is usually relieved by bending the elbow, and athletes will normally hold their injured extremity in some degree of flexion. Swelling and muscle spasms will often limit complete extension. It may be difficult to determine significant instability of the elbow joint unless there has been a complete dislocation and rupture of ligaments. There may also be an avulsion of the ligament with a fragment of bone present. It is important to recognize significant ligamentous injuries to the elbow and initiate proper treatment procedures to prevent the development of residual contractures with resultant loss of motion and chronic disability.

❖ Dislocations

Dislocations involving the elbow joint are not common but can be a serious injury. The most common type of elbow dislocation is the posterior displacement of the ulna and radius in relationship to the humerus. This normally occurs because of a fall on an outstretched hand with the elbow in extension. As the elbow is forced into hyperextension, the olecranon process is levered against the humerus, which can force the ulna backward (posteriorly) (Figure 21-14). The collateral ligaments are severely stretched or ruptured but the annular ligament often remains intact so that the head of the radius usually accompanies the ulna in its posterior displacement. In addition, there may be an associated lateral displacement, with either a varus or valgus deformity of the forearm. Elbow dislocations that remain displaced should be readily recognized as there will be obvious deformity, with the olecranon process abnormally prominent, loss of elbow function, and the athlete expressing considerable pain. The initial examination of these injuries must include an evaluation of the circulation and nerve function to the distal portion of the extremity. Determine the presence or absence of a radial pulse, as well as sensory and motor functions of the hand. All elbow dislocations should be properly immobilized and referred to a physician immediately.

❖ Fractures

Fractures about the elbow and forearm can result from any of the injury-producing mechanisms described in this chapter. Normally fractures occur as the result of either direct trauma to the forearm or elbow or indirect stresses transmitted through the upper extremity as the result of falling on an outstretched arm. In addition, excessive forces associated with throwing and swinging activities may cause an interruption in bony continuity. Fractures about the elbow are among the most frequent involving children and skeletally immature athletes. Many of these involve the epiphysis because the ligamentous structures in young athletes are much stronger than the bony and cartilaginous components of the growth plate. Therefore athletic trainers should maintain a high level of suspicion concerning fractures whenever evaluating an acute elbow injury in a young athlete. Fortunately,

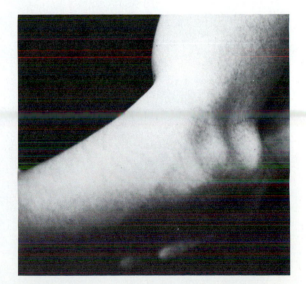

FIGURE 21-14
Posterior dislocation of an elbow.

fractures of the elbow are not common in skeletally mature athletes. All epiphyses at the elbow are normally fused by 18 years of age.

There are a wide variety of fractures that may occur about the elbow. These may involve the distal humerus, proximal ulna, or radius. These can range from simple avulsions with a small flake of bone to serious and complicated fractures. The signs and symptoms associated with these injuries are directly related to the degree of severity. There may or may not be any visible or palpable deformity. Point tenderness is normally present at the site of injury, and varying amounts of hemorrhaging or swelling are common. The athlete may also demonstrate a limited ROM, disability at the elbow or hand, and an increase in pain at the fracture site with attempted movements.

❖ **Supracondylar fracture.** The most common fracture of the elbow is the humeral supracondylar fracture, or fracture proximal to the growth plate. This fracture is caused by falling on an outstretched hand or by forced hyperextension and frequently occurs in children. The distal fragment is usually pushed upward and backward by the fracturing force and is maintained in that position by spasm of the triceps. Athletic trainers should be aware of the fact that a supracondylar fracture of the distal humerus may appear to be a posterior dislocation. However, the epicondyles of the humerus and the olecranon process maintain their normal anatomic relationship in a supracondylar fracture.

❖ **Forearm fractures.** Fractures of the forearm (radius and ulna) are common in young athletes. They are usually caused by a direct blow or falling on an outstretched hand (Figure 21-15). The signs and symp-

FIGURE 21-15
Wrestler with a fractured radius. (X-ray shows fracture near mid-point of diaphysis).

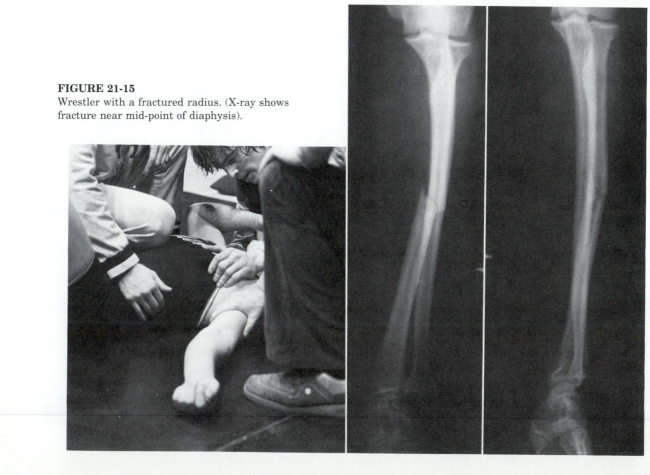

toms of forearm fractures may include point tenderness, swelling, angulation of the bone, pain on motion, disability, and crepitation. Whenever a fracture is suspected, the athlete should be referred to a physician.

❖ **Volkmann's ischemic contracture.** Potential complications resulting from fractures about the elbow or from improper management of the injuries include neurovascular compromise and faulty bony union with deformity. Direct disruption of an artery or arterial occlusion as a result of swelling in the closed relatively inelastic compartment of the forearm may result in an impairment of the distal circulation. This can cause a compartment syndrome, which may in turn result in irreparable damage to the forearm and hand musculature, a condition called Volkmann's ischemic contracture. Volkmann's contracture is considered the result of a vascular disturbance that may arise in a number of different ways. We know, for example, that trauma inflicted on any body area will have significant effects on the functioning of the sympathetic nervous system in the area involved. Sympathetic stimulation caused by elbow trauma can cause very sudden and serious changes to occur in forearm blood vessels. Vasoconstriction and segmental arterial spasm can result in paralysis and widespread degeneration of the flexor compartment forearm muscles. If this should occur, replacement of muscle by fibrous tissue results in a disabling "claw hand" syndrome. In addition to sympathetic stimulation, increased compartment pressure caused by internal swelling as a result of hemorrhage or external pressure caused by tight bandages or splints can also result in ischemic contracture. This tragic condition may develop insidiously for 6 to 12 hours after the injury. The classic signs of a compartment syndrome and impending Volkmann's contracture include pain, pallor, paralysis, and absence of pulse. The most important of these findings is deep, unremitting, and poorly localized pain, particularly when pain increases with finger motion. Always be suspicious in cases in which pain is disproportionate to the apparent seriousness of the injury. Remember,

fractures about the elbow can be extremely serious and require early recognition and prompt referral so that they can be reduced early.

❖ **Epiphyseal plate injury.** In a skeletally immature athlete, the growth plate is the weakest link in the kinetic chain. In the young athlete, throwing can produce significant shearing and compressive forces on the growth centers around the elbow. As previously mentioned, the medial epicondylar growth plate is the one most often involved (little league elbow). Symptoms include medial elbow pain, which is increased with throwing and relieved by rest. Often this pain progresses over a period of several weeks. Tenderness will be over the medial epicondyle and the athlete may express pain with passive extension of the wrist and fingers. These athletes should be referred to medical assistance for further diagnostic tests.

❖ **Osteochondritis dissecans.** Osteochondritis dissecans was discussed in more detail with the knee, but can also develop in the growth centers of the elbow. When it occurs, the most often cause is avascular necrosis produced on a epiphysis receiving repetitive compression or shearing forces. Symptoms will be similar to those described for an epiphyseal plate injury or epiphysitis. This condition will be recognized on radiographic studies.

Nerve Involvement

Neural involvement is not as common as musculotendinous and articular injuries to the elbow. However, it is important to recognize and initiate proper treatment for these conditions.

❖ **Ulnar nerve.** As previously discussed, the ulnar nerve passes through the cubital tunnel in the posterior aspect of the medial epicondyle. The floor of this tunnel is the medial epicondylar groove and the remaining components are formed by fascial bands. The repetitive movement of the ulnar nerve within the cubital tunnel and the relative lack of bony protection make this nerve vulnerable to compression forces and tension stresses at the elbow. The ulnar nerve can become irritated, compressed, or entrapped in this tunnel due to repetitive throwing and/or swinging activities. This is often referred to as **cubital tunnel syndrome.** Symptoms may include pain along the inner aspect of the elbow, tenderness over the medial epicondylar groove, and paresthesias in the distribution of the ulnar nerve in the hand. A positive Tinel's sign can be elicited in this region. Motor and sensory functions can be diminished in the ring and little finger. Atrophy and motor loss can occur if the condition progresses.

❖ **Radial nerve.** The radial nerve passes anteriorly to the lateral epicondyle and lies in a tunnel formed by several muscles and tendons. It is in this area that the radial nerve can become entrapped, especially during activities requiring repetitive pronation and supination of the forearm. This radial nerve entrapment is called **radial tunnel syndrome.** While this condition occurs infrequently, it should be considered in the assessment of lateral epicondylitis (tennis elbow) as symptoms are very similar. It can be difficult to differentiate between epicondylitis and nerve entrapment as the conditions may occur together. The athlete will exhibit pain over the lateral aspect of the elbow. However, with a nerve entrapment, the tenderness may be present over the anterior radial head instead of the common extensor tendon. Symptoms may also be reproduced by resisting supination with the elbow flexed 90° or resisting extension of the middle finger with the elbow extended. Radial tunnel syndrome should be considered a possible cause of lateral elbow pain when conservative treatment of lateral epicondylitis has failed and symptoms continue for an extended period of time.

❖ **Median nerve.** The median nerve crosses the anterior elbow and passes between the two heads of the pronator teres muscle just distal to the joint. At this point it is vulnerable to entrapment or compression due to hypertrophy of the pronator teres or activities that involve repetitive pronation of the forearm. This condition is referred to as **pronator teres syndrome.** Symptoms include pain radiating down the anterior forearm with numbness and tingling in the thumb, index, and middle fingers. Resistive pronation may increase the pain.

ATHLETIC INJURY ASSESSMENT PROCESS

The elbow and forearm are frequently injured during athletic participation. Most athletic injuries in this area result from some type of direct blow such as falling on an outstretched arm or elbow, or by overload forces associated with throwing or swinging activities (Figure 21-16). As a group, athletic injuries to the elbow are potentially serious because inadequate evaluation and inappropriate treatment may lead to functional impairment or permanent disability. Of all the large joints in the body, the elbow is the most susceptible to loss of motion after injury or insult. Therefore proper care of elbow injuries is dependent on accurate assessment and closely supervised treatment and rehabilitation programs.

Secondary survey ▬▬▬▬▬▬
Accurate determination of the severity of injury is the first step in assessment of elbow injuries. Unrecognized, a serious injury in this area can result in catastrophic complications, especially in children. Fractures and dislocations involving the elbow can cause circulatory or neural impairment that can result in irreparable damage to the forearm and hand. This is especially true in children and skeletally immature athletes. Athletic trainers must consider the age of the athlete and be cognizant of the possibility that these elbow injuries may involve the epiphysis or growth centers in young athletes. Any suspected fracture or elbow dislocation should not be manipulated in any manner. These injuries must be protected from further damage by gently splinting them in the position found and referring the athlete to medical assistance for further diagnosis and proper care. Therefore the assessment of all acute elbow injuries, especially in children and those who express much pain or remain lying on the court or field, should include an evaluation of circulation to the hand and an investigation of nerve function distal to the site of injury.

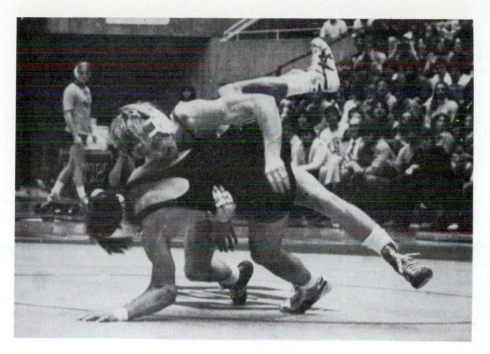

FIGURE 21-16
Elbow dislocating as the result of athletic activity.

Adequacy of hand circulation can be evaluated by checking for the radial pulse and compressing the nail beds and noting the return of normal color. Nerve impairment can be assessed by evaluating sensations over the palm, thumb, and fingers and noting the ability to contract the extrinsic and intrinsic muscles of the hand. Once the presence of adequate circulation and nerve functions has been established, the athletic injury assessment process can continue. Significant injuries to the elbow should also be reevaluated frequently after the injury to recognize the development of any circulatory or nerve impairment.

History

The comprehensive assessment of injuries to the elbow and forearm includes a careful history. Begin by inquiring about the primary complaint. What happened to the elbow or forearm? Question the athlete about the mechanism of injury to determine exactly how the injury occurred. Was there a direct blow delivered to the elbow or forearm? If a blow was delivered, was the elbow joint forced in an abnormal direction? Did the athlete fall and land on the elbow, forearm, or outstretched hand? What was the position of the elbow at the time of injury? Did the injury result from throwing or swinging activities? Did the symptoms of this injury, including onset of pain, come on very suddenly or did they develop over a period of time? The more information gained concerning the mechanism of injury and the onset of symptoms, the easier it is to accurately assess the nature and severity of the injury and determine those structures that may be involved.

Allow the athlete to describe the symptoms associated with the injury. Exactly where are the painful or tender areas? Ask the athlete to locate and describe the pain. Pain about the elbow and forearm is normally easy to localize and is seldom diffuse or radiating unless there is neural involvement. On those occasions when a nerve is compressed, a burning pain may travel the length of the nerve pathway, such as occurs when the ulnar nerve is hit. Is pain only present during activity? If so, what types of activities or movements cause the pain? The athlete may be asked to demonstrate the painful motions.

Question the athlete about any unusual sensations associated with the injury. Did he or she feel anything at the time of injury, such as a popping, clicking, or snapping sensation? Does the athlete feel any crepitation? Is there any tightness, tension, or swelling associated with the injury? Does the athlete complain of any numbness, burning, tingling, or weakness in the forearm or hand? Ask the athlete to describe his or her impressions concerning the injury.

Also inquire about previous injuries. Has the athlete suffered an injury to this area of the body before? If so, obtain as much information as possible concerning the circumstances surrounding previous injuries. When was the athlete injured? What was the nature and severity of previous injuries? Had the athlete fully recovered from prior injuries or did he or she still experience symptoms? What types of activities could the athlete participate in before the current injury? Was the athlete's elbow able to function normally? Does this injury appear to be the same or very similar to previous injuries?

Observation

The initial observations regarding injuries about the elbow must be concerned with recognizing obvious deformity. As previously discussed, it is critically important for the athletic trainer to recognize elbow dislocations and fractures early in the assessment process in order to initiate proper handling and treatment procedures. Early identification of serious injury reduces the possibility of complications. If clothing or protective equipment covers the elbow, it can generally be removed easily from this area of the body without causing additional trauma or pain to the athlete. Remember, if the athlete is unable or unwilling to move the elbow, visual inspection should be accomplished in whatever position the injured elbow is held. Begin the observation by noting the contours of the elbow and forearm. Is there any obvious deformity? Dislocations that remain displaced are normally easy to visually rec-

ognize because of the associated deformity. Note in Figure 21-14 the posterior displacement of the ulna in relation to the humerus. Remember, to the untrained observer, a supracondylar fracture may look like a posterior dislocation. However, the epicondyles and the olecranon process maintain their normal anatomic relationship in a supracondylar fracture. This would not be the case in a posterior dislocation. In this type of fracture the median nerve and blood vessels in the cubital fossa are easily injured and the possibility of Volkmann's contracture must be considered. Supracondylar or fractures of the distal humerus occur most frequently in young athletes. In addition to the presence of a growth plate, in the years before skeletal maturity the anteroposterior diameter of the humerus is quite narrow just above the condyles. Fractures about the elbow and forearm may be less obvious than a dislocation and may require close visual inspection combined with various signs and symptoms recognized and expressed during the assessment process.

When confronted with an injured elbow, inspect and compare both elbows to note any differences in symmetry. Is there any swelling? If so, note exactly where the swelling is located. Swelling about the elbow or forearm may be localized to the olecranon bursa or diffused throughout the joint. Athletes with diffuse swelling will normally hold the elbow in a flexed position to accommodate the swelling with minimal pain. Whenever you suspect bleeding into the elbow of a young athlete, consider the possibility of development of Volkmann's ischemic contracture and refer the athlete to medical assistance. In addition to swelling, carefully inspect the injured area for signs of trauma that can indicate what type of force has been applied and assist in establishing or confirming the mechanism of injury.

Note the alignment of both arms. Normally with the arm in complete extension the forearm forms a slight valgus (lateral) angle at the elbow joint in relation to the upper arm. This is called the **carrying angle** and normally ranges from approximately 5° in men to 10° to 15° in women. If the forearm bones were in straight alignment with the humerus in the anatomic position, a 180° line would result. Instead, the carrying angle reduces the 180° straight line to 175° in men and less than 170° in women. As a result, the hand is normally carried away from the sides of the body when the elbow is extended and the forearm supinated. It is important to remember when observing contours and alignment, that some athletes may have unilateral hypertrophy or range of motion compromise consistent with their sport.

Compare the carrying angle of both arms. Are they equal? An increase (**cubitus valgus**) or decrease (**cubitus varus**) in the carrying angle of the injured elbow may be caused by a fracture or epiphyseal separation. Figure 21-17 shows a cubitus varus, sometimes called a **gunstock deformity,** resulting from a malunion of a fracture to the distal end of the humerus. This type of deformity is seen more frequently than an increase in the carrying angle.

Physical Examination

The physical examination portion of the assessment process is used to perform a more detailed investigation of the musculoskeletal system. Depending upon what your impressions are up to this point in the assessment process, you may continue with palpation techniques, movement procedures, or neurological and circulatory evaluations. Not all these procedures will be used in any one athletic injury. Choose the specific tests or procedures that will assist in completing your assessment of the shoulder. Remember, physical examination is both a skill and an art, mastered only by study and experience.

Palpation

Palpation of the injured elbow or forearm is used to identify specific structures that may be involved in the injury. This is accomplished by accurately locating all areas of associated tenderness and swelling, as well as any other physical signs that may assist in recognizing the injury. The specific structures or areas to be palpated will be determined by the information gained during the history and inspection phases in the assessment process.

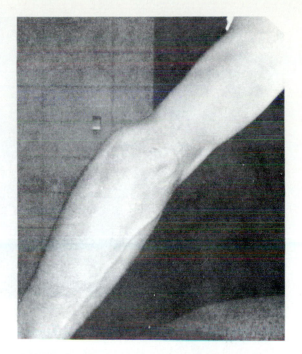

FIGURE 21-17
Gunstock deformity resulting from malunion of a fractured humerus.

As with any area of the body, palpation procedures should be conducted with the injured area as relaxed as possible. This is best accomplished by supporting the athlete's injured arm with one hand and palpating the suspected area of injury with the other hand. The athlete may be sitting, standing, or lying. Gently feel those areas suspected of being injured and correlate this information with the underlying anatomy. Procedures used to palpate the various anatomical structures of the elbow and forearm will be discussed briefly, as will the common athletic injuries which may be indicated by positive findings.

The olecranon process of the ulna is a good point of reference to begin palpating the elbow (Figure 21-18, *A*). This bony tip of the elbow feels subcutaneous although it is covered by the olecranon bursa and the insertion of the triceps. When an olecranon bursitis is present there will be varying amounts of swelling and tenderness over the olecranon. Occasionally there will be a small palpable mass in this area. This is normally

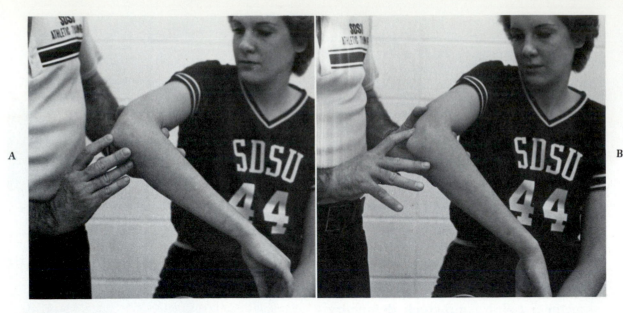

FIGURE 21-18
Palpating, **A,** the olecranon process of the ulna and, **B,** the olecranon fossa of the humerus.

a fibrinous or cartilaginous mass, but may be mistaken for a chip of bone. A physician may order radiographs to rule out a bone chip or other fracture.

Just proximal to the olecranon is the olecranon fossa of the humerus. This depression can best be felt with the elbow in about 45° of flexion and the triceps completely relaxed (Figure 21-19, *B*). If the triceps is not relaxed, the tendon of this muscle will be palpated covering the fossa. With the elbow in extension, the olecranon process will fill this depression. Distal to the olecranon process, the subcutaneous border of the ulna can be palpated along its entire length to the styloid process at the wrist (Figure 21-19).

On either side of the olecranon the epicondyles of the humerus can be palpated. The medical epicondyle, the lateral epicondyle, and the olecranon process should lie in a straight line when the elbow is completely extended. With the elbow in flexion, these three bony prominences should form an isosceles triangle. The geometric alignment of these bony prominences can best be appreciated by placing your index finger on the

olecranon process and your thumb and middle finger on either epicondyle (Figure 21-20). A noticeable deviation in this alignment when compared to the uninjured elbow may indicate a structural problem such as a condylar fracture.

The medial epicondyle of the humerus is larger and more easily palpated than its lateral counterpart. Gently palpate about this bony prominence (Figure 21-21, *A*). Various athletic injuries can cause pain or tenderness when palpating on and around the medial epicondyle. Remember, this medial epicondyle is the part of the elbow most frequently fractured, especially in young athletes whose epiphyses are not yet united. Palpating proximal to this eminence, you can feel the medial supracondylar ridge for a short distance. Lying just posterior to the medial epicondyle is the groove through which the ulnar nerve passes into the forearm (Figure 21-21, *B*). Palpating just distal to the medial epicondyle, you can feel the common flexor tendon, which is the shared origin of four muscles (Figure 21-22, *A*). Pain in this area frequently represents an acute

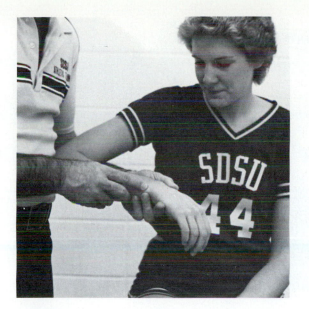

FIGURE 21-19
Palpating styloid process of the ulna.

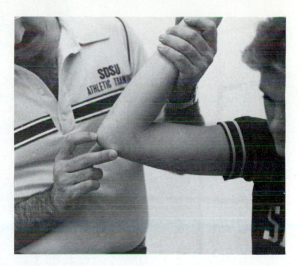

FIGURE 21-20
Palpating and noting the geometric alignment of the olecranon process, the medial epicondyle, and the lateral epicondyle.

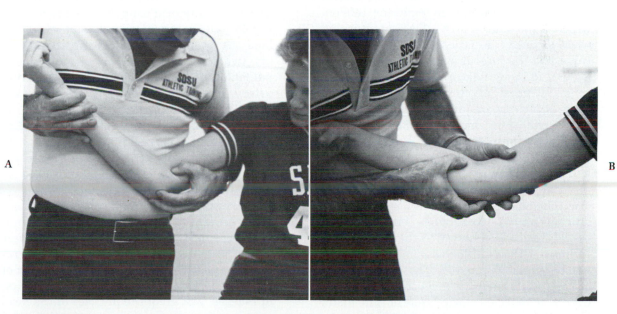

A   B

FIGURE 21-21
Palpating the, **A,** medial epicondyle and, **B,** ulnar nerve.

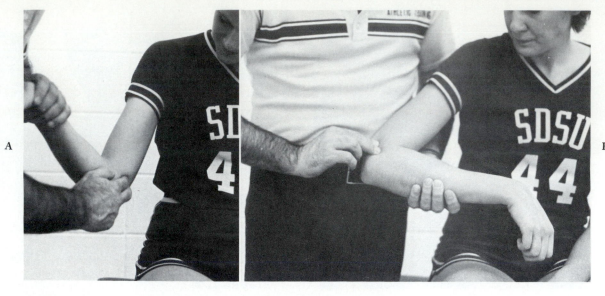

FIGURE 21-22
Palpating the, **A,** common flexor tendon and, **B,** common extensor tendon.

or chronic strain resulting from activities requiring acute or chronic pronation and wrist flexion.

The less prominent lateral epicondyle of the humerus is palpated on the outside of the elbow. The lateral supracondylar ridge can be felt running proximal to the lateral epicondyle. The common extensor tendon, which is the shared origin for supinator and wrist extensor muscles, arises along this ridge and the lateral epicondyle (Figure 21-23, *B*). Pain in this area frequently represents an acute or chronic strain resulting from activities requiring supination and wrist extension. Just distal to the lateral epicondyle, palpate the head of the radius (Figure 21-23, *A*). This is most easily felt when the elbow is in approximately 90 degrees of flexion with the surrounding muscles relaxed. Instruct the athlete to pronate and supinate the forearm as you palpate the radial head. Just distal to the head of the radius lies the annular ligament, which cannot be directly palpated. The proximal half of the radius then becomes obscured by the overlying muscles of the forearm. The distal shaft of the radius can be palpated from the radial styloid at the wrist to a point approximately half way up the forearm (Figure 21-23, *B*).

Soft tissue structures can be palpated over the anterior surface of the elbow. The hollow triangular area in front of the elbow is called the *cubital fossa* and is formed by the pronator teres muscle medially and the brachioradialis laterally. The base of the cubital triangle is formed by a line drawn between the humeral condyles. At the apex of the fossa the brachioradialis muscle overlaps the pronator teres. Within this space are two structures that are usually easily palpable, the biceps tendon and the brachial artery. The biceps tendon with its strong expansion, the **bicipital aponenrosis,** is readily palpated during mild resistance to elbow flexion (Figure 21-24 H). *A*). The brachial artery lies directly medial to the bicepts tendon (Figure 21-24, *B*). This pulse is normally used when taking blood pressure.

The muscles of the forearm should be palpated as a unit, that is, the wrist flexors and extensors as two separate groups. Support the forearm to ensure the muscles are as relaxed as possible. Attempt to locate areas of tenderness, swelling, muscle spasm, deficits, or masses. Not all of the muscles of the forearm are distinguishable by palpation, and resistive motion is normally required to complete the evaluation of muscle integrity.

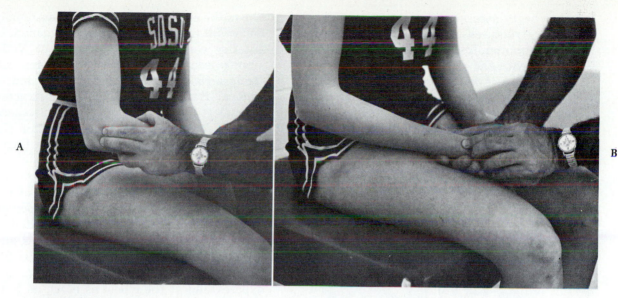

FIGURE 21-23
Palpating the radius: **A,** head of the radius and, **B,** the styloid process.

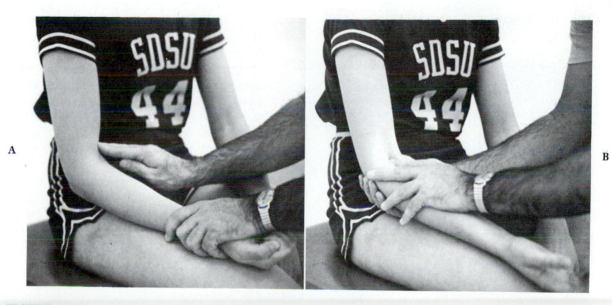

FIGURE 21-24
A, Palpating the biceps tendon during mild resistance to elbow flexion. **B,** Locating the brachial pulse.

Movement procedures

Movement procedures should never be used during the assessment of elbow injuries until you are sure there is no associated fracture or dislocation. Manipulation of the elbow when these types of injuries are present may cause additional damage and per-haps permanent disability. Therefore, all elbow injuries suspected of involving a fracture or dislocation should be protected from any movements and referred to a qualified physician.

Active movements. Active movements are normally performed to evaluate ROM and to begin assessing the integrity of contractile structures in the area of injury. A classic symptom involving the elbow, which may indicate the development of a severe complication, is an increase in pain at the elbow with finger motion. This is especially true when the fingers are actively or passively moved into extension (Figure 21-25). Therefore the initial active movements used to evaluate an injured elbow should be finger motions. These movements require no mo-

tion of the elbow joint and may be extremely important in recognizing the development of anterior compartment syndrome or Volkmann's ischemic contracture. Athletes suffering an elbow injury and not referred to medical attention should also be instructed to be alert for the development of increased swelling or tightness and pain about the elbow, especially pain increasing on finger extension.

To evaluate active ROM at the elbow, instruct the athlete to flex and extend at the elbow as far as possible. Normally a person can flex approximately 150°, being limited by the muscle mass of the front of the arm, and extend the arm straight out to 0° (Figure 21-26). Many athletes, especially women, can hyperextend at the elbow as much as 5° to 15° beyond the straight position (Figure 21-27). The active ROM of both elbows should be examined simultaneously to detect any differences. Remember, pain, swelling, muscle spasms, and previous injuries can all limit the ROM available at the elbow joint.

Active supination and pronation should also be evaluated in one continuous motion. Instruct the athlete to flex the elbow to 90° to avoid shoulder motion, and then turn the palm up and down. Normally the forearm can be rotated approximately 90° in each direction or until the palm is facing directly upward or downward (Figure 21-28). Small differences in the ROM between both forearms may be more easily noticed if the athlete is asked to hold something, such as tape

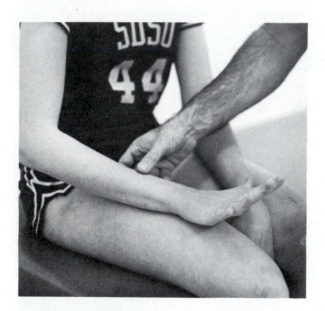

FIGURE 21-25
Instructing athlete to actively extend fingers to recognize increased pain at the elbow.

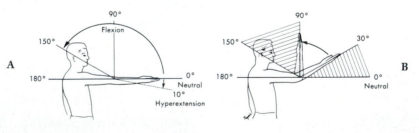

FIGURE 21-26
ROM of the elbow: flexion, extension, and hyperextension. **A,** Flexion and hyperextension. *Flexion:* zero to 150°. *Extension:* 150° to zero. *Hyperextension:* measured in degrees beyond the zero starting point. This motion is not present in all persons. When it is present, it may vary from 5° to 15°. **B,** Measurement of limited motion. (The unshaded area indicates the limited ROM). Limited motion may be expressed in the following ways: (1) the elbow flexes from 30° to 90° (30°–90°); (2) the elbow has a flexion deformity of 30° with further flexion to 90°.

scissors, in each fist as he or she supinates and pronates both forearms simultaneously (Figure 21-29).

Resistive movements. Resistive movements are used to further evaluate the integrity of contractile structures. Applying manual resistance against each of the active motions of the elbow and forearm can assist in accurately locating specific painful areas. A knowledge of the functional anatomy allows you to differentiate one muscle from another. Resistive movements are also used to compare muscular strength between extremities.

To apply resistance against elbow flexion, stabilize the arm or elbow with one hand and apply resistance to the movement proximal to the wrist with the other hand (Figure 21-30). Note any areas of pain. Although this is primarily a test for the biceps and brachialis muscles, other accessory muscles may assist elbow flexion and exhibit pain if injured. For example, those muscles originating high in the common flexor and

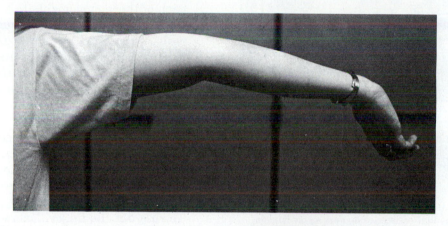

FIGURE 21-27
Athlete exhibiting hyperextension at the elbow joint.

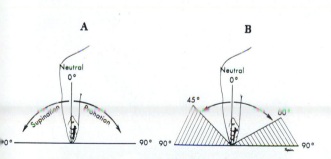

FIGURE 21-28
ROM of the forearm: pronation and supination. **A,** Pronation and supination. *Pronation:* zero to 80° or 90°. *Supination:* zero to 80° or 90°. *Total forearm motion:* 160° to 180°. Persons may vary in the range of supination and pronation. Some may reach the 90° arc, and others may have only 70° plus. **B,** Limited motion. *Supination:* 45° (0–45°). *Total joint motion:* 105°.

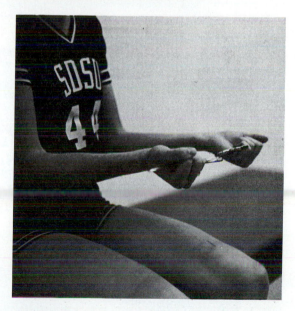

FIGURE 21-29
Active supination and pronation with athlete grasping bandage scissors in an attempt to note small differences in ROM.

common extensor tendons may also weakly assist elbow flexion. To evaluate these muscles, further resistance must be applied against their primary action.

Maintain the same position to apply re-

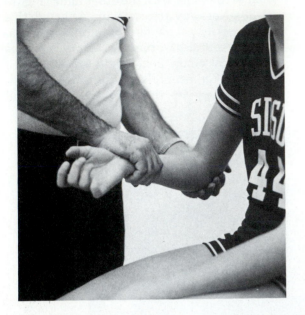

FIGURE 21-30
Applying manual resistance against elbow flexion.

sistance against elbow extension. Instruct the athlete to slowly extend the arm while you increase the resistance against extension. Again note any areas of pain on resisted movement and evaluate the relative strength of both triceps.

It is difficult, as well as unnecessary, to differentiate individual muscles of the forearm during the assessment process. These muscles act in groups and are primarily responsible for supination and pronation as well as wrist flexion and extension. Therefore resistance should be applied against each of these movements to evaluate the integrity of each functional muscle group. To resist supination, maintain the same positioning, with the athlete's forearm pronated, and instruct the athlete to supinate as you apply resistance against the dorsal surface of the distal end of the radius. Resistance to pronation is accomplished by applying resistance on the volar surface of the distal end of the radius as the athlete pronates. To test wrist flexion and extension, stabilize the athlete's forearm and apply resistance to the hand during each movement (Figure 21-31). To rule out the finger flexors and extensors

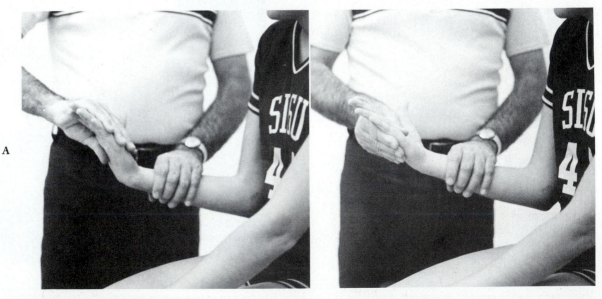

FIGURE 21-31
Applying manual resistance against **A,** wrist flexion and **B,** wrist extension.

assisting during each movement, instruct the athlete to keep the thumb and fingers relaxed.

Passive movements. Generally the only passive movements or maneuvers that are performed in conjunction with elbow injuries are those that evaluate the integrity of the medial and lateral collateral ligaments, as well as the integrity of the radius and ulna. The ROM of an injured elbow should always

be evaluated actively. Passive procedures can cause further damage and must be used with caution and restraint.

To assess the integrity of the collateral ligaments, cup the injured elbow in one hand and grasp the wrist with the other. Flex the elbow approximately 15° to 20° in order to "unlock" the olecranon process from the olecranon fossa. Instruct the athlete to relax the muscles of the upper extremity. To evaluate

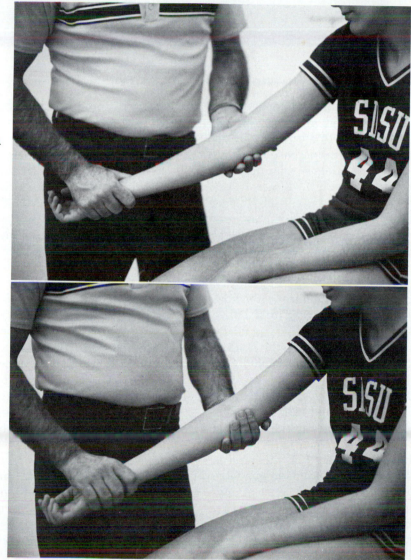

FIGURE 21-32
Stressing collateral ligaments. **A,** Valgus stress to evaluate the integrity of the ulnar collateral ligament. **B,** Varus stress to evaluate the integrity of the radial collateral ligament.

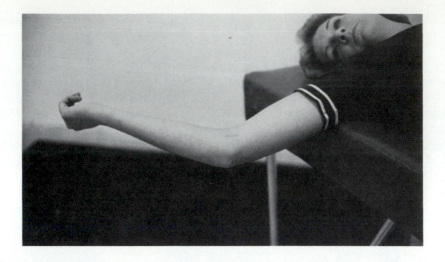

FIGURE 21-33
Gravity stress test to evaluate medial collateral instability.

the medial (ulnar) collateral ligament, apply a valgus stress to the elbow (Figure 21-32, *A*). Remember to begin this type of maneuver very gently and then increase intensity depending on the athlete's tolerance. To evaluate the lateral (radial) collateral ligament, apply a varus stress to the elbow joint (Figure 21-32, *B*). Does the athlete express any pain with these stress procedures? Note any gaping or instability with either of these movements and compare to the uninjured elbow.

Another method of demonstrating medial instability is a **gravity stress test.** Have the athlete lie supine, abduct the arm 90 degrees, externally rotate the shoulder maximally, and flex the elbow approximately 20 degrees to clear the olecranon from its fossa (Figure 21-33). If the elbow is unstable, the weight of the forearm and hand will normally exert enough valgus stress to open the medial side. In a muscular athlete, a 1 or 2 pound weight may be placed on the hand to increase the stress or a manual valgus force can be applied by the athletic trainer. A physician may use this procedure in conjunction with radiography to determine the extent of medial instability.

Passive stress procedures may also be used to assess the integrity of the two long bones of the forearm. If the signs and symptoms exhibited up to this point in the as-

sessment process cause you to suspect a possible fracture of the shaft of the radius or ulna, stress can be applied to these two bones. This can be accomplished by applying longitudinal or transverse stress. This stress should be very gentle initially and increased depending on the athlete's tolerance. Longitudinal stress can be accomplished by stabilizing the elbow with one hand and applying force or pressure directly along the long axis of both bones (Figure 21-34, *A*). Transverse stress is applied away from the site of pain and can be accomplished by squeezing the ulna and radius together (Figure 21-34, *B*) or applying a medial or lateral force. Locate the point tenderness and move away from this area to apply the transverse pressure. If the bone integrity is intact, there should be no pain or crepitation with these stress procedures. However, if these maneuvers cause additional pain at the original site of tenderness, the athlete should be treated as if there is a fracture.

Functional movements. As with shoulder injuries, functional movements or activities can prove helpful in the assessment of elbow injuries. Many injuries involving the elbow result from repetitive throwing or swinging activities, and these same movements may be required to replicate the associated symptoms. Instruct the athlete to perform the activities that produced the

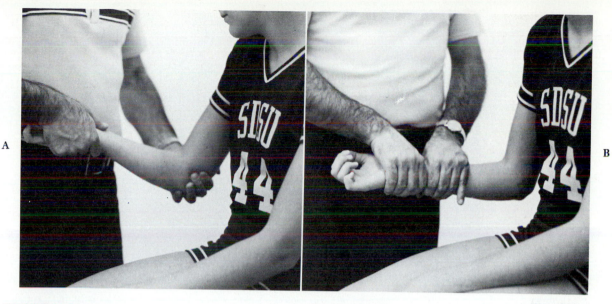

FIGURE 21-34
Applying passive stress to evaluate the integrity of the radius and ulna. **A,** Longitudinal
compression stress. **B,** Tranverse stress by squeezing radius and ulna.

symptoms in an effort to identify the mechanism of injury, as well as the anatomic structures that may be involved.

Functional movements are normally used to determine when an athlete can return to athletic activity, especially those requiring throwing or swinging. During each reevaluation, question the athlete directly or observe his or her functional abilities concerning the elbow. The intensity of these activities should be progressively increased within the athlete's tolerance.

Neurological evaluations

Sensory functions. The athletic trainer should be aware of the basic sensory distribution of the normal dermatomes of the various peripheral nerves about the elbow and forearm. The dermatomes about this area of the body are C5, which supplies the lateral side of the arm and elbow; C6, the lateral forearm; C7, the middle of the anterior forearm; C8, the medial forearm and posterior elbow; and T1, the medial arm and elbow (Figure 21-35). Run your relaxed hands and fingers over these surfaces, note any differences in sensations, and compare the sensations to the uninjured side.

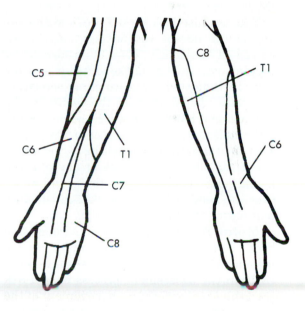

FRONT   BACK

FIGURE 21-35
Dermatomes of the elbow and forearm.

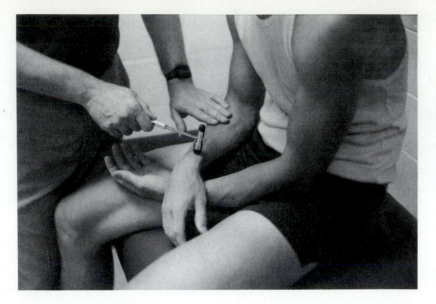

FIGURE 21-36
Test for brachioradialis reflex (C6).

You can also look for a **Tinel's sign** over any of the nerves you suspect may be involved in the injury. This is performed by tapping over the site of the nerve. A positive sign is indicated by a tingling sensation along the distribution of the nerve in the forearm and hand distal to the compression. This indicates a partial lesion or the regeneration of the nerve. To test the three nerves about the elbow, tap the ulnar nerve in the medial epicondylar groove, the radial nerve over the head of the radius, and the median nerve over the pronator muscle.

Motor functions. Motor functions have been previously discussed under active movements. These procedures may occur early in the assessment process as you ask the athlete to perform each movement of the elbow through as great a ROM as possible. The primary myotomes of the elbow and forearm are C5 and C6, biceps, brachioradialis, and supinator; C6, wrist and finger extensors; C7, triceps and flexor carpi radialis; C8 and T1, flexor carpi ulnaris, flexor digitorum profundus, pronator quadratus, opponens pollicis, and interossei; and T1, flexor pollicis.

Reflexes. The reflexes commonly checked about the elbow are the biceps (C5) and triceps (C7). These reflexes are described in Chapter 20. Another reflex that can be tested is the brachioradialis (C6). To test this reflex, place the athlete's elbow in flexion and support the forearm in the same manner as you would to elicit the biceps reflex. Using a reflex hammer, tap the brachioradialis tendon at the distal end of the radius (Figure 21-36). The normal response is slight elbow flexion. Test the opposite forearm and compare the results.

Evaluation of Findings

The elbow can be subjected to tremendous forces or stresses during many types of athletic activity. This area of the body is frequently involved in athletic injuries occurring as acute traumatic episodes (direct or muscular violence) or chronic overuse syndromes. Acute fractures and dislocations must be promptly recognized and adequately managed to avoid serious and possibly catastrophic complications. Early recognition of circulatory impairment or nerve compression syndromes is essential to preventing permanent impairment. Overuse syndromes resulting from the cumulative

When to Refer the Athlete . . .

Gross deformity about the elbow or forearm
Significant swelling about the elbow joint
Considerable pain, especially on finger extension
Significant loss of motion
Audible "click" or "pop" at time of injury
Loss of sensation below the elbow
Abnormal sensations that do not quickly subside, such as numbness, tingling, or weakness
Joint instability
Suspected fracture or dislocation
Any doubt regarding the severity or nature of the elbow or forearm injury

harmful effects associated with throwing or swinging activities must also be accurately recognized and properly treated to promote healing and allow the athlete to return to participation. Inadequate treatment may result in permanent functional disability, chronic problems, or possibly early retirement from athletic activity.

When to refer the athlete

Elbow injuries, especially acute traumatic episodes, should be evaluated and managed with caution and a high index of suspicion. You must be cognizant of epiphyseal injuries in skeletally immature athletes. With all elbow injuries, you must be concerned with circulation and nerve function to the forearm and hand. Conditions or findings that can be used to determine if medical referral is indicated are listed in the "When to Refer the Athlete . . ." box.

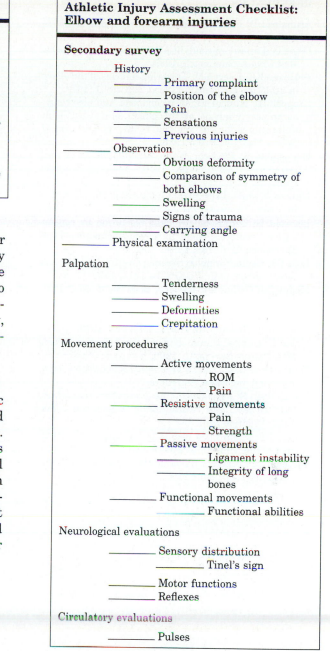

Athletic Injury Assessment Checklist: Elbow and forearm injuries

Secondary survey

——— History
  ——— Primary complaint
  ——— Position of the elbow
  ——— Pain
  ——— Sensations
  ——— Previous injuries
——— Observation
  ——— Obvious deformity
  ——— Comparison of symmetry of both elbows
  ——— Swelling
  ——— Signs of trauma
  ——— Carrying angle
——— Physical examination

Palpation
  ——— Tenderness
  ——— Swelling
  ——— Deformities
  ——— Crepitation

Movement procedures
  ——— Active movements
    ——— ROM
    ——— Pain
  ——— Resistive movements
    ——— Pain
    ——— Strength
  ——— Passive movements
    ——— Ligament instability
    ——— Integrity of long bones
  ——— Functional movements
    ——— Functional abilities

Neurological evaluations
  ——— Sensory distribution
    ——— Tinel's sign
  ——— Motor functions
  ——— Reflexes

Circulatory evaluations
  ——— Pulses

REFERENCES

Arnheim DD, Prentice WE: *Principles of athletic training,* ed 8, St. Louis, 1993, Mosby.

Davis G: Lateral epicondylitis in tennis players, *Sports Med Update* Summer:3, 1989.

DeHaven KE, Evart EM: Throwing injuries of the elbow in athletics, *Orthop Clin North Am* 3:801, 1973.

Groppel JL, Nirschl FP: A mechanical and electromyographical analysis of the effects of various joint counterforce braces on the tennis player, *Am J Sports Med* 14(3):195, 1986.

Hoppenfeld S: *Physical examination of the spine and extremities,* New York, 1976, Appleton-Century-Crofts.

Hulkko A, and others: Stress fractures of the olecranon in javelin throwers, *Int J Sports Med* 7(4):210, 1986.

Legwold G: Tennis elbow: joint resolution by conservative treatment and improved technique, *Phys Sportsmed* 12(6):168, 1984.

Lutz FR: Radial tunnel syndrome: an etiology of chronic lateral elbow pain, *JOSPT* 14(1):14, 1991.

Magee DJ: *Orthopedic physical assessment,* ed 2, Philadelphia, 1992, Saunders.

Midgley RD: Volkmann's ischemic contracture of the forearm, *Orthop Clin North Am* 4:983, 1973.

Nolan R: Cubital tunnel syndrome in athletics, *Sports Med Update* Spring:21, 1990.

O'Donoghue DH: *Treatment of injuries to athletes,* ed 4, Philadelphia, 1984, Saunders.

Roy S, Irvin R: *Sports medicine: prevention, evaluation, management, and rehabilitation,* Englewood Cliffs, 1983, Prentice-Hall.

Slager RF: From little league to big league, the weak spot is the arm, *Am J Sports Med* 5(2):37, 1977.

Zarins B and others: *Injuries to the throwing arm,* Philadelphia, 1985, Saunders.

SUGGESTED READINGS

Cooney WP: Sports injuries to the upper extremity, *Postgrad Med* 76(4):45, 1984.
Provides an overview of the many types of injury to the upper extremity that may occur during athletic activities and up-to-date techniques for their diagnosis and treatment.

Ireland ML, Andrews MR: Shoulder and elbow injuries in the young athlete, *Clin Sports Med* 7(3):473, 1988.
Discusses recognition, early activity modification, and treatment of unique injuries in the upper extremity in skeletally immature athletes.

Leach RE, Miller JK: Lateral and medial epicondylitis of the elbow, *Clin Sports Med* 6(2):259, 1987.
Describes the usual history and physical examination, and outlines a treatment plan for tendinitis of the forearm extensors and flexors.

McCue FC, editor: Injuries to the elbow, forearm, and hand, *Clin Sports Med* 5(4), 1986.
Discusses various topics related to diagnoses, treatment, and rehabilitation of injuries occuring to the elbow, forearm, and hand.

Nicholas JA, Hershman EB, editors: *The upper extremity in sports medicine,* St. Louis, 1990, Mosby.
An excellent text by many contributors discussing the various upper extremity injuries and conditions.

CHAPTER 22

Hand and wrist injuries

After you have completed this chapter, you should be able to:

- Identify the basic anatomy of the hand and wrist.
- Discuss the common athletic injuries and conditions that may occur to the hand and wrist.
- Describe the assessment process for an athlete suffering an injury to the hand or wrist.
- Discuss the various manipulative procedures and tests used to evaluate injuries and conditions about the hand and wrist.
- List the signs and symptoms that indicate an athlete with a hand or wrist injury should be referred to medical assistance.

The hand, which includes the fingers and thumb, is a functionally intricate and complex anatomic structure located at the distal end of our upper extremity. The wrist is that area of articulation between the forearm and hand. Precise functioning of the hand and wrist is essential to almost every type of athletic activity. The primary function of the proximal portion of the upper extremity is to position the hand where it can best perform its designated tasks. Functional anatomists sometimes refer to the hand and wrist as the "reason for the upper extremity." Both structures are frequently used during athletic activity and often function as a single unit. Together they permit an incredible array of intricate movements and also serve to absorb or transmit forces caused by falls or traumatic contact. Because the hand and wrist normally do not bear weight and because injuries to this area are not usually totally disabling, there is a tendency by some athletes to underestimate the severity and importance of these injuries. Many injuries to the hand and wrist are relatively minor and do not require extensive care. However, if neglected or unrecognized, they can develop into longterm impairment and possibly permanent disability and disfigurement. Hand and wrist injuries may require expert treatment to avoid these complications. It is imperative therefore that athletic trainers be able to accurately assess athletic injuries to this important area of the body, initiate proper treatment, and recognize when referral is necessary. The comprehensive evaluation of injuries to the hand and wrist begins with a well-founded knowledge of gross and functional anatomy of the area, as well as an understanding of the common athletic injuries and how they may occur.

FIGURE 22-1
Surface anatomy of the left hand and wrist. **A,** Palmar view and, **B,** dorsal view.

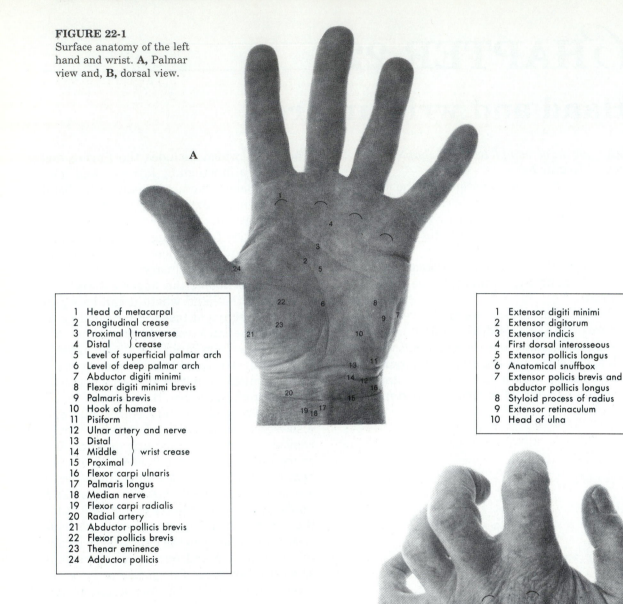

1	Head of metacarpal
2	Longitudinal crease
3	Proximal } transverse
4	Distal } crease
5	Level of superficial palmar arch
6	Level of deep palmar arch
7	Abductor digiti minimi
8	Flexor digiti minimi brevis
9	Palmaris brevis
10	Hook of hamate
11	Pisiform
12	Ulnar artery and nerve
13	Distal
14	Middle } wrist crease
15	Proximal
16	Flexor carpi ulnaris
17	Palmaris longus
18	Median nerve
19	Flexor carpi radialis
20	Radial artery
21	Abductor pollicis brevis
22	Flexor pollicis brevis
23	Thenar eminence
24	Adductor pollicis

1	Extensor digiti minimi
2	Extensor digitorum
3	Extensor indicis
4	First dorsal interosseous
5	Extensor pollicis longus
6	Anatomical snuffbox
7	Extensor policis brevis and abductor pollicis longus
8	Styloid process of radius
9	Extensor retinaculum
10	Head of ulna

ANATOMY OF THE WRIST

Begin your study of the hand and wrist anatomy by reviewing the surface anatomy (Figure 22-1). The term *wrist* is used to describe the anatomic and functional link between forearm and hand. It contains the carpal bones, the distal ends of the radius and ulna, and the proximal ends (bases) of the metacarpal bones together with the surrounding soft tissues. The wrist actually contains three sets of joints: (1) the radiocarpal, (2) the midcarpal, and (3) the carpometacarpal joints.

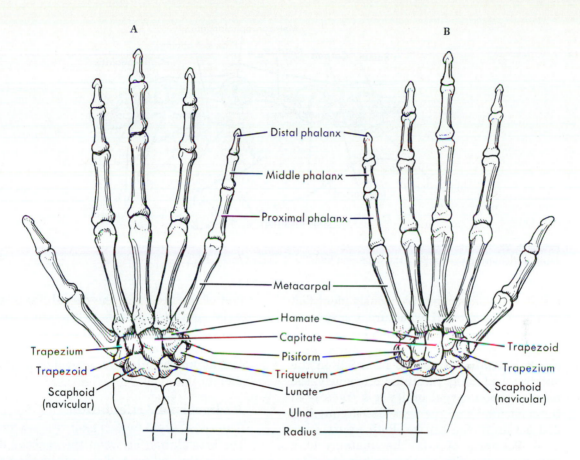

A   B

Distal phalanx

Middle phalanx

Proximal phalanx

Metacarpal

Hamate
Capitate
Trapezium   Trapezoid
Pisiform
Trapezoid   Trapezium
Triquetrum
Scaphoid   Scaphoid
(navicular)   Lunate   (navicular)
Ulna
Radius

FIGURE 22-2
Bones of the right hand and wrist. **A,** Dorsal view and, **B,** palmar view.

Carpals

The eight carpal bones of the wrist (Figure 22-2) are named according to their general appearance and shape. They are arranged in two rows, proximal and distal, each consisting of four bones. The proximal row of four carpals, from thumb (radial) side to little finger (ulnar) side, is composed of the navicular or scaphoid (boat-shaped), the lunate (moon-shaped), the triquetrum (three-cornered), and the pisiform (pea-shaped) bones. The distal row, from thumb side to little finger side, is made up of the trapezium (greater multangular), trapezoid (lesser multangular), capitate (head-shaped), and hamate (hooked) bones.

The navicular, lunate, and capitate carpals are of particular significance in the assessment of athletic injuries. The navicular is the most commonly fractured of all the carpals. The lunate (moon-shaped) carpal is the middle bone of the proximal row and is the one most frequently dislocated. The capitate is the largest of the carpals and is the most prominent bone in the central wrist. The capitate transmits the force of a fall on the hand, through the navicular and lunate bones, to the radius. The interval between the pisiform and hamate carpal bones permits the passage of the ulnar artery and nerve into the hand, which is of considerable clinical significance. The pisiform is easily located on the little finger (ulnar) side of the wrist. Anatomists consider this carpal as a sesamoid bone in the tendon of the flexor carpi ulnaris (a major flexor of the wrist). When this tendon is relaxed the pisiform can be moved about on the adjacent carpal. As a

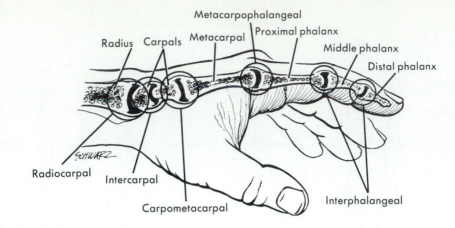

FIGURE 22-3
Joints articulating the bones of the wrist and hand.

result, it is sometimes erroneously identified as a bone fragment if a fracture is suspected after some type of wrist trauma.

The carpal bones are often injured as a result of trauma produced by a fall on the outstretched hand. As stated previously, the most common carpal injury is a fracture of the navicular, and the next most frequent is dislocation of the lunate. Both injuries are good examples of how the anatomy of a structure can influence the mechanism of injury or progression of pathology after trauma.

As a group, the posterior surfaces of the carpal bones are larger than the anterior surfaces. They resemble wedges with the bases behind (posterior). The navicular and lunate bones are exceptions. Both have anterior surfaces that are more extensive than the posterior. This explains why, when dislocations occur, the navicular and lunate almost always dislocate anteriorly whereas the other carpals dislocate posteriorly. Fracture of the navicular carpal occurs when it is brought directly under the radius as a result of a fall on the outstretched hand and is pinched between it and the capitate bone.

Distal Radioulnar Articulation

The distal, or inferior, radioulnar joint is the articulation between the head of the ulna and the ulnar notch on the lower end of the radius. A triangular fibrocartilaginous disc (articular disc) is located between the distal

end of the ulna and the carpal bones of the wrist and also serves as the chief uniting structure at the distal radioulnar joint. This distal radioulnar joint is covered by a thin, lax fibrous capsule that is lined by a synovial membrane.

Radiocarpal Articulation

The radiocarpal (wrist) joint (Figure 22-3) is the articulation between the concave distal end of the radius and its intervening articular disc with the convex proximal surfaces of the navicular, lunate, and triquetrum bones. The navicular and lunate form the primary articular surface. The proximal surfaces of these bones form the carpal articular surface in the radiocarpal (wrist) joint. The concave to convex surfaces form an ellipsoid (spindle shaped) articulation. It is a true synovial (diarthrotic) joint. The movements available are flexion and extension around the transverse axis, abduction (radial deviation) and adduction (ulnar deviation) around the anteroposterior axis, and circumduction.

Midcarpal Articulations

The principal midcarpal (intercarpal) joint is located between the bones of the proximal and distal rows of the wrist as the two rows articulate with each other. In addition, discrete articulations also exist between adjacent carpals in both the proximal and distal rows of bones. A small joint also exists be-

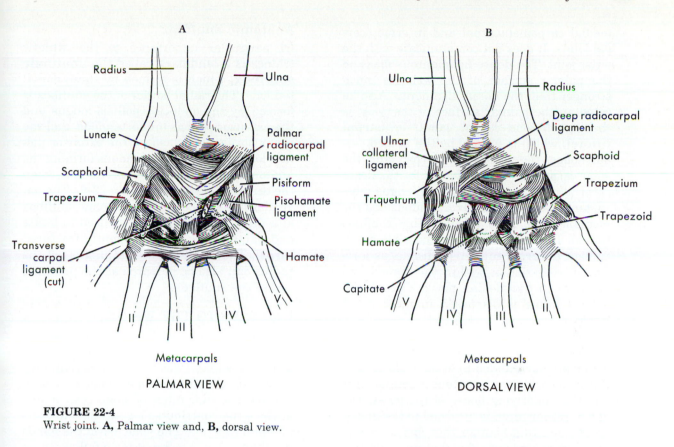

A

Radius

Ulna

Lunate

Palmar radiocarpal ligament

Scaphoid

Trapezium

Pisiform

Pisohamate ligament

Transverse carpal ligament (cut)

Hamate

I

II

III

IV

V

Metacarpals

PALMAR VIEW

B

Ulna

Radius

Deep radiocarpal ligament

Ulnar collateral ligament

Scaphoid

Triquetrum

Trapezium

Trapezoid

Hamate

Capitate

I

II

III

IV

V

Metacarpals

DORSAL VIEW

FIGURE 22-4
Wrist joint. **A,** Palmar view and, **B,** dorsal view.

tween the pisiform and the triquetrum bones. The cavity of this joint is independent of all others in the wrist. Combined movements at the midcarpal articulations increase the range of movements of the hand and supplement movements at the radiocarpal joint. Limited gliding movements also occur between adjacent carpals in both the proximal and distal rows.

Carpometacarpal Articulations

The articulation between the trapezium and the first metacarpal (of the thumb) is unique in that the joint cavity formed by this articulation is separate from all others in the area. The joint cavities of the four other carpometacarpal joints (of the fingers) communicate with the large midcarpal joint cavity.

The second metacarpal articulates with the trapezoid, the capitate with the third metacarpal, and the hamate with the fourth and fifth metacarpals. The bases of the four metacarpal bones of the fingers are united

by strong ligaments in an intermetacarpal joint. No joint or direct bony articulation exists between the first and second metacarpals.

The separate carpometacarpal joint of the thumb is a saddle-shaped articulation with reciprocally concavoconvex surfaces between the trapezium and the first metacarpal. This "thumb joint" is surrounded by a strong but loose articular capsule that permits opposition, flexion, extension, abduction, adduction, and circumduction. In contrast, only slight gliding movements are possible between the carpals and the metacarpals of the four fingers.

Ligaments

A fibrous capsule formed by a complex series of ligaments binds the carpals firmly together into a functional unit (Figure 22-4). A large and complex intercarpal synovial cavity extends between the carpals and communicates with the joint cavities of the four medial carpometacarpal and intermetacarpal joints. It does not communicate with the wrist joint. The dense ligamentous mass on the palmar surface of the wrist is much stronger than the dorsal ligaments. Also located on the palmar surface of the wrist is the osseofibrous carpal canal, or **carpal tunnel,** which is formed by the arched carpal bones, the transverse carpal, and the volar carpal ligaments. Except for the flexor carpi ulnaris and the palmaris longus muscle tendons, all of the flexor tendons and the median nerve pass through this confined tunnel. This gives rise to the possible development of carpal tunnel syndrome, as a result of constriction within the tunnel and pressure on the median nerve. Carpal tunnel syndrome is discussed in more detail later.

Crossing the dorsal surface of the wrist are the extensor tendons of the fingers, which are surrounded by tendon sheaths as they pass between the extensor retinaculum and the underlying bones of the wrist. The dorsal retinaculum is attached to the underlying bones in a manner that forms six separate compartments for the extensor tendons. Figure 22-5 illustrates the placement of the tendon sheaths in the cross section view of a wrist.

Anatomic Snuffbox

Of particular importance to the athletic trainer is a landmark called the **anatomic snuffbox,** which is formed by three dorsal tendons. The radial border of the snuffbox is formed by the abductor pollicis longus and the extensor pollicis brevis tendons, and the ulnar border is formed by the extensor pollicis longus tendon. The tendons forming the anatomic snuffbox become prominent when the thumb is extended (Figure 22-6). The navicular lies just below the anatomic snuffbox and this surface landmark is used to locate and palpate this most frequently fractured carpal. The tip of the styloid process of the radius can also be palpated at the proximal end of the snuffbox.

INJURIES TO THE WRIST

The wrist is a frequently injured area of the body. Athletic injuries often result from a direct blow to the wrist or stresses that force the wrist beyond its normal range of motion (ROM). The wide range of mobility available at the wrist contributes a great deal to overall hand function. The wide use of the hands in athletics, such as breaking a fall, warding off another player, grasping, catching, throwing, or hitting, frequently force the wrist beyond its normal ROM (Figure 22-7).

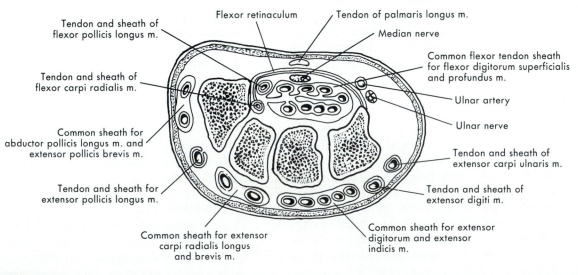

FIGURE 22-5
Cross section of the right wrist. Note the carpal canal and the arrangement of the tendon sheaths.

Structures in the wrist can also be injured as the result of chronic overuse. These mechanisms of injury can result in contusions, sprains, strains, dislocations, fractures, and carpal tunnel syndrome.

Contusions

Contusions of the wrist frequently occur as the result of a direct blow. The result is a bruise involving underlying structures such as the bones, tendons, nerves, or blood vessels. For one of the carpals to be fractured in this manner, the blow would have to be a severe crushing type. A more common injury associated with contusions involves one of the many tendons that crosses the wrist. A tenosynovitis may result from a direct blow to the wrist or repeated trauma to this area. Occasionally a nerve compression or vascular injury may develop from repeated trauma about the wrist. Therefore athletic trainers must carefully examine all wrist contusions for associated injuries to underlying structures. Athletes exhibiting sharp localized pain over a bony prominence, or pain, tingling, or numbness radiating into the fingers, should be referred to medical assistance.

Strains

Any of the many tendons that cross the wrist may be strained. This is especially true of the wrist flexors and extensors. Strains can result from a violent muscular contraction against resistance, an overstretching such as that associated with hyperflexion or hyperextension, or chronic overuse. These injuries can also be confused with a wrist sprain or carpal fracture. Strains, however, will cause increased pain on active and resistive contraction of the muscle or muscles involved.

The tendon and its synovial sheath may also become inflamed as a result of a strain and progress to a tenosynovitis. As this condition develops, the tendon swells and the synovial sheath thickens, causing discomfort and pain as the tendon slides within the tubelike sheath. As this constriction progresses, palpable and audible sensations may be exhibited in the area, such as clicking or grating. Tenosynovitis of the flexor tendons may predispose an athlete to carpal tunnel syndrome and may progress until the tendons are no longer able to move through these tunnels. This condition may also be caused by an active violent contraction, pas-

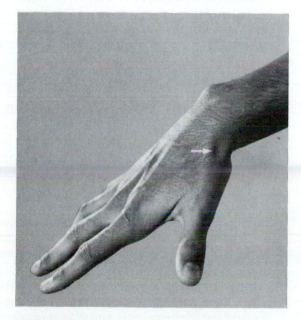

FIGURE 22-6
Anatomic snuffbox formed by dorsal tendons of the thumb.

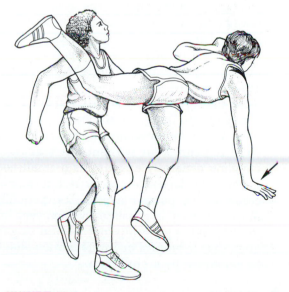

FIGURE 22-7
Common mechanism of injury to the wrist or hand as athlete breaks a fall with an outstretched arm.

sive stretching, or contusion to the area.

De Quervain's disease. De Quervain's disease is a common form of tenosynovitis of the wrist, occurring frequently in racquet sports. This is an inflammation of the tendons of the abductor pollicis longus and extensor pollicis brevis as they pass through a fibro-osseous tunnel at the level of the radial styloid. Repetitive ulnar deviation and gripping can inflame these tendons in their closed space, resulting in pain when using the thumb, stiffness, and pinch weakness. Swelling and tenderness are present along the radial aspect of the wrist and follow the course of the tendons. Evaluation is confirmed with a positive **Finkelstein's test.** Have the athlete make a fist with the thumb inside the fingers and ulnarly deviate the wrist. A positive test is indicated by pain over the abductor pollicis longus and extensor pollicis brevis tendons. Because this test may cause some discomfort in an uninjured wrist, always compare the pain on the injured side to the discomfort on the uninjured side.

✤ **Wrist ganglion.** Another condition that can involve the tendinous sheath or synovial joint capsule is a synovial hernia or knot-like mass called a wrist ganglion, which occurs most often on the back of the wrist. It is believed that a ganglion of this type results from a defect in the fibrous sheath of a tendon or joint, which permits a portion of the underlying synovium to herniate through it. This herniated sac forms a cystic enlargement that gradually fills with fluid and may become quite large. In athletics, this condition usually follows a strain or sprain of the wrist but can occur without any trauma. A ganglion generally appears as a small nodule over the dorsum of the wrist, but can also occur on the palmar aspect. Its cystic-like mass may vary in consistency from very soft to firm and is generally not painful. A ganglion that is painful or limits motion should be examined by a physician.

✤ **Sprains**
Many athletic injuries to the wrist are sprains. The most common mechanism of injury is forced hyperextension. Isolated injury to the large and very strong volar liga-

ments seldom occurs. Instead injuries in this area will involve the volar tendons or bones of the wrist. Forced hyperflexion may injure the weaker dorsal ligaments, as well as involve the tendons or bones. Therefore wrist sprains should be approached assuming an associated fracture until proved otherwise. Tenderness over the carpals or styloid processes of the radius or ulna should be referred to a physician for X-ray. If initial radiographs are negative, the athlete should be treated as if there is a sprain. In the presence of persistent pain and swelling lasting for 2 to 3 weeks a second radiograph should be requested.

Dislocations
Because of the strong ligamentous structures about the articulations of the wrist, dislocations are not common injuries and occur far less often than fractures. Dislocations of the radiocarpal, midcarpal or carpometacarpal joints are extremely uncommon in athletic activity, although they may occur as the result of violent trauma and associated fractures. These types of injuries are normally indicated by obvious disability and deformity and are readily recognized.

✤ **Lunate dislocation.** The most frequent carpal instability is scapholunate dissociation, which may be as common as scaphoid (navicular) fractures. During a fall on an outstretched hand, resulting in hyperextension, the capitate can be driven between the scaphoid and lunate. Stretched ligaments may account for dynamic instability. Any athlete complaining of radial wrist pain after a fall on an outstretched hand must be carefully evaluated for both scaphoid fracture and ligamentous injury. If the ligaments are ruptured, the lunate may eventually dislocate.

The lunate is the most commonly dislocated carpal of the wrist. This bone may be displaced by forced hyperextension because of its shape and relationship to the surrounding carpals. Dislocation of the lunate is usually caused by a self-reduced backward dislocation of the carpals and often occurs in two steps. The ligaments of the lunate attach it more firmly to the distal radius and ulna than are the other carpal bones. As a result of its shape and this strong attachment, the lunate does not dislocate backward with the wrist after trauma. Instead, ligaments connecting it with adjacent carpals are torn. The second step in the dislocation occurs as a result of spontaneous reduction of the other displaced carpals. When they return to their normal position they push the lunate forward and tend to rotate it around its dorsal ligamentous attachment to the radius. This ligament carries the most important nutrient vessel to the bone. If it is torn as a result of the dislocation, the reduced blood supply may cause progressive degeneration or necrosis **(Kienbock's disease).** Despite an impaired blood supply, early reduction of a dislocated lunate may prevent necrosis if other nutrient vessels remain uninjured.

Dislocation of the lunate may not be readily recognized. Symptoms usually include tenderness and swelling over the lunate. Palpation may detect the displaced lunate under the flexor tendons. Movements of the wrist are often painful and limited. On making a fist, the knuckle formed by the head of the third metacarpal moves proximally, so that it is on a level with the adjoining knuckles and does not project distally to them as it normally should. This is known as **Murphy's sign.** The medial nerve is normally some distance anterior to the lunate; however, forward displacement of the lunate may compress the carpal tunnel, causing pain and paresthesia in the median nerve distribution of the hand.

Fractures

Fractures about the wrist usually result from forced hyperextension such as falling on an outstretched hand. This mechanism transmits the force of the fall through the capitate, lunate, and navicular bones to the radius.

❖   **Navicular fracture.** The carpal most often fractured is the navicular or scaphoid. This is a result of its shape and location. The navicular is an oval, elongated bone that extends the most distally of those in the proximal row of carpals. The center portion, or waist, of the navicular is narrowed, making this area most vulnerable to fracture. During forced hyperextension, the navicular may be impinged between the capitate and radius, resulting in a fracture. Normally there is no displacement of fragments, and such an injury may be erroneously evaluated as a wrist sprain. A fractured navicular will cause pain just distal to the radius, and point tenderness will be elicited during palpation of the anatomic snuffbox. Therefore all wrist injuries exhibiting these symptoms should be referred for radiographic examination. If initial X-ray films are negative, the wrist should be handled as if the athlete has suffered a sprain. The wrist should be radiographed again if pain and disability persists for 2 weeks because a navicular fracture is notorious for not being readily visible on initial X-ray films. Navicular fractures frequently result in complications, such as nonunion or avascular necrosis **(Preiser's disease),** because the blood supply to the fracture fragments is not always adequate.

❖   **Fractured radius.** Falling on an outstretched hand may cause a fracture to the distal end of the radius. This type of fracture will cause tenderness over the lower end of the radius and pain on hand movement. Complete fracture of the distal radius, in which the fragment is displaced dorsally, is

❖ known as **Colles' fracture** (Figure 22-8). With this type of fracture, movement of the hand and fingers is markedly limited or absent. In Colles' fracture a so-called **silver-fork deformity** results, in which there is a prominence on the back of the wrist and a lateral or radial displacement or deviation of the hand. Dislocations of the wrist are rare. If a dorsal dislocation does occur, the deformity will resemble a Colles' fracture but will be closer to the hand. The reverse of Colles' fracture, produced by a fall on the back of the hand with the wrist flexed, is

❖ called **Smith's fracture,** in which the frag-

❖ ment is forwardly displaced. A **Barton fracture** involves a rim of the articular surface of the distal radius. Usually there is an associated subluxation of the carpal bones.

❖   **Epiphyseal plate injury.** In preadolescent and adolescent athletes, these same mechanisms may cause an epiphyseal displacement in the distal radius or ulna rather than a fracture. Epiphyseal fractures occur

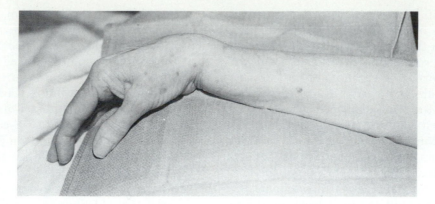

FIGURE 22-8
Colles' fracture of the wrist.

more commonly in the radius and normally result from forces applied to an extended wrist. Prognosis is excellent. Epiphyseal fractures involving the distal ulna usually occur in association with a distal fracture of the radius. Prognosis is not as good. Epiphyseal displacement is normally more difficult to recognize than a fracture. Therefore, in young athletes with tenderness around the wrist after trauma to this area, you must attempt to rule out epiphyseal plate injuries. Any suspicions of possible epiphyseal involvement should be referred to medical assistance.

✤ **Carpal Tunnel Syndrome**

As previously discussed, there is a canal in the palmar surface of the wrist, the *carpal tunnel,* that is formed by the arched carpal bones and the transverse carpal and volar carpal ligaments. These structures form a fibrous sheath that contains the median nerve and all the flexor tendons, with the exception of the palmaris longus and flexor carpi ulnaris. Review the contents of the carpal tunnel in Figure 22-5.

Constriction or narrowing within the carpal tunnel and pressure on the median nerve is called **carpal tunnel syndrome.** This condition can result from swelling secondary to trauma, such as a Colles' fracture or wrist sprain. The median nerve can also be compressed by a lunate dislocation, tenosynovitis of the flexor tendons, a ganglion, or col-

lagen disease. In carpal tunnel syndrome, compression of the median nerve can restrict motor function and sensation along the nerve distribution of the hand. Athletes suffering from this condition often complain of numbness and tingling along the median nerve distribution. These symptoms often increase with use and may occur at night.

There are two tests that may elicit altered sensory phenomena and indicate carpal tunnel syndrome. The most common test is called **Phalen's test.** Have the athlete flex both wrists maximally and hold this position for at least 1 minute (Figure 22-9). A positive test is indicated by tingling or numbness over the palmar surface of the hand, the first three fingers and part of the fourth. The symptoms resolve quickly after the hand is returned to the resting position. The other test is the **Tinel's sign.** This test consists of tapping over the volar carpal ligament, which may cause tingling along the median nerve distribution. A positive test indicates carpal tunnel syndrome.

ANATOMY OF THE HAND

The hand is an organ capable of a great variety of discrete and complicated movements. These movements, so important in numerous sports and athletic activities, are possible because of the coordinated actions of its many joints and muscles. Remember from Chapter 3 that the metacarpals form the skeleton of the major part of the hand

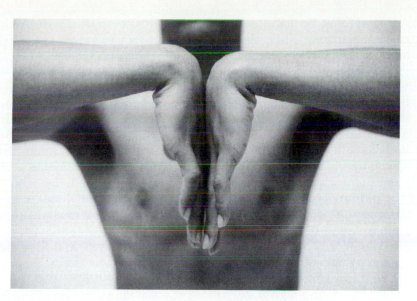

FIGURE 22-9
Phalen's test to evalute for carpal tunnel syndrome. Have the athlete flex both wrists maximally and hold this position for at least 1 minute. A positive test is indicated by tingling or numbness over the palmar surface of the hand, the first three fingers, and part of the ring finger.

and the phalanges are the bones of the digits. Anatomically, the hand can be divided into the (1) palmar region, (2) dorsal region, and (3) phalanges.

Metacarpals
The metacarpals of the hand are identified by numbers from 1 to 5, beginning on the lateral side with the metacarpal of the thumb. Each metacarpal has a slightly curved shaft and two extremities: (1) a *base,* which articulates proximally with the carpals, and (2) a *head,* which articulates distally with the proximal phalanx in the thumb or one of the digits. The heads of the metacarpals form the knuckles on the back of the hand.

Phalanges
The phalanges form the bony framework of the digits. There are 14 phalanges in each hand: two for the thumb and three for each of the remaining four fingers. The bony anatomy of all five fingers is essentially the same. Starting proximally the phalanges are identified by name or number as the proximal, middle, and distal phalanges, or as the first, second, and third phalanges. They resemble the metacarpals in shape and appearance.

Metacarpophalangeal Articulations
The metacarpophalangeal (MCP) joints are synovial articulations between the head of a metacarpal and the base of a proximal phalanx. With the digits clenched into a fist the metacarpophalangeal joint is about ½ inch distal to the prominence of the knuckle on the dorsum of the hand. Each joint is maintained by a joint capsule that is thin posteriorly (dorsally) but thickened by a palmar ligament anteriorly and by collateral ligaments laterally. Movements available at these joints include flexion, extension, adduction, abduction, and circumduction. No rotation occurs at these joints. Metacarpophalangeal joint dislocations resulting from athletic activity do occur, particularly in the thumb. In dislocations at these joints the base of the first phalanx will usually pass posteriorly (backward). Small sesamoid bones, which may be mistaken for bone fragments, are sometimes present near the metacarpophalangeal joint of the thumb. Al-

though such bones may be found around other metacarpophalangeal joints, they are not common.

Interphalangeal Articulations

The interphalangeal joints are similar in structure to metacarpophalangeal joints. Both are classified as diarthrotic (synovial) joints and both have a thin capsule and a pair of strong collateral ligaments that pass around onto the palmar aspect to fuse with the sides of the **palmar (volar) plate.** This plate is a fibrocartilaginous structure that covers the palmar aspect of the metacarpophalangeal and proximal interphalangeal (PIP) joints. Each palmar plate has a distal fibrous portion and a proximal membranous portion that shortens during digital flexion. In prolonged flexion of a finger, this proximal membranous portion can passively shorten by fibrosis, resulting in stiffness and a limiting of complete extension. Interphalangeal articulations join the head of one phalanx and the base of the more distal one. They do not permit abduction or adduction, only flexion and extension.

Of the two palmar skin creases between the first and second phalanges, the proximal crease identifies the joint. The crease between the second and third phalanges marks the distal joint. The skin creases of the proximal interphalangeal joints are closely bound to the underlying flexor sheaths. Even superficial cuts in these proximal creases can cause serious infections. Such injuries, although they appear to be minor, should be monitored very carefully for signs of developing infection.

Palmar Region

The palmar region of the hand is quadrilateral in shape and contains soft tissues located anteriorly to the metacarpals. A triangular "hollow" central portion is bounded on the lateral or radial side by the **thenar eminence** and on the medial or ulnar side by the **hypothenar eminence.** The thenar eminence at the base of the thumb contains short intrinsic muscles of the hand involved in moving the thumb, whereas the hypothenar eminence consists of muscles involved in moving the little finger. The two eminences almost approximate each other proximally as they approach the wrist. Skin of the palm is thick and coarse, especially over the heads of the metacarpals. It is firmly bound to the underlying palmar aponeurosis and is well supplied with sweat glands. No hairs or sebaceous glands are present in the skin of the palm. In most persons two transverse skin creases, proximal and distal, are present in the palm. Movements of the index finger are accommodated by the proximal crease, whereas the distal crease permits movements of the medial three digits and serves as a surface landmark for the heads of the third, fourth, and fifth metacarpals.

Dorsal Region

The dorsal region of the hand, in contrast to the palmar surface, is covered with loose skin containing numerous sweat and sebaceous glands. The skin has a fine texture and in men contains a variable number of short but visible hairs. The extensor tendons are both visible and palpable over the dorsum of the hand. They are united by oblique bands and form a thin aponeurotic sheet that attaches to the sides of the second and fifth metacarpal bones. The dorsal subcutaneous space is an extensive area of loose areolar tissue just below the skin over the dorsum of the hand. It permits dramatic swelling to occur over the back of the hand during infection or after trauma.

Fingers

The skin of the flexor surface of all the digits is thick, only slightly mobile, and devoid of hair. Some subcutaneous fat is present. Over the dorsum of the digits the skin is thinner and more mobile. Subcutaneous fat is extremely limited or absent. Transverse flexor skin creases approximate the positions of the underlying joints. The skin creases are closely bound to the underlying flexor tendon sheaths, and any penetrating wound at the crease is likely to penetrate the synovial sheath beneath it.

Muscles of the Hand

The hand is a particularly complicated organ. It contains the tendons of the long (extrinsic) muscles that were discussed in

Chapter 21, as well as a number of **intrinsic** muscles and important nerves and blood vessels. Review the extrinsic muscles of the hand in Table 21-1 and Figures 21-9 and 21-10. Review the intrinsic muscles of the hand in Table 22-1 and Figure 22-10. Figure 22-11 illustrates many of the intrinsic muscles and the flexor tendon sheaths of the hand.

Sensory Innervation of the Hand

The sensory innervation of the hand involves the median, ulnar, and radial nerves. Sensory branches of the median nerve supply the median (central) palmar area and the palmar surfaces of the lateral three and one-half fingers. It also supplies the skin over the dorsum (top) of the distal two phalanges of the thumb, index, and middle fingers. The ulnar nerve supplies sensory nerves to the palmar and dorsal surfaces of the medial third of the hand and to both surfaces of the little finger and half of the ring finger. The radial nerve transmits sensory impulses from the thenar eminence and from the lateral two thirds of the dorsum of the proximal hand and dorsal aspects of the proximal phalanges of the thumb, index,

middle, and one half of the ring finger. It is important to remember the peripheral nerve supply of the hand when performing a sensory neurologic evaluation.

Motor Innervation of the Hand

Motor control of the intrinsic hand muscles is furnished by the ulnar and median nerves. However, since these intrinsic muscles are not the sole manipulators of the hand, the radial nerve, which supplies motor control to a number of important extrinsic muscles, must also be considered when discussing control of voluntary hand movements.

The ulnar nerve supplies motor control to those muscles that abduct and adduct (spread and approximate) the fingers, whereas functioning of the median nerve is required to approximate successively the tip of the thumb to the tips of the fingers. Damage to the radial nerve results in **wrist-drop**, which is caused by paralysis of the wrist extensor muscles.

INJURIES TO THE HAND

There are few sports in which the hands are not used in some manner. An athlete's

TABLE 22-1

Intrinsic Muscles of the Hand

Muscle	Nerve	Segmental innervation	Primary action(s)
Abductor pollicis brevis	Median	C_8, T_1	Abduction of thumb
Flexor pollicis brevis (superficial head)	Median	C_8, T_1	Flexion of MCP joint of thumb
Flexor pollicis brevis (deep head)	Ulnar	C_8, T_1	Flexion of MCP joint of thumb
Opponens pollicis	Median	C_8, T_1	Opposition of thumb
Lumbricals I and II	Median	C_8, T_1	Flexion of MCP joints & extension of IP joints of digits
Lumbricals III and IV	Ulnar	C_8, T_1	Flexion of MCP joints & extension of IP joints of digits
Adductor pollicis	Ulnar	C_8, T_1	Adduction of MC and flexion of MCP joints of thumb
Abductor digiti minimi	Ulnar	C_8, T_1	Abduction of little finger
Flexor digiti minimi brevis	Ulnar	C_8, T_1	Flexion of MCP joint of little finger
Opponens digiti minimi	Ulnar	C_8, T_1	Opposition of little finger
Palmar interossei	Ulnar	C_8, T_1	Adduction of digits II, IV, & V; flexion of MCP and extension of IP joints of digits
Dorsal interossei	Ulnar	C_8, T_1	Abduction of digits II, IV, & V; flexion of MCP and extension of IP joints of digits

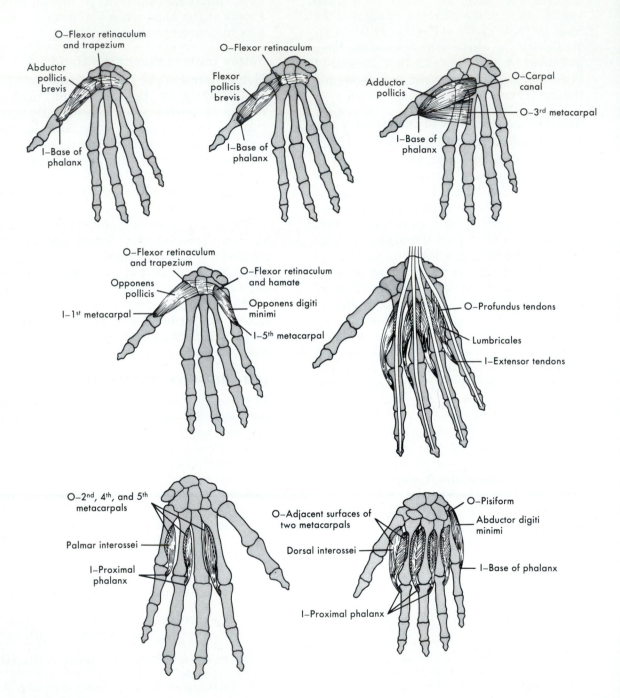

FIGURE 22-10
Intrinsic muscles of the hand.

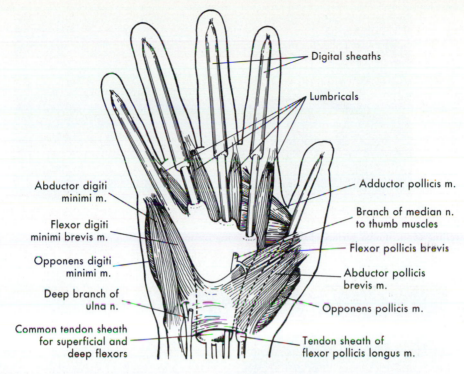

FIGURE 22-11
Intrinsic muscles and flexor tendon sheaths of the hand.

hands are constantly exposed to various types of forced movements and direct trauma. As a result, a wide variety of athletic injuries to the hands can occur. Many are relatively minor and are never reported to the athletic trainer. Because there is a tendency by many athletes to underestimate or minimize injuries to this area of the body, injuries to the hands can develop into long-term impairment and permanent disability if not recognized and cared for properly. Therefore it is important for athletic trainers to be aware of signs and symptoms associated with the various injuries to the hand to avoid possible complications.

Contusions and Abrasions

These types of injuries are normally of little consequence; however, whenever the skin is broken about the hand, infection becomes a concern. All abrasions must be thoroughly cleaned and properly cared for in an attempt to prevent contamination and subsequent infection. Contusion injuries resulting in hematoma formation about the hand are un-

common. The firmly fixed skin on the palmar surface allows little room for the pooling of blood. The loose mobile skin on the dorsum of the hand, however, permits very marked swelling (Figure 22-12), even if the initial trauma or focus of infection is located on the palm of the hand or on the fingers. This type of dorsal hand swelling, which may be marked and spectacular in appearance soon after an injury, normally subsides quickly and seldom develops into a fixed or pooled hematoma. On the palmar surface, the fleshy thenar and hypothenar eminences can be contused because of some type of direct blow. These injuries can be quite bothersome to an athlete because swelling in the confined area can produce tightness and pain, which limits hand function. Occasionally subcutaneous structures may be compressed and damaged in conjunction with contusing trauma. A careful evaluation of contused or abraded areas can generally determine if there is any associated involvement of underlying structures.

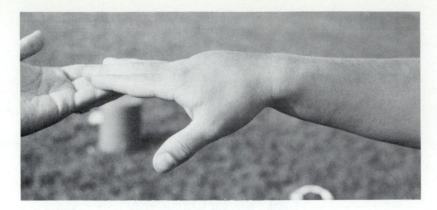

FIGURE 22-12
Marked swelling of the dorsal surface of the hand following trauma.

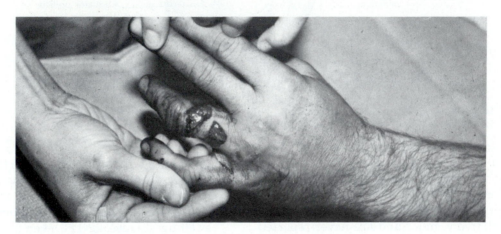

FIGURE 22-13
Example of a "ring injury."

✢   **Subungual hematoma.** Direct trauma to the tips of the fingers or fingernails can cause blood to accumulate under the nail (subungual hematoma). As the blood pools under the fingernail, a painful, throbbing pressure develops that is usually relieved by drilling a hole in the nail and releasing the blood. Every athletic trainer has a favorite method of drilling a hole in the fingernail to relieve a subungual hematoma. Common methods involve use of a nail drill designed for this purpose, drilling with a sharp-pointed scalpel blade, or applying a red-hot paper clip to the nail.

Lacerations and Punctures

Although open wounds such as lacerations or punctures are generally not serious, the potential for significant and serious consequences exists, and such wounds should never be taken lightly. An athlete wearing a ring during activity is at risk in the event of localized finger trauma. Figure 22-13 illustrates a finger injury caused by wearing a ring. Open wounds may damage subcutaneous structures such as tendons or nerves, which are often close to the surface. Therefore, after athletic injuries of this nature, a complete and careful evaluation of hand and finger function should be performed.

Infections

An important consideration of all open injuries about the hand is infection, because this too may have serious consequences, can impair performance, and may develop into permanent disability. All open injuries about the hands must be thoroughly cleaned, debrided, and protected from further injury and contamination in an attempt to avoid infections. In addition, athletes should be instructed to report any symptoms that may indicate a developing infection such as an increase in aching, soreness, or throbbing in the hand, the presence of pus, or an increase in body temperature.

❖ **Felon.** A felon, or **whitlow,** is an extremely painful infection located in the soft tissues surrounding the terminal phalanx of a finger. Accumulation of pus or fluid in the confined tissue spaces of the fingertip produces marked pressure that can shut off the blood supply and cause early necrosis of bone. Suppurative (pus filled) felons are common and dangerous and should always be referred to a physician for treatment and drainage.

❖ **Paronychia.** A paronychia is an infection involving the subepithelial folds of tissue surrounding the fingernail. It can be acute or chronic and is usually caused by staphylococci. The infection is frequently introduced as a result of picking at a hangnail or rough manicuring. In the early stages there is pain, redness, and swelling of the tissues at the side of the nail (Figure 22-14). If incised and drained early, no ill effects result. However, if neglected the infection may spread along the sides and base of the nail, forming what is called a "run around." Occasionally a subungual abscess can result.

Strains

Injuries involving the vast complex of tendons in the hand are not uncommon in athletics and are often missed on examination. The most common cause of these strains is overstretching or forcing the musculotendinous unit beyond its normal ROM. The long flexor and extensor tendons are those most often strained. Symptomatically, these tendinous strains will present tenderness at the site of injury and increased pain on active

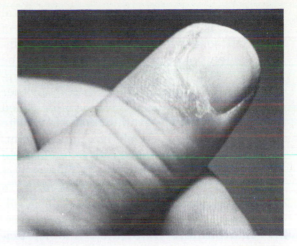

FIGURE 22-14
Infection involving the subepithelial folds of tissue around a thumbnail (paronychia).

and resistive contraction or passive stretching of the musculotendinous unit.

❖ **Baseball finger.** Occasionally there will be a tendon rupture or avulsion of the tendinous attachment to the bone. This occurs most often at the distal phalanx, because the tendinous slip becomes narrow at the point of attachment. The extensor tendon may be injured by a blow to the tip of the finger, forcing the distal interphalangeal joint into flexion and rupturing or partially rupturing the extensor tendon slip at the point of its insertion into the base of the terminal phalanx. This injury, called a **baseball finger** or **mallet finger,** is characterized by the athlete's inability to extend the distal phalanx. The distal attachment of the flexor digitorum profundus muscle can also be ruptured or avulsed. This type of injury occurs often in a contact sport in which an actively flexed finger is violently extended. If the extending force is too great, the flexor digitorum profundus may be avulsed from its insertion into the distal phalanx. This injury is characterized by pain, swelling, and tenderness at the distal interphalangeal joint, as well as the inability of the athlete to actively flex at this joint while the proximal and middle finger joints are held straight.

❖ **Profundus tendon rupture.** Rupture or avulsion of the flexor digitorum profundus tendon from its attachment to the distal phalanx, is caused by a sudden extension of the DIP joint while held in flexion. This injury often occurs when an athlete gets the tip of a finger caught in a jersey or equipment as he or she attempts to grab another player. Therefore, this injury is often called **jersey finger.** On examination the athlete will be unable to actively flex the DIP joint. These athletes should be referred to medical attention. The avulsed tendon may retract to the PIP joint or possibly into the palm. To avoid any permanent functional deficit, adequate treatment and/or repair is necessary.

❖ **Boutonnière deformity.** Another tendon injury with which athletic trainers should be familiar involves the central slip of the extensor tendon. This tendon can be avulsed from its insertion in the dorsal lip of the middle phalanx by a severe flexion force or crushed by a direct blow to the proximal interphalangeal (PIP) joint. Initially the athlete may be able to extend the PIP joint and straighten this finger. However, this extension is very weak when tested against resistance. Without proper recognition and adequate care, the soft tissues surrounding the joint or the central slip itself begin to stretch, and the finger may gradually stiffen in a flexed position. Finally, like a button going through a buttonhole, the PIP joint will extrude through the defect in the tendon, forming the **boutonnière deformity** (Figure 22-15). This classic deformity is characterized by hyperextension of the MCP joint, flexion of the PIP joint, and hyperextension of the DIP.

The tendon of the extensor pollicis longus muscle inserts into the terminal phalanx of the thumb. This muscle, which originates from the ulna and interosseous membrane, extends the terminal phalanx of the thumb and assists in extending the hand at the wrist. It is this tendon that is most often ruptured in a Colles'-type fracture. The rupture may occur at the time of the fracture or 6 to 7 weeks after the injury. Anytime an athlete cannot fully and strongly flex and extend at each joint of the finger, tendon rupture should be suspected and the athlete referred to a physician.

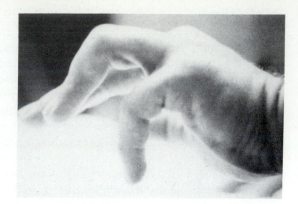

FIGURE 22-15
Boutonnière deformity of a finger.

Strains may occur to the intrinsic muscles of the hand because of excessive overuse. This happens often in sports requiring constant gripping such as gymnastics or rowing. Symptoms of these injuries are cramping and fatigue of the involved muscles and an increase in pain against resistive movements. Symptoms normally subside when activity is reduced or discontinued.

❖ **Sprains**

Injuries involving the ligaments or ligamentous capsules surrounding the various joints of the hand are very common in athletic activity. This is especially true of the interphalangeal joints and the metacarpophalangeal joint of the thumb. Sprains are normally the result of forced motion at a joint that stresses the supporting ligaments, causing varying degrees of damage. This forced motion is usually lateral motion, which stresses the collateral ligaments, or hyperextension, which stresses the anterior capsule. If this displacing force is strong enough or continuous, the joint will sublux (dislocate).

Symptoms of sprains about the hand or digits are tenderness at the site of injury and an increase in pain on reproduction of the stress that caused the injury. In addition, there are normally varying amounts of swelling, stiffness, and soreness surrounding the articulation that may take months

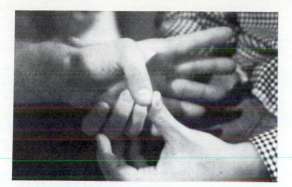

FIGURE 22-16
Torn ulnar collateral ligament of the metacarpophalangeal joint of the thumb. Note abnormal abduction of the joint.

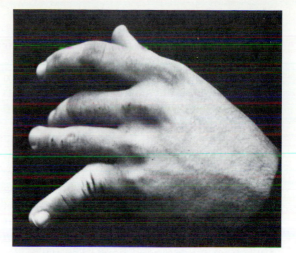

FIGURE 22-17
Finger dislocation.

to resolve. Depending on the amount of ligamentous damage, there may be varying amounts of instability associated with sprain injuries. If instability is recognized, the athlete should be referred to medical assistance.

The most common sprain of the hand is to the proximal interphalangeal joints. When a finger is pulled or forced to the side, the supporting collateral ligaments or volar plate may be injured. This type of injury will exhibit tenderness over the collateral ligament involved, rapid swelling, and pain on passive stressing. Instability will be present with severe sprains. Inadequate evaluation and treatment of these injuries may lead to prolonged swelling, stiffness, pain, and loss of motion.

Forced hyperextension may actually tear the volar plate away from its insertion at the middle phalanx. With this type of injury, the athlete will complain of pain in the PIP joint area with and without motion, hold the affected finger in a mildly flexed position, and express pain on active and passive extension. There will be definite local tenderness at the volar aspect of the PIP joint. Suspected volar plate injuries should be X-rayed for a small avulsion fracture from the middle phalanx. Unless a volar plate injury is appropriately recognized and treated, a permanent limitation of motion may result.

Skier's thumb. A sprain of the ulnar collateral ligament of the MCP joint of the thumb is called a **skier's thumb** or **gamekeeper's thumb.** This commonly sprained ligament provides the stability necessary for normal grip and pinch. This type of injury is often overlooked or dismissed as a sprained thumb. If the ulnar collateral ligament is torn and inadequately cared for, continued instability, weakness of pinch, and recurrent effusion will probably occur. Injury characteristics are local tenderness over the ligament, joint effusion, and increased pain on attempted abduction of the thumb. Instability will be present if the ligament is torn (Figure 22-16).

❖ **Dislocations**

The same mechanisms causing sprains may result in dislocations of the many joints of the hand. Dislocations involving the fingers occur more commonly than those in any other area of the body (Figure 22-17). These dislocations may remain displaced or may reduce spontaneously and appear as sprains on assessment. Finger dislocations are often readily reduced by the player, coach, or athletic trainer. It is good practice to refer all athletes with dislocations, no matter how minor the injury may seem, to medical assistance. Radiographic studies may be necessary to evaluate the presence of gross instability, ligament avulsion, or articular fracture. All too often athletes suffering dislocated fingers are treated casually and never seen by a physician. Inadequate treatment can lead to permanent instability and deformity of the joint.

Complete dislocations of the metacarpophalangeal joint of the thumb presents another problem in that the flexor tendons may loop around the metacarpal head, making closed reduction impossible. Dislocation of the thumb most often results from a fall that produces forceful hyperextension of the thumb on an extended hand. The usual deformity permits the phalanx to pass backward and rest upon the dorsal aspect of the thumb metacarpal. Dislocated thumbs should be reduced by a physician.

Fractures

Fractures of the hand frequently occur in athletics and result from the same mechanisms of injury previously described. Because these fractures involve small bones, they are often thought to be minor injuries and thus treated casually. However, finger stiffness, malunion, and functional disability may be disturbing consequences of hand fractures. Fractures of the metacarpals, which are more common than phalangeal fractures, usually result from a direct blow to the area or to the metacarpal head, which transmits the force down the shaft of the bone. In metacarpal fractures exclusive of the thumb, the typical deformity is characterized by bowing of the fragments and shortening of the bone. The result is an inverted V-type deformity with a dorsal projection at the fracture site and a palmar or volar displacement of the metacarpal head (Figure 22-18, *A*). A fracture of the neck of the fifth metacarpal is often referred to as a

✢ **boxer's fracture.**

Fractures of the proximal and middle phalanges can result from a direct blow or the same mechanisms that cause dislocations, that is, forced lateral motion or hyperextension. A fracture of the shaft of a proximal phalanx, which is more commonly fractured than the other two phalanges, may result in a V-shaped deformity or angulation (Figure 22-18, *B*). A fracture at the base of

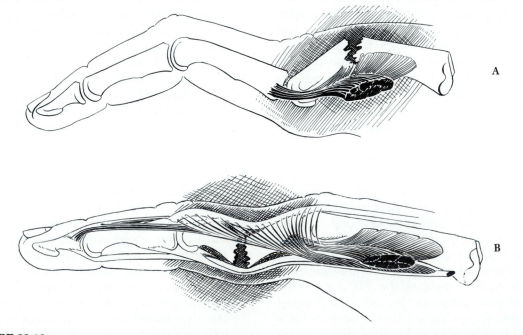

FIGURE 22-18
A, Midshaft fracture of a metacarpal with deformity. **B,** Fracture of proximal phalanx with deformity.

a proximal phalanx may be a combination fracture-dislocation. The distal phalanx is fractured most often by a crushing-type of mechanism.

❖ **Bennett's fracture.** A Bennett's fracture is a fracture of the proximal end (base) of the first metacarpal with an associated subluxation of the metacarpal and the trapezium. The result is an oblique intra-articular fracture or the bone splits as part of it remains in place by the intact volar ligament while the remaining shaft of the metacarpal is displaced radially and dorsally by the pull of the abductor pollicis longus tendon. The dislocation component of this injury is of most importance. If the displacement is not accurately reduced and maintained, malunion or nonunion may result which may lead to significant pain, weakness, and disability. An athlete with a Bennett's fracture will express pain and tenderness at the base of the first metacarpal with possible crepitus. X-rays are necessary to confirm the injury.

Because of the subcutaneous nature of the long bones of the hand, athletic trainers should be able to readily recognize the presence of a fracture. Remember, approach significant hand injuries as if there is a fracture until proven otherwise. Symptomatically, fractures will be tender at the site of injury, with pain elicited at the fracture site during longitudinal or transverse stress. In addition, deformity, crepitation, and a false joint may be present. All suspected fractures should be examined by a physician.

ATHLETIC INJURY ASSESSMENT PROCESS

The hands and wrists are exceedingly vulnerable to athletic injuries. There are few sports in which the fingers, hands, and wrists are not used in some manner, thereby exposing them to a wide variety of possible injuries. Many of these injuries are relatively minor and do not require extensive treatment; unfortunately, too many potentially serious injuries to the hands, wrists, and especially the fingers are regarded as insignificant and neglected by the athlete, coach, or athletic trainer. Remember that even seemingly minor injuries can be extremely disabling to certain athletes, depending on their sport. For example, finger injuries on the throwing hand of a pitcher can prevent the athlete from competing, whereas such an injury may be only a minor annoyance to athletes in other sports. Injuries to the hand and wrist can develop into long-term impairment and permanent disability or disfigurement. The key to proper care of injuries to this area of the body is an early, accurate assessment followed by proper care and referral as indicated.

Secondary survey ▬▬▬▬▬▬

Evaluation procedures are used during the assessment of hand and wrist injuries to recognize an injury that has the potential to result in dysfunction or permanent deformity. Athletic trainers must maintain a high level of suspicion during the assessment process so an injury is not neglected or dismissed as minor when in fact a more serious injury is involved. The significant role of the intricate movements performed by the hands and wrists in regular daily functions, as well as in many athletic activities, makes the accurate evaluation of these injuries extremely important. Therefore careful attention must be exercised by the athletic trainer to ensure that a proper and thorough evaluation is performed.

Circulatory and neurologic assessment

An important consideration mentioned throughout this unit is the value of assessing circulation and neurologic involvement with any significant injury involving the upper extremities. These evaluations are normally performed about the wrist, hand, and fingers and must be considered with any upper extremity injury. Circulation can be evaluated by feeling for a radial or ulnar pulse. The nail beds can be temporarily compressed to check the return of normal color. Once the presence of adequate circulation and nerve functions has been established, the athletic injury assessment process can continue.

Most athletic injuries to the hand and wrist result from acute trauma or direct impact. This can occur during any athletic activity as an athlete hits another athlete or object, or falls on an outstretched hand. The instinctive reaction to any fall is to thrust out the hand in an attempt to break the fall. When this occurs, the outstretched hand may receive the entire stress or force of the fall. This can result in injury to the hand or wrist and can transmit injurious forces throughout the upper extremity, as described in the previous two chapters. An accurate assessment of hand and wrist injuries includes a detailed history of the causative trauma accompanied by systematic physical examination.

History

Because most athletic injuries to the hand and wrist result from direct trauma, the initial history procedures should be concerned with the primary complaint and mechanisms of injury. Question the athlete to get a detailed description of how the injury occurred. Did the athlete fall on the hand? If so, what was the position of the wrist and fingers at the time of impact? Was the wrist forced into flexion or extension? Were the fingers extended or flexed into a fist? Was there a direct blow delivered to the hand? If so, exactly where on the hand and by what? Attempt to determine the severity of the blow or force. Were the fingers forced through an excessive ROM or in an abnormal direction? Was there a blow delivered to the tip of a finger? Occasionally injuries to the hand or wrist result from overuse or repetitive trauma. In other instances an athlete will consider the injury trivial and not report it for a period of time or until it begins to impair function. When these situations occur, inquire about the onset of symptoms. Attempt to find out what happened and how the symptoms have progressed since the athlete first noticed the injury. The more information gained concerning the mechanisms of injury, the better you can assess the nature and determine those structures that may be involved.

Instruct the athlete to describe the symptoms associated with the injury. Where exactly are the painful or tender areas? Pain is not referred appreciably from tissues lying at the distal extent of a limb; therefore tenderness is usually felt exactly at the site of the lesion. Ask the athlete to locate and describe the pain. Is there pain only during movement of the fingers, thumb, or wrist? If so, ask the athlete to demonstrate these movements. The athlete should also be asked about any other sensations associated with the injury. Did he or she feel anything at the time of the injury, such as a popping or snapping sensation? Does the athlete experience any crepitation? The athlete's descriptions of any sensations and impressions concerning the injury should never be ignored, as they often yield valuable information.

Question the athlete carefully concerning any previous injuries to the hand or wrist in an attempt to determine if the current complaint is an aggravation or recurrence of a previous injury. If the area has been injured before, obtain as much information as possible concerning the circumstances surrounding previous injuries. Are symptoms of the current injury similar to those of any previous injuries? Had symptoms completely subsided and full function been restored before the onset of the present injury? The more information gained concerning previous injuries, the better you can evaluate the nature and severity of the current complaint.

Observation

Observations concerning hand and wrist injuries should commence with looking for obvious deformity. This area of the body is primarily subcutaneous, which often allows for the visual recognition of any irregularities such as those associated with an unreduced dislocation or angulated fracture. Note the contours of the hand and wrist. Is there any obvious deformity? If so, note the exact location of the deformity and plan your strategies for caring for the injury.

Notice the positioning and functioning of the injured hand as you talk with the athlete. Is the athlete holding or supporting the hand in such a manner as to protect the area and guard against any movements? If so,

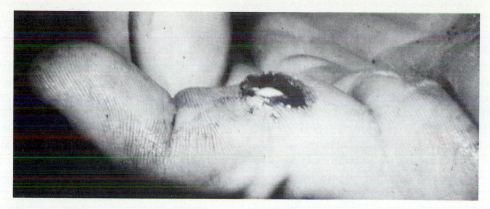

FIGURE 22-19
Skin is split on the volar surface of a finger after a proximal interphalangeal joint
dislocation.

note the position of the wrist, hand, fingers, and thumb. Do they all appear to be held in a normal position of function, that is, slight extension or dorsiflexion of the wrist, all joints of the fingers partially flexed, and the thumb lying parallel to the forearm? Are all fingers parallel to each other, or is one finger held in an abnormal position? Does the hand appear to be hanging limp? Is the athlete voluntarily moving the wrist, thumb, and fingers? If so, do the movements appear to be normal and performed freely, or unnatural and guarded? Is there any indication of pain on movement?

Carefully inspect the injured hand for signs of trauma that can indicate what type of force has been applied and assist in establishing or confirming the mechanism of injury. Is there any bleeding? Since this area is mainly subcutaneous, fractures and dislocations may split the skin, especially on the volar surface (Figure 22-19). Because this area commonly is subjected to direct impact, lacerations, abrasions, and contusions are common. Injuries involving the fingertips may cause tearing of the fingernail or blood pooling under the nail (*subungual hematoma*).

In the absence of obvious deformity, inspect and compare the injured hand or wrist to the uninjured hand or wrist to note any differences in symmetry. Do the metacarpophalangeal joints (knuckles) appear to line up normally and symmetrically on both hands? Is there an obvious difference between corresponding knuckles? If the MCP joints are not symmetrical and/or do not line up, it may indicated a metacarpal fracture. Is there any swelling? If so, note exactly where the swelling is located. As previously explained, the loose skin over the back of the hand allows this area to swell quickly. Blood accumulated in the dorsum of the hand also readily infiltrates out of the area; thus hematoma formation is not common. On the palmar surface of the hand there is not much room for the accumulation of fluid, therefore any bleeding into the front of the hand readily shows up as an ecchymosis. Periarticular swelling around the joints of the fingers can impair function and take months to be absorbed. It may never completely disappear.

Physical Examination

The physical examination portion of the assessment process is used to perform a more detailed investigation of the musculoskeletal system. Depending upon what your impressions are up to this point in the assessment process, you may continue with palpation techniques, movement procedures, or neurological and circulatory evaluations. Not all these procedures will be used in any one athletic injury. Choose the specific tests or procedures that will assist in completing your assessment of the hand and wrist. Remember, physical examination is both a skill and an art, mastered only by study and experience.

Palpation

In the absence of obvious deformity, the assessment of injuries to the hand and wrist should include palpation techniques. The subcutaneous nature of this area makes underlying structures readily accessible to palpation. Athletic trainers should always approach hand and wrist injuries as if there is a fracture until indicated otherwise. Frequently, fractures can be recognized by careful palpation and gentle manipulation described later in this chapter. Gently palpate those areas suspected of being injured to accurately locate such physical signs as tenderness, deformity, swelling, or crepitation. Correlate this information with the underlying anatomy. Procedures used to palpate the various anatomic structures of the hand and wrist are discussed briefly, as are the common athletic injuries that may be indicated by positive signs. Specific structures to be palpated are determined by the information gained up to this point during the assessment process.

The radial and ulnar styloid processes are good points of reference to begin palpating the wrist. Place your thumb on one of these processes and your index finger on the other (Figure 22-20). Note that the radial styloid

process is located more distally than the ulnar. The two rows of small carpal bones lie just distal to these points of reference. With careful palpation techniques, athletic trainers can palpate each of the carpals individually. However, in most athletic injuries involving the wrist, it is not necessary to be able to distinguish each carpal bone by touch. When evaluating wrist injuries, signs and symptoms that indicate the athlete should be referred to medical assistance include point tenderness over a carpal bone, pain on forced motion, and local swelling. These signs and symptoms can be confusing because they may indicate a sprain, strain, fracture, or dislocation.

Athletic trainers should be able to locate and palpate the two primary carpals that articulate with the radius and are the most commonly injured, the navicular and the lunate. The navicular, which is the carpal most frequently fractured, is situated just distal to the radial styloid process. When the wrist is ulnarly deviated, this bone will slide out from beneath the radial styloid, making it easily palpable. The navicular also forms the floor of the anatomic snuffbox and can be felt by pressing into this depression during ulnar deviation (Figure 22-21). Any time

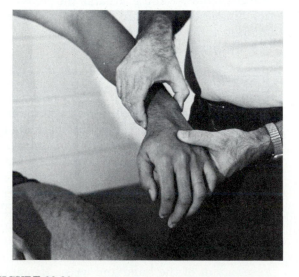

FIGURE 22-20
Palpating the radial and ulnar styloid processes. Note the radial styloid is more distal.

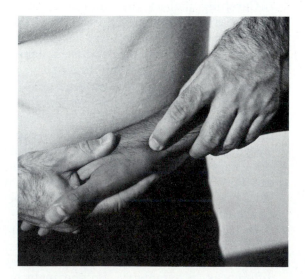

FIGURE 22-21
Palpating the navicular bone during ulnar deviation.

point tenderness is elicited during palpation of the navicular, the athlete should be referred to a physician. The lunate, which is the carpal most frequently dislocated, lies next to the navicular and distal to the radius. It can be palpated just distal to the radial tubercle, which is the bony prominence lying approximately one third of the way across the dorsum of the wrist from the radial styloid process. Palpating just distal to the radial tubercle, a slight depression can be felt. Ask the athlete to flex his or her wrist so that you can feel the lunate as it becomes more prominent on sliding out from under the radius (Figure 22-22, *A*).

The full length of the metacarpals can be palpated because these bones are mainly subcutaneous, especially on the dorsum of the hand. Gently palpate from the base of each of these bones to their distal ends or heads (Figure 22-22, *B*). Note the areas of pain. Point tenderness along the shaft of one of these bones suggests a possible fracture. Tenderness expressed around the articulations suggests a possible sprain. Additional stress maneuvers discussed later will assist in differentiating these symptoms.

The phalanges can also be palpated individually and along their entire length. Gently palpate each digit, including the shaft of the phalanges, the metacarpophalangeal joints, the proximal interphalangeal joints, and the distal interphalangeal joints. Note areas of tenderness, swelling, deformity, or crepitation. Are physical defects felt along the shaft of one of the phalanges or about an articulation? Additional stress procedures may be indicated to complete the assessment.

Palpating soft tissues about the wrist and hand is generally not as extensive as in other areas of the body. The numerous tiny ligaments surrounding the various joints are palpated in conjunction with the bony anatomy. The intrinsic muscles are for the most part indistinguishable from each other through palpation techniques. These muscles and the structures within the palm are palpated as a group in an attempt to localize the injured area. The extrinsic muscles of the hand are tendons of attachment by the time they cross the wrist. Each of these tendons can be palpated if suspected of being injured. These tendons become more pronounced and easier to palpate during active and resistive movements of the hand and

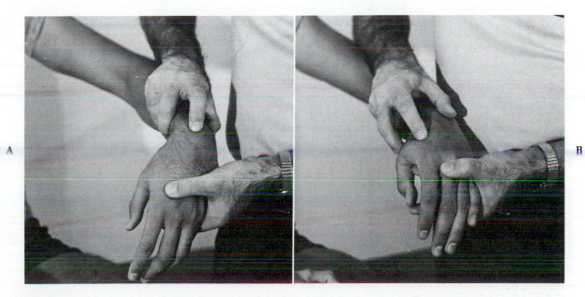

FIGURE 22-22
A, Palpating the lunate bone during wrist flexion. **B,** Palpating the second metacarpal bone.

digits. To palpate individual tendons about the hand and wrist, review the location of the muscles and the action each performs.

Movement procedures

Movement procedures are used to facilitate the assessment of athletic injuries of the wrist and hand. Because of the delicate and intricate makeup of this area of the body, various types of movement techniques are usually necessary to complete the assessment process. These techniques are used to apply stress to various structures in and around the injury site in an attempt to implicate or rule out involvement of specific anatomic structures. Remember, these stressful procedures should be performed gently so as not to cause additional trauma or unnecessary pain.

Active movements. Active movements are performed first to evaluate the ROM and to begin assessing the integrity of specific contractile units. These movements can be performed with the athlete sitting, standing, or supine. Instruct the athlete to execute each movement through as great a ROM as possible and to express any sensations or symptoms that are experienced. It is helpful to have the athlete perform each movement on both sides simultaneously for a bilateral comparison.

To evaluate the active ROM available at the wrist, instruct the athlete to flex and extend, as well as radially and ulnarly deviate, as far as possible, Normally a person can flex (palmar flexion) approximately 80 degrees and extend (dorsiflexion) approximately 70 degrees (Figure 22-23, *A*). An athlete can deviate the wrist farther toward the ulnar side than the radial because the ulna does not extend distally as far as the radius and does not articulate directly with the carpals. Normally a person can ulnar deviate approximately 30 degrees, whereas radial deviation is limited to about 20 degrees (Figure 22-23, *B*).

The finger active ROM is usually evaluated en masse, that is, each finger and all joints collectively in continuous motion. For example, ask the injured athlete to make a tight fist and then straighten the fingers. Notice whether each digit moves easily

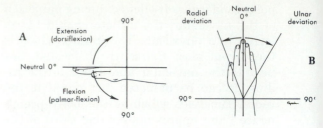

FIGURE 22-23
ROM of the wrist. **A,** Flexion and extension. *Flexion* (palmar flexion): zero to ±80°. *Extension* (dorsiflexion): zero to ±70°. **B,** Radial and ulnar deviation. *Radial deviation:* zero to 20°. *Ulnar deviation:* zero to 30°.

through a complete ROM at each joint. If one of the fingers does not move through a complete ROM, that digit can be evaluated separately. Particular attention must be paid to the distal phalanx where the narrow flexor and extensor tendons insert. Make sure the athlete can actively and strongly flex and extend the distal phalanx. Abduction and adduction can be evaluated by instructing the athlete to spread his or her fingers apart and then bring them back together again. Observe if the fingers move consistently in comparison to the uninjured hand. Each of the digits and each motion of the finger can be evaluated separately if necessary. Refer to Figure 22-24 for a description of the ROM for the fingers.

The active ROM for the thumb consists of flexion and extension, abduction and adduction, and opposition. Instruct the athlete to perform each of these motions and observe the movement. Refer to Figure 22-25 for a description of the ROM for the thumb.

Resistive movements. After evaluating the active ROM, apply resistance against these same movements to further assess the integrity of the contractile units. Manual resistance against each of these motions can assist in accurately identifying specific painful areas and in comparing muscular strengths between extremities. Remember, various muscles can enter into different actions about the wrist and hand, which can make it difficult to evaluate each muscle separately.

To apply resistance against wrist flexion, stabilize the athlete's forearm with one hand

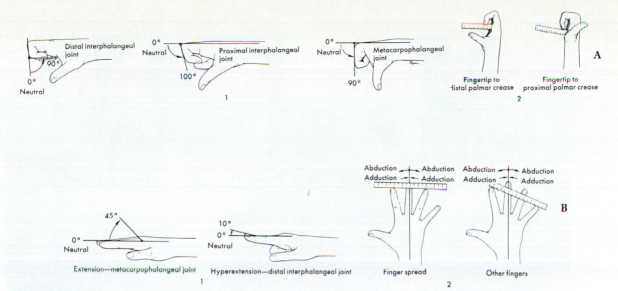

FIGURE 22-24

ROM of the fingers. **A**, Flexion. *1*, Motion can be estimated or measured in degrees. *2*, Motion can be estimated by a ruler as the distance from the tip of the finger to the distal palmar crease *(left)* (measures flexion of the middle and distal joints) and the proximal palmar crease *(right)* measures the distal, middle, and proximal joints of the fingers). **B**, Extension, abduction, and adduction. *1*, Extension and hyperextension. *2*, Abduction and adduction. These motions take place in the plane of the palm away from and to the long, or middle, finger of the hand. The spread of fingers can be measured from the tip of the index finger to the tip of the little finger *(right)*. Individual fingers spread from tip to tip of indicated fingers *(left)*.

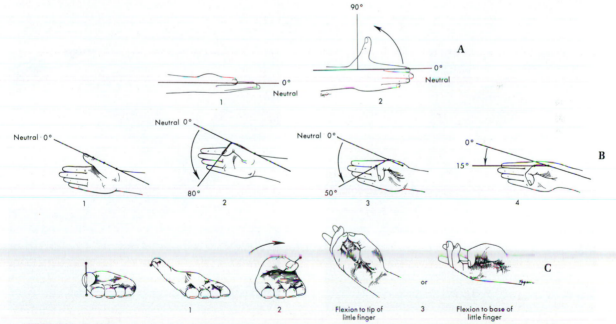

FIGURE 22-25

ROM of the thumb. **A**, Abduction. *1*, zero starting position: the extended thumb alongside the index finger, which is in line with the radius. *Abduction* is the angle created between the metacarpal bones of the thumb and index finger. This motion may take place in two planes. *2*, Radial abduction or *extension* takes place parallel to the plane of the palm. **B**, Flexion. *1*, Zero starting position: the extended thumb. *2*, Flexion of the interphalangeal joint: zero to ±80°. *3*, Flexion of the metacarpophalangeal joint: zero to ±50°. *4*, Flexion of the carpometacarpal joint: zero to ±15°. **C**, Opposition. Zero starting position *(far left)*: the thumb in line with the index fingers. *Opposition* is a composite motion consisting of three elements: (1) abduction; (2) rotation, and (3) flexion. Motion is usually considered complete when the tip of the thumb touches the tip of the fifth finger. Some consider the arc of opposition complete when the tip of the thumb touches the base of the fifth finger. Both methods are illustrated.

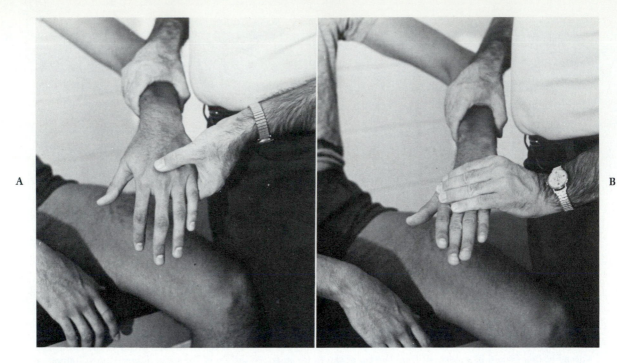

FIGURE 22-26
Applying manual resistance against wrist motion. **A**, Flexion and, **B**, extension.

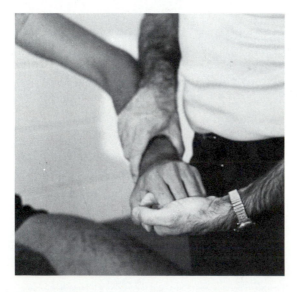

FIGURE 22-27
Applying manual resistance against flexion of the
fingers as a functional unit.

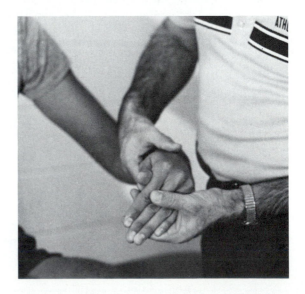

FIGURE 22-28
Applying manual resistance against flexion of the
metacarpophalangeal joints.

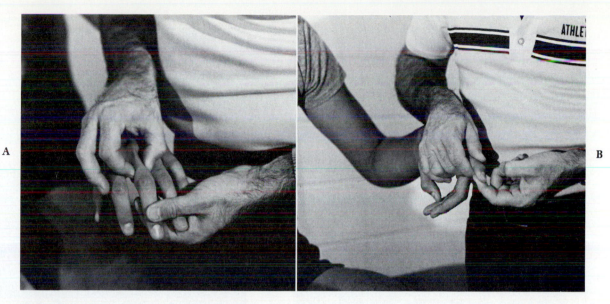

FIGURE 22-29
Applying manual resistance against flexion of an individual finger. **A**, Proximal interphalangeal
(PIP) joint and, **B**, distal interphalangeal (DIP) joint.

and apply resistance to movement against the palm of the athlete's hand with your other hand (Figure 22-26, *A*). Instruct the athlete to keep the muscles of the thumb and fingers relaxed to ensure they do not assist wrist flexion. To evaluate wrist extension, apply resistance against the dorsum of the athlete's hand (Figure 22-26, *B*). Again, the muscles of the thumb and fingers should remain relaxed. It is not necessary to resist radial and ulnar deviation because these muscles are evaluated during flexion or extension. However, specific muscles may be isolated and evaluated by adding radial or ulnar deviation to the resistance sequence. For example, to specifically test the flexor carpi radialis muscle, apply resistance in the direction of wrist flexion and radial deviation.

Finger flexion is often resisted as a functional unit. Instruct the athlete to flex all fingers into a fist as you curl and lock your fingers into his or hers and attempt to pull the fingers into extension (Figure 22-27). Can the athlete resist your attempt to straighten the fingers? Each joint can also be resisted separately. The motion at the metacarpophalangeal joints is resisted by

having the athlete flex these joints while keeping the interphalangeal joints extended as resistance is applied to the proximal row of phalanges (Figure 22-28). Resistance can be applied to each finger if strength appears to be unequal. Flexion of the proximal interphalangeal joints can be resisted by stabilizing the proximal phalanges and instructing the athlete to flex these joints while resistance is applied to the middle phalanges. The distal interphalangeal joints should remain extended. Flexion of the distal interphalangeal joints can be resisted by stabilizing the middle phalanges and asking the athlete to flex the tips of the fingers while resistance is applied to the distal phalanges. It may be easier to perform these last two resistive procedures on the fingers individually (Figure 22-29).

The muscles involved with finger extension can be resisted in the same manner as the flexors, that is, all at one time, each separate joint, or each individual finger. A quick and easy method to resist gross finger extension is to curl your fingers over the athlete's fist and instruct the athlete to extend the fingers as you apply resistance (Figure 22-30). Note any differences in strength or in-

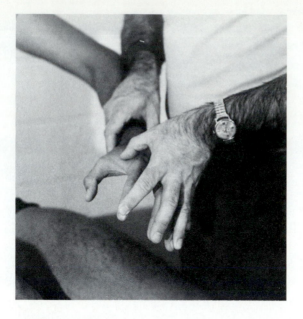

FIGURE 22-30
Applying manual resistance against extension of all the fingers.

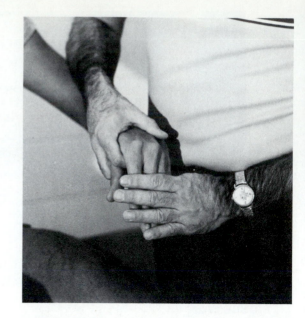

FIGURE 22-31
Applying manual resistance against extension of the metacarpophalangeal joints.

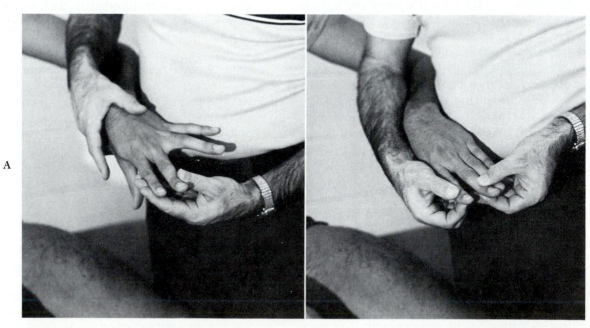

FIGURE 22-32
Applying manual resistance against, **A**, finger abduction and, **B**, finger adduction.

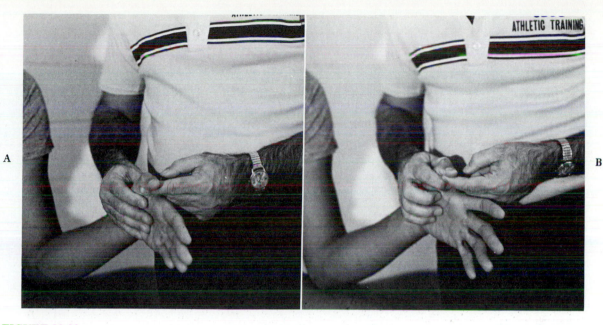

FIGURE 22-33
Applying manual resistance against thumb flexion. **A**, Metacarpophalangeal joint and, **B**, interphalangeal joint.

creases in pain. To resist MCP extension, stabilize the metacarpals and apply resistance against the proximal row of phalanges (Figure 22-31). Resistance can be applied in a similar manner to each individual joint.

To resist finger abduction, instruct the athlete to spread the fingers as far apart as possible. Resistance is then applied to the outside surfaces of those fingers being tested (Figure 22-32, A). To test finger adduction, instruct the athlete to keep the fingers together as you attempt to pull them apart (Figure 22-32, B).

Resistance is applied against thumb movement similar to those techniques used on the fingers. To test thumb flexion at the metacarpophalangeal joint, stabilize the first metacarpal and apply resistance to the volar surface of the proximal phalanx (Figure 22-33, A). To test the interphalangeal joint of the thumb, stabilize the proximal phalanx and resist flexion on the distal phalanx (Figure 22-33, B). Resisting thumb extension is performed in the same manner, with the resisting force applied on the dorsal surface of the thumb.

Thumb abduction is accomplished by sta-

bilizing the hand and wrist with your hand and applying resistance against the lateral border of the proximal phalanx of the thumb during abduction (Figure 22-34, A). Reverse your resistance to the medial border of the proximal phalanx and instruct the athlete to adduct the thumb to test thumb adduction. To test opposition of the thumb, instruct the athlete to touch the top of the little finger with the tip of the thumb. Resistance is then applied to the palmar surfaces of the thumb and little finger (Figure 22-34, B)

Passive movements. Passive movements are frequently used to facilitate the assessment of hand and wrist injuries. These include evaluating the bony integrity, assessing the integrity of the supporting ligaments, and performing passive ROM tests. The specific maneuvers used depend on the type of injury suspected or indicated up to this point in the assessment process.

When the signs and symptoms cause you to suspect a possible fracture in the hand or fingers, passive stress can be applied to each bone. Applying this type of passive stress can be extremely helpful in evaluating bony integrity. The metacarpals and phalanges

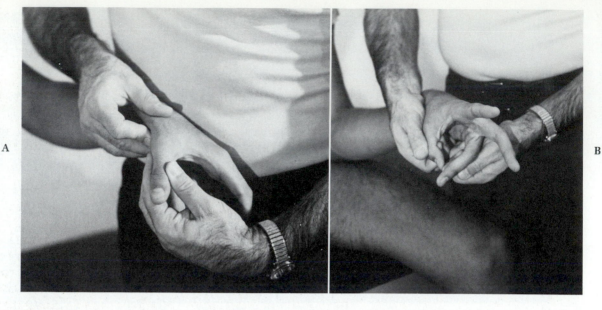

FIGURE 22-34
Applying manual resistance against thumb. **A**, Abduction and adduction and, **B**, opposition.

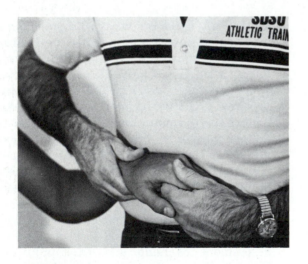

FIGURE 22-35
Applying passive longitudinal compression stress to evaluate the bony integrity of the second metacarpal.

are all long bones and mainly subcutaneous. Longitudinal stress can be applied, beginning very gently and then gradually increased depending on the athlete's tolerance. This stress is accomplished by applying force or pressure directly along the long axis of the bone being evaluated (Figure 22-35). If the bony integrity is intact, there should be no increase in pain. When the pain is located about a joint, this same longitudinal stress can be used to assess the bony integrity at the articulation. Stabilize both bones involved and apply longitudinal pressure directly along the long axis of the bones (Figure 22-36). Again, if the bony integrity is intact, there should be no increase in pain. If this longitudinal stress causes additional pain or crepitation at the original site of tenderness, the athlete should be treated as if there is a fracture.

Once the bony integrity is assured, the athletic trainer should evaluate the supporting ligaments. This is accomplished by applying transverse stress to those joints suspected of being injured. Again, begin very gently and increase pressure according to the athlete's tolerance. Stabilize the bones on either side of the injured joint and apply lateral, medial, or hyperextension stress to the articulation. For example, Figure 22-37 shows a method for testing the stability of the supporting ligaments around the proximal interphalangeal joint of the index finger. Note any increase in pain or instability with these passive maneuvers. Note in Fig-

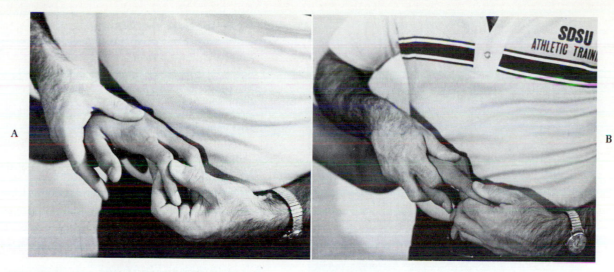

FIGURE 22-36
Applying passive longitudinal compression stress to evaluate the bony integrity of, **A**, metacarpophalangeal (MCP) joint and, **B**, proximal interphalangeal (PIP) joint.

ure 22-38 the instability of the index finger during passive transverse stress.

Passive ROM can also be used to evaluate the integrity of a joint. Whenever active ROM is limited or restricted in a joint or joints, passive motion may be implemented to evaluate the available range. As with all areas of the body, passive ROM must be performed gently and cautiously so no further damage results. All motions described under active movements can be evaluated passively.

Functional movements. Functional movements or activities can be beneficial to the comprehensive assessment of wrist and hand injuries. Often observing an athlete perform those activities that reproduce painful symptoms will be helpful. Observing such activities assists the athletic trainer in identifying the mechanism of injury and the anatomic structures that may be involved. However, for the most part, functional movements are used to determine when an athlete with a wrist or hand injury can return to full activity. As an athlete recovers from an injury to this area of the body, assessment of functional activity becomes increasingly important on each reevaluation. Can the athlete perform skills required of his or her sport effectively and without an increase

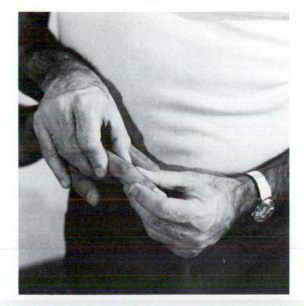

FIGURE 22-37
Applying passive transverse stress to evaluate the supporting ligaments around the proximal interphalangeal joint of the index finger.

in injury symptoms? The intensity of functional activities should be continually increased within tolerable levels until the athlete is functioning at or near optimum capacity.

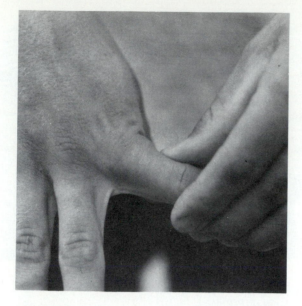

FIGURE 22-38
Subluxation of metacarpophalangeal joint of the index finger during transverse stress.

Neurological evaluations

Sensory functions. To evaluate sensations, remember the sensory distribution of each nerve. The radial nerve supplies sensation mainly to the radial side of the dorsum of the hand, and the median nerve supplies sensation to the radial side of the palm and fingers. The ulnar nerve supplies sensation mainly to the ulnar side of the hand, little finger, and half of the ring finger. The normal dermatome pattern of the hand is C6, which supplies sensation to the thumb and index finger, C7, which supplies the middle finger, and C8, which supplies the ring and little finger. Review these dermatomes in Figure 19-22. Run your relaxed fingers over these surfaces and note any differences in sensations when compared to the uninjured hand.

Motor functions. To evaluate motor function, it is again important to remember nerve distribution. The radial nerve supplies motor function to the extrinsic wrist and finger extensors (C6 to C8). The median nerve supplies the thenar muscles (C8, T1); its function is evaluated by resisting opposition or abduction of the thumb. The ulnar nerve provides motor supply to most of the intrinsic muscles of the hand (C8, T1), with the exception of the thenar muscles. Its function is easily evaluated by resisting finger abduction.

Circulatory evaluations

As previously discussed, circulation can be evaluated by feeling for a radial or ulnar pulse. The nail beds can be temporarily compressed to check the return of normal color.

Evaluation of Findings

Injuries involving the wrist and hand commonly occur in athletics. Most of these injuries occur because of direct trauma to the exposed area or overload forces associated with absorbing direct impacts. The many small bones and articulations may not be able to withstand the numerous and accumulative stresses that can be associated with all the various functions of the hand in athletic activity. Many athletic injuries to the hand and wrist are relatively minor and do not require extensive treatment. However, because even potentially serious injuries to this area of the body are usually not disabling to an athlete, there is a tendency to underestimate the severity and importance of injuries to the hand and wrist. If neglected or unrecognized, these injuries can develop into long-term impairment and possibly result in permanent disability and disfigurement. It is therefore important that athletic trainers not ignore injuries involving the hand and wrist and be able to accurately assess injuries to this important area of the body.

When to Refer the Athlete

Many hand and wrist injuries can be accurately evaluated and properly managed

Athletic Injury Assessment Checklist: Hand and wrist injuries

Secondary survey

_____ History
    _____ Primary complaint
    _____ Mechanism of injury
    _____ Pain
    _____ Previous injuries
_____ Observation
    _____ Obvious deformity
    _____ Positioning and functioning of injured hand
    _____ Signs of trauma
    _____ Symmetry comparison
    _____ Swelling
_____ Physical examination

Palpation

    _____ Tenderness
    _____ Deformity
    _____ Swelling
    _____ Crepitation

Movement procedures

_____ Active movements
    _____ ROM
    _____ Associated symptoms
_____ Resistive movements
    _____ Pain
    _____ Strength
_____ Passive movements
    _____ Bony integrity
    _____ Ligament instability
    _____ ROM
_____ Functional movements
    _____ Functional abilities

Neurological evaluations

    _____ Sensory function
    _____ Motor function

Circulatory evaluations

    _____ Pulses

without seeking additional medical assistance. However, these injuries also have the potential of resulting in dysfunction or permanent deformity. Hand and wrist injuries may require expert medical attention to avoid complications. Conditions or findings that can be used to determine if medical referral is indicated are listed in "When to Refer the Athlete . . ." box.

REFERENCES

Alexander AH, Lichtman DM: Kienbocks disease, *Orthop Clin North Am* 17(3):461, 1986.

Burton RI, Eaton RG: Common hand injuries in the athlete, *Orthop Clin North Am* 4:809, 1973.

Conwell HE: Injuries to the wrist, *CIBA Clinical Symposia* 22:1, 1970.

Drewniany JJ, Palmer AK: Injuries to the distal radioulnar joint, *Orthop Clin North Am* 17(3):451, 1986.

Flatt AE: *The care of minor hand injuries,* ed 4, St. Louis, 1979, Mosby.

Giachino AA: Injury to the scapholunate ligaments: avoiding sequelae in one type of wrist sprain, *Phys Sportsmed* 21(5):51, 1993.

Hoppenfeld S: *Physical examination of the spine and extremities,* New York, 1976, Appleton-Century-Crofts.

Knight B: DeQuervain's syndrome in golfers, *Sports Med Update* 5(2):12, 1990.

Lichtman DM, editor: The wrist, *Orthop Clin North Am* 15(2), 1984.

McCue FC, editor: Injuries to the elbow, forearm, and hand, *Clin Sports Med* 5(4), 1986.

McCue FC and others: Hand and wrist injuries in the athlete, *Am J Sports Med* 7:275, 1979.

O'Donoghue DH: *Treatment of injuries to athletes,* ed 4, Philadelphia, 1984, Saunders.

Rettig AC: Hand injuries in football players: getting a grip on fractures, *Phys Sportsmed* 19(11):55, 1991.

Rettig AC: Hand injuries in football players: soft-tissue trauma, *Phys Sportsmed* 19(12):97, 1991.

Riester JN and others: A review of scaphoid fracture healing in competitive athletes, *Am J Sports Med* 13(3):159, 1985.

Shea KG, Shumsky IB, Shea OF: Shifting into wrist pain: DeQuervain's disease and off-road mountain biking, *Phys Sportsmed* 19(9):59, 1991.

Simmons BP, Lovallo JL: Hand and wrist injuries in children, *Clin Sports Med* 7(3):495, 1988.

Tubiana R and others: *Examination of the hand and upper extremity,* Philadelphia, 1984, Saunders.

Wadsworth LT: How to manage skier's thumb, *Phys Sportsmed* 20(3):69, 1992.

SUGGESTED READINGS

Brunet ME and others: How I manage sprained finger in athletes, *Phys Sportsmed* 12(8):99, 1984.
Discusses aggressive, closed treatments for finger injuries that includes early management, intensive therapy, and protection during athletic participation.

Gelberman RH and others: Carpal tunnel syndrome, *Orthop Clin North Am* 19(1):115, 1988.
Reviews the four classifications of median nerve compression at the wrist, and discusses management approaches based on clinical findings.

Melchioda AM, Linburg RM: Volar plate injuries, *Phys Sportsmed* 10(1):77, 1982.
Discusses the functional anatomy of the PIP joint, mechanism of injury, treatment, possible complications, and rehabilitation.

Nicholas JA, Hershman EB, editors: *The upper extremity in sports medicine,* St. Louis, 1990, Mosby.
An excellent text by many contributors discussing the various upper extremity injuries and conditions.

Osterman AL and others: Soft-tissue injuries of the hand and wrist in racquet sports, *Clin Sports Med* 7(2):329, 1988.
Discusses various injuries that may occur to the hand and wrist as the result of racquet sports and the importance of prompt diagnosis.

Ruby LK: Common hand injuries in the athlete, *Orthop Clin North Am* 11(4):819, 1980.
Discusses the importance of recognizing and properly treating the injuries that commonly occur to the hand.

GLOSSARY

A

abdomen Body area between the diaphragm and pelvis

abduction Movement of a body part away from the midline of the body, 60

abduction stress test Passive procedure used to evaluate medial stability of the knee, 490

abrasion Break in skin continuity occurring when epidermis and a portion of dermis is scraped or rubbed away, 151

acetabular labrum Triangular ring of fibrocartilage attached to the rim of the acetabulum, increasing the depth of the cavity, 510

acetabulum Socket in the hip bone into which the head of the femur fits

acne vulgaris A chronic inflammatory disease of the sebaceous glands characterized by any combination of noninflamed comedones (blackheads and whiteheads) to inflammatory papules, pustules, and cysts, 162

Acquired Immune Deficiency Syndrome (AIDS) End stage of HIV infection. HIV cripples the immune system and leaves the body vulnerable to a variety of viral, bacterial, and parasitic diseases, 164

acromion Bony projection of the scapula, forming point of shoulder, 547

active movements Those movements that can be initiated and completed by the athlete without assistance of any kind

acute Of short duration, 127

acute traumatic injury Injury occurring instantaneously as a result of some type of trauma, 146

Page numbers are given for key terms in text.

adduction Movement of a body part toward the midline of the body, 60

adduction stress test Passive procedure used to evaluate lateral stability of the knee, 490

adhesions Fibrous bands that may connect or unite two adjacent surfaces or parts

adhesive capsulitis (frozen shoulder) Inflammation of the rotator cuff and capsular area, which develops because of immobility and results in loss of ROM, 562

Adson's maneuver Test used to evaluate for thoracic outlet syndrome. Feel the radial pulse as you passively extend and outwardly rotate the arm. If there is compression of the subclavian artery, you will feel a marked diminution or absence of the radial pulse, 585

adventitious bursae New bursae developed by our body in response to trauma or friction, 466

agonists (prime movers) Muscles whose contractions produce movement, 74

amenorrhea Absence or abnormal stoppage of the menses, 381

anorexia nervosa An eating disorder with symptoms of self-starvation, a refusal to maintain normal bodyweight, and an intense fear of gaining weight or becoming fat, 378

amphiarthroses Slightly movable joints having a pad of either hyaline or fibrocartilage located between adjoining bony surfaces

anaphylactic shock The most severe form of allergic reaction of the body to an allergen, something to which the athlete is extremely allergic, 128

657

anatomic position   Position in which the body is upright, the feet are parallel, and the palms of the hands face forward, 18

anatomic snuffbox   Surface landmark for the navicular bone. The radial border is formed by the abductor pollicis longus and the extensor pollicis brevis tendons, and the ulnar border is formed by the extensor pollicis longus tendon. These tendons become prominent when the thumb is extended, 626

anesthesia   Loss of feeling or sensation, 113

angiography   Radiographic study of the vascular system, using a contrast medium injected either intra-arterially *(arteriogram)* or intravenously *(venogram),* 207

annulus fibrosus   Circumferential portion of an intervertebral disc, composed of fibrocartilage and fibrous tissue, 207

anserine bursitis   Inflammation of the bursa between the pes anserine tendon insertion and the medial collateral ligament, 467

antagonists   Muscle or muscles that oppose action of other muscles or gravity, 74

anterior (ventral)   Front, 18

anterior drawer test (ankle)   Test to evaluate the integrity of the anterior talofibular ligament—with the athlete's ankle in a relaxed position, the athletic trainer stabilizes the leg with one hand and lifts anteriorly with the other while cupping the calcaneus, 452

anterior drawer test (knee)   Test to evaluate the anterior cruciate ligament—with hip flexed approximately 45° and the knee flexed 90°, the tibia is lifted anteriorly

anterograde amnesia   Loss of memory for events occurring immediately after awakening, 276

anterolateral rotatory instability   Instability represented by anterior displacement of the lateral tibial plateau with re-

spect to the femur during testing of the knee

anteromedial rotatory instability   Instability represented by anterior displacement of the medial tibial plateau with respect to the femur during testing of the knee

aphasia   Loss of speech or comprehension of spoken or written language, 277

Apley's compression test   Test to evaluate the integrity of the menisci—with the athlete lying prone and the injured knee flexed 90°, pressure is applied to the heel in an attempt to entrap a torn meniscus between the articular surfaces, 503

Apley's distraction test   Test to differentiate between a meniscal and ligamentous injury—with athlete lying prone and injured knee flexed 90°, pull up and rotate on the tibia in an attempt to distract the knee joint; in case of ligamentous injury, this maneuver should elicit pain, whereas if it is a meniscal injury, there should be no increase in pain, 504

Apley's scratch test   Method to evaluate active ROM of the shoulder by asking athlete to place hand behind the back and neck, 575

apnea   Temporary cessation of breathing, 225

apophysis   A bony projection or outgrowth, 427

apophysitis   Inflammation of an apophysis, 427

appendicitis   Inflammation of the appendix, 374

appendicular   Pertaining to the appendages of a structure; in the body this refers to the upper and lower extremities, 18

apprehension test   Test to evaluate possible subluxations—often used in the assessment of patellofemoral and glenohumeral integrity, 480

arcuate complex   An anatomic complex that consists of the arcuate ligament, the popliteal tendon, the lateral collateral ligament, and the posterior third of the capsular ligament of the knee, 494

areflexia Absence of a reflex, 245

arousal The extent of the physiological activation of the various organs of the body that are under control of the autonomic nervous system, 183

arthrography Radiographic study of joints using a contrast medium to outline the soft tissue structures; the resulting radiograph is called an *arthrogram,* 204

arthrology A specialized area of anatomy that deals with the study and description of joints or articulations, 50

arthroscopy Surgical procedure that allows the surgeon to view the interior of a joint through a series of small lenses with a fiberoptic light source, 220

articular Refers to a joint

articulation Joint

asthma Respiratory disease characterized by intermittent episodes of airway obstruction caused by bronchospasm, excessive bronchial secretion, or edema of bronchial mucosa, 367

ataxia Failure of muscular coordination or irregularity of muscular action, 272

athletic injury Disruption in tissue continuity that results from athletic activity and causes a cessation of participation or restriction of usual activity

athletic injury assessment Comprehensive evaluation of an athletic injury beginning when the injury occurs and continuing through the healing process until the injured area has been rehabilitated to its fullest extent, 196

athletic trainer Provider of athletic training services, which can be divided into six major functions: (1) prevention, (2) assessment, (3) management and treatment, (4) rehabilitation, (5) organization and administration, and (6) education and counseling, 4

athletic training Sports medicine subspecialty that provides a wide array of health care support services for athletes, 3

athlete's foot (tinea pedis) A very common skin infection characterized by redness, scaling, cracking, and itching of the skin of the feet, 162

atrophy Wasting away or deterioration of a tissue, organ, or part, 125

attentional focus The ability to concentrate on relevant information during competition while ignoring or "gating out" irrelevant information, 184

autonomic nervous system (ANS) Portion of the motor nervous system that controls the activities of smooth muscles, cardiac muscle, and certain glands, 89

avascular Without blood vessels, 54

avascular necrosis Death of cells or groups of cells as a result of loss of blood supply, 523

avulsion Tearing away of part of a structure, which may be torn completely free or remain partially attached, hanging as a flap, 154

avulsion fracture Fracture in which a piece of bone is pulled loose at the attachment of a tendon, ligament, or muscle, normally occurring with a sudden violent contraction or stress, 178

axial Pertaining to the axis of a structure; in the body this refers to the head, neck, and trunk, 18

B

Baker's cyst Swelling in popliteal space on the posterior part of the knee, 467

ballotable patella Palpatory procedure for evaluating marked effusion of the knee; when the patella is pressed down and released quickly, the large amount of fluid under it causes the knee cap to rebound or appear to be floating, 479

Barton fracture A fracture involving a rim of the articular surface of the distal radius, with an associated subluxation of the carpal bones, 629

baseball finger Deformity resulting from rupture of the extensor tendon slip at the point of its attachment into the base of the distal phalanx. Also known as *mallet finger*, 637

Battle's sign Discoloration appearing over the mastoid area, 259

Bennett fracture Fracture of the proximal end or base of the first metacarpal, often associated with subluxation of the carpometacarpal joint, 641

bicipital aponeurosis A strong expansion of the biceps tendon, which blends with the fascia over the flexor muscles of the forearm, 610

bioelectrical impedance Method of measuring body composition, designed to detect changes in electrical impedance between electrodes placed on the body, 17

blocker's spur Name given to an irritative exostosis that develops near the deltoid muscle insertion caused by repeated blows to the area; it is most frequently seen in football players, 556

blood pressure Pressure caused by blood exerting force on the walls of blood vessels, 261

boil (furuncle) Localized skin infection formed by staphylococci invading skin through sebaceous glands or hair follicles, 161

bone scan Nuclear imaging technique used to detect particular areas of abnormal metabolic activity within a bone, 214

boutonnière deformity Deformity that results from an injury to the central slip of the extensor tendon; the proximal interphalangeal joint is flexed, and the distal interphalangeal and metacarpophalangeal joints are in a hyperextended position, 638

boxer's fracture A fracture of the neck of the fifth metacarpal, 640

brachial Pertaining to the arm

brachial plexus Network of nerves found within the shoulder and axilla that innervate the lower part of the shoulder and all the arm, 104

bronchitis Inflammation of bronchial tubes and can be acute or chronic, 368

bulimia Eating disorder that includes episodes of binge eating followed by self-induced vomiting, use of laxatives or diuretics, strict dieting and fasting, or vigorous exercise to undo the effects of the binge episode and to prevent weight gain, 378

bunion (hallux valgus) An inflammation and thickening of the bursa of the metatarsophalangeal joint of the great toe, usually associated with abnormal enlargement of the joint and lateral displacement of the toe, 409

bunionette Bunionlike enlargement of the metatarsophalangeal joint of the little toe (also called a *tailor's bunion)*, 409

bursa Fluid-containing sac lined with synovial membrane, 466

bursitis Inflammation of a bursa, 466

C

calcaneal apophysitis, *(Sever's disease)* An inflammation of the bony projection at the attachment of the Achilles tendon in young, adolescent athletes, 427

carbuncle An extensive infection of several adjoining hair follicles that drains with multiple openings onto the skin's surface. A cluster of boils commonly seen on the back of the neck, upper back, and lateral thighs, 161

cardiogenic shock Shock caused by inadequate functioning of the heart, 128

carpal tunnel Passageway for the median nerve and flexor tendons, formed by the arched carpal bones, the transverse carpal, and the volar carpal ligaments, 626

carpal tunnel syndrome Symptoms resulting from constriction in carpal tunnel and pressure on median nerve, 630

carrying angle Angle formed by the axes of the arm and forearm when the elbow is extended, 606

cauda equina Latin equivalent for horse's tail; the lower spinal nerve roots descending in the spinal canal from their point of attachment to the spinal cord to the site of their emergence between the vertebrae, 318

cauliflower ear (hematoma auris) Repeated contusions and twisting or friction-type injuries to external ear that may result in a hematoma formation between skin and underlying cartilage, 300

cavities Depressions, openings, and grooves within bones, 31

cavus foot (pes cavus) Inflexible high-arched foot that does not adequately absorb shock or easily adapt to various surfaces, 405

celiac Pertaining to the abdomen

celiac plexus (solar plexus) Largest of the abdominal plexuses, it supplies the viscera in the abdominal cavity and lies in the upper middle region of the abdomen

celiac plexus syndrome Most common intraabdominal injury is a blow to the celiac plexus (solar plexus), commonly known as having "wind knocked out", 373

cellulitis An inflammation of the dermis and subcutaneous tissue that is usually caused by a bacteria (group A streptococcus and *Staphylococcus aureus*), 162

centering The process of bringing one's focus of attention on an important task-relevant cue or suggestion, 192

central nervous system (CNS) Brain and spinal cord, 89

cerebellum Second largest portion of brain occupying the most inferior and posterior aspect of the cranial cavity, 99

cerebrum Largest and most superficial area of the brain, 98

cervical lordosis Increased concavity in the curvature of the cervical spine, 339

cervical plexus Network of nerves found deep in the neck and innervating the muscles and skin of the neck, upper shoulders, and part of the head, 104

charley horse Term usually restricted to injuries of the quadriceps muscle group caused by a contusion, or possibly a strain producing soreness and stiffness, 519

chicken pox (varicella) A mild, highly contagious viral infection marked by an eruption of vesicles on the skin and mucous membranes. It is characterized by a rash that begins on the trunk and spreads to the face and extremities, 164

chondral fracture Break involving the articular cartilage, 54

chondrocytes Cartilage cells, 54

chondromalacia patellae Degenerative process that results in a softening or degeneration of the articular surface of the patella, 472

chondrosternal separation Injury to or separation of the cartilage between the ribs and the sternum, 365

chronic Of long duration, 127

chronic overuse syndrome Athletic injury resulting from forces or stresses applied to a structure or tissues over a considerable period of time, 146

circumduction Composite movement that combines flexion, abduction, extension, and adduction in which the body segment describes a cone, 62

closed fracture Fracture that does not break the skin, 177

closed kinematic chain Distal end of the extremity is fixed and motion at one joint will cause predictable movement in adjacent joints, 58

chlamydia A genus of microorganisms that are intracellular parasites that cause a wide variety of diseases in man. Chlamydia trachomatis causes genital infections in males and females and is the most common sexually transmitted pathogen, 383

coccidioidomycosis   A disease caused by infection of the lungs by a fungus (*Coccidioides immitis*), 369

cognitive state anxiety (cognitive A-state)   A state which is characterized by worry, fear, apprehension, and self-doubt. It is always accompanied by heightened levels of physiological arousal, 184

colitis   An inflammation of the colon, 376

collagen   Main supportive protein in skin, tendon, bone, cartilage, and connective tissue, 123

Colles' fracture   Fracture of the distal end of the radius in which the fragment is displaced dorsally, 629

coma   State of unconsciousness from which the athlete cannot be aroused, even by powerful stimulus

comminuted fracture   Break in which three or more bone fragments are produced, 178

compartment syndromes   Conditions in which increased tissue pressure compromises the circulation of the muscles and nerves within one of the osseofascial compartments; these may be acute or chronic in nature, 430

competitive trait anxiety (competitive A-trait)   A feature of personality that can be described as a predisposition to perceive competitive situations as threatening and to respond with heightened levels of state anxiety (A-state), 184

compression fracture   Impacted break characterized by crushed bone tissue such as to the body of a vertebra, 179

computed tomography (CT scan)   Sophisticated procedure using computerized radiographic equipment to get a three-dimensional image of the area, 207

concentric contraction   Muscle shortens during contraction, 73

concussion   Syndrome involving immediate and transient impairment in the ability of the brain to function properly, 276

condyle   Rounded projection at the end of a bone

conduction   Process of transfer by direct contact, 131

conjunctivitis   An inflammation or infection of the conjunctiva, 310

consensual light reflex   Similar reaction of both pupils to a light stimulus applied to only one eye, 286

constipation   An infrequent or difficult evacuation of the feces, 376

contact dermatitis   An acute inflammatory reaction of the skin resulting from direct contact with a substance to which the skin is sensitive, 160

contralateral   Pertaining to the opposite side, 18

contrecoup (counterblow)   Injury resulting from a blow on the opposite side, such as an intracranial injury, 275

contrecoup fracture   Break of the skull at a distance away from the point of impact

contusion (bruise)   Skin or soft tissue injury that usually results from a direct blow or impact delivered to some area of the body, 167

convection   Transfer of heat from one place to another by motion or circulation, 131

corn   A localized hardening and thickening of the skin produced by friction and pressure. The most common location is over the dorsal aspect of the proximal interphalangeal joint of the fifth toe. A corn has a conical shaped core extending into the dermis, causing pain and irritation

corneal abrasion   Abrasion on the corneal surface, 307

corneal laceration Cut or laceration on the eyeball, 309

coronal (frontal) plane Runs from side to side and divides the body into front and back, 19

coryza Nasal mucous discharge, 367

costal Pertaining to the ribs

costochondral separation A separation or actual dislocation at the articulation between the rib and its cartilage, 365

cranial nerves Twelve pairs of nerves which arise from the undersurface of the brain, 99

crepitation Grating, grinding, or sticking sensations that may be produced by various conditions, 240

crossover maneuver Actively or passively bringing the abducted arm across the front of the body, compressing the acromioclavicular joint. The presence of superior pain or discomfort may confirm an injury to this joint, 584

cubital Pertaining to the forearm

cubital tunnel syndrome Ulnar nerve becomes irritated, compressed, or entrapped in the cubital tunnel due to repetitive throwing or swinging activities, 604

cubitus valgus Increase in the carrying angle of the elbow, 607

cubitus varus Decrease in the carrying angle of the elbow, 607

cyanosis Bluish discoloration of skin caused by poor oxygenation of the circulating blood, 259

D

decerebrate rigidity Postural attitude characterized by extension of all four extremities, 260

decorticate rigidity Postural attitude characterized by extension of the legs and marked flexion of the elbows, wrists, and fingers, 260

deep Away from the body surface, 18

deep fascia Sheet of fibrous connective tissue investing the trunk, limbs, and various muscles, 70

deep frostbite Freezing of the entire tissue depth, including muscles and bone, 143

delayed union fracture Fracture that has not united successfully within expected period of time although the healing process continues, 180

dens Conical pivot process that projects from the superior surface of the axis, 56

dental caries Tooth decay or cavities and is the most frequent cause for pain originating from the teeth, 303

depression Return of movement from an elevated position, 62

depressed fracture Fracture in which part of a flat bone, such as the skull or cheek bone, is depressed inward or below the surface, 179

de Quervain's disease Tenosynovitis of the tendons of the abductor pollicis longus and extensor pollicis brevis as they pass through a fibro-osseous tunnel at the level of the radial styloid, 628

dermatitis Inflammation of the skin evidenced by itching, redness, and various skin lesions, 160

dermatome Segment or strip of skin supplied by a given spinal nerve, 104

dermis Inner and thicker layer of the skin, 147

detached retina A condition in which the inner layers of the retina are separated from the pigment layer

deviated septum An angulation or variation in the partition separating the two nasal cavities, 295

diabetes mellitus A disorder of carbohydrate and fat metabolism that is due to an absolute or relative lack of insulin, 377

diabetic coma A slowly developing condition caused by an increase in blood sugar levels and the loss of body fluids. Individual may become listless, dehydrated, breathe rapid and deep, have a weak and rapid pulse, and have a sweet or fruity odor on their breath. Without treatment the individual will eventually become unresponsive and comatose. This individual needs medical attention and insulin, 377

diapedesis Movement or migration of blood or its elements through the intact vessel wall, 121

diaphysis Long shaftlike portion of the bone, 27

diarrhea A condition of abnormally frequent and liquid bowel movements, 376

diarthroses Freely movable joints, often called synovial joints

diastolic blood pressure Force with which blood is pushing against the artery walls when ventricles are relaxed, 262

diplopia Double vision, 286

discography Radiographic study of the spine using a contrast medium injected into an intervertebral disc; the resulting radiograph is called a *discogram,* 206

discoid meniscus A round or disk shaped meniscus found in a small percent of the population, 470

dislocation Luxation or displacement of contiguous surfaces of bones comprising a joint, 174

dislocation of the peroneal tendons Dislocation or subluxation of the peroneal tendons as they pass in a groove posterior to the fibula beneath the superior peroneal retinaculum

displaced fracture Fracture in which a bone fragment is out of normal alignment, 180

distal Farther from the point of attachment of an extremity to the trunk or the point of origin of a part, 18

distended Inflated, swollen, or stretched

dorsal Posterior; pertaining to back, 18

dorsiflexion Movement of the top of the foot upward, 60

drop arm test Test that evaluates the status of the supraspinatus tendon. Athlete abducts the arm past 90° and then slowly lowers it to the side. A positive test is indicated if the athlete is unable to return the arm to the side slowly or has pain when attempting the movement, 576

duodenal ulcer An ulcer in the duodenum next to the stomach, 376

dura mater Outermost layer of the meninges, 273

dysmenorrhea Painful menstruation, 381

dysphagia Difficulty in swallowing, 357

dyspnea Difficult or labored breathing, 226

dysuria Sensation of pain, burning, or itching while urinating, 381

E

eccentric (negative) contraction Muscle is exerting tension but is being lengthened by some outside force or by gravity, 73

ecchymosis Discharge or escape of blood into the tissues under the skin (black & blue mark), 147

echocardiography Technique that uses echoes or reflected high-frequency sound waves to visualize the heart, 214

ectomorph Type of body build in which there is a relative predominance of linearity over fat and muscle, 12

eczema A common inflammatory skin disease caused by contact with an allergen and can vary from moderate to intense. Eczema develops with a bright red swollen plaque and pebbly surface that may develop into vesicles and blisters, 166

edema Accumulation of excessive amounts of body fluids in the tissue spaces, 121

electrocardiography Study of electrical activity of the heart; the graphic recording is called an *electrocardiogram* (ECG or EKG), 214

electromyography Study of electrical potentials generated in muscles; the graphic recording is called an *electromyogram* (EMG), 220

electroencephalography Study of electrical currents developed by the brain; the graphic recording is called an *electroencephalogram* (EEG), 214

elevation Upward movement, 62

empty can position The arm is horizontally abducted 30 degrees with the arm internally rotated and the thumb pointing downward. Used to test the supraspinatus muscle, 576

endomorph Type of body build in which there is a relative predominance of roundness and softness of the body, 12

endomysium Connective tissue between individual muscle fibers, 69

endosteum Fibrous membrane that lines the marrow cavity of long bones, 28

epicondylitis Chronic strains occurring in the region of the medial and/or lateral epicondyles of the humerus, 600

epidermis Outer and thinner layer of the skin, 147

epidural hematoma Hematoma outside the dura, 277

epilepsy Disorder of the brain characterized by a tendency for recurrent seizures, 251

epimysium Connective tissue sheath that envelops a skeletal muscle, 69

epiphyseal fracture Break at the growth plate of long bones that occurs in growing children, because this is the weakest link along the bone, 525

epiphyseal (growth) plate Thin plate of cartilage separating the diaphysis from each epiphysis in growing bones, 28

epiphyses Extremities, or ends, of long bones, 27

epistaxis (nosebleed) Hemorrhage from the nose, 296

evaporation To dissipate in the form of vapor, 132

eversion Sole of the foot is turned outward, 62

exercise-induced asthma (EIA) Exercise can provoke the symptoms of asthma or bronchospasms, 368

exostosis Bony growth projecting outward from the surface of a bone, 169

exposed injury Athletic injuries or conditions that disrupt the continuity of the skin, 147

extension Return from the flexed position, 60

external rotational recurvatum test Test for posterolateral rotatory instability in which both legs are held extended by the heels; a positive test results in the tibia showing excessive hyperextension and external rotation, 500

extravasate Process of escaping or passing out of a vessel into the tissues, 120

extrinsic muscles Long flexor and extensor muscles that take origin within the forearm or leg and are entirely tendinous in the hand or foot

exudate Fluid that has escaped from a tissue or its vessels, 121

F

fascia Sheet of connective tissue

fasciculi Groups of individual muscle fibers bound into discrete bundles, 69

felon (whitlow) Painful infection located in the soft tissues surrounding the terminal phalanx of a finger, 637

fibroblast Connective tissue cells that form collagen fibers, 123

fibroplasia Production of fibrous tissue, 123

fibroplastic phase Initial phase of the healing process in which fibrous tissue is produced

Finkelstein's test Used to evaluate *de Quervain's disease*. Instruct the athlete to make a fist with the thumb inside the fingers and ulnarly deviate the wrist. A positive test is indicated by pain over the affected tendons, 628

fissure Groove

fixators Muscles that fix or stabilize joints to assist prime movers, 75

flexion Decreasing the size of the angle between the anterior or posterior surfaces of articulated bones, 60

folliculitis A common infection of the hair follicles, which can be caused by a staphylococci, chemical irritation, or physical injury, 161

footdrop A condition in which the foot hangs in a plantar flexed position because of a lesion of the peroneal nerve

forefoot Area of the foot composed of the metatarsals and phalanges, 411

forward head Deviation from normal alignment in which the head is carried in an abnormal anterior position, 339

forward shoulders Deviation from normal alignment in which shoulders are carried in an abnormal forward position, 339

fossa Cavity or hollow

fracture Disruption in the continuity of bone,

fracture-dislocation Fracture near a joint that occurs simultaneously with a dislocation, 180

frostbite Localized freezing of a part of the body, 142

frostnip Initial stage of frostbite involving only the surface of the skin, 143

functional movements Series of active movements or activities performed by the athlete that simulates the type of activity required in a particular sport

furunculosis A self-limiting infection in which one or several furuncles are present, 161

G

gamekeeper's thumb Sprain of the ulnar collateral ligament of the metacarpophalangeal joint of the thumb. Also called *skier's thumb*, 639

ganglion Cluster of nerve cell bodies outside the central nervous system, 628

gaster Central fleshy or "meaty" contractile portion of a muscle, 68

gastritis An inflammation of the lining of the stomach, 376

gastroenteritis An inflammation of the stomach and intestines. It is usually of viral or bacterial origin and a very common cause of vomiting, 376

genu Pertaining to the knee

genu recurvatum (knee hyperextension) Angulation of leg is posterior, or backward, from midline of the body, 477

genu valgus (knock knees) Angulation of lower leg is away from the midline of the body, 477

genu varum (bowlegs) Angulation of lower leg is toward the midline of the body, 477

gingivitis Inflammation of gingiva, 304

glenohumeral translation test Applying anterior and posterior force to the humeral head in an attempt to recognize the degree of glenohumeral translation. Translation up to 50% of the humeral head diameter is considered normal

glycosuria Glucose escapes into the urine, 377

gomphosis Type of synarthrotic joint in which a conical peg or projection fits into a socket

goniometer Instrument used to objectively measure ROM. Consists of two rigid shafts connected by a hinge joint, with a protractor fixed to one shaft to accurately read the ROM in degrees, 58

gonorrhea Commonly called the *clap,* caused by the gonococcal bacteria and is normally spread through sexual intercourse, 383

grand mal seizure Classic type of seizure in which the person will fall down and display uncontrollable jerking or shaking movements of the extremities, 251

graphesthesia The ability to recognize numbers or letters written on the skin, 113

gravity stress test Passive test using gravity and the weight of the hand and forearm to stress the medial side of the elbow; place the athlete supine, externally rotate the shoulder, and flex the elbow approximately 20° (weights can be added to increase the stress), 616

greenstick fracture Incomplete break of a long bone that occurs in adolescent athletes whose bones are still pliable; a common example would be a greenstick fracture of the clavicle in children, 179

gunstock deformity (cubitus varus) Decrease in carrying angle of arm, 607

H

hammertoe Toe permanently flexed at midphalangeal joint, resulting in clawlike appearance, 409

Hawkins-Kennedy Impingement Test Forcibly rotate the proximal humerus inwardly when the arm is flexed 90°, 581

hay fever An allergic rhinitis, occurring in sensitive individuals in a seasonal pattern depending on the allergens involved (pollen for example), 295

healing by first intention Primary union by fibrous adhesions without the formation of infection and pus

healing by second intention Secondary union accompanied by infection and delayed healing

heat acclimation Process of becoming accustomed to athletic activity in hot weather, 133

heat cramps Painful muscle spasms resulting from a fluid volume problem, 134

heat exhaustion Heat stress condition characterized by profuse sweating, which makes the skin cool and clammy, 135

heatstroke (sunstroke) Heat stress condition characterized by lack of sweating, resulting in hot dry skin and a rising body temperature, 136

heel spur Bony projection at the plantar aspect of the calcaneal tuberosity, which may accompany or result from severe cases of plantar fasciitis, 411

hemarthrosis Accumulation of blood in joint cavity

hematemesis Vomiting of blood, 367

hematoma Accumulation of extravasated blood that becomes organized into a localized mass, 120

hematoma auris (cauliflower ear) End result of keloid formation between the skin and underlying cartilage of an injured external ear, 300

hematuria Blood in the urine, 375

hemorrhoids (piles) A condition in which the veins at the lower end of the rectum become varicose (swollen) and enlarged, 376

hemopneumothorax Presence of both blood and air in the pleural cavity, 366

hemopoiesis Process of blood cell formation

hemoptysis Coughing up blood or blood-stained sputum, 367

hemorrhage Internal or external bleeding

hemothorax Blood in pleural cavity, 366

hepatitis Inflammation of the liver, 377

hernia Protrusion of abdominal viscera through portion of abdominal wall, 373

herpes simplex This is commonly called a fever blister or cold sore and is an acute infection of the mucous membranes and skin by herpes virus Type 1, 163

herpes zoster (shingles) A viral infection that almost always affects the skin of a single dermatome, 164

hindfoot Area of the foot composed of the calcaneus and talus, including the ankle joint

hip pointer Contusion to the crest of the ilium

history procedures Process of finding out as much information as possible about the injury itself and the circumstances surrounding its occurrence

hives (urticaria) A localized eruption of itchy wheals, caused by some type of allergen, such as foods, drugs, plants, or physical stimulation, 166

horizontal abduction Movement of the upper limb through the transverse plane at shoulder level away from the midline of the body, 60

horizontal adduction Movement of the upper limb through the transverse plane at shoulder level toward the midline of the body, 60

hyaline (articular) cartilage Thin layer of gristle-like material firmly fixed to the layer of compact bone covering the joint surfaces of the epiphyses, 28

hydrocele Fluid in the tunica vaginalis which is the membrane covering the front and sides of the testis and epididymis, 382

hyperesthesia Abnormal increase in sensitivity to pain, touch, or other sensory stimuli, 113

hyperextension Continuation of extension beyond the anatomic position, 60

hyperglycemia Blood sugar levels rise above normal, 377

hyperhidrosis Excessive sweating or perspiration, 149

hyperreflexia Exaggeration of a reflex (increased amplitude of a muscle contraction to an evoked reflex), 245

hypertension High blood pressure, 263

hyperventilation Overbreathing or very rapid deep breathing, resulting in abnormally lowered carbon dioxide levels in the blood, 226

hyphema Hemorrhage into anterior chamber of eye, 310

hypoesthesia Abnormal decrease in sensitivity to pain, touch, or other sensory stimuli, 113

hypoglycemia Insufficient sugar in the blood, 378

hyporeflexia Weakening of a reflex (decreased amplitude of a muscle contraction to an evoked reflex), 245

hypothenar eminence Prominence at the base of the little finger containing the intrinsic muscles involved in moving the little finger

hypothermia Systemic condition in which the core temperature falls below 95° F (35° C), 142

hypotonia Condition of abnormally diminished tone, tension, or activity, 272

hypovolemic shock Shock caused by the loss of body fluids or blood. Dehydration due to diarrhea, vomiting, or heavy perspiration can lead to its development. When caused by blood loss, this type of shock is called *hemorrhagic shock,* 128

hypoxia Inadequate or reduced oxygen content, 121

I

iliotibial band or tract Strong lateral portion of the deep fascia of the thigh that is the insertion of the tensor fascia latae muscle, 466

iliotibial band friction syndrome Inflammatory process that develops over the lateral femoral condyle during repetitive activity

impacted cerumen A firmly lodged accumulation of earwax in the external auditory canal, 299

impacted fracture Fracture in which one fragment of bone has been driven into and embedded in another fragment, 179

impetigo A highly contagious bacterial (streptococcal or staphylococcal) inflammation of the skin. It is characterized by the appearance of small vesicles that form pustules and eventually honey-colored, weeping crustations, 161

impingement sign Passively bringing the arm into complete flexion, driving the greater tuberosity against the anteroinferior surface of the acromion which will compress the irritated tissues and is frequently positive in impingement syndrome, 581

impingement syndrome Chronic conditions or injuries involving the soft tissues comprising the subacromial space, 558

incision Open wound caused by cutting the skin with a sharp object, such as a knife, 152

inferior Away from the head; lower, 18

infectious mononucleosis A condition due to an infection, most probably a virus, occurring between the ages of 10 and 35 years of age, that is spread by intimate oral contact and may be transmitted by asymptomatic individuals after a symptomatic or asymptomatic infection, 368

inflammation Basic response of vascularized tissues to an injurious agent, whether the source is physical, bacterial, thermal, or chemical, 120

influenza (flu) A viral bronchitis due to influenza viruses A or B, 367

infrapatellar bursitis Inflammation of one of the two infrapatellar bursae. The *superficial infrapatellar bursa* lies between the proximal patellar tendon and the skin, and the *deep infrapatellar bursa* lies between the distal patellar tendon and the tibia, 466

ingrown toenail Occurs when the skin of the nail fold receives pressure from the nail edge, causing inflammation and pain, 410

inguinal Of the groin

insertion More movable end of a muscle attachment, 68

insulin shock Seen in an individual who has taken too much insulin, not enough food, or has exercised too much and used up all available glucose. In this situation, not enough sugar remains in the blood to provide the continuous supply needed for the brain. Develops quickly and individual needs sugar immediately, 378

intertrigo A red, macerated, half moon-shaped plaque occurring in skin folds. The most common area is in the groin area where moisture accumulates in the crural folds, 163

intervertebral disc herniation Condition in which the nucleus pulposus herniates through the annulus fibrosus and presses against the spinal cord or the spinal nerve roots

intracerebral hematoma Hematoma within the cerebrum, 277

intrinsic muscles All musculotendinous units contained within the hand or foot

inversion Sole of the foot turned inward, 62

ipsilateral Pertaining to the same side, 18

ischemia Local anemia; temporary lack of blood supply to an area, 430

isometric Muscle contraction that produces no change in length of muscle, 74

isotonic Muscle contraction that produces movement at a joint, 73

J

jerk test Test for anterolateral rotatory instability in which the knee is flexed to 90°, the tibia is internally rotated, and a valgus stress is applied to the knee; if positive, as the knee is passively extended, the lateral tibial plateau will audibly and palpably sublux at approximately 30° to 40° and relocate as it approaches complete extension, 497

jersey finger Rupture or avulsion of the flexor digitorum profundus tendon from its attachment to the distal phalanx, 638

jock itch (tinea cruris) A fungal infection that affects the groin area. The infection usually starts near the crural folds and becomes fan-shaped as it spreads peripherally in the medial thighs, 162

joint capsule Tough but flexible sleeve-like structure that encloses the space that exists between opposing bone surfaces of a synovial joint, 52

joint effusion The accumulation of fluid in a joint cavity, 467

Jones fracture Fracture to the base of the fifth metatarsal distal to the tuberosity, 415

jumper's knee (patellar tendinitis) Inflammatory response to repeated stress or irritation at the patellar tendon insertion, 472

K

Kehr's sign Referred pain to the left shoulder and upper arm resulting from an injury to the spleen, 374

keloid New growth or tumor of the skin consisting of whitish ridges, nodules, and plates of dense tissue, 300

keratitis An inflammation or infection of the cornea, 310

ketoacidosis Acid waste products in the blood, 377

Kienbock's disease Slow progressive avascular necrosis of the carpal lunate bone resulting from a circulatory disturbance, 629

kinematic chain In our extremities, the series of bones connected by joints to form a linkage system, 58

knocked-down shoulder Separation of the acromioclavicular joint resulting in obvious deformity, with the clavicle displaced upward and the acromion remaining down, 559

kyphosis Increased convexity in the curvature of the thoracic spine, 339

L

laceration Open wound or cut made by tearing the skin, which usually results from some type of direct blow to the skin; lacerations are especially common over bony prominences, 152

Lachman's test Passive procedure used to evaluate anterior and posterior stability with the knee flexed 10° to 15°

lacunae Small cavity or space in cartilage or bone, 54

laryngitis Inflammation or irritation of the larynx indicated by hoarseness, dryness, soreness, and difficulty in swallowing, 357

larynx (voice box) Anatomic structure between the root of the tongue and the upper end of the trachea, 355

Lasègue's test Following a straight leg raising with radicular symptoms, drop the leg down slightly until there is no pain or discomfort and dorsiflex the foot. This places additional pull on the sciatic nerve trunk and increased pain indicates possible sciatic nerve involvement, 349

lateral Away from the midline of the body, 18

lateral pivot shift test Test for anterolateral rotatory instability that begins with the leg extended, the tibia internally rotated, and a valgus stress at the knee; as the knee is passively flexed, the lateral tibial plateau subluxes immediately and relocates again at approximately 30° to 40° if the test is positive, 497

lethargic   Condition of drowsiness, 280

lever   Mechanical device consisting of a bone (force arm), fulcrum (joint), weight arm (resistance), and force or effort movement (muscle contraction)—*first-class lever,* lever system in which the fulcrum lies between the effort and resistance; *second-class lever,* lever system in which the resistance lies between a long force and a short weight arm; *third-class lever,* lever system in which the effort is exerted between the fulcrum and resistance, 66

life stress   An increase in stress brought about by certain life events. Such events can be perceived to be positive (e.g., birth of a child, marriage, purchasing a house), or negative (e.g., divorce, death of a loved one, losing a job), 183

ligament   Band of fibrous tissue that connects bone to bone,

locomotion   Movement of the body as a whole,

locus of control   A psychological construct pertaining to one's belief that he or she can control what happens to her or him, 184

lumbar lordosis   Increased concavity in the curvature of the lumbar spine, 339

lumbar puncture   Piercing of the subarachnoid space in the lumbar region, usually between the third and fourth lumbar vertebrae, for the purpose of withdrawing cerebrospinal fluid, 326

lumbosacral plexus   Nerve network formed by intermingling of fibers from both the lumbar and sacral plexuses, 104

luxatio erecta   Inferior dislocation of the shoulder in which the arm stands straight above the head, 561

luxation   Complete dislocation, 174

M

magnetic resonance imaging   A noninvasive and highly accurate method of diagnosing a broad spectrum of musculoskeletal disorders. Involves placing the body part in a strong magnetic field, which causes the various protons to spin about their axis and emit energy. These signals can be detected by a receiver and interpreted by a computer that distinguishes among the variations and represents them as a spatial arrangement of a spectrum of white, grey, and black—known as *MRI,* 211

Maisonneuve fracture   A severe eversion and external rotation injury of the ankle resulting in a deltoid ligament injury, with an intact tibiofibular syndesmosis causing an associated fracture of the proximal shaft of the fibula, 432

malleolus   Projection at the distal end of the tibia and fibula

mallet finger (dropped finger)   Deformity resulting from rupture of the extensor tendon slip at the point of its attachment into the base of the distal phalanx. Also known as *baseball finger,* 637

malunion   Fracture that has united with faulty alignment of the fragments, 180

manual muscle testing   Subjective grading of muscle strength by applying resistance against active movements, 242

manubrium   Upper part of the sternum

march fracture   Stress fracture of one of the metatarsals; this name caught on during World War II when many soldiers unaccustomed to being on their feet received fatigue fractures after walking long distances, 415

margination   Accumulation of white blood cells on the inner surface of blood vessels near the site of an injury, 121

marrow (medullary) cavity   Tubelike hollow in the diaphysis of long bones, 28

maturation phase   Final phase of the repair process, in which the newly formed fibrous connective tissue matures and becomes stronger

McMurray test   Test to evaluate the integrity of the menisci; the athlete's hip and knee are flexed maximally, and as the leg is passively extended the tibia is rotated, and valgus or varus force is applied to the knee, 500

measles (rubeola) A highly contagious viral disease transmitted by respiratory droplets. It typically has an incubation period of 10 to 14 days and lasts from 7 to 14 days. Symptoms begin much like the common cold, followed by cutaneous eruptions of small, irregular, bright red spots with bluish-white centers. These eruptions begin to fade in 2 to 3 days and are gone in 1 to 2 weeks

mechanism of injury Manner and location by which excess forces or stresses are applied to the body, resulting in athletic injuries, 146

medial Toward the midline of the body, 18

medial-lateral grind test Test used to evaluate possible meniscal injury. With the athlete supine, a circular motion is produced at the knee by applying valgus and varus stresses as the knee is passively flexed to 45° and extended. A torn meniscus may produce a grinding sensation, as well as joint line pain, 50

mediastinum Central portion of chest cavity containing the heart, its great vessels, part of the esophagus, and part of the trachea

meninges Three membranes surrounding the brain and spinal cord

meningitis An inflammation of the membranes (meninges) of the spinal cord or brain, 318

menisci Crescent-shaped discs of fibrocartilage, 55

mesomorph Type of body build in which there is a relative predominance of muscle, bone, and connective tissue, 12

metabolic shock Shock associated with a profound fluid loss from an uncontrolled disease such as diabetes mellitus. Other possible causes could be diarrhea, vomiting, and excessive urination, 128

metabolism Chemical process by which energy is produced, 131

metatarsalgia Pain or tenderness beneath the metatarsal head, more commonly the second and occasionally the third

metatarsus Consists of the five metatarsal bones, 400

midfoot Area of the foot composed of the navicular, cuboid, and three cuneiform bones

Morton's foot Characterized by a short first metatarsal and a longer second metatarsal, 406

Morton's neuroma (plantar neuroma) Swelling of one of the digital nerves, which is squeezed or pinched between the metatarsal heads; the nerve between the third and fourth metatarsal heads is involved most often, 409

motorneuron Nerve fiber that transmits nerve impulses away from the brain or spinal cord (to a muscle), 71

motor unit One neuron plus the muscle fibers it innervates, 71

mumps An inflammation of the parotid glands which lie just beneath each ear. This is a contagious disease caused by a virus, 357

Murphy's sign Sign evident on a dislocation of the lunate; the third metacarpal moves proximally so that it is on a level with adjoining knuckles and does not project distally to them, 629

myelography Radiographic study of the spinal cord and canal, using a contrast medium injected into the spinal canal; the resulting radiograph is called a *myelogram,* 206

myology Study of muscles, 65

myositis ossificans Formation of bone within or around a muscle (commonly called a calcium deposit), 169

myotome Muscle or group of muscles supplied by the ventral or motor root fibers from a specific spinal nerve, 104

N

necrosis Death of one or more cells, or of a portion of tissue or organ, 120

neurapraxia The cessation of function of a nerve without degenerative changes occurring, 324

neurogenic shock Shock caused by a failure of the nervous system to control the size and muscular tone of the blood vessels. This type of shock may be seen with spinal injuries, 129

neurology Study of the nervous system

neuroma A tumor or mass growing from a nerve and normally consisting of nerve fibers, 409

neuromuscular junction (motor end-plate) Area of contact between a nerve and muscle fiber, 71

Noble compression test Procedure to evaluate for an *iliotibial band friction syndrome*. With the knee flexed 90°, apply pressure with your thumb to the lateral femoral epicondyle, and maintain pressure as the athlete slowly extends the knee. A positive test is indicated if the athlete expresses pain as the iliotibial band slides over the epicondyle at about 30° of flexion

nociceptors Pain receptors. Those located in the skin and mucosa are stimulated by any kind of intense stimuli. Those in the viscera are stimulated only by marked changes in pressure and by certain chemicals, 91

nondisplaced fracture Fracture in which pieces of bone lie in relatively normal alignment; occasionally this type of break may be difficult to see on X-ray films, 180

nonunion Failure of the ends of a fracture to unite, 180

nuclear imaging Radiographic study using short-term radioactive substances injected into the body and recorded on a scanner, 214

nucleus pulposus Semifluid mass of fine white and elastic fibers that forms the central portion of an intervertebral disc, 316

nystagmus Involuntary rapid movement of the eyeball, 283

O

Ober's test Used to assess for iliotibial band tightness. With the athlete sidelying, passively abduct and extend athlete's upper leg and slowly lower limb. If there is any iliotibial band tightness or shortening, the hip will remain abducted, 485

oblique fracture Fracture in which the break line crosses the bone at an oblique angle to its long axis

observation procedures Process that involves the recognition, notice, and inspection of an injured area and the circumstances associated with its occurrence

olecranon Proximal bony projection of the ulna at the elbow

olecranon bursitis Inflammation of the olecranon bursa, 598

olfactory Pertaining to the sense of smell

oligomenorrhea Abnormally infrequent or scanty menstruation, 381

open fracture Fracture associated with a break in the skin, 177

open kinematic chain Distal end of the extremity is not fixed allowing a joint to function independently without necessarily causing motion at another joint, 58

open wound Wound in which the skin is broken, 150

optimum angle of pull Right angle to the long axis of a bone to which a muscle is attached, 66

origin More fixed end of a muscle attachment, 68

Osgood-Schlatter syndrome Condition involving the epiphysis of the tibial tuberosity in adolescents

osteitis pubis An inflammation of the pubic bones in the region of the symphysis, 524

osteochondral fracture Break involving the articular cartilage and underlying bone

osteochondritis dissecans Condition of unknown cause in which a segment of subchondral bone undergoes avascular necrosis,

osteology Study of bones

otitis externa (swimmer's ear) Common infection of the external ear in swimmers, 301

otitis media Infection of the middle ear, 301

otorrhea Discharge from the ear, 259

overriding fracture Fracture in which bony fragments overlap, resulting in shortening of the bone, 180

P

painful arc Pain caused by tender tissue being squeezed as a joint passes midpoint during the ROM, 574

pallor Paleness or absence of skin coloration, 258

palmar (volar) plate Fibrocartilaginous structure that covers the flexor aspect of the metacarpophalangeal and proximal interphalangeal joints

palpation Examination by touch, 237

pancreatitis An inflammation of the pancreas which can be mild and lead to vague abdominal symptoms, or severe, presenting with intense pain often referred to as an "acute abdomen," 377

paralysis Loss or impairment of motor function, 332

paraplegia Paralysis of the lower extremities, 332

paresis Slight or incomplete paralysis, 332

paresthesia An abnormal sensation such as burning, itching, or prickling, 91

paronychia Acute infection involving the subepithelial folds of tissue surrounding a fingernail, 637

passive movements Procedures performed entirely by the athletic trainer

patella femoral grinding test Test to evaluate the integrity of the underside of the knee cap; the patella is pushed manually against the femoral condyles, and the athlete is asked to contract the quadriceps as pressure is maintained,

pectoral Pertaining to the chest or breast, 360

pedal pulse Foot pulse

pediculosis An infestation with lice, 164

peptic ulcer An ulcer of the stomach, 376

pericoronitis Inflammation and swelling of the gingiva due to the eruption of the third molars or "wisdom teeth", 305

periodontal membrane Fibrous membrane located between the root of a tooth and its socket, 52

periodontitis Continuing inflammation of the gingiva where there is ultimately loss of alveolar bone, 304

perimysium Connective tissue between bundles of muscle fibers, 69

periorbital contusion Black eye, 310

periosteum Dense fibrous membrane covering the outer surface of long bones except at the joint surfaces, 28

peripheral Pertaining to the outward surface

peripheral nervous system (PNS) Nervous structures which lie outside of the central nervous system (CNS), 89

peritonitis An intense, painful, inflammatory reaction to the peritoneum, 374

peritoneum   Membrane that lines the abdominal cavity, 371

peroneal nerve contusion   A direct blow to the peroneal nerve as it passes just below the head of the fibula and can result in a contusion and injure the nerve, 473

pes cavus   A high longitudinal arch, 405

pes planus (flatfoot)   Static structural abnormality in which the relative position of the foot bones have been altered, resulting in a lowering of the longitudinal arch, 404

petechiae   Small, nonelevated, pinpoint, purplish or red discolorations resulting from localized hemorrhage into the skin or mucous membranes, 147

phagocytosis   Ingesting and disposing of unwanted substances such as elements of a hematoma, 122

Phalen's test   Athlete flexes both wrists maximally and holds for at least one minute. Tingling or numbness over the palmar surface of the hand and fingers is indicative of *carpal tunnel syndrome*

pharyngitis   Inflammation of the pharynx or throat, indicated by pain on swallowing, dryness, burning, and hoarseness, 357

pharynx   Throat

physical examination   The third phase of the secondary survey, which involves the selective use of a variety of assessment procedures and maneuvers designed to further locate and evaluate the integrity of the structures involved in the injury

physis (epiphyseal plate)   The segment of bone concerned mainly with growth, 416

pia mater   Vascular innermost covering (meninges) of the brain or spinal cord, 273

piano key sign   High-riding clavicle resulting from a third-degree sprain of the acromioclavicular joint; it can be pushed down but will spring back up when pressure is released, similar to a piano key, 559

pigment labile   Area of the body that may show abnormal changes in skin color, 258

piriformis syndrome   A condition of tension pain in the pelvic floor, with possible involvement of the sciatic nerve, 523

pityriasis rosea   A common, self-limiting skin eruption of young adults. It is of unknown etiology and appears as round-to-oval patches most frequently on the trunk or proximal extremities, 166

plain-film radiography   Procedure that uses no contrast material to enhance the various structures of the body; these are the most common types of radiographic procedures used in sports medicine, 202

plantar   Pertaining to the sole of the foot

plantar aponeurosis   Strong band of fibrous connective tissue originating on the calcaneal tuberosity and inserting near the metatarsal heads, which acts as one of the primary supports for the longitudinal arch; also called *plantar fascia*

plantar fasciitis   Overuse syndrome that involves an inflammatory reaction at the insertion of the plantar fascia or aponeurosis into the calcaneus, 411

plantar flexion   Movement of the sole of the foot downward, 60

plantar warts (verruca plantaris)   Plantar warts develop on the sole of the foot and may cause pain and disability, especially if they are located on a weight-bearing surface, 164

pleura   Double membrane sac; the outer layer lines the chest wall and the inner layer covers the outside of the lungs, 363

plexus   Network, 104

plica   Remnants of embryonic tissue that appear in the knee as folds or plications in the joint lining

plica syndrome   These normally thin, elastic, pliable tissues may become inflamed and edematous, making them inelastic, which can progress to thickening or fibrosis of the plica, 469

pneumocephalus   Presence of air in the intracranial cavity, 295

pneumonia   An inflammation of the lower respiratory tract that involves the airways of the lungs, 369

pneumothorax   Air in pleural cavity, 366

polyuria   Increased secretion of urine, 377

popliteal   Behind the knee

popliteal cyst   A swelling in the popliteal space on the posterior part of the knee, also called *Baker's cyst*

popliteus tendinitis   Inflammation of the popliteus tendon caused by running, especially down hills, 462

post-concussion syndrome   Consists of headache (especially with exertion), dizziness, fatigue, irritability, and impaired memory and concentration. These symptoms may persist for days or weeks and indicate altered brain functioning, 277

posterior (dorsal)   Back, 18

posterior drawer test (knee)   Test to evaluate the posterior cruciate ligament. With hip flexed approximately 45° and the knee flexed 90°, the tibia is pushed posteriorly, 494

posterolateral rotatory instability   Instability represented when the lateral tibial plateau displaces backward in relation to the lateral femoral condyle

posture   Position or attitude of the body

Pott's fracture   Fracture of the lower fibula that involves the tibial articulation and usually a chipping off of a portion of the medial malleolus or a rupture of the deltoid ligament; also called *Dupuytren's fracture,* 432

Preiser's disease   Avascular necrosis of the carpal navicular (scaphoid) caused by trauma or a fracture that has not been kept immobilized, 629

prepatellar bursitis   Inflammation of the prepatellar bursa, which lies between the front of the patella and the skin, 466

prickly heat   An inflammation of noncontagious eruptions of red pimples, with intense inching and tingling around the sweat ducts, usually seen in hot weather, 150

primary injury   Initial insult or injury resulting directly from the trauma, 120

primary lesions   Lesions that appear initially in response to some changes in the internal or external environment of the skin, 157

primary survey   Portion of the athletic injury assessment process concerned with evaluation of the basic life support mechanisms of airway, breathing, and circulation, 223

processes   Prominences and projections on bones, 31

pronated foot   Flexible foot that exhibits excessive pronation, which is a combination of dorsiflexion, eversion, and abduction at the subtalar joint, 404

pronation   Palms-downward position, 62

pronator teres syndrome   The median nerve becomes entrapped or compressed as it crosses the anterior elbow and passes between the two heads of the pronator teres muscle, 604

protraction   Motion moving a body part forward, 62

proximal   Nearer the point of attachment of an extremity to the trunk or the point of origin of a part, 18

psoriasis   A chronic disease that fluctuates in intensity and occurs as sharply demarcated erythematous plaques with a dry, silvery scale, 166

psychogenic shock   Shock caused by a sudden, temporary dilation of the blood vessels to the brain, causing the individual to faint. This is also known as *syncope,* 129

pulse   Alternate expansion and contraction of arterial walls as the heart pumps blood, 260

pump bump A bony growth in the area of the posterior calcaneal tuberosity, which is the attachment of the Achilles tendon. These bumps usually result from local irritation caused by rigid, poorly-fitting heel counters, 428

puncture wound Open lesion occurring as a result of direct penetration of the skin with a pointed object, 154

pupillary reflex Contraction of the pupil on exposure of the retina to light, 258

Q

Q angle Angle formed by the intersection of a line from the anterior superior iliac spine to the midpatella and another line from midpatella to the tibial tuberosity; an angle of 15° or less is considered normal

quadriparesis Partial or incomplete quadriplegia, 324

quadriplegia Paralysis of all four extremities, 332

R

racoon eyes Discoloration around the eyes indicative of a skull fracture, 259

radial flexion Movement at the wrist of the thumb side of the hand toward the forearm

radial tunnel syndrome The radial nerve becomes entrapped, especially during activities requiring repetitive pronation and supination of the forearm, 604

radiation Process of emitting radiant energy in the form of waves, 131

receptors Specialized sensory components of the nervous system that generate nerve impulses, 91

referred pain Pain felt in a part of the body other than where the source or cause of the pain is located, 374

reflex Involuntary action, 95

reflex arc The nervous routes traveled in a reflex arc. An impulse travels inward over an afferent nerve to a nerve center, and the response then travels outward over an efferent nerve, 94

rehabilitation After an injury, restoration of optimum form and function in the shortest possible time, 8

relocation test A test for instability of the glenohumeral joint. When pain and apprehension is increased by an anterior force applied to the humeral head during external rotation and abduction of the shoulder, a posterior translation force is applied to note any differences

resistive movements Resistance applied against active movements

retraction Return of a protracted body part, 64

retrocalcaneal bursitis Inflammation of the retrocalcaneal bursa, which is located between the Achilles tendon insertion and the calcaneus

retrograde amnesia Loss of memory for events leading up to the injury, 276

rhinitis An inflammation of the mucosa of the nasal cavity commonly caused by a viral infection, as in the common cold or flu, 295

rhinorrhea Discharge from the nose, 259

ringworm (tinea corporis) Generally involves the upper extremities and trunk and is characterized by reddened, ringlike areas that may be scaly or crusted, 163

Romberg's sign Sign elicited by having the athlete stand with his or her feet together, arms at the side, and eyes closed; normally a person can stand still in this position, 285

rotated fracture Fracture in which one of the bony fragments has rotated in relation to the other, 180

rotation Pivoting of a body part on its own central or longitudinal axis, 60

rotator cuff Group of four muscles whose tendons surround and attach about the head of humerus and are primarily responsible for the integrity of the shoulder joint, that is, maintaining the head of the humerus within the glenoid cavity, 549

rotatory instabilities (knee) Abnormal anteroposterior movements combined with inward or outward rotation of the tibia, 258

rubor Redness of the skin, 258

runner's nipple A term given to an irritating and sometimes painful condition caused by the nipple rubbing against a shirt or uniform top, 364

S

sacralization Fusion of the fifth lumbar vertebra to the first segment of the sacrum, 327

sagittal plane Plane that runs from front to back and divides the body into right and left, 19

sarcomere Contractile unit of muscle tissue, 72

scabies A contagious disease caused by a mite, which is characterized by extreme nocturnal itching and elevated burrows, 166

sciatica Pain along the course of the sciatic nerve, with possible associated paresthesia of the thigh and leg and atrophy of calf muscles, 327

scoliosis Lateral curvature or deviation of the spine, 337

sebaceous cyst A cyst filled with sebaceous material from a distended sebaceous gland, 149

second impact syndrome. Occurs when an athlete sustains a second head injury before symptoms associated with a previous injury have cleared, 278

secondary injury Additional responses or damage occurring secondary to the primary injury, 120

secondary lesion Lesion that does not appear initially but results from a primary lesion, 157

secondary survey Portion of the athletic injury assessment process that examines the athlete in an attempt to recognize and evaluate all athletic injuries and conditions; it consists of an ordered sequence of procedures used to assess the nature, site, and severity of an athletic injury, 157

self-concept Refers to the hierarchy or organization of all of the beliefs, attributes, and opinions that a person believes to be true about him or herself, 185

self-esteem How the individual feels about who and what they are. The degree to which an individual feels positive about herself or himself, 185

septal hematoma Blood trapped in the space between the septum and mucous membrane of the nose, 297

septic shock A type of shock almost always associated with some form of serious illness and is caused by severe infection. Toxins are released into the bloodstream and cause blood vessels to dilate, 129

shin splints Catch-all term for chronic pain and discomfort in the leg, generally limited to musculotendinous involvement

shock State of collapse or depression of the cardiovascular system

shoulder pointer Contusion to the tip of the shoulder or over acromion process, 556

shoulder separation Sprain of the acromioclavicular joint, 559

sickle cell anemia A hereditary, genetically-determined, sometimes fatal disease that is characterized by an abnormal type of hemoglobin, 377

sign Objective evidence of an injury, something the athletic trainer can see, hear, or feel, 201

silver-fork deformity Particular deformity associated with a Colles' fracture in which the distal fragment of the radius is displaced dorsally, 629

Sinding-Larsen-Johansson disease Resembles Osgood-Schlatter disease except that the pathology involves the proximal rather than the distal end of the patellar tendon, 473

sinus tarsi Concavity just in front of the lateral malleolus, 436

sinusitis An inflammation of the mucous lining of the sinuses, 296

skier's thumb A sprain of the ulnar collateral ligament of the metacarpophalangeal joint of the thumb. Also known as a *gamekeeper's thumb,* 639

Slocum test Test for anterolateral rotatory instability similar to the pivot shift test except the athlete is placed on his or her uninjured side, 497

Smith's fracture Fracture of the distal end of the radius in which the fragment is displaced forward; also called *reversed Colles' fracture,* 629

snapping hip Chronic trochanteric bursitis with thickening of the bursal walls, causing an audible and palpable snap as the tensor fascia lata slides back and forth over the greater trochanter, 521

SOAP note A common format for writing notes used for documentation. The acronym stands for subjective, objective, assessment, and plan, 229

soft corn Thickening of the epidermis between toes caused by pressure between two prominent phalangeal condyles. This type is kept softened by moisture and maceration, and often leads to painful inflammation beneath the corn, 409

somatic state anxiety (somatic A-state) The physiological component of state anxiety. Conceptually equivalent to the idea of arousal, 184

somatotype Particular category of body build, determined on the basis of certain morphologic traits, 11

somatotyping System of objectively classifying body build or physique, 11

spina bifida occulta Defect in the bony spinal canal without involvement of the spinal cord or meninges, 329

spinal cord concussion The spinal cord is concussed, which may cause transitory paralysis and symptoms, but complete recovery is usual, 324

spinal cord contusion The spinal cord is compressed, which can cause edematous swelling within the cord, resulting in various degrees of temporary or permanent damage, 324

spinal cord transection The spinal cord is cut across the long axis, 324

spiral fracture Fracture in which the break twists around and through the bone, caused by a twisting injury, 180

spondylitis Inflammation of vertebrae, 329

spondylolisthesis Forward displacement or slippage of one vertebra on another, usually occurring between L_4 and L_5 or L_5 and the sacrum, 328

spondylolysis Defect in the pars interarticularis or that part of the vertebra between the superior and inferior articular processes, 328

spondylosis Refers to degenerative changes of the vertebrae and can include bony (osteophyte) formation at the disc spaces, 329

spontaneous pneumothorax Pneumothorax occurring without apparent cause, 366

sports medicine Multifaceted term encompassing all phases of medical concerns as they relate to the biomechanical, psychological, nutritional, environmental, pathological, and physiological nature of the athlete, 3

sprain Athletic injury involving a ligament, 172

squinting patellae Patellae that appear to face inward when the feet are pointed straight ahead, 477

status epilepticus Successive seizures occurring within a short period of time, 251

stereognosis Ability to identify familiar objects by the sense of touch, 113

stone bruise Persistent contusion on the plantar aspect of the foot; also called a *heel bruise* when located under the calcaneus, 410

strain Athletic injury involving the musculotendinous unit, 171

strangulated hernia Herniated portion of viscera that has become incarcerated or tightly constricted and is likely to become gangrenous, 373

stress fracture Incomplete break in a bone occurring after prolonged repetitive activity, 177

stress procedures Involves the use of manipulative techniques to locate and define the structures involved in the injury, 240

stress radiograph Radiographic procedure performed while stress is being applied to the joint; may be performed with the athlete under anesthesia, 202

stuporous Partial or nearly complete unconsciousness, 250

sty Inflammation of one or more of the sebaceous glands of the eye lid, 305

subconjunctival hemorrhage (red eye) Rupture of the tiny blood vessels in the conjunctiva, 305

subcutaneous Beneath the skin; usually refers to the fatty and connective tissue layer found beneath the dermis

subdeltoid bursitis Inflammation of the subdeltoid bursa, 558

subdural hematoma Hematoma beneath the dura, 277

subluxation Incomplete dislocation, 174

substrate phase Initial phase of the acute inflammatory response characterized by localized vascular changes, 120

sulcus sign Pulling down the relaxed arm and noting inferior migration of the humeral head. If there is a "hollowing out" just distal to the acromion, this is a positive test for inferior instability of the shoulder, 584

subungual hematoma Accumulation of blood under the fingernail

superficial Near the surface, 18

superficial fascia Sheet of fibrous connective tissue just below the skin, 70

superficial frostbite Freezing of the skin and subcutaneous tissue, 143

superior Toward the head end of the body, 18

supination Palms-upward position, 62

supine Lying on the back

supracondylar fracture Fracture proximal to the growth plate of the humerus, 602

sustentaculum tali Medially projecting ledge on the upper surface of the calcaneus; it is the largest articular facet for the talus, 399

suture Type of synarthrotic joint united into rigid, immovable joints by a series of jagged, interlocking processes, 30

swimmer's shoulder Overuse syndrome associated with repetitive swimming. The most significant symptom is pain about the shoulder and is usually associated with the impingement process, 558

symphysis Type of amphiarthrotic joint in which a pad of fibrocartilage joins one bone to another, 52

symptom Subjective evidence of an injury or something the athlete relates, 201

synapse Joining; point of contact between adjacent neurons, 95

synarthroses Immovable joints

synchondrosis Type of amphiarthrotic joint in which a pad of hyaline cartilage joins one bone to another

syncope Fainting, 129

syndesmosis Type of synarthrotic (fibrous) joint characterized by the presence of a dense fibrous membrane that binds the articular surfaces together

syndesmosis ankle sprain This injury occurs as the tibia and fibula are forced apart, most often by forced dorsiflexion, injuring the ligaments that bind these bones together

synergists Muscles that assist prime movers, 74

synovial joint Diarthrotic or freely movable joint, 52

synovitis An inflammation of the synovial membrane, 467

syphilis A sexually transmitted disease caused by the spirochete, *Treponema pallidum,* which is a slender, spiral, parasitic microorganism, 383

systolic blood pressure Force with which the blood is pushing against the artery walls when the ventricles are contracting, 262

T

talotibial exostoses Bone spurs developing about the foot and ankle secondary to direct trauma, avulsion of ligaments, chronic synovitis, and fractures

tarry stool Blood in the fecal discharge from the bowels, 374

tarsal tunnel syndrome An entrapment of the posterior tibial nerve within the tarsal tunnel, 410

tarsus Collective term used to describe the seven bones that constitute the mid- and rear foot: talus, calcaneus, navicular, cuboid, and the three cuneiforms, 399

temporomandibular joint dysfunction Pain and limitation of jaw movement, which can occur as a result of trauma to the mouth, chin, or side of the head, 294

tendon Band or cord of fibrous connective tissue that attaches a muscle to a bone or other structure, 69

tendon reflex An involuntary contraction of a muscle in response to a brisk tap on its tendon, 245

tension pneumothorax Condition in which air continues to be drawn into the pleural cavity and cannot escape; pressure continues to rise on the affected side, pushing the collapsed lung against the heart and unaffected lung, 366

tetanic contraction A sustained and steady muscle response produced by a series of stimuli, 73

tetanus An acute infection disease due to a toxin growing at the site of injury. Characterized by severe uncontrolled skeletal muscle spasms. Normally begins with stiffness of the jaw, esophageal muscles, and muscles of the neck. The jaw can become rigidly fixed (*lockjaw*), 73

thenar eminence Prominence at the base of the thumb, containing the intrinsic muscles involved in moving the thumb, 83, 632

thigh compartment syndrome A rare but limb-threatening condition that can result when an athlete sustains a serious thigh contusion to one of the three major compartments in the thigh, 521

Thomas test Evaluating tightness in hip flexor muscles by having the athlete pull one thigh up against the chest. The opposite leg should remain on the table. Compare both legs, 345

Thompson test Test to indicate the integrity of the Achilles tendon. With the athlete lying prone, legs extended, and feet hanging over the table, each calf muscle is squeezed, and normally, the foot will react by plantar flexing; if the Achilles tendon is ruptured, there will be no movement of the foot, 358

thoracic cavity Body cavity above the diaphragm, 358

thoracic outlet syndrome Group of symptoms resulting from compression of the thoracic neurovascular bundle, which includes the brachial plexus and subclavian artery and vein, 563

thorax Chest, 354

thought stoppage The act of stopping a negative thought and replacing it with a success-oriented positive thought, 192

tibial stress syndrome A recurrent discomfort along the medial border of the middle and distal tibia caused by a stress reaction of the fascia, periosteum, and/or bone along the posteromedial aspect of the tibia, 429

Tinel's sign This test consists of tapping over the site of a nerve. A positive sign is indicated by a tingling sensation along the distribution of the nerve distal to the compression, 630

tinnitus Ringing in the ears, 276

tomography Radiographic technique using a specialized computer to give a view of one particular area of tissue at any depth; the resulting radiograph is called a *tomogram,* 204

tonsillitis An inflammation of the tonsils, which are small almond-shaped masses located in the back of the throat and composed mainly of lymphoid tissue, 357

tooth abscess Dental decay which progresses to form a pocket of pus

tooth extrusion A tooth that in protruding or extending outward more than normal, 304

tooth intrusion A tooth that in projecting inward or upward more than normal, 304

torticollis (wryneck) Contracted state of the cervical muscles, producing an unnatural position of the head, 338

trachea Windpipe

transverse (horizontal) plane Crosswise section that divides the body into upper and lower portions, 19

transverse fracture Fracture in which the break is across the bone at a right angle to its long axis and is often caused by a direct blow, 180

trauma Injury

Trendelenburg (abductor) gait An exaggerated shift of the trunk towards the stance leg in an attempt to maintain the center of gravity closer to the base of support, 528

Trendelenburg sign The pelvis on the unsupported side drops, indicating a weak gluteus medius muscle or an unstable hip on the stance side, 528

Trendelenburg test To assess the ability of the hip abductors to stabilize the pelvis on the femur, ask the athlete to stand on one leg. Normally the pelvis on the opposite side should rise slightly, 527

triceps surae Name given to the gastrocnemius and soleus muscles, which share the same tendon of insertion, 399

trochlea Pulley-shaped surface of the talus that articulates with the tibia and fibula

turf toe Sprain of the metatarsophalangeal joint of the great toe, normally caused by extreme dorsiflexion or plantar flexion, 411

twitch contraction A quick, jerky muscle response to a stimulus, 72

U

ulcer A disintegration and necrosis of the mucous membrane of the gastrointestinal tract caused by the acid gastric juices

ulnar flexion Movement at the wrist of the little finger side of the hand toward the forearm

unconsciousness Unresponsiveness, or the inability to respond to any sensory stimuli, with the possible exception of those causing pain, 251

unexposed injury Internal athletic injury with no associated disruption or break in the continuity of the skin, 147

unhappy triad Classic knee injury described by O'Donoghue, is a sprain of the medial collateral and anterior cruciate ligaments and damage to medial meniscus, 465

urethritis An inflammation of the urethra, 383

urography Radiographic study of the urinary tract using a contrast medium injected intravenously; the resulting radiograph is called an *intravenous pyelogram* (IVP), 207

V

vaginitis Inflammation of the vagina, common and usually caused by a yeast or parasitic infection, 381

valgus Bent outward; denoting a deformity in which the angulation of the distal part is away from the midline of the body

Valsalva maneuver Increase of intrathoracic and intra-abdominal pressure by forcible exhalation against the closed glottis, 345

vaporization Conversion of a liquid or solid into a vapor, 131

varicocele Varicose condition of veins from testicle and epididymis forming a swelling that feels like "bag of worms", 382

varus Bent inward; denoting a deformity in which the angulation of the distal part is toward the midline of the body

vastus Wide, of great size

ventral Front or anterior, 18

vertigo Sensations of movements, 299

viscarious experience Experiencing an event through another individual. In athletics, a parent may re-live sports participation through their child. In a rehab setting, watching an individual rehabilitate an injury may give you confidence and motivation to rehabilitate your injury, 193

viscera Internal organs; usually refers to the abdominal organs, 354

vital signs Important indicators of the health status of an individual

volar Pertaining to the palm of the hand or the sole of the foot; palmar; plantar

Volkmann's ischemic contracture Condition that may develop after a severe injury in the region of the elbow and is caused by the loss of blood supply to the musculature of the forearm; this catastrophic complication is characterized by permanent flexion of the fingers and sometimes of the wrist, 603

W

wart (verruca vulgaris) Small tumor caused by a virus may appear anywhere on the skin. Characterized by small dark spots in the center and distinct border at which all skin lines end, 164

water warts (molluscum contagiosum) More contagious than warts, particularly in activities requiring direct body contact, such as wrestling; viral infections appear as small, skin-colored, dome-shaped papules, 164

wen Sebaceous cyst, 267

winged scapula Marked projection and upward tilt of the lower angle of the scapula

wristdrop Condition resulting from paralysis of the wrist extensor muscles

wrist ganglion Cystic enlargement or knotlike mass formed by the synovial herniation of a tendon sheath on the back of the wrist

X

xiphoid Inferior process of the sternum

Y

Yergason test Evaluates status of long head of biceps tendon; flex elbow at side of body as resistance is applied against elbow flexion and external rotation, 580

Z

zygoma bone Cheek bone, 36

Index

A

A bands, 70, 73
ABCs of life support, 223-227
Abdomen, 369-370, 371
  "acute," 377
  injuries and conditions of, 371-378, 384-394
  strains of, 371-372
Abdominal cavity, 371, 372
Abdominal muscles, 347-348, 372
Abdominal oblique muscle, external, 78
Abdominal reflexes, 114
Abdominal viscera, injuries to, 374
Abdominal wall, 370-373
  anterior, muscles moving, 77
Abdominopelvic quadrants, 19, 20, 22
Abdominopelvic regions, 19, 22
Abducens nerve, 100, 101, 286-287
Abduction, 60
  horizontal, 60
  scapular, 64
Abduction stress test of knee, 490, 491
Abductor digiti minimi muscle, 83, 87, 633, 634, 635
Abductor gait, 528
Abductor hallucis muscle, 87
Abductor pollicis brevis muscle, 83, 633, 634, 635
Abductor pollicis longus muscle, 594, 597
Abrasions, 151-152
  eye, 307-309
  facial, 291
  hand, 635-636
Abscess
  dental, 303
  septal, 297
Absorptiometry to assess body composition, 14
Accessory bones of foot, 401
Accessory nerve, 109
Accessory organs of skin, 149-150
Acclimation, heat, 133-134
Acetabular labrum, 510
Acetabular notch, 512
Acetabulum, 42, 47
Acetylcholine, 71, 97
Acetylcholine receptor sites, 72
Achilles reflex, 114, 351
Achilles tendinitis, 427
Achilles tendon, 85, 406, 408, 420-421
  curvature of, 424
  palpation of, 443, 444
  rupture of, 428
Achilles tendon reflex, test of, 453-454
Achilles tenosynovitis, 427
Acne vulgaris, 162
Acoustic nerve, 100, 101-102, 286
Acquired immune deficiency syndrome, 164-165
Acromioclavicular joint, 547-548, 569
Acromioclavicular ligament, 547
Acromioclavicular sprain, 558-559
Acromion, 547
Acromion process of scapula, 29, 31, 39, 78, 81
Active range of motion of injured extremity, 242
"Acute abdomen," 377
Adam's apple, 355, 356
Adduction, 60
  horizontal, 60
  scapular, 64
Adduction stress tests of knee, 490-493
Adductor brevis muscle, 84, 513, 516
Adductor gracilis muscle, 84
Adductor longus muscle, 84, 85, 513, 516
Adductor magnus muscle, 84, 85, 513, 516

Adductor pollicis muscle, 83, 633, 634, 635
Adhesive capsulitis, 562-563
Adson maneuver, 585
Adult-onset diabetes, 377
Adventitious bursae, 466
Afferent nerves, 89
Afferent neurons, 93
Agonists, 74
AIDS, 164-165
AIDS-related complex, 164
Airway, 224, 225-226
  inflammation of, 368
  of unconscious athlete, care of, 252
Ala, 295
Alert, 280
Alienation following injury, 189-190
Alignment
  of lower extremity, 421-423
  spinal, wall test to observe, 339, 340
Allergic rhinitis, 295
Alveoli, 363
Amenorrhea, 381
Amnesia, anterograde and retrograde, 276
Amphiarthroses, 50, 52
Amphiarthrotic joints, 50, 52
Anaphylactic shock, 128
Anatomic snuffbox, 626, 627
Anconeus muscle, 81, 594
Anemia, sickle cell, 377
Anesthesia, 113, 244
  following spinal injury, 332
Angiography, 207, 209
Angle
  carrying, of elbow, 606
  of pull, optimum, 66
  Q, 471, 477, 479
  sternal (Louis'), 358, 360
Angular movements, 60, 61
Ankle, 29, 406-407, 408; see also Foot and ankle
  dislocations of, 414
  fractures of, 415
  injured, support for, 126
  mechanics of, 423-425
  motion of, evaluation of, 445, 447
  palpation of, 437-445
  sprains of, 173, 412-413
    syndesmosis, 407, 413-414
  stress film of, 204
  stress radiographs of, 452
  traumatic injury to, 436
Annular ligament of elbow, 595
Annulus fibrosus, 316-317
Anorexia nervosa, 378, 379
Anserine bursitis, 467
Antagonists, 74
Antebrachial cutaneous nerve, 107, 108
Anterior, 18
Anterior commissure, 98
Anterior compartment, 417, 420
Anterior compartment muscles, evaluation of, 448
Anterior drawer test, 452, 453, 493, 496
Anterior instability of knee, tests for, 493-494
Anterior superior iliac spine, 29, 79, 85
Anterograde amnesia, 276
Anxiety, 184
  competitive trait, assessing, 187
Aphasia, 277, 282
Apley scratch test, 575-576
Apley's compression test, 503-504
Apley's distraction test, 504
Apnea, 225, 257
Aponeurosis, 69
  bicipital, 81, 610
  of epicranius muscle, 267-268
  palmar, 81
  plantar, 87, 410
    palpation of, 442, 443

Apophysis, 427
Apophysitis, 427, 525
  calcaneal, 427
Appendicitis, 374
Appendicular division of body, 18, 19
Appendicular skeleton, bones of, 31
Appendix, referred pain from, 374
"Apple-shape" fat distribution and risk of disease, 13-14
Apprehension test, 480, 482, 483
  for shoulder injuries, 584
Arachnoid membrane of meninges, 273
ARC; see AIDS-related complex
Arches of foot, 46, 47, 401-402, 412
Arcuate complex, 494
Areflexia, 245
Areola, 360
Arm; see also Upper extremity
  muscles moving, 80, 81
  upper, 320, 586
Arrector pili muscles, 149
Arteriogram, 207, 209
Artery; see specific artery
Arthrogram, 204
Arthrography, 204, 206
Arthrology, 23, 50-64
Arthroscopy, 220-222
Articular capsule, 511-512, 591-592
Articular cartilage, 28, 53, 54-55
Articular discs, 53, 54-55, 624
Articular facets, 321
Articular processes between vertebrae, 57
Articulation(s); see also Joint(s)
  carpometacarpal, 625
  costosternal, 37
  of femur, 44
  humeroradial, 589
  humeroulnar, 589
  interphalangeal, 632
  metacarpophalangeal, 631-632
  midcarpal, 624-625
  radiocarpal, 624
  radioulnar, 624
  between ribs and sternum, 53
  tibiofibular, distal, 51
Asthma, 367-368
Ataxia, 272
Ataxic breathing, 257
ATC; see Certified athletic trainer
Athlete, 187, 190
  unconscious, 250-265
Athlete's foot, 162
Athletic footwear and overuse syndromes of lower extremity, 435-436
Athletic injuries; see specific injury(ies)
Athletic Life Event Scale, 187
Athletic trainer, 4, 5-10
  AIDS guidelines for, 165
  protection of, from athlete's body fluids, 150-151
Athletic training, 3-10
Athletic-related trauma, 116-193
Atlantoaxial joint, 56, 322
  rotation of, 62
Atlantooccipital joint, 56, 322
Atlas cervical vertebra, 38, 55-56, 322
Atrophy following injury, 125
Attentional focus and predisposition to injury, 184
Attitudes and predisposition to injury, 185
Auditory branch of acoustic nerve, 102
Auditory canal, 298-299, 300
  external, 36
Auditory meatus, 35, 298-299
Auditory nerve, assessment of, 286, 287
Auricle, 298, 299
Auricular nerve, 109
Autonomic nervous system, 89

Avascular necrosis of femoral head, 523-524
Avascular tissue, 54
"AVPU" method of determining level of consciousness, 281
Avulsion fracture, 178
Avulsion injuries, periosteal, 28
Avulsions, 151, 154-155
  tibial tuberosity, 473
  tooth, 304
Axial division of body, 18, 19
Axial region, athletic injuries of, 248-395
Axial skeleton, 31, 34-39
Axillary line, 359, 360
Axillary nerve, 107, 108, 109
  injury to, 560
Axis cervical vertebra, 38, 322
Axons, 71, 92, 93

B

Babinski reflex, 114
Back, 320, 327, 335
  muscles of, 358
Back knee, 423
Backbone, 34
Bacterial skin lesions, 160-162
Baker's cyst, 467, 485
Balance of athlete with head injury, 284-285
Ball-and-socket joints, 55, 56-57
Ballotable patella, 479, 480
Bargaining following injury, 188
Bartholin's glands, 380
Barton fracture, 629
Baseball finger, 637
Battle's sign, 259
Bench-warmer's bursitis, 521
Bending, lateral, 342, 343
  cervical, evaluation of, 345, 346
  of trunk, evaluation of, 347-348
Bennett's fracture, 641
Biaxial joints, 55, 56
Biceps brachii muscle, 81, 82, 551, 553, 572, 573, 594
  myositis ossificans from contusion injury of, 169
  rupture of, 170
  rupture of long head of, 558
Biceps femoris muscle, 83, 85, 461-462, 513, 515
Biceps reflex, 114, 351, 586
Biceps strain, 557
Biceps tendon, 610, 611
  dislocation/subluxation of, 557-558
  rupture of, 599
Bicipital aponeurosis, 81, 610
Bicipital groove, palpation of, 570, 571
Bicipital tenosynovitis, 557
Bicuspids, 302
Bilateral symmetry of body, 17-18
Bioelectrical impedance to assess body composition, 16, 17
Biot's respirations, 257
Bipartite patella, 470
Bipennate muscle fibers, 68, 69
Bite lesions of skin, 166
Black eye, 310
Bladder, referred pain from, 374
Bleeding, control of, 150, 151
Blisters, 157-158, 159
Blocker's spur, 556
Blood, extravasated, 120
Blood pressure, 261-263
  of athlete with head injury, monitoring, 283
Blow-out fracture, orbital, 311-312
Blunt-blow injuries to eye, 310-312
Body, 11-24
  normal alignment of, 336, 338
  response of
    to cold exposure, 140-145
    to heat, 130-140
    to trauma and environmental stress, 118-145
  temperature regulation by, 132-133

Body composition, 12-17
Body fat distribution patterns, 13-14
Body-fat percentages, 13
Boil, 161
Bone(s), 25, 26-27, 28; see also specific bone
  "crazy," hitting, 599
  of face, 291
  of foot, 46
    accessory, 401
  of hand, 42
  of hip girdle and lower extremities, 42-48
  of lower extremities, 47
  study of, 25-49
  of upper extremities, 39
  of vertebral column, 38
  of wrist, 41, 42
Bone bruises of tibia, 42
Bone density, lifespan changes in, 49
Bone markings, 28-31
Bone marrow, 28
Bone scan, 214, 215
Bony landmarks, palpable, 28-29
Bony levers, muscles and, 66-68
Borderline hypertension, 263
Boutonnière deformity, 638
Bowlegs, 477
"Bowler's elbow," 600
Boxer's fracture, 640
Brachial cutaneous nerve, 107, 108, 109
Brachial plexus, 90, 104, 109, 554
  injuries of, 563
Brachial pulse, locating, 610, 611
Brachialis muscle, 81, 82, 594
  contraction of, 66
Brachioradialis muscle, 81, 82, 594, 596
Brachioradialis reflex, 114
  testing, 351, 618
Brain, 89, 270-278
  right half of, 98
Brain case, 34
Brain stem, 270-272
  concussion of, 270, 276
  contusion of, 270, 276
  twisting injuries of, 275-276
Breasts, 360, 361-362
  contusions of, 364
Breathing, 225-226, 257
  of unconscious athlete, assessment of, 252-253
Breathing patterns, abnormal, 257
Bronchi, 363
Bronchial spasm, 367
Bronchial tree, 363
Bronchioles, 363
Brozek's equation to determine body fatness, 16
Bruises, 167-169, 171; see also Contusions
  of brain, 277
  stone, 410
Bucket handle tear, 469
Bulimia, 378, 379
Bulla, 156, 158
Bunion, 409
  tailor's, 440
Bunionette, 409, 440
"Burner," 323, 563
Bursa(e)
  adventitious, 466
  of knee, 466-467
  shoulder, 550, 572
  subcutaneous, of elbow, 592-593
  subdeltoid, inflamed, 550
Bursitis, 466
  anserine, 467
  bench-warmer's, 521
  iliopectineal, 521
  infrapatellar, 466-467
  ischial, 521
  olecranon, 598-599
  retrocalcaneal, 427, 443, 444
  shoulder, 558
  subdeltoid, 558
  trochanteris, 521

C

Calcaneal apophysitis, 427
Calcaneal nerve, 108
Calcaneal tendon; see Achilles tendon
Calcaneocuboid joint, 402
Calcaneofibular ligament, 408, 441
Calcaneonavicular joint, 403
Calcaneus, 29, 31, 46, 47, 399
  palpation of, 442, 443
Calcium deposit following contusion, 169
Calf strains, 428
California Pyschological Inventory, 184
Calluses, 158, 160
Calor, 122
Cancellous bone, 27
Cancer, testicular, 382-383
Canines, 301-302
Capital femoral epiphysis, slipped, 525
Capitate bone, 42, 623
Capitulum, 40, 590, 591
Capsulitis, adhesive, 562-563
Carbuncle, 161
Cardiac arrest, 226
Cardiogenic shock, 128
Cardiopulmonary resuscitation for unconscious athlete, 253
Caries, 303
Carotid artery(ies), 226, 227
Carpal bones, 30, 39, 41, 42, 623-624
Carpal tunnel, 626
Carpal tunnel syndrome, 626, 630
Carpet layer's knee, 467
Carpometacarpal articulations, 625
Carpometacarpal joint of thumb, 56
Carrying angle of elbow, 606
Cartilage
  articular (hyaline), 28, 53, 54-55
    costal, 30, 37, 38
    cricoid, 355, 356
    thyroid, 356
Catecholamines, 97
Cattell 16PF Questionnaire, 184
Cauda equina, 90, 318
Cauliflower ear, 300-301
Cavity(ies), 30, 31
  abdominal, 371, 372
  cranial, floor of, 35
  glenoid, 39
  marrow (medullary), 28
  nasal, 295
  pelvic, 47, 371
  pleural, 360, 362, 363
  synovial, 53, 467-468
  thoracic, 358; see also Chest; Thoracic cavity
Cavus foot, 405-406
Celiac plexus syndrome, 373-374
Cell(s)
  death of, from trauma, 120
  nerve; see Neurons
  nervous system, 91-97
  Schwann, 72
Cell body
  motor neuron, synaptic knobs on, 96
  neuron, 92, 93
Cellulitis, 162
Centering, 192
Central nervous system, 89, 90
Central sulcus, 98
Cerebellum, 90, 98-99, 272
Cerebral aqueduct, 98
Cerebral concussion, 275, 276
Cerebral contusion, 275
Cerebral cortex, 99, 272
Cerebrospinal otorrhea, 300
Cerebrospinal rhinorrhea, 296
Cerebrum, 90, 98-99, 272-273
Certified athletic trainer, 4
Cerumen, impacted, 299
Ceruminous glands, 150
Cervical compression, 348-349
Cervical curve, 37
Cervical distraction, 348-349
Cervical extension, 345, 346
Cervical flexion, 345, 346

Cervical lordosis, 339
Cervical nerve syndrome, 323
Cervical nerves, 103, 109
Cervical plexus, 90, 104, 109
Cervical spine, 321-324
  active range of motion of, 341
Cervical vertebrae, 31, 34, 38
Chaddock reflex, 114
Chancre of syphilis, 384
Charley horse, 519
Cheek, 29
Cheekbone, fractures of, 293-294
Chest 358-364; see also Thoracic cavity
  injuries and conditions of, 364-369,
    384-394
  palpation of, 387-388
Chest wall
  anterior, 358-360
  contusions of, 364
  muscles moving, 79
  strains of, 364-365
Cheyne-Stokes respirations, 257
Chicken pox, 164
Chlamydia, 383
Chondral fracture, 178, 415-416, 473-
  474
Chondrocytes, 54
Chondromalacia patellae, 472
Chondrosternal separation, 365
Chronic, 127
Chronic compartment syndrome, 430
"Cinder burns," 151
Circular muscle fibers, 68, 69
Circulation, 226-227
  of leg, 425-426
  of unconscious athlete, assessment of,
    253
Circumduction, 62
"Clap," 383
Clavicle, 30, 37, 38, 39, 79, 81
  fractures of, 39, 561, 562
  palpation of, 568-569
Claw toes, 409
Clicking from meniscal injuries, 469
Clitoris, 380
Clonus, 113
Closed athletic injuries, 166-181
Closed fracture, 177
Clothing
  to prevent heat loss, 142
  to prevent heat stress, 138
Cluster breathing, 257
Cluster pattern of skin lesions, 156
Coach
  behavior of, toward injured athlete,
    190
  as manager for injured athlete, 4-5
Coccidioidomycosis, 369
Coccygeal nerve, 103
Coccyx, 30, 31, 34, 37, 38
  and sacrum, 329-330
Cochlear branch of acoustic nerve, 102
Cognitive restructuring for treatment
  and rehabilitation of injuries, 192
Cognitive state anxiety, 184
Cold exposure
  body's response to, 140-145
  physiological basis of, 140, 142
Cold sore, 163
Cold-related conditions, 142-145
Colitis, 376
Collagen in repair-regeneration
  following trauma, 123
Collapsed lung, 366
Collar bone; see Clavicle
Collateral ligaments
  of ankle, 407
  of elbow, 591-592
  of knee, 464-466
Colles' fracture, 629, 630
Color, skin, 147
  of unconscious athlete, observation of,
    258-259
Coma, 250-251
  diabetic, 377-378
Comatose, 280

Comminuted fracture, 178
Common cold, 367
Compartment syndrome, 426, 430
  of elbow, 603
  thigh, 521-522
Competitive trait anxiety, 184, 187
Compression
  cervical, evaluation of, 348-349
  for immediate treatment of athletic
    injury, 126
  nerve root, 328-329
  to rib cage to evaluate injury, 392
Compression fracture, 179
  of lumbar vertebrae, 328
  of thoracic vertebra, 325
Compression test
  Apley's, 503-504
  on leg, 431
Computed tomography, 207, 211, 212
  to assess body composition, 14
Concentric contraction, 73
Conchae, 34, 36
Concussion, 276-277
  brain stem, 270, 276
  cerebral, 275, 276
  myocardial, 367
  of spinal cord, 324
Conditioning of athletes, 7
Conduction
  and heat gain, 131-132
  and heat loss, 132, 142
  saltatory, 93
Conduction test, ulnar nerve, 219
Condyle(s), 30
  tibial, 45, 416, 417
Condyloid joints, 56
Condyloid process, 35, 292
Conjunctiva, 305
Conjunctivitis, 310
Connective tissue of scalp, 267, 268
Connective tissue components of
  skeletal muscle, 69-70
Conoid ligament, 547-548
Consciousness, level of, 256
  of athlete with head injury, 279-281
Consensual light reflex, 286
Constipation, 376
Contact dermatitis, 160
Contact lenses, displaced, 312-313
Contractile components of skeletal
  muscle, 70
Contraction
  of brachialis muscle, 66
  muscle, types of, 72-74
Contracture, Volkmann's ischemic, 603
Contrast-enhanced radiography, 204,
  206-207
Contrecoup fracture, 177, 180
Contrecoup injury, 275
Control, locus of, 184
Contusion(s), 167-169, 171, 277
  of abdominal muscles, 372
  brain stem, 270, 276
  of breast, 364
  cerebral, 275
  of chest wall, 364
  elbow and forearm, 598-599
  facial, 291
  of foot, 410
  hand, 635-636
  of iliac crest, 372-373
  infrapatellar fat pad, 472
  leg, 426-427
  of lower back, 327
  myocardial, 367
  periorbital, 310
  peroneal nerve, 473
  of scalp, 268
  shin, 426
  shoulder, 556
  of spinal cord, 324
  of testicles, 381-382
  thigh and hip, 519-522
  of thoracic spine, 325
  ulnar nerve, 599
  of vulva, 381
  wrist, 627

Convection
  and heat gain, 131
  and heat loss, 132, 142
Convulsions causing unconsciousness,
  251
Coordination of athlete with head
  injury, testing, 284-285
Coordination exercises, 284-285
Coping resources of athletes, depletion
  of, 190
Coping strategies of athletes, 187
Coracoacromial ligament, 550
Coracobrachialis muscle, 80, 551, 552
Coracoclavicular ligament, 547-548
Coracohumeral ligament, 550
Coracoid process, palpation of, 570, 571
Corn, 409-410
Cornea, 307-309
Corneal reflex, 113
Coronal plane of body, 19, 20
Coronal suture, 35, 51
Coronoid fossa, 40
Coronoid process, 35, 292, 591
Corpora cavernosa penis, 380
Corpus callosum, 98, 272
Corpus cavernosum urethrae, 380
Corpus spongiosum, 380
Corpuscle
  Meissner's, 92
  pacinian, 92, 148
  Ruffini's, 92
Cortex, cerebral, 99
Cortical sensory system tests, 113
Coryza, 367
Costal angle, 369
Costal cartilage, 30, 37, 38
Costal facets of thoracic vertebra, 325
Costochondral separation, 365
Costoclavicular ligament, 546
Costosternal articulation, 37
Costovertebral joints, sprain of, 365
Cracked ribs, 365
Cramps, heat, 134-135
Cranial cavity, floor of, 35
Cranial nerves, 89, 98-99, 100-102, 273
Cranium, 34, 268, 270
"Crazy bone," hitting, 599
Cremaster muscle, 79
Cremasteric reflex, 114
Crepitation, 180, 240
Crest, 30
Cribriform plate, 35, 295
Cricoid cartilage, 355, 356
Crista galli, 35
Cross bridges, 70
Crossover maneuver, 584
Cruciate ligaments, 462-464
Crust, 157, 158
CT scan, 207, 211
Cubital fossa, 595, 610
Cubital tunnel, 599
Cubital tunnel syndrome, 604
Cubitus valgus, 607
Cubitus varus, 607
Cuboid bone, 46, 47, 399
Cuboid ligament, 408
Cullen's sign, 367
Cuneiform bones, 46, 47, 399
Curves of spine, 37
Cutaneous nerves, 107, 108
  lateral femoral, 90
Cutaneous rami, 107
Cyanosis, 147, 259
Cyclic pattern of skin lesions, 156
Cyst, 156, 158
  Baker's, 467, 485
  popliteal, 467, 485
  sebaceous, 149
  of scalp, 267

D

Daily Hassles Scale, 187
De Quervain's disease, 628
Decerebrate rigidity, 259-260
Decorticate rigidity, 260, 261

Deep, 18
Deep fascia, 70
Deep frostbite, 143
Deep peroneal nerve, 90, 107
Deep posterior compartment, 420
Deep receptors, 91
Deep reflexes, 114, 115
Deep tendon reflexes, testing, 351
Deformity(ies)
  boutonnière, 638
  gunstock, 607
  Haglund's, 428
  after spinal injury, 334
Delayed union of fracture, 180
Deltoid ligament of ankle, 407, 408, 439
Deltoid muscle, 78, 79, 80, 81, 551, 552
  fiber arrangement of, 68
  palpation of, 570, 572
Deltoid tuberosity, 40
  palpation of, 570, 571
Dendrites, 92, 93
Dens of cervical vertebra, 56
Dental abscess, 303
Dental caries, 303
Dental injuries, 302-304
Depressed fracture, 179
Depression, 62, 63, 188
Dermatitis, contact, 160
Dermatomes, 104, 110-112, 320
  of elbow and forearm, 617
  of foot, ankle, and leg, 454
  of shoulder and upper arm, 586
  of thigh and hip, 537
Dermis, 147, 148
"Desert fever," 369
Deviated septum, 295, 297
Diabetes mellitus, 377-378
Diabetic coma, 377-378
Diagnostic procedures, 201-214
Diapedesis, 121
Diaphragm, 79
  and inspiration, 364
  referred pain from, 374
Diaphysis, 27
Diarrhea, 376
Diarthroses, 50, 52-57
  range of motion and type of
    movement in, 57-64
  structural features of, 52-55
  types of, 55-57
Diarthrotic joints, 50, 52-57
Diastolic blood pressure, 262
Diet to prevent heat stress, 139
Diploic venous system, 268
Diplopia, assessment for, 286
Directional terms related to body, 18
Discogram, 207, 208
Discography, 206-207, 208
Discoid meniscus, 470
Discriminatory tests, 113
Dislocations, 167, 174-177
  ankle, 414
  biceps tendon, 557-558
  elbow, 601, 605
  finger, 639-640
  foot, 414
  glenohumeral, 560-561
  hand and wrist, 639-640
  hip, 524
  incomplete, 174
  joint, 52
  knee, 464
  lunate, 629-630
  patellar, 470-471
  shoulder, 560-561
  sternoclavicular joint, 560
  temporomandibular joint, 294
  wrist, 628-629
Displaced contact lenses, 312-313
Displaced fracture, 180
Distal, 18
Distraction, cervical, evaluation of, 348-
    349
Distraction test, Apley's, 504
Documentation of findings after athletic
  injury assessment, 229

Dolor, 122
Dopamine, 97
Dorsal, 18
Dorsal root of spinal nerve, 99, 104
Dorsalis pedis, 425
Dorsiflexion, 60
Dorsoscapular nerve, 109
Drawer test
  anterior, 493, 496
  posterior, 494
Drop arm test, 576, 577
Duodenal ulcer, 376
Dura mater of meninges, 273
Dural sheath, 103
Dysmenorrhea, 381
Dyspepsia, 376
Dysphagia with tonsillitis, 357
Dyspnea, 226
Dysuria, 381

E

Ear, 298-299
  cauliflower, 300-301
  examination of, 299-300
  injuries to, 299-301
  ossicles of, 34, 36
  swimmer's, 301
Eardrum, 298, 301
Earwax, 299
Eating disorders, 378, 379
Eccentric contraction, 73
Ecchymoses, 147, 168
  from hip contusion, 520-521
ECG; see Electrocardiogram
Echocardiography, 214, 218
Ectomorph, 12, 13
Eczema, 166
Edema, 121
Education and counseling, athletic
    trainer's role in, 8-9
EEG; see Electroencephalography
Effector, 95
Efferent nerves, 89
Efferent neurons, 93
Effusion
  joint, 467
  in knee, palpating for, 481
EKG; see Electrocardiogram
Elbow, 56
  anatomy of, 589-595
  bones of, 591
  contusions of, 598-599
  dislocation of, 175, 601, 605
  fractures of, 601-603
  hyperextension of, 613
  ligaments of, 592
  muscles and movements of, 593-595
  sprains of, 600-601
  strains of, 599-600
  "tennis," 600
Elbow and forearm injuries, 589-620
Electrocardiogram, 214, 217, 218
Electrocardiography, 214, 217
Electroencephalogram, 214, 216
Electroencephalography, 214, 216
Electromyogram, 219, 220
Electromyography, 219, 220
Eleidin, 148
Elevation, 62, 63
  for immediate treatment of athletic
    injury, 126
EMG; see Electromyogram
Emissary veins of scalp, 268
Empty can position, 576
Enamel of teeth, fracture of, 303
Encapsulated nerve endings, 91, 92
Encircling pattern of skin lesions, 156
Endomorph, 12, 13
Endomysium, 69
Endorphins, 97
Endosteum, 28
Enkephalins, 97
Environmental stress, body's response
  to, 120-145
Environmentally produced skin lesions,
  165-166

Epicondyle(s), 30
  of elbow, 589-590
  of femur, 44
  of humerus, 29, 40
Epicondylitis, 600
Epicranius muscle, aponeurosis of, 267-
  268
Epidermal ridges, 149
Epidermis, 147, 148
Epididymis, 378
Epidural hematoma, 277
Epidural hemorrhage, 270
Epigastrium, 369
Epilepsy, 251
Epimysium, 69
Epiphyseal fracture, 171, 179, 525
  of foot and ankle, 416
  proximal humerus, 561-562
Epiphyseal (growth) plates, 28
  injury to, 603, 629-630
Epiphyseal injuries, 474
Epiphyses, 27-28
  femoral, slipped capital, 525
Epistaxis, 296-297
Epstein-Barr virus, 368
Erector spinae muscle, 76
Erosion, 157, 158
Erythema, 160
  from sunburn, 165
Esophagus, 356, 356
  referred pain from, 374
Ethmoid bone, 34, 36
Ethmoid sinus, 36
Evaporation and heat loss, 132, 142
Eversion, 62, 63
Exercise stress test, 217
Exercise-induced asthma, 368
Exercises, coordination, 284-285
Exhaustion, heat, 135-136
Exostosis, shoulder, 556
Experience, vicarious, 193
Expiration, 364
Exposed injuries, 147, 150-166
Extension, 60, 61
  cervical, evaluation of, 345, 346
Extensor carpi radialis brevis muscle,
  81, 82, 594, 596
Extensor carpi radialis longus muscle,
  81, 82, 594, 596
Extensor carpi ulnaris muscle, 81, 82,
  594, 596
Extensor digiti minimi muscle, 81, 594,
  596
Extensor digitorum longus muscle, 85,
  86, 418, 420, 448
Extensor digitorum muscle, 81, 82, 594,
  596
Extensor hallucis longus muscle, 85, 86,
  418, 420, 448
Extensor indicis muscle, 594, 596
Extensor muscles of knee, 460-461
Extensor pollicis brevis muscle, 594,
  596
Extensor pollicis longus muscle, 594,
  596
Extensor retinaculum, 81, 85
Extensor tendon, common, 595, 610
External abdominal oblique muscle, 78
External auditory canal, 36
External auditory meatus, 35
External ear, 298
External hemorrhoids, 376
External intercostal muscles, 79
External oblique muscle, 77, 79
External occipital protuberance, 270
External rotational recurvatum test,
  500
Externally palpable bony landmarks,
  28-29
Exteroceptors, 91
Extravasated blood, 120
Extremity(ies)
  lower; see Lower extremity(ies)
  posturing of, 259-260
  upper; see Upper extremity(ies)

Extrusion, tooth, 304
Exudate, 121
Eye(s), 305, 306, 307-310
  injuries to, 305-313
  raccoon, 259
Eye teeth, 301-302
Eyelashes, 305
Eyelids, 305, 309-310

F

Face guard, removing, 252, 253
Face, 290-315
  bones of, 34, 36, 291
  laceration of, 153
Facet, 30
Facial nerve, 100, 101, 286, 287
Fallen arches, 46, 47, 402
False ribs, 37, 38, 39
Fascia, 70, 78, 147-148
Fasciculi, 69
Fasciitis, plantar, 411
Fatigue fracture, 177
Fear following injury, 189
Fear hierarchy, 192
Felon, 637
Femoral artery, 425
Femoral cutaneous nerves, 107, 108, 110
Femoral epiphysis, slipped capital, 525
Femoral nerve, 110
Femur, 30, 31, 42, 43, 44, 45, 47, 509
  epiphyseal fracture of, 171
  fracture of, 524-525
  stress fractures of, 525
Fever blister, 163
Fibroblasts, 123
Fibrocartilage, 55
Fibroplasia, 123
Fibrous capsule of hip joint, 511-512
Fibrous joint capsule, 52, 53
Fibula, 29, 30, 31, 42, 43, 44, 45, 46, 47,
    416, 417
  fracture of, 430-432
Fibular notch, 45
Filaments of skeletal muscle, thick and
    thin, 70
Filum terminale, 103
Finger(s), 632
  baseball, 637
  bones of, 30, 39, 41, 42
  dislocations of, 176, 639-640
  mallet, 637
Finger-to-nose test, 272
Finkelstein's test, 628
First-class levers, 67
Fissure(s), 157, 158
  of cerebrum, 272
  palpebral, 305
Fixators, 75
Flaccid muscles, 72
Flat bones, 26-27
Flatfoot, 46, 47, 401, 402, 404
Flexibility, 57
Flexible cavus foot, 405
Flexible tape measurement of spinal
    motion, 342
Flexion, 60, 61
  cervical, evaluation of, 345, 346
  plantar, 60
  trunk, evaluation of, 347-348
Flexor carpi radialis muscle, 81, 82,
    594, 596
Flexor carpi ulnaris muscle, 81, 82, 594,
    596
Flexor digiti minimi brevis muscle, 83,
    87
Flexor digiti minimi muscle, 633
Flexor digitorum brevis muscle, 87
Flexor digitorum longus muscle, 86,
    419, 420, 449, 450
Flexor digitorum profundus muscle, 82,
    594, 596
Flexor digitorum profundus tendon,
    avulsion of, 637-638

Flexor digitorum sublimis muscle, 81,
    596
Flexor digitorum superficialis muscle,
    82, 594
Flexor digitorum superficialis tendon,
    83
Flexor hallucis brevis muscle, 87
Flexor hallucis longus muscle, 86, 419,
    420, 449, 450
Flexor muscles of knee, 461-462
Flexor pollicis brevis muscle, 83, 633,
    634
Flexor pollicis longus muscle, 594
Flexor retinaculum, 81, 83, 85
Flexor tendon, common, 595, 610
Flexor tendon sheaths of hand, 635
Floating ribs, 37, 38
"Floor burns," 151
Flu, 367
Fluid, synovial, 52, 53
Fluid replacement to prevent heat
    stress, 138
Flushed skin color, 147
Focus stretch, 187
Follicle, hair, 148, 149
Folliculitis, 161
Foot, 29, 401-406
  and ankle, 398-407
    dislocations of, 414
    fractures of, 414-416
    injuries/conditions of, 407-416
    joints of, 402-403
    and leg injuries, 398-456
  contusions of, 410
  mechanics of, 423-425
  Morton's, 406
  palpation of, 437-445
  sprains of, 411-414
  strains of, 410-411
  traumatic injury to, 436
Football helmet, removing, from
    unconscious player, 252-253, 254
Football jersey, cutting off, 253, 255
Footwear and overuse syndromes of
    lower extremity, 435-436
Foramen (foramina), 30
  infraorbital, 34
  interventricular, 98
  intervertebral, 37
  jugular, 35
  mental, 34, 35
  nutrient, 41
  optic, 34, 35
  sacral, 329, 330
  supraorbital, 34
  vertebral, 321
Foramen lacerum, 35
Foramen magnum, 35, 36
Foramen ovale, 35
Foramen rotundum, 35
Forearm; *see also* Elbow and forearm
  abrasion of, 152
  fractures of, 602-603
  muscles moving, 82
  muscles of, 595, 596
Forefoot
  fractures of, 415
  sprains of, 411-412
Forehead, lacerations of, 291
Foreign bodies in eye, 307-309
Foreskin, 380
Forward head, 339
Forward shoulders, 339
  testing for, 343
Fossa, 30
  coronoid, 40, 590
  cubital, 595, 610
  olecranon, 40, 41, 590, 608
Fourth ventricle, 98
Fovea, 30
Fracture(s), 167, 177-181
  ankle, 415
  avulsion, 178

Fracture(s)—cont'd
  Barton, 629
  Bennett's, 641
  boxer's, 640
  cervical, 323-324
  cheekbone, 293-294
  chondral/osteochondral, 178, 179, 415-
    416, 473-474
  clavicular, 39, 561, 562
  closed, 177
  Colles', 629, 630
  comminuted, 178
  compression, 179
    of lumbar vertebrae, 328
    of thoracic vertebra, 325
  contrecoup, 177, 180
  delayed union of, 180
  depressed, 179
  displaced, 180
  elbow, 601-603
  epiphyseal, 171, 179, 525
    of foot and ankle, 416
    proximal humerus, 561-562
  femur, 524-525
  of foot and ankle, 414-416
  forearm, 602-603
  forefoot, 415
  greenstick, 179
  hand and wrist, 640-641
  humerus, 561, 562
  impacted, 179
  jaw, 292-293
  Jones', 415
  of larynx, 357
  leg, 430-432
  Maisonneuve, 432, 433
  malunion of, 180
  mandible, 292-293
  march, 415
  maxilla, 294
  nasal, 297
  navicular, 629
  nondisplaced, 180
  nonunion of, 180
  oblique, 179
  open, 177, 178
  orbital blow-out, 311-312
  overriding, 180
  patellar, 471-472
  pelvic, 525
  Pott's, 432
  radius, 629
  rib, 365
  rotated, 180
  shoulder, 561-562
  skull, 259, 270
  Smith's, 629
  of spinous and transverse processes of
      lumbar vertebrae, 328
  spiral, 180
  of sternum, 365-366
  stress; *see* Stress fractures
  supracondylar, 602
  tooth, 303-304
  of trachea, 357
  transverse, 180
  trimalar, 293
  tripod, 293
  wrist, 629-630
  zygoma, 293-294
Fracture-dislocation, 180
Free nerve endings, 91, 92
Freely movable joints; *see* Diarthroses
Friction blisters, 157, 159
Frontal bone, 30, 34, 35, 36
Frontal lobe of cerebrum, 272
Frontal sinuses, 36, 295
  skull fracture involving, 296
Frostbite, 142-143, 165-166
  of ears, 301
Frostnip, 143
"Frozen shoulder," 562

Functio laesa, 122
Function, loss of, from inflammation, 122
Fungal skin lesions, 162-163
Furunculosis, 161

G

Gait, 424-425
 following spinal injury, 334
 Trendelenburg (abductor), 528
Galea aponeurotica, 267-268
Gamekeeper's thumb, 639
Ganglion(ganglia), 89
 posterior root, 96
 wrist, 628
Gaster of muscle, 68
Gastritis, 376
Gastrocnemius muscle, 85, 86, 418, 419, 420, 461, 462
 evaluation of, 449, 451
 palpation of, 443, 444
 strain of, 429
Gastroenteritis, 376
Gastrointestinal conditions, 375-377
Genital herpes, 163
Genitalia
 female, 380
 injuries and conditions involving, 381-384
 male, 378-380
Genitofemoral nerve, 107, 110
Genu recurvatum, 423, 477
Genu valgum, 477
Genu valgus, 477
Genu varum, 477
Genu varus, 477
Gerdy, tubercle of, 466, 482
Gingivitis, 304-305
Girdle pattern of skin lesions, 156
Glabella, 34, 291
Gladiolus, 36
Gland(s)
 Bartholin's, 380
 ceruminous, 150
 sebaceous, 148, 149
 Skene's, 380
 skin, 149-150
 sweat, 148, 149-150
 thyroid, 355, 356-357
Glans penis, 380
Glasgow Coma Scale, 280-281
Glass fragment causing incision, 153
Glenohumeral dislocation, 560-561
Glenohumeral joint, 548-550
Glenohumeral ligament, 550
Glenohumeral sprain, 559
Glenohumeral translation test, 584-585
Glenoid cavity, 39
Glenoid labrum, 549
Gliding joints, 55, 57
Gliding movements, 62
Globe of eye, 305
Glossopharyngeal nerve, 100, 102, 286, 287
Gluteal nerve, 110
Gluteal reflex, 114
Gluteus maximus muscle, 78, 84, 85, 513, 517
Gluteus medius muscle, 84, 513, 517
Gluteus minimus muscle, 84, 513, 517
Glycosuria with diabetes mellitus, 377
Goal setting for treatment and rehabilitation of injuries, 192
"Golfer's elbow," 600
Golgi tendon organs, 71
Golgi tendon receptors, 92
Gomphosis, 51, 52
Goniometer, measuring joint range of motion with, 58, 59
Gonorrhea, 383
"Goose egg" hematoma of scalp, 268
Gooseflesh, 149
Gordon reflex, 114
Gracilis muscle, 85, 461, 462, 513, 516
Grand mal seizures, 251

Graphesthesia, 113
Gravity stress test, 616
Gray matter, 96
Great toe sprain, 411-412
Greater trochanter, 30, 44, 509, 530
Greater tubercle of humerus, 40
Greater tuberosity, palpation of, 570, 571
Greenstick fracture, 179
Grey-Turner's sign, 387
Grief response following injury, 187-188
Grind test, medial-lateral, 502-503
Groin muscles, 523, 529
Groove, 30
 bicipital, palpation of, 570, 571
Grouped skin lesions, 156
Growth plates of epiphyses, 28
Gunstock deformity, 607

H

H zone, 70
Haglund's deformity, 428
Hair, 148, 149
Hair follicle, 148, 149
Hallux valgus, 409
Hamate bone, 42, 623
Hammertoe, 409
Hamstring muscle, tightness of, evaluation of, 344, 345
Hamstring muscles, 83, 461-462, 513, 515, 530
Hamstring reflex, medial, test of, 505, 506
Hamstring strain, 170, 522-523
Hand, 630-637
 dislocations of, 639-640
 fractures of, 640-641
 injuries of, 633-641
 muscles moving, 82
 sprains of, 638-639
 strains of, 637-638
 and wrist, 622
Hand and wrist injuries, 621-655
Hawkins-Kennedy Impingement Test, 581
Hay fever, 295
Head injuries, 266-289
Head tilt, jaw thrust without, to open airway, 224-225
Head tilt-chin lift to open airway, 224-225, 226
Headache as symptom of head injury, 281-282
Healing, wound, stages of, 120-125
Heart
 contusion or concussion of, 367
 referred pain from, 374
Heat
 body's response to, 130-140
 from inflammation, 122
 prickly, 150
Heat acclimation, 133-134
Heat cramps, 134-135
Heat dissipation, 132
Heat exhaustion, 135-136
Heat exposure, physiologic basis of, 130-134
Heat gain, 131-132
Heat loss, 131, 132
Heat preservation, 142
Heat production, 131
 in cold weather, 140, 142
 role of skeletal muscle in, 66
Heat stress, prevention of, 136-139
Heat transmission, 142
Heath-Carter somatotype, 12
Heatstroke, 135, 136
Heel bone; see Calcaneus
Heel bruise, 410
Heel spur, 411
Helmet, football, removing, from unconscious player, 252-253, 254
Hematemesis, 367
Hematocele, 382

Hematoma, 120, 167
 epidural, 277
 intracerebral, 277
 safety-valve, 268
 septal, 297
 subdural, 277
 subungual, 636, 643
Hematoma auris, 300-301
Hematuria, 375
Hemopneumothorax, 366
Hemopoiesis, role of skeleton in, 26
Hemoptysis, 367
Hemorrhage
 brain, 277-278
 epidural, 270
 intracranial, 277-278
 petechial, 147
 subconjunctival, 305, 310
Hemorrhagic shock, 128
Hemorrhaging from trauma, 120
Hemorrhoids, 376-377
Hemothorax, 366-367
Hepatitis, 377
Hernia, 373
Herniated intervertebral disc, 317
Herniation, intervertebral disc, 328-329
Herpes simplex virus, 163
Herpes zoster, 164
Herpesvirus, 163-164
Hindfoot, 412-414, 415
Hinge joints, 55
Hip(s), 57, 510-519; see also Thigh and hip
 dislocations of, 524
 injuries to; see Thigh and hip injuries
 level of, difference in, 421
 snapping, 521
 traumatic synovitis of, 523
Hip flexor muscles, tightness of, evaluation of, 343-345
Hip girdle and lower extremities, bones of, 42-48
Hip pointer, 372, 520
HIV, 164
Hives, 166
Holding strength of muscle, 84
Horizontal abduction, 60
Horizontal adduction, 60
Horizontal plane of body, 19, 20
"Hot shot," 323, 563
"Hot spot," 157
Housemaid's knee, 467
Hughston test, 497
Human immunodeficiency virus, 164
Humeroradial articulation, 589
Humeroulnar articulation, 589
Humerus, 30, 31, 38, 39, 40, 41
 epicondyles of, 29
 fractures of, 561, 562
 olecranon fossa of, palpation of, 608
 palpation of, 570-571
 proximal, epiphyseal fracture of, 561-562
Humidity and temperature, monitoring, to prevent heat stress, 137-138
Hyaline cartilage; see Articular cartilage
Hydration and body composition, relationship of, 16
Hydrocele, 382
Hyoid bone, 34, 36, 355, 356
Hyperesthesia, 113, 244
Hyperextension, 58, 60, 61
 elbow, 613
 of knee, 423
 of spine, testing, 342-343
 trunk, evaluation of, 347-348
Hyperglycemia, 377
Hyperhidrosis, 149
Hyperpnea, 257
Hyperpronated foot, 404
Hyperreflexia, 245
Hypertension, 263
Hyperventilation, 226, 257
Hyphema, 310-311
Hypoesthesia, 113, 244

Hypoglossal nerve, 100, 102, 109, 286, 287
Hypoglycemia, 378
Hyporeflexia, 245
Hypothenar eminence, 83, 632
Hypothermia, 143-144
Hypotonia, 272
Hypovolemic shock, 128
Hypoxia after trauma, 121-122

I

I bands, 70, 73
Ice for immediate treatment of athletic injury, 125
ICERS, 125
Iliac crest, 29, 369, 529-530
  contusion of, 372-373, 520-521
Iliac spine, 529
  anterior superior, 29, 79, 85
Iliacus muscle, 84
Iliocostalis cervicis muscle, 76
Iliocostalis lumborum muscle, 76
Iliocostalis thoracis muscle, 76
Iliofemoral ligament, 511, 512
Iliohypogastric nerve, 90, 108, 110
Ilioinguinal nerve, 107, 110
Iliopectineal bursitis, 521
Iliopsoas muscle, 84, 85, 513, 517
Iliotibial band, 466
Iliotibial band friction syndrome, 466, 484
Iliotibial tract, 85
Ilium, 29, 30, 31, 44, 47
Imagery for treatment and rehabilitation of injuries, 191-192
Immovable joints; see Synarthroses
Impacted cerumen, 299
Impacted fracture, 179
Impetigo, 161-162
Impingement sign, 581
Impingement syndrome, 558
Impingement test, Hawkins-Kennedy, 581
Impulses, nerve, 93-94
Incisions, 151, 152-154
Incisors, 301
Incus, 36
Indigestion, 376
Infectious mononucleosis, 368-369
Inferior concha, 34
Inferior extensor retinaculum, 85
Inferior turbinate, 36, 291
Infestation, skin, 166
Inflammation, 120, 122, 127
Inflammatory process, 120-125
Influenza, 367
Infraorbital foramen, 34
Infrapatellar bursitis, 466-467
Infrapatellar fat pad contusion, 472
Infraspinatus muscle, 78, 80, 320, 549, 551
Infundibulum, pituitary, 98
Ingrown toenail, 410
Inguinal canals, 379
Inguinal ligament, 85, 369
Initial insult, 120
Injury(ies), 146; see specific body part; specific injury
Injury assessment, 196
  checklist for, 246
  considerations in, 197-200
  evaluations of findings of, 245-247
  factors related to, 196-222
  history in, 230-234
  introduction to, 2-10
    and anatomic basis for, 1-115
  movement procedures in, 240-243
  observation in, 234-237
  place for, 197
  plan of action for, 199-200
  procedures for, 223-247
  process for, 2, 7-8, 194-247
  referral after, 199
  skills needed for, 197-199
  time for, 197

Inner ear, 298
Innominate bone, 30, 42
Insertion of muscle, 68
Inspiration, 364
Instability of knee, 490-500
Insulin shock, 378
Insulin-dependent diabetes, 377
Integrative functions of cerebrum, 272-273
Intercellular matrix, 54
Interclavicular ligament, 546
Intercostal muscles, 79, 358
Intercostal nerves, 90
Intermetatarsal joint, 402, 403
Internal auditory meatus, 35
Internal hemorrhoids, 376
Internal intercostal muscles, 79
Internal oblique muscle, 77, 79
Internal receptors, 91
Interneurons, 92, 93
Interosseous membrane of elbow, 596-598
Interosseous muscles, 83, 633, 634
Interphalangeal articulations, 632
Interphalangeal joint, 402
  dislocation of, 643
Interspinous ligaments, 317
Intertarsal joint, 403
Intertransverse ligaments, 317
Intertrigo, 163
Interventricular foramen, 98
Intervertebral disc, 37, 316-317
  herniated, 317, 328-329
Intervertebral foramen, 37
Intestines, referred pain from, 374
Intraabdominal injuries, 373-375
Intracapsular ligaments, 52
Intracerebral hematoma, 277
Intracranial hemorrhage, 277-278
Intrathoracic injuries, 366-367
Intravenous pyelogram, 207, 210
Intrinsic muscles of back, 320-321
Intrusion, tooth, 304
Inversion, 62, 63
Invincibility, sense of, and predisposition to injury, 184
Involuntary nerves, 91
Irregular bones, 26, 27
Ischemia, 430
Ischemic contracture, Volkmann's, 603
Ischial bursitis, 521
Ischiofemoral ligament, 511, 512
Ischium, 30, 31, 44, 47
Isometric contractions, 74
Isotonic contractions, 73-74
Isotope dilution to assess body composition, 14

J

Jaundice, 377
"Javelin thrower's elbow," 600
Jaw, 292-294
Jaw thrust without head tilt to open airway, 224-225
Jerk test, 497
Jersey, football, cutting off, 253, 255
Jersey finger, 638
Jock itch, 162-163
Joint(s), 50-64
  acromioclavicular, 547-548
    palpation of, 569
  ankle, 406-407; see also Foot and ankle
  atlantooccipital, 322
  calcaneocuboid, 402
  calcaneonavicular, 403
  costovertebral, sprain of, 365
  of foot and ankle, 402-403
  glenohumeral, 548-550
  hip; see Hip joint
  intermetatarsal, 402, 403
  interphalangeal, 402
    dislocation of, 643
  intertarsal, 403
  lumbosacral, 326-327

Joint(s)—cont'd
  metacarpophalangeal, subluxation of, 654
  metatarsocuneiform, palpation of, 439
  metatarsophalangeal, 402
    palpation of, 438, 439, 441, 442
  patellofemoral, 457; see also Knee
  sacroiliac, 329-330
    passive stress to evaluate, 349-350, 351
  sternoclavicular, 39, 546-547
  subacromial, internal derangement of, 558
  subtalar, 399, 402-403
  talocalcaneonavicular, 402, 403
  talonavicular, 402
  tarsal, 402
  tarsometatarsal, 402, 403
  temporomandibular, 292
  tibiofemoral, 457; see also Knee
  tibiofibular, 416-417, 457; see also Knee
Joint capsule, fibrous, 52, 53
Joint disarticulations of shoulder girdle, 39
Joint effusion, 467
Joint mice, 474
Jones' fracture, 415
Jugular foramen, 35
Jumper's knee, 472
Juvenile-onset diabetes, 377

K

Kehr's sign, 374
Keloid from hematoma auris, 300
Keratin, 148
Keratitis, 310
Ketoacidosis, 377-378
Kidney
  injuries of, 375
  referred pain from, 374
Kienbock's disease, 629
Kinematic chains, 58, 60
Knee, 457-470
  arthroscopy of, 220
  back, 423
  effusion in, palpating for, 481
  hyperextension of, 423
  instability of, tests for, 490-500
  jumper's, 472
  knock-, 477
  magnetic resonance imaging of, 213
Knee injuries, 457-508
Kneecap, 29
Knock-knees, 477
Knocked-down shoulder, 559
Krause's end-bulbs, 92
Kyphosis, 339

L

Labia majora, 380
Labia minora, 380
Laboratory evaluations, 214
Labrum, acetabular, 510
Labrum, glenoid, 549
Lacerations, 151, 152, 153
  of brain, 275
  of eye, 309-310
  facial, 291
  forehead, 291
  hand, 636
  perineal, 381
  of scalp, 268
Lachman's test, 493-494, 495
Lacrimal bone, 34, 35, 36, 291
Lacunae, 54
Lambdoidal suture, 35
Lamina of cervical vertebra, 321
Laryngitis, 357
Larynx, 355, 356, 357
Lasegue's test, 349, 350
Lateral, 18
Lateral bending, 342-348
Lateral compartment, 420
Lateral compartment muscles, evaluation of, 448-449

Lateral pivot shift test, 497, 498
Latissimus dorsi muscle, 78, 80, 320, 358, 551, 553
  palpation of, 572, 573
Leg, 416-432, 437-445
  ankle, and foot injuries, 398-456
  lower, muscles moving, 83
  varus and valgus angulation of, 477
Lenses, contact, displaced, 312-313
Lesions, skin; see Skin, lesions of
Lethargic, 280
Lethargy, 250
Levator scapulae muscle, 75, 78, 320, 551
Lever systems, 66-68
Leverage, basic principle of, 66
Levers, types of, 67-68
Lice, 166
Life stress, 183
Life stress events and predisposition to injury, 183-184, 185
Life support, ABCs of, 223-227
Ligament(s); see specific ligament
Ligamentum flavum, 317
Ligamentum nuchae, 317
Ligamentum nuchae muscle, 78
Ligamentum teres, 511, 512
Light reflex, consensual, 286
Line, 30
Linea alba, 370
Linea semilunares, 370
Linear pattern of skin lesions, 156
"Little League elbow," 600, 603
Liver, 374, 375
Locking from meniscal injuries, 469
Locomotion and skeletal muscle, 66
Locus of control, 184
Long bones, 26
Long intrinsic muscles of back, 320
Longissimus capitis muscle, 76
Longissimus thoracis muscle, 76
Longitudinal arch of foot, 47, 401
  sprains of, 412
Longitudinal fissure of cerebrum, 272
Longitudinal ligaments of vertebral column, 317
Lordosis, 339
Louis, angle of, 358, 360
Low back pain, 327
Lower abdominal reflex, 114
Lower extremity(ies), 396-541
  hip girdle and, bones of, 42-48
Lumbar curve, 37, 326
Lumbar lordosis, 339
Lumbar nerves, 103
Lumbar plexus, 90, 104
Lumbar puncture, 326
Lumbar spine, 326-329
  active range of motion of, 341-342
Lumbar vertebrae, 31, 34, 38, 326
  compression fractures of, 328
Lumbodorsal fascia, 78
Lumbosacral joint, 326-327
Lumbosacral plexus, 104, 110
Lumbosacral trunk, 110
Lumbrical muscles, 633, 634, 635
Lumbricales, 83, 87
Lunate bone, 42, 623, 624
  dislocation of, 628-629
  palpation of, 644-645
Lungs
  collapsed, 366
  and pleura, 363
Lunula, 149
Luxatio erecta, 561
Luxation, 174; see also Dislocations
  joint, 52
Lymph nodes in neck, 357

M

MacIntosh test, 497
Macule, 156, 158
Magnetic resonance imaging, 211-214
  to assess body composition, 14
Maisonneuve fracture, 432, 433

Malar bone, 36, 291
Male and female skeletons, differences between, 48
Male genitalia, 378-380
Malleoli of tibia and fibula, 29, 45, 47, 406
  palpation of, 439, 441
Mallet finger, 637
Malleus, 36
Malunion of fracture, 180
Mandible, 30, 34, 35, 36, 291, 292-293
Manual muscle testing, 242
  grading for, 243
Manual resistance of injured extremity, 242
Manubrium, 36, 37
March fractures, 415
Margination, 121
Marrow cavity, 28
Martens' Sport Competition Anxiety Test, 187
Mastoid process of temporal bone, 35, 270
Mastoid sinus, 36
Maturation, remodeling and, following trauma, 123-125
Maturation phase of wound healing, 123
Maxilla, 30, 34, 35, 36, 294
Maxillary bones, 291
Maxillary sinus, 36
McMurray test, 500-502
Meatus, 30
  auditory, 35
  urinary, 380
Mechanical advantage, law of, 66
Mechanically produced skin lesions, 157-160
Mechanism of injury, 146
Medial, 18
Medial-lateral grind test, 502-503
Median nerve, 90, 107, 109
  involvement of, in elbow and forearm injuries, 604
Mediastinum, 360, 362, 363
Medicine, sports, 3, 4
Medulla oblongata, 270, 271
Medullary cavity, 28
Meissner's corpuscles, 92
Membrane
  interosseous, of elbow, 596-598
  periodontal, 52
  plasma, 96, 97
  polarized, 93
  synovial, 52, 53, 54
    of elbow, 592-593
    of hip joint, 512
  tympanic, 298
Meninges, 273, 274
  of spinal cord, 318, 319
Meningitis, 318
Meniscal tear, 469
Menisci of knee, 55, 468-470
Meniscus tests, 500-504
Menstrual dysfunctions, 381
Mental foramen, 34, 35
Mental toughness and predisposition to injury, 185, 186
Mesomorph, 12, 13
Metabolic shock, 128
Metabolism and heat production, 131
Metacarpal bones, 30, 39, 41, 42, 631
  fracture of, 640
  palpation of, 645
Metacarpophalangeal articulations, 631-632
Metacarpophalangeal joint, subluxation of, 654
Metatarsal arch of foot, 47, 402
Metatarsal bones, 29, 30, 43, 46, 47, 48, 398-399, 400
  palpation of, 438, 442
Metatarsalgia, 440, 443
Metatarsocuneiform joint, palpation of, 439

Metatarsophalangeal joint, 402
  palpation of, 438, 439, 441, 442
Metatarsus, 400
Microscopic hematuria, 375
Midbrain, 271
Midcarpal articulations, 624-625
Midclavicular line, 359
Midfoot, 412, 415
Midsternal line, 359
Mixed cranial nerves, 99
Molars, 302, 303
Molluscum contagiosum, 164
Mononucleosis, infectious, 368-369
Mons pubis, 380
Morton's foot, 406
Morton's neuroma, 409
Motor cranial nerves, 89, 99
Motor endplate, 71, 72
Motor function tests, 245
Motor nervous system, 89
Motor neuron cell body, synaptic knobs on, 96
Motor neuron fiber, 72
Motor neurons, 71, 92-93
Motor root of spinal nerve, 99, 104
Motor unit, 71
Movement(s)
  angular, 60, 61
  elbow, 593-595
  gliding, 62
  role of skeletal muscle in, 66
  role of skeleton in, 26
  special, 62-64
  following spinal injury, 334-335
  types of, 60-64
Movie sign, 472
MRI; see Magnetic resonance imaging
Multiaxial joints, 55, 56-57
Multipennate muscle fibers, 68, 69
Multipolar neuron, diagram of, 93
Mumps, 357-358
Murphy's sign, 629
Muscle(s); see specific muscle
Muscle spasm
  palpation to recognize, 240
  following trauma, 122-123
Muscle spindles, 71, 92
Muscle tone, 72
Musculocutaneous nerve, 109
Myelinated nerve fibers, 93
Myelogram, 206, 207
Myelography, 206, 207
Myocardial contusion or concussion, 367
Myofibrils, 73
Myology, 65-87
Myositis, 172
Myositis ossificans, 520
  following contusion, 169, 171
Myotomes, 104, 110-112, 320
  important, 112

N

Nails, 149
Nares, 295
Nasal bones, 30, 34, 35, 36, 291, 295
Nasal cavity, 295
Nasal septum, 295
  abscess of, 297
  deviated, 295, 297
  examination of, 297
  hematoma in, 297
Nasion, 291, 295
NATA; see National Athletic Trainer's Association
NATABOC; see National Athletic Trainer's Association Board of Certification
National Athletic Trainer's Association, 5
National Athletic Trainer's Association Board of Certification, 5
Navicular bone, 42, 46, 47, 399, 400, 623, 624
  fractures of, 629
  palpation of, 644-645

Navicular tubercle, palpation of, 439
Neck, 355-356, 357
  anterior; see Throat
  and back, alignment of, following
    spinal injury, 335
Necrosis, 120
  avascular, of femoral head, 523-524
Negative work, 73
Nerve cells; see Neurons
Nerve endings, 91, 92
Nerve fibers, myelinated, 93
Nerve impulses, 93-94
Nerve involvement in elbow and
    forearm injuries, 603-604
Nerve plexuses, 104-112
Nerve root of spinal nerves, 318-319
Nerve root compression, 328-329
Nerve root distributions, segmental, 332
Nerve supply of leg, 425-426
Nerve tissue, 70-71
Nerves, 89
  cranial, 89, 99, 100-102, 273
    assessment of, 98-99, 285-287
    sensory, 71
  spinal, 89, 99, 103-104, 318-320
    peripheral branches of, 105
    segmental distribution of, 111
  ulnar, 81
Nervous system, 88-115
Neurapraxia, 324
Neurilemma, 93
Neurogenic shock, 129
Neuroglia, 91-92
Neurological assessment, 97-112
Neurological evaluations, 243-245
Neurology, 88-115
Neuroma, 409
  Morton's (plantar), 409
Neuromuscular junction, 71, 72
Neurons, 91, 92-93, 96
  motor, 71
    fiber of, 72
Neurotransmitter, 96-97
Neutron activation to assess body
    composition, 14
Nipples, 360
  runner's, 364
Noble Compression Test, 466, 484
Nociceptors, 91
Nodes
  lymph, in neck, 357
  of Ranvier, 93
Nodule, 156, 158
Nondisplaced fracture, 180
Non-insulin-dependent diabetes, 377
Nonunion of fracture, 180
Norepinephrine, 97
Nose, 295-296
  fractures of, 297
  injuries to, 296-297
Nosebleeds, 296-297
Nostrils, 295
Nuclear imaging, 214, 215
Nucleus pulposus, 316-317
Nutrient foramine, 41
Nystagmus, 283, 286

O

Ober's test, 485, 486
Oblique fracture, 179
Oblique muscles, 77, 78, 79, 358, 370,
    371
Obturator nerve, 90, 107, 108, 110
Occipital bone, 31, 35, 36
Occipital lobe of cerebrum, 272
Occipital nerve, 109
Occipital protuberance, external, 270
Oculomotor nerve, 100, 101
  assessment of, 286-287
Odontoid process, 322
Olecranon bursa, 592-593
Olecranon bursitis, 598-599
Olecranon fossa, 40, 41
  palpation of, 608
Olecranon process, 29, 31, 39, 591
  palpation of, 607-608, 609

Olfactory nerve, 100, 101, 285
Oligomenorrhea, 381
Open fracture, 177, 178
Open wounds, 124, 150-155
Oppenheim reflex, 114
Opponens digiti minimi muscle, 83, 633,
    634, 635
Opponens pollicis muscle, 83, 633, 634,
    635
Optic chiasm, 98
Optic foramen, 34, 35
Optic nerve, 100, 101, 285-286
Optimum angle of pull, 66
Orbicularis oris muscle, fiber
    arrangement of, 68
Orbit, 30
Orbital blow-out fracture, 311-312
Orbital margins, lateral, 291
Os coxae, 30, 42, 47
Osgood-Schlatter disease, 472-473, 482
Osteitis pubis, 524
Osteoblasts, 28
Osteochondral fracture, 179, 415-416,
    473-474
Osteochondritis dissecans, 416, 474
  of elbow, 603
Osteoclasts, 28
Osteology, 25-49
Otitis, external, 301
Otitis media, 301
Otorrhea, 259, 260
  cerebrospinal, 300
Overriding fracture, 180
Overuse syndromes of lower extremity,
    434-436

P

Pacinian corpuscles, 92, 148
Pain
  anterior knee, 470
  following spinal injury, 333
  from inflammation, 122
  locating areas of, 234
  low back, 327
  palpation to localize, 239
  reaction to, of unconscious athlete,
    monitoring, 263-264
  type of, 234
  visceral, referred, 374-375
Pain-spasm cycle, 122-123
Painful arc, 574
Painful arc syndrome, 558
Palatine bone, 36, 291
Pallor, 147, 258-259
Palmar aponeurosis, 81
Palmar plate of interphalangeal
    articulations, 632
Palmaris longus muscle, 81, 82, 594,
    596
Palpable bony landmarks, 28-29
Palpation of injured area, 237-240
  of unconscious athlete, 260-264
Palpebrae, 305
Palpebral fissure, 305
Pancreas, referred pain from, 374
Pancreatitis, 377
Papilla, hair, 148, 149
Papule, 156, 158
Paraaminobenzoic acid sunscreens to
    prevent sunburn, 165
Parallel muscle fibers, 68, 69
Paralysis from spinal injury, 332
Paranasal air sinuses, 295
Paraplegia, 332
Parasympathetic nervous system, 91
Paresis, 332
Paresthesias, 91, 113
  following spinal injury, 333
Parietal bone, 31, 34, 35, 36
Parietal layer of abdominal cavity, 371
Parietal lobe of cerebrum, 272
Parietal pleura, 363
Parietooccipital sulcus, 98
Paronychia, 637
Partial sit-up to stress abdominal
    muscles, 391

Patch, 156, 158
Patella, 29, 30, 43, 44, 45, 47, 85, 470-
    472
  ballotable, 479, 480
  plain film radiography of, 203
  squinting, 477, 478
  tendinitis of, 477, 484
Patellar ligament, 85
Patellar reflex, 114
  neural pathway in, 95, 96
  testing, 351, 505, 506
Patellar tendon rupture, 472
Patellofemoral dysfunction, 470
Patellofemoral joint, 457; see also Knee
Pathologic reflexes, 114, 115
"Pear-shape" fat distribution and risk of
    disease, 13-14
Pectineus muscle, 85, 513, 516
Pectoral nerve, 109
Pectoralis major muscle, 79, 80, 81, 358,
    360, 551, 553
  fiber arrangement of, 68
  palpation of, 570, 572
  rupture of, 170
Pectoralis minor muscle, 75, 551
Pediculosis, 166
Pelvic cavity, 47, 371
Pelvic fractures, 525
Pelvic inlet, 47
Pelvis, 369-371
  injuries to, 384-394
  level of, observation for, 335-336, 337
  male and female, differences in, 48
  stress fractures of, 525
  tilted, 422
  true, 47
Penis, 378, 379-380
Peptic ulcer, 376
Perforations, eardrum, 301
Performance, effects of athletic injury
    on, 9
Pericoronitis, 305
Pericranium of scalp, 268
Perimysium, 69
Perineum, lacerations of, 381
Periodontal membrane, 52
Periodontitis, 304
Periorbital contusion, 310
Periosteal avulsion injuries, 28
Periosteum, 28, 69
  of scalp, 268
Peripheral nervous system, 89, 90
Peritoneum, 371
Peritonitis, 374-375
Peroneal nerve, 90, 107, 110
  common, 425, 426
  contusion of, 473
  injury to, 426-427
Peroneal retinaculum, 85, 408
Peroneal tendons, subluxation of, 429
Peroneus brevis muscle, 86, 418, 420
  evaluation of, 449
Peroneus brevis tendon, 408
Peroneus longus muscle, 85, 86, 418,
    420
  evaluation of, 449
Peroneus longus tendon, 408
Peroneus tertius muscle, 86
Perpendicular plate of ethmoid bone, 34
Personality factors and predisposition
    to injury, 184
Pes anserinus, 462
Pes cavus, 405
Pes planus, 404
Petechiae, 147
Phagocytosis, 122
Phalanges
  of hand, 30, 39, 41, 42, 631
    palpation of, 645
  of foot, 29, 30, 43, 46, 47, 48, 398-399,
    400-401
    fracture of, 640-641
Phalen's test, 630, 631
Pharyngitis, 357
Pharynx, 356, 356, 357
Phrenic nerve, 109

Physical trauma, body's response to, 118-128
Physis, 416
Pia mater of meninges, 273
Piano key sign, 559
Pigment labile, 258
"Piles," 376-377
"Pinched nerve," 323, 563
Pinna, 298, 299
Piriformis muscle, 84
Piriformis syndrome, 523
Pisiform bone, 41, 42, 623
"Pitcher's elbow," 600
Pituitary infundibulum, 98
Pityriasis rosea, 166
Pivot joints, 55-56
Pivot shift test, lateral, 497, 498
Plain film radiography, 202-204
Plantar aponeurosis, 87, 410
    palpation of, 442, 443
Plantar calcaneonavicular ligament, 408
Plantar fasciitis, 411
Plantar flexion, 6,
Plantar ligament, 408
Plantar neuroma, 409
Plantar reflex, 114
Plantar warts, 164
Plantaris muscle, 85, 419, 420
    rupture of, 429
Plaque, 156, 158
Plasma membrane, 96, 97
Pleura, 362, 363
Pleural cavities, 360, 362, 363
Pleural sac, 363
Plexus(es), 104
    brachial, 90, 554
        injuries to, 563
    cervical, 90
    lumbar, 90
    nerve, 104-112
    sacral, 90, 103
Plica syndrome, 469-470
Pneumocephalus, 295, 296
Pneumonia, 369
Pneumothorax, 366
Point localization, 113
Point tenderness, 239
Polarized membrane, 93
Polyuria with diabetes mellitus, 377
Pons, 271
Popliteal artery, 425
Popliteal cyst, 467, 485
Popliteal vein, 425
Popliteus muscle, 461, 462
Popliteus tendinitis, 462
Position(s) 18, 19, 58
    empty can, 576
    following spinal injury, 334-335
Post-concussion syndrome, 277
Posterior, 18
Posterior compartment muscles, evaluation of, 449, 450
Posterior drawer test, 494
Postsynaptic neuron, 96
Posture
    after spinal injury, 334, 335-339
    lifespan changes in, 49
    role of skeletal muscle in, 66
Posturing of extremities, 259-260
Pott's fracture, 432
PQRST technique, questions using, 232
Preiser's disease, 629
Premolars, 302
    fractures of, 303
Prepatellar bursitis, 466
Prepuce, 380
Presynaptic neuron, 96
Prevention of injuries, athletic trainer's role in, 6-7
Prickly heat, 150
Primary injury, 120
Primary sensory system tests, 113
Primary skin lesions, 156, 157, 158
Primary survey, 223-227
    basic steps of, 228

Prime movers, 74
Process(es), 30, 31; see also specific process
    of skull, 35
Profundus tendon rupture, 637-638
Pronated foot, 404-405
Pronation, 62, 63
Pronator quadratus muscle, 82, 594, 595, 596
Pronator teres muscle, 81, 82, 594, 595
Pronator teres syndrome, 604
Proprioceptors, 91
Protraction, 62, 63, 64
Psoas major muscle, 84, 517
Psoas minor muscle, 517
Psoriasis, 166
Psychogenic shock, 129
Psychological aspects of injury, 182-193
Psychrometer, sling, to monitor environmental conditions, 138
Pterygoid process, 35
Pubic bone, 47
Pubis, 30, 44
Pubofemoral ligament, 511, 512
Pudendal nerve, 110
Pull, optimum angle of, 66
Pulls; see Strains
Pulmonary function test, 221, 222
Pulmonary ventilation, mechanism of, 363-364
Pulse, 226, 227
    of athlete with head injury, monitoring, 283
    of unconscious athlete, monitoring, 260-261
    brachial, locating, 610, 611
Pump bump, 428
Puncture(s)
    hand, 636
    lumbar, 326
Puncture wounds, 151, 154
Pupil response
    in athlete with head injury, 282-283
    of unconscious athlete, observation of, 258, 259
Pupillary reflex of unconscious athlete, observation of, 258, 259
Pupils of unconscious athlete, observation of, 257-258
Pustule, 156, 158
Pyelogram, intravenous, 207, 210
Pyramidalis muscle, 79

Q

Q angle, 471, 477, 479
Quadratus lumborum muscle, 76
Quadriceps contusion, 519
Quadriceps femoris muscle, 83, 460-461, 514
Quadriceps mechanism, 461
Quadriceps muscles, 513, 514
    strength of, 84
Quadriceps strain, 522-523
Quadriparesis, 324
Quadriplegia, 324, 332

R

Raccoon eyes, 259
Radial artery, palpating, to take pulse, 261
Radial collateral ligament, 592
Radial nerve, 90, 107, 108, 109
    injury to, 561
    involvement of, in elbow and forearm injuries, 604
Radial notch, 591, 595
Radial tunnel syndrome, 604
Radiate muscle fibers, 68, 69
Radiation
    and heat gain, 131
    and heat loss, 132, 142
Radiocarpal articulation, 624
Radiograph, sunrise view," 471

Radiography
    contrast-enhanced, 204, 206-207
    plain film, 202-204
    stress, 202, 204
Radiology, 202-214
Radioulnar articulation, 624
Radius, 29, 30, 31, 38, 39, 40, 41, 42
    fractures of, 602-603, 629
    palpation of, 610, 611
    styloid process of, palpation of, 644
Rami, cutaneous, 107
Range of motion
    active, of injured extremity, 242
    in diarthroses, 57-58
    knowledge of muscles and bony levers and, 66
Ranvier, nodes of, 93
Rearfoot varus, 405
Rebound tenderness, 389
Receptors, 91, 92, 95
Rectus abdominis muscle, 77, 79, 358, 370-371
    fiber arrangement of, 68
Rectus femoris muscle, 83, 84, 85, 460-461, 514
    fiber arrangement of, 68
Recurvatum test, external rotational, 500
Red bone marrow, 28
Red eye, 305, 310
Redness from inflammation, 122
Referred visceral pain, 374-375
Reflex arcs, 94-97
    testing, 113
Reflex center, 95
    of brain stem, 271
Reflex status tests, 113-115
Reflex, 95
    Achilles tendon, test of, 453-454
    biceps, testing, 586
    brachioradialis, testing, 618
    consensual light, 286
    deep tendon, testing, 351
    of elbow and forearm, assessment of, 618
    of foot, ankle, and leg, evaluation of, 453-454
    hamstring, medial, test of, 505, 506
    patellar
        neural pathway in, 95, 96
        test of, 505, 506
    pupillary, of unconscious athlete, observation of, 258, 259
    in shoulder injuries, 586
    tendon, 245
    testing, 245
        with knee injuries, 506
        in spinal injury assessment, 351
    triceps, testing, 586
Regeneration, repair and, following trauma, 123
Regions, abdominopelvic, 19, 22
Rehabilitation program, 127
Remodeling and maturation following trauma, 123-125
Repair and regeneration following trauma, 123
Repolarization, 94
Resistance, manual, of injured extremity, 242
Respirations
    of athlete with head injury, 283
    Biot's, 257
    Cheyne-Stokes, 257
    symmetry of, feeling for, 388
    of unconscious athlete, observation of, 256-257
Respiratory tract, conditions affecting, 367-369
Rest for immediate treatment of athletic injury, 126
Rest periods to prevent heat stress, 138-139
Resting potential of neuron, 93
Resuscitation, cardiopulmonary, for unconscious athlete, 253

Reticular activating system, 271-272, 274
Retinaculum
    extensor, 81, 85
    flexor, 81, 83, 85
    of foot, 406
    peroneal, 85, 408
Retinal detachment, 312
Retraction, 63, 64
Retrocalcaneal bursitis, 427, 443, 444
Retrograde amnesia, 276
Rhinitis, 295-296
Rhinorrhea, 259
    cerebrospinal, 296
Rhomboid muscles, 551, 552
Rhomboideus major muscle, 75, 78, 320
Rhomboideus minor muscle, 320
Rib cage, 358
    compression to, to evaluate injury, 392
Ribs, 30, 36-39, 78, 79
    articulation between sternum and, 53
    cracked, 365
    fracture of, 365
Rigid cavus foot, 406
Rigidity
    decerebrate, 259-260, 261
    decorticate, 260, 261
"Ring injury," 636
Ring-shaped pattern of skin lesions, 156
Ringworm, 163
Risk-taking behavior and predisposition to injury, 184
ROM; see Range of motion
Romberg's sign, 285
Root of tooth in socket, 51
Rotated fracture, 180
Rotation, 60, 62
    cervical, evaluation of, 345, 346
    of spine, testing, 342, 343
    trunk, evaluation of, 347-348
Rotator cuff, 549
Rotator cuff impingement, 558
Rotator cuff muscles, 549
Rotator cuff strains, 557
Rotatory instability of knee, tests for, 494-500
Rubor, 122, 258
Ruffini's corpuscles, 92
Running gaits, phases of, 424-425
Rupture; see also Strains
    Achilles tendon, 428
    biceps tendon, 599
    of eardrum, 301
    of long head of biceps, 558
    patellar tendon, 472
    plantaris muscle, 429
    profundus tendon, 637-638
    of quadriceps mechanism, 461
    of spleen, 375

S

Sacral foramina, 329, 330
Sacral nerves, 103
Sacral plexus, 90, 103, 104
Sacral promontory, 329, 330
Sacral vertebrae, 329
Sacralization, 327
Sacroiliac joints, 329-330
    passive stress to evaluate, 349-350, 351
Sacroiliac ligaments, 330
Sacroiliac sprains, 330
Sacrospinalis muscle, 76, 78
Sacrum, 30, 31, 34, 37, 38, 43
    and coccyx, 329-330
Saddle joints, 55, 56
Safety-valve hematoma, 268
Sagittal plane of body, 19, 20
Saltatory conduction, 93
Saphenous nerve, 90, 107, 108
Saphenous vein, 425
Sarcolemma, 73
Sarcomere, 70, 72
Sarcoplasm, 72

Sartorius muscle, 83, 85, 461, 462, 513
    fiber arrangement of, 68
Saunas and thermoregulatory controls, 133
Scabies, 166
Scale, 157, 158
Scalp, 267-268
    examination of, for signs of trauma, 259
Scaphoid bone, 42, 623
Scapholunate dissociation, 628
Scapula, 29, 31, 38, 39, 78, 81
    abduction of, 64
    adduction of, 64
    palpation of, 569, 570
    positioning of, observation for, 337-338
    winged, 338, 580
Scapular line, 360
Scapulohumeral rhythm, 550
Scar, 157, 158
Scar formation, 123
Schwann cell, 72
Sciatic nerve, 90, 425
Sciatica, 327
Sclera, 305
Scoliosis, 337, 338
Scratch test, Apley, 575-576
Scrotum, 378-379
Sebaceous cyst, 149
    of scalp, 267
Sebaceous gland, 148, 149
Sebum, 149
Second impact syndrome, 278
Secondary injury, 120
Secondary response to trauma, 122
Secondary skin lesions, 157, 158
Secondary survey, 227-245
    basic steps of, 229
Second-class levers, 67-68
Segmental nerve root distributions, 332
Seizures
    grand mal, 251
    causing unconsciousness, 251
Self, structure and organization of, 186
Sella turcica, 35, 36
Semicomatose, 280
Semiflexible cavus foot, 405
Semilunar notch, 591
Semimembranosus muscle, 83, 85, 461-462, 515
Semispinalis capitis muscle, 78, 320
Semitendinosus muscle, 83, 85, 461-462, 515
    rupture of, 170
Sensory cranial nerves, 99
Sensory function testing, 243-245
Sensory nerves, 71, 89
Sensory nervous system, 89
Sensory neurons, 92
Sensory root of spinal nerve, 99, 104
Sensory system, 112-115
Sensory system tests, 113
Separation, shoulder, 559
Septal hematoma, 297
Septic shock, 129
Serotonin, 97
Serratus anterior muscle, 75, 358, 360, 551, 552
Serratus inferior muscle, 78
Serratus posterior muscle, 78
Sesamoid bones, 27
Sever's disease, 427
Severe sprain, 174
Severe strain, 172
Sexually transmitted diseases, 383-384
SHARP and wound infection, 150
Sharpey's fibers, 28
Sheldon somatotyping system, 12
Shift test, lateral pivot, 497, 498
Shin, 416; see also Tibia
    contusion of, 426
Shin splints, 429, 445
Shingles, 164
Shock, 128-130
    insulin, 378

Shoes and overuse syndromes of lower extremity, 435-436
Short bones, 26
Short intrinsic muscles of back, 320
Shoulder, 57, 554-561
    bursae of, palpation of, 572
    circumduction at, 62
    dislocation of, 176, 560-561
    forward, 339
        testing for, 343
    muscles of, 550-554
    positioning of, observation for, 337-338
    skeletal components of, 546
Shoulder blade; see Scapula
Shoulder girdle
    muscles moving, 75
    and upper extremity, bones of, 38, 39-41
Shoulder injuries, 544-588
Shoulder pointer, 556
Sickle cell anemia, 377
Sickle cell trait, 377
Side ache, 373
Sign
    of athletic injuries, 201
    Battle's, 259
    Cullen's, 387
    Grey-Turner's, 387
    impingement, 581
    Kehr's, 374
    movie, 472
    Murphy's, 629
    piano key, 559
    Romberg's, 285
    sulcus, 584
    Tinel, 630
    Trendelenburg, 528
    vital, of unconscious athlete, monitoring, 256
Silver-fork deformity, 629
Sinding-Larsen-Johansson disease, 473
Sinus, 30
    ethmoid, 36
    frontal, 36, 295
        skull fracture involving, 296
    mastoid, 36
    maxillary, 36
    paranasal, 295
Sinus tarsi, swelling in, 436
Sinusitis, 296
Siri's equation to determine body fatness, 16
SITS muscles, 549
Situational factors and predisposition to injury, 184-185
Sit-up, partial, to stress abdominal muscles, 391
Skeletal muscle(s), 68-75
Skeleton, 25
    anterior view of, 32
    appendicular, bones of, 31
    axial, 34-39
        bones of, 31
    functions of, 25-26
    lifespan differences in, 48-49
    male and female, differences between, 48
    organization of, 31-48
    posterior view of, 33
Skene's glands, 380
Skier's thumb, 639
Skin, 147-150
    bite lesions of, 166
    common lesions of, 155-166
    infestations of, 166
    injury to, 124
    of scalp, 267
Skin lesions, 155-166
Skull, 34, 35, 268-270
    bones of, 29
    bony anatomy of, 292
    fracture of, 259, 270
Slightly movable joints; see Amphiarthroses
Sling psychrometer to monitor environmental conditions, 138

Slipped capital femoral epiphysis, 525
Slocum test, 497, 499
Smith's fracture, 629
Snapping hip, 521
SOAP note, 229
Social support for injured athlete, 190-191
Soft corn, 409-410
Soft tissue injuries of face, 291-292
Solar plexus, blow to, 374
Soleus muscle, 85, 86, 418, 419, 420
  evaluation of, 449
Somatic nerves, 89
Somatic state anxiety, 184
Somatotype, 11-12, 13
Spasm
  bronchial, 367
  muscle
    following trauma, 122-123
    palpation to recognize, 240
  testicular, 381
    reducing, 382
Spastic muscles, 72
Spermatic cord, 79, 378
  torsion of, 381-382
Sphenoid bone, 34, 35, 36
Spina bifida occulta, 329
Spinal accessory nerve, 100, 102
  assessment of, 286, 287
Spinal cord, 90, 318, 319
  concussed, 324
  contused, 324
  myelography of, 206, 207
  transected, 324
Spinal meningitis, 318
Spinal nerves, 89, 99, 103-104, 318-320
  peripheral branches of, 105
  segmental distribution of, 111
Spinalis thoracis muscle, 76
Spine, 30, 34, 316-353
  cervical, 321-324; see also Cervical spine
  curves of, 37
  iliac, anterior superior, 29, 79, 85
    palpation of, 529
  injuries to, 316-353
  lumbar, 326-329; see also Lumbar spine
  thoracic, 324-326; see also Thoracic spine
Spinous process, 30, 37, 317, 321
  of lumbar vertebrae, fracture of, 328
Spiral fracture, 180
Spleen, 374, 375
Splenius capitis muscle, 78, 320
Spondylitis, 329
Spondylolisthesis, 328
Spondylolysis, 328
Spondylosis, 329
Spongy bone, 27
Spontaneous pneumothorax, 366
Sport Competition Anxiety Test, 187
Sports medicine, 3, 4
Sprains, 167, 172-174
  acromioclavicular, 558-559
  ankle, 412-413
    syndesmosis, 407, 413-414
  cervical, 323
  of collateral ligaments of knee, 465
  of costovertebral joints, 365
  cruciate ligament, 462, 463
  elbow and forearm, 600-601
  of foot, 411-414
  glenohumeral, 559
  great toe, 411-412
  hand, 638-639
  longitudinal arch, 412
  of lower back, 327
  of lumbosacral joint, 327
  sacroiliac, 330
  shoulder, 558-560
  sternoclavicular, 559-560
  thigh and hip, 523-524
  of thoracic spine, 325
  transverse arch, 412
  wrist, 628

Spring ligament, 403
Spur
  blocker's, 556
  heel, 411
  talotibial, 411
Squamous suture, 35
Squinting patellae, 477, 478
Stapes, 36
Status epilepticus, 251
Steam baths and thermoregulatory controls, 133
Stereognostic function, 113
Sternal angle, 358, 360
Sternoclavicular joint, 39, 546-547
  dislocation/subluxation of, 560
Sternoclavicular ligaments, 546
Sternoclavicular sprain, 559-560
Sternocleidomastoid muscle, 78, 79, 320, 355, 356
Sternum, 30, 36, 37, 38, 79
  articulation between ribs and, 53
  fracture of, 365-366
Stimulus, 91, 93
"Stinger," 323," 563
"Stitch in the side," 373
Stone bruise, 410
Stools, tarry, 374
Straight-leg raising to evaluate spinal injury, 349
Strains, 167, 170, 171-172
  abdominal, 371-372
  biceps, 557
  calf, 428
  cervical, 323
  of chest wall, 364-365
  elbow and forearm, 599-600
  of foot, 410-411
  gastrocnemius, 429
  groin muscle, 523
  hand, 637-638
  leg, 427-430
  of lower back, 327
  plantaris muscle, 429
  quadriceps mechanism, 461
  rotator cuff, 557
  severe, 172
  shoulder, 556-558
  thigh and hip, 522-523
  of thoracic spine, 325
  wrist, 627-628
Strangulated hernia, 373
Stratum corneum, 148
Stratum germinativum, 148-149
Stratum granulosum, 148
Stratum lucidum, 148
Stratum spinosum, 148
"Strawberry," 151
Strength, muscle, 84, 86
Strep throat, 357
Stress
  environmental, body's response to, 120-145
  heat, prevention of, 136-139
  passive, for elbow, 616, 617
  and predisposition to injury, 183-184, 185
Stress Audit Questionnaire, 187
Stress fracture, 177, 180
  of foot and ankle, 415
  nuclear imaging of, 215
  of pelvis and femur, 525
  of tibia and fibular, 432
Stress procedure, applying, to injured area, 240, 241
Stress radiograph, 202, 204
  of ankle, 452
Stress test(s)
  adduction, of knee, 490-493
  exercise, 217
  gravity, 616
  for knee, abduction, 490, 491
  valgus, 490, 491
Stretch, focus, 187
Stuporous, 280
Stuporous athlete, 250
Sty, 305, 307

Styloid process, 35
  palpation of, 441, 610, 611
  of radius, 29, 41
    palpation of, 644
  of ulna, 29, 41
    palpation of, 608, 609, 644
Subacromial bursa, palpation of, 572
Subacromial joint, internal derangement of, 558
Subaponeurotic space, 268
Subclavian nerve, 109
Subconjunctival hemorrhage, 305, 310
Subcoracoid dislocation, 560
Subcutaneous bursae of elbow, 592-593
Subcutaneous tissue, 147-148
Subdeltoid bursa
  inflamed, 550
  palpation of, 572
Subdeltoid bursitis, 558
Subdural hematoma, 277
Subluxation, 52, 174
  of biceps tendon, 557-558
  cervical, 323-324
  metacarpophalangeal joint, 654
  of patella, 470-471
  of peroneal tendons, 429
  sternoclavicular joint, 560
  tooth, 304
Subscapularis muscle, 80, 549, 551
Substrate phase of inflammatory process, 120-123
Subtalar joint, 399, 402-403
Subtalar motion, evaluation of, 445
Subungual hematoma, 636, 643
Sulcus, 30
  central, 98
  parietooccipital, 98
Sulcus sign, 584
Sunburn, 165
"Sunrise view" radiograph, 471
Sunscreens, 165
Sunstroke, 136
Superficial, 18
Superficial fascia, 70, 147-148
Superficial frostbite, 143
Superficial peroneal nerve, 90, 107
Superficial posterior compartment, 420
Superficial receptors, 91
Superficial reflexes, 114, 115
Superior, 18
Superior extensor retinaculum, 85
Supination, 62, 63
Supinator muscle, 82, 594, 595
Support
  for immediate treatment of athletic injury, 126
  role of skeletal muscle in, 66
  role of skeleton in, 26
Supraclavicular nerve, 107, 108, 109
Supracondylar fracture, 602
Supraorbital foramen, 34
Supraorbital margin, 290
Suprascapular nerve, 109
Supraspinatus muscle, 78, 80, 320, 549, 551
Supraspinatus syndrome, 558
Supraspinous ligament, 317-318
Sural nerve, 107, 108
Surface anatomy, 22-23
Surgical repair of wounds, 124
Sustentaculum tali, 399, 408
Suture, 30
  coronal, 51
  for incisions and lacerations, 154
  lambdoidal, 35
  of skull, 35, 51-52
  squamous, 35
Swallowing reflex, 113
Swayback, 339
Sweat gland, 148, 149-150
Sweating to promote heat loss, 132, 133
Swelling
  from inflammation, 122
  palpation to recognize, 239
Swimmer's ear, 301
Swimmer's shoulder, 558

Symmetry, bilateral, of body, 17-18
Sympathetic nervous system, 91
Symphysis, 52, 53
Symphysis pubica, 53
Symphysis pubis, 47
Symptoms of athletic injuries, 201
Synapse, 94, 95, 97
Synaptic cleft, 72, 96, 97
Synaptic knobs, 96, 97
Synaptic vesicles, 72
Synarthroses, 50, 51-52, 53
Synarthrotic joints, 50, 51-52, 53
Synchondrosis, 52, 53
Syncope, 129
Syndesmosis, 51, 407
Syndesmosis sprains of ankle, 407, 413-414
Synergists, 74
Synovial cavity, 53, 467-468
Synovial fluid, 52, 53
Synovial joints, 52; see also Diarthroses
  angular movements at, 60
Synovial membrane, 52, 53, 54
  of elbow, 592-593
  of hip joint, 512
Synovitis, 467-4368
  traumatic, of hip, 523
Syphilis, 383-384
Systolic blood pressure, 262

T

Tailor's bunion, 409, 440
Talocalcaneal ligament, 408
Talocalcaneonavicular joint, 402, 403
Talofibular ligament, 408
  palpation of, 441
Talonavicular joint, 402
Talotibial spurs, 411
Talus bone, 45, 46, 47, 399-400
Tarry stools, 374
Tarsal bones, 30, 43, 46, 47, 48, 398-399
Tarsal joints, 402
Tarsal plate, 305
Tarsal tunnel syndrome, 410
Tarsometatarsal joint, 402, 403
Tarsus, 399
"Tattoo, traumatic," 151-152
Tear
  bucket handle, 469
  meniscal, 469
Teeth, 301-305
Temporal bone, 35, 36
Temporal lobe of cerebrum, 272
Temporomandibular joints, 292
  dislocation of, 294
  dysfunction of, 294
Tendinitis, 172
  Achilles, 427
  patellar, 472, 484
  popliteus, 462
Tendon organs, Golgi, 71
Tendon receptors, Golgi, 92
Tendon reflex, 245
Tendon sheaths, 69
  of wrist, 626
Tendon(s), 69; see also specific tendon
"Tennis elbow," 600
Tenosynovitis, 172
  Achilles, 427
  bicipital, 557
Tension pneumothorax, 366
Tensor fasciae latae muscle, 84, 85, 513
Teres major muscle, 78, 80, 320, 551, 553
Teres minor muscle, 78, 80, 320, 549, 551
Test(s); see specific test
Testicles
  cancer of, 382-383
  contusion of, 381-382
  self-examination of, 383
  spasm of, 381
    reducing, 382
  tumors of, 383
Tetanic contractions, 73
Tetanus, 73

Tetanus toxoid booster for puncture
    wounds, 154
Texture, skin, 147
Texture discrimination, 113
Thenar eminence, 83, 632
Thermal exposure, body's response to, 130-140
Thermoregulatory system of body, 132-133
Thick filament, 70
Thigh and hip, 509-541
  contusions of, 519-522
  dermatomes of, 537
  muscles moving, 84
Thigh compartment syndrome, 521-522
Thighbone; see Femur
Thin filament, 70
Third ventricle, 98
Third-class levers, 68
Thomas test, 344, 345
Thompson test, 443, 444
Thoracic cavity, 358; see also Chest
  visceral structures contained in, 360, 362, 363
Thoracic curve, 37
Thoracic nerves, 103, 109
Thoracic outlet syndrome, 563
Thoracic spine, 324-326
  active range of motion of, 341-342
  injuries to, 325-326
Thoracic vertebrae, 31, 34, 38
  compression fracture of, 325
  typical, 325
Thorax, 36-39, 354
  lines of reference of, 359, 360
  topographic anatomy of, 358-360
  and ventilation, 363-364
  visceral structures contained in, 360, 362, 363
Thought stoppage, 192
Three-neuron reflex arc, 94
Throat, 354-394
Thumb, 625
  carpometacarpal joint of, 56
  gamekeeper's, 639
  skier's, 639
Thyroid cartilage, 356
Thyroid gland, 355, 356-357
Tibia, 29, 30, 31, 42, 43, 45, 46, 44, 45, 47, 416, 417
  avulsion injury to, 155
  bone bruises of, 42
  condyles of, 45
  fracture of, 430-432
  tomograms of, 205
Tibial artery, 425
Tibial nerve, 90, 110, 425-426
Tibial plateau, 482
Tibial stress syndrome, 429-430
Tibial tuberosity, 416, 417
  avulsion of, 473
Tibialis anterior muscle, 85, 86, 418, 420
  evaluation of, 448
Tibialis anterior tendon, 408
Tibialis muscle, palpation of, 442
Tibialis posterior muscle, 86, 419, 420
  evaluation of, 449, 450
Tibialis posterior tendon, 408
Tibialis tendon, palpation of, 442
Tibiocalcaneal ligament, 408
Tibiofemoral joint, 457; see also Knee
Tibiofibular articulation, distal, 51
Tibiofibular joint, 416-417, 457; see also
    Knee
Tibiofibular ligament, 408
Tibiofibular syndesmosis, 407
Tibionavicular ligament, 408
Tibiotalar ligament, 408
Tinea corporis, 163
Tinea cruris, 162-163
Tinea pedis, 162
Tinel sign, 630
Tinnitus, 276

Toe(s)
  palpation of, 438, 439
  phalanges of, 29, 30, 43, 46, 47, 48
  range of motion of, evaluation of, 445
  turf, 411
Toenail, ingrown, 410
Tomography, 204, 205
  computed, 207, 211, 212
  to assess body composition, 14
Tongue blocking airway, 225
Tonic muscle contraction, 72
Tonsillitis, 357
Tonsils, 357
Tooth; see Teeth
Torsion of spermatic cord, 381-382
Torticollis, 338
Toughness, mental, and predisposition
    to injury, 185, 186
Trachea, 355, 356
  blockage of, 224
  fracture of, 357
Traction apophysis, 472
Trainer, athletic; see Athletic trainer
Training, athletic, 3-10
  competencies, in, 6-7
Transection of spinal cord, 324
Transudate, 121
Transverse arch of foot, 47, 401, 402
  sprain of, 412
Transverse fracture, 180
Transverse ligament of axis, 322
Transverse plane of body, 19, 20
Transverse processes, 37, 321
  of lumbar vertebrae, fracture of, 328
Transverse ridges of sacrum, 329, 330
Transversus abdominis muscle, 77, 79, 370, 371
Trapezium bone, 42, 623
Trapezius muscle, 75, 78, 79, 81, 355, 356, 358, 551
  palpation of, 572
Trapezoid bone, 42, 623
Trapezoid ligament, 547-548
Trauma, 119
  acute vascular response to, 120-123
  anterior neck, 357
  athletic-related, 116-193
  body's response to, 118-128
  signs of
    in athlete with head injury, 283
    with spinal injury, 334
    in unconscious athlete, 259, 263, 264
Traumatic injury, 230, 436
Traumatic pneumothorax, 366
Traumatic shock, continuous cycle of, 129
Traumatic synovitis of hip, 523
"Traumatic tattoo," 151-152
Treatment of athletic injuries
  athletic trainer's role in, 8
  follow-up, 126-127
  immediate, 125-126
  psychological considerations in, 190-193
Trendelenburg gait, 528
Trendelenburg sign, 528
Trendelenburg test to assess hip
    stability, 527-528
Triceps brachii muscle, 78, 81, 82, 551, 553, 594, 595
  palpation of, 572, 573
Triceps reflex, 114
  testing, 351, 586
Triceps surae, 399
Tricuspids, 302
Trigeminal nerve, 100, 101
  assessment of, 286, 287
Trimalar fracture, 293
Tripartite patella, 470
Tripod fracture, 293
Triquetrum bone, 42, 623, 624
Trochanter, 30
  greater, 30, 44, 509
    palpation of, 530
  lesser, 509

Trochanteric bursitis, 521
Trochlea, 40, 399-400, 590, 591
Trochlear nerve, 100, 101
  assessment of, 286-287
Trochlear notch, 591
True pelvis, 47
True ribs, 36, 37, 38, 39
Trunk
  movements of, evaluation of, 347-348
  muscles of, 78, 79
Tubercle, 30
  of Gerdy, 466, 482
  of humerus, 40
  navicular, palpation of, 439
Tuberosity, 30
  deltoid, 40
    palpation of, 570, 571
  greater, palpation of, 570, 571
  tibial, 416, 417
    avulsion of, 473
Tumor, 156, 158
  from inflammation, 122
  testicular, 383
Turbinate bones, 36
"Turf burns," 151
Turf toe, 411
Twitch contractions, 73
Two-neuron reflex arc, 94
Two-point discrimination, 113
Tympanic membrane, 298

U

Ulcer, 157, 158, 376
Ulcerative colitis, 376
Ulna, 29, 30, 31, 38, 39, 40, 41, 42, 590-591
  fractures of, 602-603
  and interosseous membrane, 596-598
  olecranon process of, palpation of, 607-608, 609
  open fracture of, 178
  styloid process of, palpation of, 608, 609, 644
Ulnar collateral ligament, 592
Ulnar nerve, 81, 90, 107, 108, 109
  contusion of, 599
  involvement of, in elbow and forearm injuries, 603-604
Ulnar nerve conduction test, 219
Ulnar nerve entrapment, 219
Umbilicus, 370
Unconscious athlete, 250-265
  physical examination of, 260-264
  primary survey of, 251-255
  referral of, 265
  secondary survey of, 255-264
Unconsciousness, 250-251
  causes of, in athletic activity, 251
Underwater weighing to assess body composition, 14-15
Unexposed athletic injuries, 147, 166-181
"Unhappy triad," 465-466
Uniaxial joints, 55-56
Uniforms to prevent heat stress, 138
Unipennate muscle fibers, 68, 69
Upper abdominal reflex, 114
Upper extremity(ies)
  athletic injuries of, 542-655
  bones of, 39
  shoulder girdle and, bones of, 38, 39-41

Ureter, referred pain from, 374
Urethritis, 383
Urinary meatus, 380
Urination, painful, 383
Urography, 207, 210
Urticaria, 166

V

Vaginal orifice, 380
Vaginitis, 381
Vagus nerve, 100, 102
  assessment of, 286, 287
Valgus, cubitus, 607
Valgus angulation of leg, 477
Valgus instability of knee, 490
Valgus stress test, 490, 491
"Valley fever," 369
Valsalva maneuver, 345
  to reduce testicular spasm, 381
Vaporization and heat production, 131
Varicella, 164
Varicocele, 382
Varus
  cubitus, 607
  rearfoot, 405
Varus angulation of leg, 477
Varus instability of knee, tests for, 490-493
Vas deferens, 379
Vascular response, acute, to trauma, 120-123
Vasoconstriction, 120-121
  to prevent heat loss, 142
Vasodilation, 120-121
  to promote heat loss, 132-133
Vastus intermedius muscle, 83, 460-461, 514
Vastus lateralis muscle, 83, 85, 460-461, 514
Vastus medialis muscle, 83, 85, 460-461, 514
Veins of scalp, 268
Venogram, 207
Venous system, diploid, 268
Ventilation, pulmonary, mechanism of, 363-364
Ventral, 18
Ventral root of spinal nerve, 99, 104
Ventricle
  fourth, 98
  third, 98
Verruca plantaris, 164
Verruca vulgaris, 164
Vertebra(e), 34, 37, 316, 317
  articular processes between, 57
  cervical, 31, 34, 38, 321
  lumbar, 31, 34, 38, 326
    compression fractures of, 328
  sacral, 329
  thoracic, 31, 34, 38, 325
    compression fracture of, 325
Vertebra prominens, 322
Vertebral column, 30, 34
  bones of, 38
  lateral view of, 37
  ligaments of, 317-318
  muscles acting on, 320-321
  muscles moving, 76
  sagittal section of, 318
Vertebral foramen, 321
Vertebral line, 360
Vertebrochondral ribs, 39

Vertebrosternal ribs, 36, 39
Vertigo, 299
Vesicle, 156, 158
  synaptic, 72
Vestibular branch of acoustic nerve, 101
Vicarious experience, 193
Viral skin lesions, 163-164
Viscera, abdominal, injuries to, 374
Visceral injuries, 366-367
Visceral layer of abdominal cavity, 371
Visceral nerves, 91
Visceral pain, referred, 374-375
Visceral pleura, 363
Visceroceptors, 91
Vital centers of brain stem, 271
Vital signs of unconscious athlete, monitoring, 256
Volar plate of interphalangeal articulations, 632
Volkmann's ischemic contracture, 603
Voluntary nerves, 89
Vomer, 34, 36, 291
Vomiting, 375
Vulva, 380-381

W

Waist-to-hip ratio and assessment of somatotype, 14
Walking gaits, phases of, 424-425
Wall test to observe spinal alignment, 339, 340
Warts, 164
Water warts, 164
Weather guide to prevent heat stress, 137
Weighing, underwater, to assess body composition, 14-15
Wens, 267
Wheal, 156, 158
Whirlpools and thermoregulatory control, 133
White matter, 93
Whitlow, 637
Wind Chill Index, 140, 141
Windpipe, blockage of, 224
Winging of scapula, 338, 580
"Winking" reflex, 113
Wisdom teeth, 302
Women and men, differences in body form of, 21, 22
Wounds, 120-125
  open, 150-155
Wrist, 622-630; see also Hand and wrist
Wryneck, 338

X

Xiphoid process, 30, 36, 37, 38

Y

Yellow bone marrow, 28
Yergason test, 580-581

Z

Z line, 70, 73
Zygoma, 36, 293-294
Zygomatic arch, 291
Zygomatic bone, 29, 34, 35, 291

CREDITS

CHAPTER 2

2-3 from Prentice W: Fitness for College and Life, ed 3, St. Louis, 1991, Mosby–Year Book, Inc; 2-12, Terry Cockerham/Synapse Media Production.

CHAPTER 3

3-1, 3-4, 3-5, Ernest Beck; 3-2, Joan M Beck; 3-3, Terry Cockerham/Synapse Media Production; 3-10, David Mascaro & Associates.

CHAPTER 4

4-4, McMullen CR, Department of Biology, South Dakota State University; 4-5, 4-6, 4-7, Rusty Jones.

CHAPTER 5

5-2, Barbara Stackhouse; 5-5, Laurie O'Keefe/John Daughtery; 5-6, George Wassilchenko; 5-8, Rolin Graphics; 5-13, 5-16, John Hagen.

CHAPTER 6

6-1, 6-3, 6-4, 6-7, Beck EW; 6-5, 6-6, Joan M Beck; 6-9, Rolin Graphics; 6-10A, 6-11, George Wassilchenko; 6-10B, 6-12, 6-13, 6-14, Michael Schenk; Tables 6-1, 6-2, 6-3, from Anthony CP and Thibodeau GA: Anatomy and physiology, ed 14, St. Louis, 1992, Times Mirror/Mosby College Publishing.

CHAPTER 7

7-5, from Brennan WT and Ludwig DJ: Guide to problems and practices in first aid and emergency care, ed 3, Dubuque, Iowa, 1976, William C. Brown Co.; 7-8, from Fox EL et al: Physiological basis of education and athletics, ed 4, 1988, WB Saunders Co. Reprinted by permission of Holt, Rinehart and Winston, CB5 College Publishing; Table 7-2, from Parcel GS: Basic emergency care of the sick and injured, ed 3, St. Louis, 1986, Times Mirror/Mosby College Publishing.

CHAPTER 8

8-7, courtesy Dr. James Garrick, Center for Sports Medicine, St. Francis Memorial Hospital, San Francisco; 8-12, 8-19, courtesy Steve Yoneda, California Polytechnic State University; 8-15B,C, courtesy Rob Williams A.T., C.; 8-15D, 8-16 courtesy Bruce Johnson, A.T.,C., Orthopedic Clinic, Grand Forks, ND; 8-17, courtesy Neal Dutton, A.T.,C. Bethel College, St. Paul, Minn.; 8-18, 8-20 courtesy A.G. Edwards, A.T.,C.

Skin disorders color insert, courtesy Thomas P Habif, M.D. (from Clinical Dermatology, ed 2, 1990, St. Louis, Mosby–Year Book, Inc).

CHAPTER 12

12-14, from Judd RL and Ponsell DD: The first responder: the first critical minutes, St. Louis, ed 2, 1986, Mosby–Year Book, Inc.

CHAPTER 13

13-6, from McClintic JR: Human anatomy, St. Louis, 1983, Mosby–Year Book, Inc.

CHAPTER 14

14-3, McMinn RH: Color atlas of human anatomy, Wolfe Publishing; 14-24, from Barber JM and Budassi SA: Mosby's manual of emergency care, St. Louis, 1979, Mosby–Year Book, Inc; 14-28, from Camp RH et al: In Gerard LJ, ed: Corneal contact lenses, ed 2, St. Louis, Mosby–Year Book, Inc.

CHAPTER 15

15-1, Joan M Beck; 15-4, John Hagen; 15-15, courtesy Steve Yoneda, California Polytechnic State University; 15-21, from Malasanos Health assessment, ed 4, 1989, St. Louis, Mosby–Year Book, Inc.

Unit V Opener, courtesy Cramer Products, Inc, Gardner, Kansas.

CHAPTER 16

16-1, 16-4, McMinn RH: Color atlas of human anatomy, Wolfe Publishing; 16-7, George Wassilchenko; 16-10, John Hagen; 16-8, Joel Gordon/Lisa Cheuk Kastner from Denney NW and Quadagno D: Human sexuality, ed 2, 1992, St. Louis, Mosby–Year Book, Inc.

CHAPTER 17

17-1, McMinn RH: Color atlas of human anatomy, Wolfe Publishing; 17-4, from Arnheim DD: Modern principles of athletic training, ed 7, St. Louis, 1989, Times Mirror/ Mosby College Publishing; 17-11, 17-21, courtesy Dr. James Garrick, Center for Sports Medicine, St. Francis Memorial Hospital, San Francisco; 17-12, courtesy Bruck Johnson, A.T.,C., Orthopedic Clinic, Grand Forks, ND.

CHAPTER 18

18-10, courtesy Bill Oakes, Northern Iowan.

CHAPTER 19

19-15, courtesy Dr. James Garrick, Center for Sports Medicine, St. Francis Memorial Hospital, San Francisco.

Unit VI Opener, courtesy Bettman Archive.

CHAPTER 20

20-1, McMinn RH: Color atlas of human anatomy, Wolfe Publishing; 20-15, from Crafts PC: Textbook of human anatomy, ed 2, New York, 1979, Wiley Medical; 20-18, courtesy Bruce Johnson, A.T.,C., Orthopedic Clinic, Grand Forks, ND; 20-19, courtesy A.G. Edwards, A.T.,C., University of Nevada-Las Vegas; 20-32, from Malasanos L et al, ed 3, St. Louis, 1986, Mosby–Year Book, Inc; 20-38, from Prior JA, Silberstein JS, and Stang JM: Physical diagnosis, ed 5, St. Louis, 1977, Mosby–Year Book, Inc.

CHAPTER 21

21-1, McMinn RH: Color atlas of human anatomy, Wolfe Publishing; 21-5, 21-6, 21-7, 21-8, 21-10, 21-27, 21-29 from Malasanos L et al, Health assessment, ed 3, St. Louis, 1986, Mosby–Year Book, Inc; 21-9, from Thibodeau GA: Anatomy and physiology, ed 14, St. Louis, 1992, Times Mirror/Mosby College Publishing; 21-14, courtesy A.G. Edwards, A.T.,C.

CHAPTER 22

22-1, McMinn RH: Color atlas of human anatomy, Wolfe Publishing; 22-3, 22-10, 22-24, 22-25, from Malasanos L et al: Health assessment, ed 3, St. Louis, 1986, Mosby–Year Book, Inc; 22-13, courtesy Gregg Voigt, A.T.,C.; 22-15, courtesy Bruce Johnson, A.T.,C., Orthopedic Clinic, Grand Forks, ND: 22-17, 22-19, courtesy A.G. Edwards, A.T.,C.; 22-18, from Flatt AE: Care of minor injuries, ed 4, St. Louis, 1979, Mosby–Year Book, Inc.